The Zuckerman Parker Handbook of Developmental and Behavioral Pediatrics for Primary Care

Third Edition

The Zuckerman Parker Handbook of Developmental and Behavioral Pediatrics for Primary Care

Third Edition

Edited by

Marilyn Augustyn, MD

Associate Professor of Pediatrics
Boston University School of Medicine;
Director, Division of Developmental and
Behavioral Pediatrics
Boston Medical Center
Boston, Massachusetts

Barry Zuckerman, MD

Joel and Barbara Alpert Professor of
Pediatrics,
Boston University School of Medicine;
Chief, Department of Pediatrics
Boston Medical Center
Boston, Massachusetts

Elizabeth B. Caronna, MD

Assistant Professor of Pediatrics
Boston University School of Medicine;
Director, Pediatric Assessment of
Communication Clinic
Boston Medical Center
Boston, Massachusetts

Wolters Kluwer | Lippincott Williams & Wilkins
Health
Philadelphia · Baltimore · New York · London
Buenos Aires · Hong Kong · Sydney · Tokyo

Acquisitions Editor: Sonya Seigafuse
Product Manager: Nicole Walz
Vendor Manager: Bridgett Dougherty
Senior Manufacturing Manager: Benjamin Rivera
Marketing Manager: Lisa Lawrence
Design Coordinator: Doug Smock
Production Service: Aptara, Inc.

© **2011 by LIPPINCOTT WILLIAMS & WILKINS, a WOLTERS KLUWER business**
© **2005 by Lippincott Williams & Wilkins**
© **1995 by Steven Parker and Barry Zuckerman**
Two Commerce Square
2001 Market Street
Philadelphia, PA 19103
LWW.com

Printed in China

Library of Congress Cataloging-in-Publication Data

The Zuckerman Parker handbook of developmental and behavioral pediatrics for primary care : a handbook for primary care / edited by Marilyn Augustyn, Barry Zuckerman, Elizabeth B. Caronna. – 3rd ed.
    p. ; cm.
    Other title: Handbook of developmental and behavioral pediatrics for primary care
    Rev. ed. of: Developmental and behavioral pediatrics / edited by Steven Parker, Barry Zuckerman, Marilyn Augustyn. 2nd ed. c2005.
    Includes bibliographical references and index.
    Summary: "The thoroughly updated Third Edition of The Zuckerman Parker Handbook of Developmental and Behavioral Pediatrics for Primary Care provides practical guidance on diagnosing and treating children with developmental and behavioral problems in the primary care setting. Written in outline format, this popular handbook enables readers to easily find the information they need to make diagnostic and management decisions. Recommended readings for both physicians and parents are included. Coverage ranges from everyday problems such as biting and social avoidance to serious and complex psychiatric disorders such as anorexia and depression. This edition includes new chapters on dealing with difficult child behavior in the office; alternative therapy for autism spectrum disorders; treatment of autism spectrum disorders; oppositional defiant disorder; bilingualism; health literacy; incarcerated parents; and military parents. A companion website includes the fully searchable text"—Provided by publisher.
    ISBN 978-1-60831-914-5 (pbk. : alk. paper)
    1. Behavior disorders in children–Handbooks, manuals, etc. 2. Child development deviations–Handbooks, manuals, etc. 3. Pediatrics–Psychological aspects–Handbooks, manuals, etc. 4. Primary care (Medicine)–Handbooks, manuals, etc. I. Zuckerman, Barry S. II. Augustyn, Marilyn. III. Caronna, Elizabeth B. IV. Developmental and behavioral pediatrics. V. Title: Handbook of developmental and behavioral pediatrics for primary care.
    [DNLM: 1. Developmental Disabilities–diagnosis–Handbooks. 2. Developmental Disabilities–therapy–Handbooks. 3. Child Behavior Disorders–diagnosis–Handbooks. 4. Child Behavior Disorders–therapy–Handbooks. WS 39]
    RJ47.5.B37 2011
    618.92'89—dc22

                                        2010026305

To purchase additional copies of this book, call our customer service department at (800) 638-3030 or fax orders to (301) 223-2320. International customers should call (301) 223-2300.

Visit Lippincott Williams & Wilkins on the Internet: at LWW.com. Lippincott Williams & Wilkins customer service representatives are available from 8:30 am to 6 pm, EST.

RRS1007

DEDICATION

To George, Henry, and Clare Westerman, who have made every milestone along the way an adventure.

To Pam, Jake, and Katherine for their love, support, and humor, which makes everything possible, and to Elliot, whose life is a force for my work.

To David, Sam, and Natalie Jones for their enthusiasm, energy, and instruction through example.

And to Steve, whose spirit and passion are the heart of this book.

CONTENTS

III
Family Issues

Marianne San Antonio, DO

Fellow
Developmental and Behavioral
Pediatrics
Yale University
New Haven, Connecticut

Marie E. Anzalone, ScD, OTR, FAOTA

Assistant Professor
Department of Occupational Therapy
Virginia Commonwealth University
Richmond, Virginia

Marilyn Augustyn, MD

Associate Professor
Department of Pediatrics
Boston University;
Director, Division of Developmental
and Behavioral Pediatrics
Department of Pediatrics
Boston Medical Center
Boston, Massachusetts

Christine E. Barron, MD

Assistant Professor
Department of Pediatrics
Warren Alpert Medical School at
Brown University;
Clinical and Fellowship Director, Child
Protection Program
Department of Pediatrics
Hasbro Children's Hospital
Providence, Rhode Island

Nerissa S. Bauer, MD, MPH

Assistant Professor
General Community Pediatrics
Indiana University
Indianapolis, Indiana

Joseph Biederman, MD

Chief, Clinical and Research Programs
in Pediatric Psychopharmacology and
Adult ADHD
Massachusetts General Hospital;
Professor of Psychiatry
Harvard Medical School
Boston, Massachusetts

James A. Blackman, MD, MPH

Professor of Pediatrics
University of Virginia;
Medical Director, Kluge Children's
Rehabilitation Center and Research
Institute
Charlottesville, Virginia

Peter A. Blasco, MD

Associate Professor
Department of Pediatrics
Oregon Health and Science University;
Director, Neurodevelopmental
Programs
Child Development and Rehabilitation
Center
Portland, Oregon

Stephanie Blenner, MD

Assistant Professor
Department of Pediatrics
Boston University School of Medicine;
Developmental Behavioral
Pediatrician
Department of Pediatrics
Boston Medical Center
Boston, Massachusetts

Robert J. Boyle, MD

Professor
Department of Pediatrics
University of Virginia;
Attending Neonatologist
Neonatal Intensive Care Unit
University of Virginia Health Sciences
Center
Charlottesville, Virginia

T. Berry Brazelton, MD

Emeritus
Department of Pediatrics
Harvard Medical School;
Founder
Brazelton Touchpoints Center
Children's Hospital Boston
Boston, Massachusetts

Margaret J. Briggs-Gowan, PhD

Assistant Professor
Department of Psychiatry
University of Connecticut Health
Center
Farmington, Connecticut

Robert B. Brooks, PhD

Assistant Clinical Professor of
Psychology
Department of Psychiatry
Harvard Medical School;
Consultant
Department of Psychology
McLean Hospital
Belmont, Massachusetts

John C. Carey, MD, MPH

Professor and Vice Chair, Academic
Affairs
Department of Pediatrics
University of Utah Health Sciences
Center
Salt Lake City, Utah

Elizabeth B. Caronna, MD

Assistant Professor
Department of Pediatrics
Boston University;
Director, Pediatric Assessment of
Communication Clinic
Department of Pediatrics
Boston Medical Center
Boston, Massachusetts

Alice S. Carter, PhD

Professor
Department of Psychology
University of Massachusetts Boston
Boston, Massachusetts

Molinda Chartrand, MD

Associate Professor
Department of Pediatrics
Uniformed Services University of
Health Sciences
Bethesda, Maryland;
Lieutenant Colonel
United States Air Force

Jonathan M. Cheek, PhD

Professor
Department of Psychology
Wellesley College
Wellesley, Massachusetts

Edward R. Christophersen, PhD, FAAP (Hon)

Professor of Pediatrics
University of Missouri at Kansas City
School of Medicine;
Pediatric Psychologist
Children's Mercy South Clinic
Kansas City, Missouri

Joanna Cole, PhD

Child Psychologist
Child and Adolescent Psychiatry
Boston Medical Center
Boston, Massachusetts

William Lord Coleman, MD

Professor of Pediatrics
Department of Pediatrics
University of North Carolina School of
Medicine
Chapel Hill, North Carolina

James Coplan, MD

Adjunct Associate Professor
School of Nursing
University of Pennsylvania
Philadelphia, Pennsylvania;
President, Neurodevelopmental
Pediatrics of the Main Line
Rosemont, Pennsylvania

Eileen M. Costello, MD

Southern Jamaica Plain Health Center
Brigham and Women's Hospital
Executive Advisory Committee,
Asperger's Association of New England
Boston, Massachusetts

David L. Coulter, MD

Associate Professor of Neurology
Harvard Medical School
Boston, Massachusetts

Howard Dubowitz, MD, MS

Professor of Pediatrics
University of Maryland School of
Medicine;
Chief, Division of Child Protection
Department of Pediatrics
University of Maryland Hospital
Baltimore, Maryland

Paul H. Dworkin, MD

Professor and Chair
Department of Pediatrics
University of Connecticut School of
Medicine
Farmington, Connecticut;
Physician-in-Chief
Connecticut Children's Medical Center
Hartford, Connecticut

Laura Edwards-Leeper, PhD

Instructor in Psychology
Department of Psychiatry
Harvard Medical School;
Assistant in Psychology
Department of Medicine
Children's Hospital Boston
Boston, Massachusetts

Margorie Engel, MA, MBA, PhD

Stepfamily Expert Council
National Stepfamily Resource Center
Auburn University
Auburn, Alabama

Ilgi Ozturk Ertem, MD

Professor of Pediatrics
Developmental Behavioral Pediatrics
Unit
Department of Pediatrics
Ankara University School of Medicine
Ankara, Turkey

Deborah A. Frank, MD

Professor of Pediatrics
Department of Pediatrics
Boston University School of Medicine;
Director, Grow Clinic for Children
Department of Pediatrics
Boston Medical Center
Boston, Massachusetts

Frances Page Glascoe, PhD

Professor of Pediatrics
Department of Pediatrics
Vanderbilt University
Nashville, Tennessee

Leandra Godoy, MA

Department of Psychology
University of Massachusetts
Boston, Massachusetts

Richard D. Goldstein, MD

Assistant Professor
Department of Pediatrics
Boston University School of Medicine;
Attending Physician
Department of Psychosocial Oncology
and Palliative Care
Dana Farber Cancer Institute
Department of Medicine
Children's Hospital of Boston
Boston, Massachusetts

Linda Grant, MD, MPH

Associate Professor of Pediatrics
Department of Pediatrics
Boston University School of Medicine;
Attending physician
Department of Pediatrics
Boston Medical Center
Boston, Massachusetts

Ross W. Greene, PhD

Associate Clinical Professor
Department of Psychiatry
Harvard Medical School;
Associate Clinical Professor
Department of Psychiatry
Cambridge Health Alliance
Cambridge, Massachusetts

Betsy McAlister Groves, MSW, LICSW

Associate Professor
Department of Pediatrics
Boston University School of Medicine;
Director, Child Witness to Violence
Project
Department of Pediatrics
Boston Medical Center
Boston, Massachusetts

Angela S. Guarda, MD

Associate Professor
Department of Psychiatry and
Behavioral Sciences
Johns Hopkins University;
Director, Eating Disorders Program
Department of Psychiatry and
Behavioral Sciences
Johns Hopkins Hospital
Baltimore, Maryland

Barry Guitar, PhD

Professor of Communication Sciences
University of Vermont
Burlington, Vermont

Randi Hagerman, MD

Endowed Chair in Fragile X Research
and Professor of Pediatrics
Department of Pediatrics
University of California at Davis
Medical Center;
Medical Director MIND Institute
Department of Pediatrics
UCDMC
Sacramento, California

Elizabeth Harstad, MD

Fellow
Developmental Medicine Center
Children's Hospital Boston
Boston, Massachusetts

Gregory F. Hayden, MD

Professor
Department of Pediatrics
University of Virginia;
Head, Division of General Pediatrics
Department of Pediatrics
University of Virginia Children's
Hospital
Charlottesville, Virginia

Phillip Hernandez, MD

Boston University School of Medicine
Boston, Massachusetts

Wilhelmina Hernandez, MD

Fellow
Department of Developmental and
Behavioral
Boston Medical Center
Boston, Massachusetts

L. Kari Hironaka, MD, MPH

Associate Professor
Department of Pediatrics
Boston University;
Development and Behavioral
Pediatrician
Department of Pediatrics
Boston Medical Center
Boston, Massachusetts

Alexander H. Hoon Jr, MD

Associate Professor of Pediatrics
Johns Hopkins University School of
Medicine
Kennedy Krieger Institute North
Broadway;
Director Phelps Center for Cerebral
Palsy
Kennedy Krieger Institute North
Broadway
Baltimore, Maryland

Barbara Howard, MD

Assistant professor
Department of Pediatrics
The Johns Hopkins University School
of Medicine;
Faculty
Department of Pediatrics
Baltimore, Maryland

Carol Hubbard, MD, MPH, PhD

Clinical Assistant Professor
Department of Pediatrics
Tufts University School of Medicine
Boston, Massachusetts
Director, Developmental and
Behavioral Pediatrics
Department of Pediatrics
Maine Medical Center
Portland, Maine

Michael Jellinek, MD

Chief, Child Psychiatry
Professor, Harvard Medical School
Department of Psychiatry
Massachusetts General Hospital
Boston, Massachusetts;
President
Newton Wellesley Hospital
Newton, Massachusetts

Carole Jenny, MD, MBA

Professor
Department of Pediatrics
Warren Alpert Medical School at
Brown University;
Division Director, Child Protection
Program
Department of Pediatrics
Hasbro Children's Hospital
Providence, Rhode Island

Alain Joffe, MD, MPH

Associate Professor
Department of Pediatrics
Johns Hopkins University School of
Medicine;
Director
Student Health and Wellness Center
Johns Hopkins University
Baltimore, Maryland

Margot Kaplan-Sanoff, EdD

Associate Professor of Pediatrics
National Program Officer, Healthy
Steps
Division of Developmental and
Behavioral Pediatrics
Department of Pediatrics
Boston University School of Medicine;
Boston Medical Center
Boston, Massachusetts

Theodore A. Kastner, MD, MS

President
Developmental Disabilities Health
Alliance, Inc.
Bloomfield, New Jersey;
Associate Professor of Clinical
Medicine
Robert Wood Johnson Medical School
University of Medicine and Dentistry
of New Jersey
New Brunswick, New Jersey

Aasma A. Khandekar, MD

Instructor
Department of Pediatrics
Boston University School of Medicine;
Fellow
Division of Developmental and
Behavioral Pediatrics
Boston Medical Center
Boston, Massachusetts

Krista Kircanski, MA

Clinical Coordinator
Child and Adolescent Psychiatry
Boston Medical Center
Boston, Massachusetts

Perri Klass, MD

Professor of Journalism and Pediatrics
New York University
Arthur L. Carter Journalism Institute
New York University School of
Medicine and
Bellevue Hospital Center Department
of Pediatrics
New York, New York

John R. Knight, MD

Associate Professor
Department of Pediatrics
Harvard Medical School;
Senior Associate in Medicine,
Associate in Psychiatry
Children's Hospital Boston
Boston, Massachusetts

Barbara Korsch, MD

Professor of Pediatrics
University of Southern California
Keck School of Medicine;
Attending Physician
General Pediatrics
Children's Hospital of Los Angeles
Los Angeles, California

Brian Kurtz, MD

Assistant Professor
Child and Adolescent Psychiatry
Tufts University School of Medicine;
Attending Physician
Child and Adolescent Psychiatry
Tufts Medical Center and Floating
Hospital for Children
Boston, Massachusetts

Carine Lenders, MD, MS, ScD

Assistant Professor
Department of Pediatrics
Boston University School of Medicine;
Medical Director, NFL Program
(Pediatric Obesity)
Department of Pediatrics
Boston Medical Center
Boston, Massachusetts

John M. Leventhal, MD

Professor of Pediatrics
Yale University School of Medicine;
Medical Director, Child Abuse
Programs
Yale-New Haven Hospital
New Haven, Connecticut

Melvin D. Levine, MD

Director and Chief Executive Officer of
Bringing Up Minds
Rougemont, North Carolina

Yi Hui Liu, MD, MPH

Clinical Instructor
Department of Pediatrics
University of California San Diego;
Medical Director
Developmental–Behavioral Pediatric
Clinic
Rady Children's Hospital San Diego
San Diego, California

Catherine Logan, MSPT

Medical Student
School of Medicine
Tufts University School of Medicine;
Consultant
Department of Pediatrics
Boston Medical Center
Boston, Massachusetts

Julie Lumeng, MD

Assistant Professor
Department of Pediatrics
University of Michigan School of
Medicine;
Assistant Research Scientist
Center for Human Growth and
Development
University of Michigan

Deborah Madansky, MD

Behavioral Pediatrician
Santa Rosa, California

Tracy Magee, PhD, RN, CPNP

Assistant Professor
Department of Family Nursing
Indiana University;
Adjunct Clinical Assistant Professor
Department of Child Development
Riley Hospital for Children
Indianapolis, Indiana

Nili E. Major, MD

Instructor
Department of Pediatrics
Yale University School of Medicine;
Attending Physician
Department of Pediatrics
Yale-New Haven Hospital
New Haven, Connecticut

Margaret Marino, PhD

Adjunct Assistant professor
Department of Pediatrics
Boston University School of Medicine;
Psychologist, NFL Clinic (Pediatric
Obesity)
Department of Pediatrics
Boston Medical Center
Boston, Massachusetts

Kevin P. Marks, MD

Clinical Assistant Professor
Department of Pediatrics, Division of
General Pediatrics
Oregon Health & Science University
Eugene, Oregon

Rebecca McCauley, PhD

Professor
Department of Speech and Hearing
Science
The Ohio State University
Columbus, Ohio

Alan Meyers, MD, MPH

Associate Professor
Department of Pediatrics
Boston University School of Medicine;
Attending Physician
Department of Pediatrics
Boston Medical Center
Boston, Massachusetts

Hannah Milch, BA

Medical Student
Boston University School of Medicine;
American Society for Nutrition Intern,
NFL Clinic (Pediatric Obesity)
Department of Pediatrics
Boston Medical Center
Boston, Massachusetts

Claudio Morera, MD

Assistant Professor
Department of Pediatrics
Boston University;
Clinical Director
Pediatric Gastroenterology
Boston Medical Center
Boston, Massachusetts

Vivien Morris, MS, RD, MPH, LDN

Assistant Professor
Department of Pediatrics
Boston University School of Medicine;
Director of Community Initiatives,
Nutrition and Fitness for Life Program
Department of Pediatrics
Boston Medical Center
Boston, Massachusetts

Michael E. Msall, MD

Professor of Pediatrics
Department of Developmental and
Behavioral Pediatrics
The University of Chicago;
Chief of Developmental Pediatrics
Kennedy Research Center on
Intellectual Disability
Comer Children's Hospital
La Rabida Children's Hospital
Chicago, Illinois

Robert Needlman, MD

Associate Professor of Pediatrics
Department of Pediatrics
Case Western Reserve University
School of Medicine;
Attending Pediatrician
Department of Pediatrics
Metro Health Medical Center
Cleveland, Ohio

Sarah S. Nyp, MD, FAAP

Assistant Professor of Pediatrics
University of Missouri at Kansas City
School of Medicine;
Developmental–Behavioral
Pediatrician
Department of Pediatrics
Children's Mercy South Clinics
Kansas City, Missouri

Anna Maria S. Ocampo, MD, MPH

Fellow
Developmental Medicine
Harvard Medical School;
Fellow
Developmental Medicine
Children's Hospital Boston
Boston, Massachusetts

Lauren Oliver, MS, RD, LDN

Instructor, Advanced Nutrition
Elective
Department of Pediatrics
Boston University School of Medicine;
Program Coordinator, NFL Clinic
(Pediatric Obesity)
Department of Pediatrics
Boston Medical Center
Boston, Massachusetts

Karen Olness, MD

Professor
Department of Pediatrics
Case Western Reserve University
Cleveland, Ohio

Judith A. Owens, MD

Associate Professor of Pediatrics
Brown Medical School;
Director, Learning, Attention, &
Behavior (LAB) Program at the Child
Development Center
Rhode Island Hospital
Providence, Rhode Island

Lee M. Pachter, DO

Chief, Section of General Pediatrics
Associate Chair for Community
Pediatrics
St. Christopher's Hospital for
Children;
Professor, Pediatrics
Drexel University College of Medicine
Philadelphia, Pennsylvania

Frederick B. Palmer, MD

Shainberg Professor
Department of Pediatrics
University of Tennessee Health
Science Center;
Director
Boling Center for Developmental
Disabilities
University of Tennessee Health
Science Center
Memphis, Tennessee

Ellen C. Perrin, MD, MA

Professor
Department of Pediatrics
Tufts University School of Medicine;
Director of Research
Developmental–Behavioral Pediatrics
Floating Hospital at Tufts Medical
Center
Boston, Massachusetts

Lisa Albers Prock, MD, MPH

Assistant Professor
Department of Pediatrics
Harvard Medical School;
Director of Adoption Program
Division of Developmental Medicine
Children's Hospital
Boston, Massachusetts

Siegfried M. Pueschel, MD, PhD, MPH

Professor Emeritus of Pediatrics
The Warren Alpert Medical School of
Brown University
Providence, Rhode Island

Leonard Rappaport MD, MS

Mary Deming Scott Professor of
Pediatrics
Department of Pediatrics
Harvard Medical School;
Chief, Division of Developmental
Medicine
Department of Medicine
Children's Hospital Boston
Boston, Massachusetts

Michele Rock, DO

Associate Professor
Department of Pediatrics
Tufts University School of Medicine
Boston, Massachusetts;
Attending
Department of Pediatrics
Maine Medical Center
Portland, Maine

Adrian Sandler, MD
Adjunct Associate Professor
Department of Pediatrics
University of North Carolina Chapel
Hill
Chapel Hill, North Carolina;
Medical Director
Olson Huff Center
Mission Children's Hospital
Asheville, North Carolina

Jodi Santosuosso, NP
Division of Developmental and
Behavioral Pediatrics
Boston Medical Center
Boston, Massachusetts

Celine A. Saulnier, PhD
Training Director, Autism Program
Yale Child Study Center
Yale University School of Medicine
New Haven, Connecticut

Glenn Saxe, MD
Chairman
Department of Child and Adolescent
Psychiatry;
Director
NYU Child Study Center, New York
University
New York, New York

Nell L. Schechter, MD
Professor and Head of Division of Pain
Medicine
Development of Pediatrics
University of Connecticut School of
Medicine;
Director, Pain Relief Program
Connecticut Children's Medical Center
Hartford, Connecticut

David J. Schonfeld, MD
Thelma and Jack Rubinstein Professor
of Pediatrics
Division of Developmental and
Behavioral Pediatrics
Cincinnati Children's Hospital Medical
Center;
Director, Division of Developmental
and Behavioral Pediatrics
Director, National Center for School
Crisis and Bereavement
Department of Pediatrics
Cincinnati Children's Hospital Medical
Center
Cincinnati, Ohio

Alison Schonwald, MD
Assistant Professor
Harvard School of Medicine
Boston Children's Hospital
Center for Developmental Medicine
Boston, Massachusetts

Barton D. Schmitt, MD
Professor of Pediatrics
University of Colorado School of
Medicine;
Medical Director
After Hours Call Center and Care
Program
The Children's Hospital
Aurora, Colorado

Yasmin Senturias, MD

Assistant Professor
Department of Pediatrics
University of Louisville;
Fetal Alcohol Spectrum Disorders
Clinic Director
Weisskopf Child Evaluation Center
University of Louisville
Louisville, Kentucky

Prachi E. Shah, MD

Assistant Professor
Department of Pediatrics
University of Michigan;
Developmental–Behavioral
Pediatrician
Department of Pediatrics
University of Michigan Health System
Ann Arbor, Michigan

Jan Harold D. Sia, MD

Clinical Fellow
Department of Pediatrics
Section of Developmental–Behavioral
Pediatrics
Yale University School of Medicine
New Haven, Connecticut

Laura Sices, MD, MS

Assistant Professor
Department of Pediatrics
Boston University School of Medicine;
Director, Fellowship training in
DBPeds
Department of Pediatrics
Boston Medical Center
Boston, Massachusetts

Benjamin S. Siegel, MD

Professor of Pediatrics and Psychiatry
Boston University School of Medicine;
Senior Pediatrician
Primary Care Pediatrics
Boston Medical Center
Boston, Massachusetts

Nicola J. Smith, MD

Clinical Associate
Department of Pediatrics
Tufts University;
Fellow, Developmental–Behavioral
Pediatrics
Department of Pediatrics
Tufts Floating Hospital
Boston, Massachusetts

Norman P. Spack, MD

Assistant Professor
Department of Pediatrics
Harvard Medical School;
Associate
Endocrine Division
Children's Hospital Boston
Boston, Massachusetts

Joshua Sparrow, MD

Assistant Professor
Department of Psychiatry
Harvard Medical School;
Director of Special Initiatives
Brazelton Touchpoints Center
Children's Hospital Boston
Boston, Massachusetts

Terry Stancin, PhD

Professor
Departments of Pediatrics, Psychiatry
and Psychology
Case Western Reserve University;
Head, Pediatric Psychology
Department of Psychiatry
Metro Health Medical Center
Cleveland, Ohio

Martin T. Stein, MD

Professor of Pediatrics (Division of
Child Development and Community
Health)
Department of Pediatrics
University of California San Diego;
Rady Children's Hospital San Diego
San Diego, California

Naomi Steiner, MD

Assistant Professor Pediatrics
Department of Pediatrics
Tufts University;
Developmental and Behavioral
Pediatrician
Department of Pediatrics
Floating Hospital for Children
Boston, Massachusetts

Victor C. Strasburger, MD

Professor of Pediatrics
Professor of Family & Community
Medicine
Chief, Division of Adolescent Medicine
Department of Pediatrics
University of New Mexico School of
Medicine
Albuquerque, New Mexico

Peter Stringham, MD, SM

Assistant Professor of Clinical
Pediatrics
Department of Pediatrics
Boston University Medical School;
East Boston Neighborhood Health
Center
Pediatrics and Adolescent Medicine
(Retired)
Boston, Massachusetts

Moira Szilagyi, MD, PhD

Associate Professor
Department of Pediatrics
University of Rochester School of
Medicine and Dentistry
Rochester, New York

J. Lane Tanner, MD

Clinical Professor of Pediatrics
University of California, San Francisco
San Francisco, California;
Associate Director
Division of Mental Health and Child
Development
Children's Hospital & Research Center
at Oakland
Oakland, California

Maria Trozzi, MEd

Department of Pediatrics
Boston University School of Medicine;
Department of Pediatrics
Boston Medical Center
Boston, Massachusetts

Stanley Turecki, MD
Attending Psychiatrist
Lenox Hill Hospital;
Associate Attending Psychiatrist
Beth Israel Medical Center
New York City, New York

Douglas Vanderbilt, MD
Assistant Professor of Clinical
Pediatrics
Department of Pediatrics
Keck School of Medicine
University of Southern California;
Developmental Behavioral Pediatrics
Fellowship Program Director
Children's Hospital Los Angeles
Los Angeles, California

Fred R. Volkmar, MD
Director
Child Study Center
Yale University;
Chief
Child Psychiatry
Yale-New Haven Hospital
New Haven, Connecticut

Kevin K. Walsh, PhD
Developmental Disabilities Health
Alliance, Inc.
Vineland Area Office
Vineland, New Jersey

Heather Walter, MD, MPH
Professor
Psychiatry and Pediatrics
Boston University School of Medicine;
Chief
Child and Adolescent Psychiatry
Boston Medical Center
Boston, Massachusetts

Laura Weissman, MD
Instructor in Pediatrics
Department of Pediatrics
Harvard Medical School;
Assistant in Medicine
Developmental Hospital Center
Children's hospital Boston
Boston, Massachusetts

Carol C. Weitzman, MD
Associate Professor
Pediatrics and Child Study Center
Yale University School of Medicine;
Attending Pediatrician
Pediatrics and Child Study Center
Yale-New Haven Children's Hospital
New Haven, Connecticut

Karen E. Wills, PhD, LP
Neuropsychologist
Psychological Services
Children's Hospitals and Clinics of
Minnesota
Minneapolis, Minnesota

Laurel M. Wills, MD
Assistant Professor
Department of Pediatrics
University of Minnesota;
Developmental–Behavioral
Pediatrician
Department of Pediatrics
Hennepin County Medical Center
Minneapolis, Minnesota

Janet Wozniak, MD

Director, Pediatric Bipolar Disorder
Clinical and Research Program
Massachusetts General Hospital
Associate Professor of Psychiatry
Harvard Medical School Boston
Boston, Massachusetts

William T. Zempsky, MD

Professor of Pediatrics
Division of Pain Medicine/Department
of Pediatrics
University of Connecticut School of
Medicine
Farmington, Connecticut;
Associate Director
Pain Relief Program
Connecticut Children's Medical Center
Hartford, Connecticut

Barry Zuckerman, MD

Joel and Barbara Alpert Professor of
Pediatrics
Boston University School of Medicine;
Chief, Department of Pediatrics
Boston Medical Center
Boston, Massachusetts

Pamela M. Zuckerman, MD

Clinical Assistant Professor
Boston University School of Medicine
Private Practice
Brookline, Massachusetts

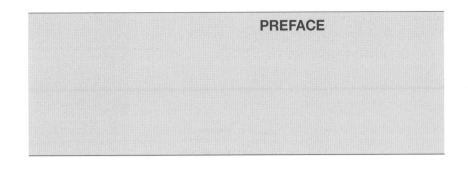

PREFACE

It is impossible to pinpoint exactly when the field of Developmental and Behavioral Pediatrics (DBP) was born. Was it with the birth of the first "second child" and temperament? Was it the child with failure to thrive whose laboratory evaluations were all normal? Was it with the revolution in toileting from "training" to a child-centered approach? Was it the first time the phrase "trust yourself" entered the rubric of modern parenting? Regardless of the timing, it is clear that parents' concerns about their children are on a rocketing trajectory. The challenges that face families today can be overwhelming, and likewise the support they request from their pediatric clinicians can at times seem too much to fit into a 17.5-minute visit.

As a field, the specialty of DBP has expanded into new areas to fill the demands of primary care clinicians and, more importantly, families. From highly specialized centers for the evaluation of children on the autism spectrum, to complex evaluations examining gene–environment interactions, to tertiary evaluations of learning style versus disability, the field has branched into exciting areas of higher specialization and complexity. Nonetheless, at its core, how DBP is translated into the primary care visit for families is the base of all DBP work. It is to this spirit that this edition, like the prior two, is focused. Toward this goal, we have added many new topics and updated all of the original chapters in this volume. We hope it will serve as a succinct, accurate, up-to-date, and practical reference, the starting point from which the interested clinician can find immediate support, timely information, and wise counsel.

MA
BZ
EBC

The Fundamentals of Developmental and Behavioral Pediatrics

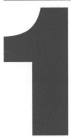

Talking with Parents

Barbara Korsch

I. **Description.** It has been documented consistently for the last five decades that the doctor–patient relationship and communication are the strongest predictors of the outcome of a medical visit. The therapeutic alliance is achieved in large measure during the interview. Rapport building; engaging the patient; eliciting psychosocial and personal aspects of the patient's experiences; supporting the parents in their roles as parents; and including the child, grandparent, and significant others—all of these are essential to establish a therapeutic relationship.

In many communities today, the clinician is faced with cultural and language barriers that complicate the interview. There are no easy solutions for this problem. For language problems, a skilled professional interpreter (preferably not a family member) is the only desirable approach. In the presence of an interpreter, it is essential that the physician maintain eye contact with the patient, continue to address the patient and family directly, and not discuss problems with the interpreter instead of the patient or caretaker (avoid saying "tell her that" or "ask him what"). Cultural sensitivities also pose unique challenges to effective healthcare and require the clinician to employ all his skills for assessing not only the individual patient's perceptions, value systems, and health beliefs, but also those that are prevalent in his or her culture. This holds especially true when offering advice and counsel.

Although there are no techniques that work for all patients or all clinicians, there are some basics that virtually always strengthen the therapeutic alliance (Table 1-1), which has become even more important in the era of the electronic medical record (EMR) and assistive technology in the examination room.

II. **Optimal communication with parents.**

A. **Listening.** Letting the parent know that you are listening is basic. Body language—sitting down, looking at the parent, leaning forward, and showing appropriate concern—is effective in conveying a listening attitude and does not require extra time in the interview. Responding to nonverbal expressions of parent affect is also essential. For example, if the mother's face falls when the clinician suggests the use of a pacifier for a colicky baby, the responsive clinician needs to inquire, *"You do not seem to like that idea. Is there any special reason why you do not want your baby to use the pacifier?"* He or she may find out that the mother had difficulty in weaning her firstborn from the pacifier or that she finds pacifiers disgusting. When screening, behavioral checklists have been used (see Appendices A and B); the parental responses can provide the topics for discussion.

B. **Facilitating the dialogue.** The parent's story should be facilitated by appropriate empathetic responses, such as, "Tell me more about that" or "I can see that it did not work out so well for you," or *"That must be hard for you."* The clinician should avoid interruptions, subject changes, and judgmental comments and not prematurely pursue other diagnostic hypotheses, which can derail the parent's narrative. Attentive listening during the opening of an interview promotes communication and rarely takes more than a couple of minutes. Yet it has also been shown that, on average, physicians interrupt the patients within a few seconds or minutes. The reason is conflicting agendas: patients want to tell their story, and clinicians want to pursue their medical task (diagnosis, prescription, or therapeutic recommendation). There are other strategies to facilitate a successful pediatric visit.

C. **Elicit the parent's concerns early in the interview.** *"What worried you especially when you brought John in to see us today? Why did that worry you?"*

D. **Elicit the parent's expectations for the visit and acknowledge them.** *"What had you hoped we might be able to do for your child today? What would you like to have us explain to you today?"* These inquiries may reveal unrealistic expectations for specific therapies or magical cures. At other times, such questions make the clinician's job simple if what the family desires is reassurance. Once the parent's expectations have been

Table 1-1. How to enhance the therapeutic alliance

Process steps	Sample comments

Greet
  Introduce self
  Set agenda jointly	

Listen
  Allow pauses
  Maintain eye contact	

Facilitate
  Do not judge
  Do not interrupt
	"Tell me more about that."

Elicit and acknowledge parent's concern	"You thought the high fever might bring on a seizure?"
Elicit and acknowledge parent's expectations	"What are you hoping we will do for her today?"
Involve the child	"What has this been like for you?" "Do you understand why you are here?"
Be family centered	
Guide (not dominate) discourse	
Elicit the parent's solutions	"What have you tried so far?" "What would you like to try at this time?"
Make treatment decisions jointly	"Do you think you will be able to give him the medicine four times a day?"
Make closure and agenda setting explicit	

acknowledged, the clinician, the parents, and the child can set an agenda for the visit, which synthesizes the parent's concerns and biomedical issues. It is only after this opening—after listening attentively to the parent—that the clinician can afford to pursue his or her line of questions and fact finding. The first phase of the interaction has taken care of urgent concerns, relaxed the parent, and made her or him realize that the clinician is interested. The parent will now be a better historian and partner in the task-oriented portion of the interview. Experience shows that the above suggestions will make the interview more effective and so lead to earlier closure, which is becoming more and more important these days, will the economic pressures and changes in healthcare delivery systems.

E. Guide but do not dominate the discourse. General questions allow parents to broach subjects of interest to them. For routine healthcare maintenance visits, clinicians can use simple questions: *"How are things going?"*, "What are some new things the baby is doing?", "How do things work out at bedtime?", "What is the hardest part of taking care of him now?", "What is most enjoyable about taking care of him?", "Is the baby's father (or mother) able to give you any help?" Open-ended, nonjudgmental questions are essential for this phase of the interview. In this context, we are often asked "What do I do when the patient takes up a lot of time in reciting irrelevant information he or she has obtained from the Internet?" A contemptuous remark, such as "Where did you go to medical school" is sure to rupture the therapeutic alliance. Courteous respectful reminders that the time for the visit is limited and the need to focus on the child's problems could be more effective.

F. Use common courtesy. All the amenities of human interaction in nonmedical contexts must also be observed. Even clinicians who usually have good manners will, in the task-oriented medical encounter, omit greetings, introductions, and courtesies (such as knocking on the door before entering the examination room or explaining the reasons for keeping someone waiting). These courtesies should include a few appropriate remarks acknowledging the parent as a person, such as, "You sure have your hands full today," to the parent who comes with several children and all the attending paraphernalia, or, "I bet you are impatient with us for having kept you waiting so long. I had to deal with an emergency upstairs." This is also critically important if one is using an EMR. Acknowledge from the beginning of the visit that at times you will need to type information in the record to ensure patient safety and accuracy.

III. Talking with the child. Early in the visit, an appropriate approach must be made to the child; this is especially important when the social distance between practitioner and family is great or when communication is difficult because of the parent's anxiety, suspicion, or hostility. The awareness of a mutual interest in helping the child creates a bond between parent and clinician. Throughout the interview, in spite of the demands of the EMR, the practitioner must maintain eye contact with the child and the parent and watch for non-verbal signs of distress or disagreement or of reassurance and relief.

IV. Dealing with acute illnesses. During an acute illness, the interview must be focused. As the parent tells the story of the illness, the practitioner can facilitate responsively: *"So the fever has been high for almost 3 days now ... What are some of the other things you have noticed? ... How did you handle that? ... How did that work out? ... What about feeding? .... Sleep? .... Any other changes?"*

- If the parents have used any complementary and alternative therapies, it is essential not to make judgmental statements. If the treatment was harmless and the parent feels it was effective (even when the practitioner would not have chosen it), it is best to support the parent's approach.
- If a parent has attempted an intervention that is potentially harmful (e.g., giving aspirin for a viral infection), the clinician should not use this moment to give alarming warnings (e.g., about Reye's syndrome). Yet the family needs to be informed. Our approach is "I am glad she is feeling better, but I need to give you some new information. Aspirin has been around a long time, and it has provided relief for many patients. However, we have learned that aspirin can have side effects that involve severe liver damage and can be very serious, although rare. Your baby is obviously fine, but I feel strongly that, from now on, you should avoid aspirin and use acetaminophen instead."
- After the episode is over and the parent is less likely to be overwhelmed by guilt and anxieties, more complete and forceful information can be given. Alternatives and additional treatments can be suggested without undermining the parent's self-confidence and self-esteem.
- To avoid embarrassment and fractures of the clinician–parent alliance, at all times the clinician should ask, *"How have you handled that? What have you been doing or giving her so far?"*, before launching into medical advice. Whenever possible, the parent's own solution should be supported. When developing other approaches, it is best to involve the parent. For example, *"Has anyone suggested to you that it is time to give up the bottle feeding? Have you yourself contemplated making a change? How ready are you to make the necessary changes?"* Before giving what seems to be appropriate advice, the clinician must assess the families' readiness to change, their conviction that change is necessary, and their confidence that they can, indeed, change. A therapeutic plan has to be a joint venture; rarely should it be imposed without parental input.

V. Redirecting the interview. The clinician needs to keep control of the interview, even while being supportive and accepting. When the discussion gets off track, the clinician needs to redirect the discourse—for instance, *"We must sit down and discuss that on another occasion after he is over this illness,"* or "There is some other information I need right now so we can decide about the treatment for this illness." If the parent makes an unreasonable request, such as, "You will give him a shot of antibiotics today, won't you?", the clinician can back off and state, *"I do not know whether that will be necessary today. We will talk about that after I have examined your son."*

VI. Counseling and reassurance. Advising and counseling the patient and family can be a continuing process. Some concerns may be addressed at the first mention. For example, if the mother says, "He still wakes up once in the night and calls for me," the clinician may reassure promptly that this is not unusual at his age: *"He misses you in the dark alone in his bedroom. Just comfort him, but do not start a night bottle again."* Other concerns may best be allayed during the physical examination: "The arches of the foot normally do not develop before the child has been weight bearing for a while." Other topics require a discussion at the end of the visit or even at another scheduled conference time: *"I can see you are having real difficulty in setting limits for his behavior at this time."* We need to take some time to see what we can work out to help him accept your discipline and to make your life a little easier.

VII. Closure.
- **A.** Summarize the relevant points the parent has raised and information he or she has given toward the end of the encounter.
- **B.** Offer other educational materials, such as handouts, and individualize them by underlining certain specific issues or relating them to the parent's concerns.
- **C.** Invite questions from caregivers, family, and child. Even when there is no time for full responses, they can be included in jointly setting the agenda for subsequent visits and follow-up healthcare.

BIBLIOGRAPHY

Beckman H, Frankel R. The effect of physician behavior on the collection of data. *Ann Intern Med* 101:692–696, 1984.

Johnson KB, Serwint JR, Fagan LA, et al. Computer-based documentation: effects on parent-provider communication during pediatric health maintenance encounters. *Pediatrics* 122(3):590–598, 2008.

Korsch B, Harding C. *The Intelligent Patient's Guide to the Doctor-Patient Relationship.* New York: Oxford University Press, 1997.

Roter D, Hall J. *Doctors Talking With Patients; Patients Talking With Doctors.* Westport, CT: Auburn House, 1997.

Stewart M, Roter D (eds). *Communicating with Medical Patients.* Newbury Park, CA: Sage Productions Inc., 1989.

2

Talking with Children

Yi Hui Liu
Martin T. Stein

I. **The importance.**
   A. **Pediatric clinicians acknowledge the significance of nurturing an independent and trusting relationship with the child.** As a child's primary care provider, the pediatric clinician has the unique opportunity to develop such a bond over time. Even short encounters with children can benefit from the skills required to sustain a longitudinal relationship.
   B. **The child must be recognized and valued as an equal partner and active participant in his care.** This enhances his self-esteem as he learns about and develops responsibility for his own health. The child must view his pediatric clinician as a source not only of treatment but also of guidance and support. He should recognize the pediatric clinician as *his* physician, not his parent's. These experiences mold the child's view of himself and may contribute to his response to health and illness in adulthood.
   C. **The establishment of a therapeutic alliance with the child allows the pediatric clinician to ascertain important information about the child and his environment** such as the child's strengths, stressors, developmental status, and place in the family and community. Children may also reveal information that the parent is unaware of or may have omitted. At the same time, the pediatric clinician is able to assess language, speech, and auditory functioning.
   D. **The pediatric clinician models for parents the art of listening to and respecting the views of their child from as early as infancy.** The pediatric clinician's response to the child's feelings or misbehavior may illustrate to the parent appropriate management techniques (e.g., reflection, limit setting).
II. **Creating the environment: promoting effective communication.**
   A. **The reception area.** A child-friendly environment conveys to the child that this place is for children. If possible, provide separate areas for children of different ages with age-appropriate décor and materials. Toys, a fish tank, books, a drawing board, room to crawl and walk, child-sized furniture, children's drawings, and children's pictures all impart a welcoming environment. Paper and crayons allow the child to draw pictures that may be used to facilitate conversation or to illustrate the child's perception of himself, his family, or his situation. Consider not having a television in the waiting room as this does not support the message that families should be selective in television viewing and does not encourage parents to interact with their children. A literacy-rich waiting room is a more positive slant on how children and adults can interact around a book.
   B. **The examination/interview room.** Toys, books, drawing materials, child-sized furniture, and child-friendly décor are useful in making the child feel at ease. A quiet, appealing, and private environment encourages the child to interact with the pediatric clinician. There should be no barriers (such as a large desk) between the pediatric clinician and the child, and the pediatric clinician should place herself at the child's eye level.
   C. **The greeting.** When appropriate, speak to the child first. This promotes the message that the child is the patient. Approach the child in a calm and friendly manner and ask him what he would like to be called. Commenting on a toy or a book that he has brought or the clothes he is wearing can be a pleasant icebreaker. If you use a computer-based electronic medical record, acknowledge to the child that sometimes you will need to type during the visit.
III. **Communication tools.**
   A. **Open-ended questions.** Start with open-ended questions to allow the child to express his thoughts and concerns for the visit. Further questions may elicit the child's personal and culturally influenced perception of his situation, helping his pediatric clinician understand his frame of reference. Closed-ended questions may follow open-ended questions to generate additional specific information. Members of some cultures will not respond to or be comfortable with an open-ended question if they are expecting the physician to act in a more directive manner.

B. **Pauses and silence.** Allowing the child time to organize his thoughts or regain composure and then to express his feelings without pressure shows him respect and concern.

C. **Reflection (repetition).** If the child makes a puzzling or significant comment, repeat the key words or phrases back in a neutral or questioning tone to encourage him to clarify or elaborate further.

D. **Empathy.** Acknowledge and respond to the child's feelings to convey warmth and sympathy. Listen for the message behind his words.

E. **Active listening.** Provide undivided attention and facilitate the conversation through open-ended questions, silences, and repetition to communicate to the child respect and concern. Both body language (leaning forward, eye contact) and verbal expressions (e.g., "tell me more") can convey support and interest, allowing the child to feel comfortable in expressing his feelings and thoughts and thus to participate in the visit more fully.

F. **Tracking.** Allow the child to set the interview's style, pace, and language.

G. **Summarizing.** After explaining the assessment and plan to the child, review the major points. Avoid using medical jargon. Asking the child to summarize what has been said will ensure that the information has been understood. It is helpful to make the recommendations practical and concrete.

IV. **Communication techniques for different age groups.**

A. **In general.**

1. Engage the child early in the visit with talk, play, or other activities to lessen anxiety. Be mindful of the child's temperament and approach the child accordingly.

2. Use age-appropriate words and eye contact. Children younger than 2 years may find eye contact to be threatening and may be comforted by watching their parents respond to the pediatric clinician in a friendly manner. In addition, questions about "when" and "why" may not be useful in young children who do not yet understand time and causality.

3. Start with casual questions about familiar and comfortable subjects in an encouraging manner before moving on to more difficult ones. Talk about a child's interests (sports, music), family, friends, or school to develop rapport with him. Use special interests as an opener for subsequent visits.

4. Approach difficult questions in a nonjudgmental and matter-of-fact manner. Indirect statements and questions can be effective in opening discussions about potentially sensitive areas (bullying, fears, school failure, drug use, sex, suicide risk, family conflicts). Starting the discussion about children in general, followed by acquaintances, and then the child is less threatening. *"Some kids tell me that they have a tough time with other kids at school. Do you know anyone with this problem? What has been your experience?"*

5. Humor can dispel anxieties and make the visit enjoyable at all age levels.

6. The **TEACHER** method can enhance communication with children and their parents (Table 2-1).

Table 2-1. TEACHER: A method for enhancing communication with pediatric patients and their parents

T	Trust	Build trust and rapport with the child by asking nonthreatening questions not related to illness
E	Elicit	Elicit information from parent(s) and child regarding parental fears and concerns and the child's understanding of the reason for the visit
A	Agenda	Set an agenda early in the visit to help ensure that the parents' concerns are addressed
C	Control	Help the child feel control over the visit (e.g., knowing what will and will not happen) to help decrease fear and increase cooperation
H	Health plan	Establish a health plan with the child and the parent to meet the child's needs and limitations
E	Explain	Explain the health plan to the child in a way he can understand
R	Rehearse	Have the child rehearse the health plan as a way of assessing understanding; reinforce the child's jobs related to healthcare; and explore any potential problems in the plan with the child and the parent

B. Communicating with children younger than 6 months.
1. Developmental stage: Symbiotic. The infant and the primary caregiver have a strong attachment. The child is not significantly fearful of strangers.
2. At this age, the pediatric clinician can model for the parent appropriate ways of speaking to and encouraging language development in babies.

C. Communicating with children 6 months to 3 years of age.
1. Developmental stage: Separation–individuation. The child often has stranger awareness and may cling to parents as she gradually loosens early attachment and develops a sense of her own autonomy.
2. The child should be allowed to stay close to the parent (sitting on parent's lap) for reassurance.
3. Avoid direct, prolonged eye contact with the child younger than 2 years as this may be perceived as threatening.
4. Approach the child gently and gradually. Watch his body language to judge his acceptance. Wait until he is willing to leave his parent's lap.
5. Use play (peekaboo, keys, flash light, or toy) to capture the child's attention and ease his anxiety.
6. Prepare the child for physical contact. Imitation with the parent or a doll/stuffed animal will ease the child's anxiety during the physical examination and any procedures.

D. Communicating with children 3–6 years of age.
1. Developmental stage: Preschool age–age of initiative. The child has increasing language skills and engages in fantasy play. The child's understanding of illness is mediated by magical thinking.
2. Use simple language. Expressive and receptive language skills starting at 3 years of age allow the pediatric clinician to begin use of the communication techniques described earlier to elicit the child's concerns and thoughts. Remember, a child's receptive language is more advanced than his expressive language.
3. Encourage the child to ask questions.
4. Engage the child by explaining procedures and allowing him to participate in the examination. Offer choices when possible and talk to him about his healthcare.
5. As these children enter school age, some time alone with the pediatric clinician can further the development of an independent relationship.

E. Communicating with children 6–12 years of age.
1. Developmental stage: School age–age of industry. The child has improved cognitive skills and develops the ability to understand cause and effect. Concrete thinking characterizes younger school-aged children, whereas the ability to generalize and begin to understand causes of illness occurs in older preadolescents.
2. School-aged children enjoy talking about family, friends, school, and other facets of their lives. Their interests and strengths are easily determined.
3. Explanation of procedures, assessments, and plans becomes important and helpful in eliciting the preadolescent's cooperation.
4. Spend some time alone with the school-aged child to determine any further concerns and to continue to foster a relationship with the child.

F. Communicating with adolescents.
1. Developmental stage: Age of identity. The adolescent is focused on changing body features and is developing abstract reasoning. He is able to understand the general principles of illness and recovery.
2. Interview the adolescent separate from the parent to respect growing independence, to recognize his individuality, and to cultivate the therapeutic alliance.
3. Elicit and address the adolescent's concerns.
4. Emphasize and clarify confidentiality issues as adolescents may withhold information that they believe will be relayed to their parents. Obtain the adolescent's permission to share information or discuss certain issues with others.
5. Do not pressure the adolescent to talk. Be patient and respect the adolescent's privacy. It is better to revisit difficult topics on a later date after trust has been gained.
6. Address difficult topics (drugs, sex, depression, anxiety, eating disorders) in a nonjudgmental manner after rapport has been developed. Indirect questions and statements as well as asking first about the experience of the adolescent's friends are helpful.
7. Talking about "stress" may be easier than asking directly about depression and anxiety. This is less threatening since "stress" is perceived as a normal part of life.
8. Always be truthful.
9. Acknowledge that the adolescent is responsible for personal healthcare and advocate for the adolescent with parents.

V. Clinical pearls and pitfalls.

   A. Cultural sensitivity.

   1. Respecting a child and family's cultural values, beliefs, and attitudes is essential in facilitating communication and cooperation. Ask about cultural interpretations of medical and social issues. *"What do you call this problem? What do you think caused it? How do you treat it? What do you expect the treatment to do?"*

   2. Knowledge about cultures is useful in avoiding unintentional distress. For example, Southeast Asians will show respect to a physician by avoiding direct eye contact. Being overly complimentary about a child may elicit fears in the Hmong who feel this may bring unwanted attention from malevolent spirits.

   B. Nonverbal communication/information. Body language (posture, facial expressions) and quality and tone of speech are important clues to the psychological state of a child. With clinical practice, nonverbal clues may provide crucial information about the veracity or full disclosure of information by a child/adolescent and receptivity to the clinician's assessment and advice. Motor, social, and adaptive skills as well as temperament can be assessed through observation of the child's activity during the encounter.

   C. The parent–child interaction. Assess parent–child interactions that may provide insights to attachment, parenting style, parenting skills, and family dynamics. Model appropriate use of language, soothing behaviors, and discipline techniques when a teachable moment presents.

   D. Procedures. Developmentally appropriate explanations of procedures (e.g., immunizations, venapuncture, operations) are critical and rehearsal of the sequence of events helps to ease a child's anxieties. The parent's presence during a procedure usually lessens the stress to the child; separation should generally be avoided. Be truthful if a procedure will cause any pain. Offer choices to the child as possible (which arm to draw blood from, what color cast he or she would like).

   E. Illness and hospitalization.

   1. Anticipatory guidance about diagnostic/therapeutic procedures and an elective hospitalization help both child and parent. A preschool child's magical thinking, a school-aged child's concrete thinking, and an older school-aged child's emerging ability to understand causality moderate their response to illness and the clinician's language and content of information.

   2. Hospitalization is associated with a sudden environmental change, loss of independence, and separation from primary caretakers. Provide the child with a description of the hospital environment and the procedures encountered. Keep some familiar toys, books, or attachment objects with the child if separation is unavoidable.

   F. Common pitfalls.

   1. **Communication only with parents.** When the pediatric clinician communicates primarily with the parents, an opportunity to uncover important information and to nurture an independent relationship with the child may be missed. As a preventive measure, start an encounter by greeting the child; the implied message is that the child is the patient.

   2. **Simultaneous examination and interview.** This technique does not allow the physician to establish eye contact, communicate effectively, or promote a trusting relationship with the child.

   3. **Distractions.** With the increasing use of electronic medical records, the pediatric clinician is cautioned to be aware of how much eye contact is made with the screen rather than with the family. Pagers and cell phones should be set on vibration, and a room-in-use sign can prevent unnecessary interruptions.

BIBLIOGRAPHY

For parents

Brazelton TB. Your child's doctor. In Brazelton TB (ed), *Touchpoints: Your Child's Emotional and Behavioral Development.* Reading, MA: Perseus Publishing, 1992, pp. 451–461.

Web site

www.kidshealth.org

For professionals

American Academy of Pediatrics. *Bright Futures: Guidelines for Health Supervision of Infants, Children, and Adolescents.* Elk Grove Village, IL: American Academy of Pediatrics, 2008.

Beresin EV. The doctor-patient relationship in pediatrics. In Kaye DL, Montgomery ME, Munson SW (eds),*Child and Adolescent Mental Health*. Philadelphia: Lippincott Williams & Wilkins, 2002.

Stein MT. Developmentally based office: setting the stage for enhanced practice. In Dixon SD, Stein MT (eds), *Encounters with Children: Pediatric Behavior and Development*. Philadelphia: Mosby, 2006, pp. 73–97.

Stein MT. Encounters with illness: coping and growing. In Dixon SD, Stein MT (eds), *Encounters with Children: Pediatric Behavior and Development*. Philadelphia: Mosby, 2006, pp. 649–673.

Taylor L, Willies-Jacobo L. The culturally competent pediatrician: respecting ethnicity in your practice. *Contemp Pediatr* 20:83, 2003.

Wender EH. Interviewing: a critical skill. In Carey WB, Crocker AC, Coleman WL, Elias ER, Feldman HM (eds), *Developmental-Behavioral Pediatrics*. Philadelphia: Saunders, 2009, pp. 747–755.

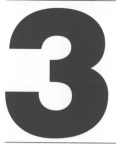

Teachable Moments in Primary Care

Barry Zuckerman
Steven Parker
Margot Kaplan-Sanoff

I. **Description.** Teachable moments (TM) represent a strategy to help pediatric clinicians provide effective education for parents within the time constraints of a typical office visit. By using the basic assessments of the pediatric visit—history taking, physical examinations, and developmental surveillance—as potent TM, one can exploit the educational opportunities they present for intervention. The strategy of TM is to use the behavior of the child and the clinician–parent interactions in the office as compelling, shared experiences that further parents' insights into their child and enhance their sense of competence as parents. Using everyday questions and experiences in the office as a shared context for discussion as the visit progresses is an efficient way to address such issues without appreciably lengthening the visit.

The goals of using TM are to:
- Enhance parents' understanding of the child's needs
- Promote "goodness of fit" between parent and child
- Model constructive interactions with the child
- Improve the relationship between the pediatric clinician and the parent

A. **Using behavior in the office as a TM.**

1. Discussions of the infant's or child's behavior in the office provide a fruitful context for TM. Newly emerging and developed skills and behaviors can challenge the equilibrium between parent and child. Frequently, a specific behavior that parents find disturbing—for example, mouthing toys at 6 months of age, throwing blocks or food at 8 months of age, refusing to lie down to be diapered at 10 months of age, irrepressible exploration at 18 months of age, playing with his penis at 3 years of age—is developmentally normal and expectable. Parents' concerns about these issues create a special opportunity to promote parental understanding of typical health and development.

   a. Concerns that new parents bring to pediatric visits in the first months of a child's life provide a wealth of TM (Table 3-1). The infant's behavior creates a special opportunity to promote parental understanding and support. For example, if the infant cries inconsolably during the visit or her cues are difficult to read, the clinician can explore how parents feel and empathize with their frustration at not being able to calm the baby. The goal of this TM is to blend information about development with the message that the parents are "experts" on their baby and doing a good job caring for their child.

2. When a child's behavior in the office provides a TM, it is up to the clinician to capitalize on it. During these TM, one might infer or "read" the child's behavior or temperament together with the parents and offer constructive interpretations of its significance. The clinician should then ask parents how they feel about the behavior or use their own reactions to explore parental concerns. If the clinician finds the child's behavior frustrating, chances are so do the parents.

3. If child behaviors do not produce TM spontaneously, the clinician may employ specific strategies to engage the child and discuss the implications for behavior and development (Table 3-2). Parents tend to watch carefully as the pediatric clinician engages the child in activities—for example, handing the child a toy or a book, rolling a ball back and forth, listening to the heart, or looking into the ears—that demonstrate a particular behavioral or temperamental quality or developmental skill. In some cases, a pediatric clinician can direct his comments to the child rather than to the parents: "You like seeing the pictures of babies in the books, don't you? This book is making you very excited" as you show parents that even 6-month-olds get fascinated by picture books. If this serves to encourage parents to start sharing books with babies, the first step in learning to read has been taken. When children push the clinician's hand away as he attempts to listen to the heart, the clinician can talk about other behaviors in which the child is "uncooperative" for the parent.

Table 3-1. Eliciting teachable moments: Exploring relationships

Birth to 4 months of age

Maneuver	Comment
Rock a fussy newborn in your arms and speak softly to console him. Hold a drowsy newborn in a vertical position on your shoulder to bring him to an alert state.	Whether or not your tactics work, explain what you are trying to do and draw the parents' attention to the infant's reactions. If their baby is unresponsive or difficult to arouse or console, they may be feeling rejected. By showing them that this is difficult for you too, you help them understand that they are not to blame. Explaining about temperament as an inherent characteristic can encourage them to try new approaches to arousing and consoling their child.
Draw parents' attention to the reciprocal interaction you see going on between parents and 2- to 3-month-old child as they take turns smiling and cooing at each other.	Tell parents that this playful exchange shows normal emotional development (baby's smiling, happy face), the beginning of language (vowel sounds, ahs and coos), and cognitive ability (taking turns).
Smile at the 3- or 4-month-old child and try to get the baby to smile back and then ask the parents to try.	Point out that parents got a quicker, bigger smile. Explain that while infants at this age smile at everyone, they smile more readily and more fully at the people to whom they feel closest. This can lead to a discussion of who else gets big smiles (grandparents, the babysitter) and help prepare parents for the next stage when the baby's general friendliness will be replaced by stranger anxiety.

4. By observing and commenting on the child's behavior, the pediatric clinician encourages the parents to step back and speculate about its meaning. Unrealistic expectations, which can contribute to parental frustration and lead to child abuse or neglect, can be gently corrected. If parents' reactions are negative, the clinician can reframe the child's behavior in a more positive light. The more mobile 12- to 18-month-old child can be described as "exuberant" or "exploratory" rather than "disobedient." The child who is "uncooperative" with the physical examination is really "asserting his independence."

   a. For example, parents often describe how their 7–8 month old child throws his food off the high chair tray, making a mess for the parents to clean. They then respond by controlling the feeding and not allowing the child to feed himself. The clinician can join with the parents around how messy babies can be. The clinician can reframe the throwing behavior, explaining how shaking and throwing are the infant's way of exploring objects to discover what the objects can do. This can easily be demonstrated by giving the child a toy in the office and watching him bang, shake, and throw it. The clinician can create a TM by narrating the child's actions, reframing them as acts of exploration rather than as deliberate attempts to make a mess. The clinician can explain how seemingly unimportant tasks, such as using a pincer grasp to pick up a cheerio, are important windows into a baby's development and learning.

   b. Another example of reframing behavior involves stranger anxiety. Many children are visibly upset by the 12- to 15-month visit because of their heightened stranger and separation anxiety. They may express this anxiety by actively refusing to cooperate with the examination and by protesting when the pediatric clinician tries to examine them. This behavior, often embarrassing to parents, can be used as a TM to discuss stranger anxiety and its developmental function and to explore its ramifications for the families. Parents are usually relieved to understand why it is a developmental inevitability and a sign of positive emotional and cognitive growth for their baby to become wary of strangers and actively and loudly resist separation. They are also pleased to learn that these behaviors are linked to cognitive growth in object permanence.

Table 3-2. Eliciting teachable moments: Exploring the world

With each maneuver, comment on the child's interest, attention, and excitement. Point out that these attributes will serve the child well in future learning situations.

Teachable moments 6–12 months

Maneuver	Comment
1. Put a cheerio in front of the baby within reach. Ask parents to observe how the baby tries to get it.	At 6 months, the baby will use her thumb and all her fingers in an uncoordinated, raking movement. Explain to parents that babies at this age do not have the fine motor coordination to pick up a small object. Have them keep watching. At 9 months, when her nervous system is more mature, she will pick up a cheerio with a pincer movement of the thumb and forefinger and put it into her mouth. Use this behavior as a teachable moment to point out that a baby who can do this with a cheerio can pick up other small objects as well, not all of them edible or safe. Warn about keeping small objects out of reach.
2. Give the child a toy car, about 2 inches long.	What the baby does with the car will change over time. At 5–6 months, he will probably put it in his mouth. Tell parents that mouthing is the first stage in a sequence of learning about the nature of objects. By 7–8 months, they can expect him to be into throwing and banging, and at 9 months he will inspect the car intently, turning it over and over in his hand and feeling its contours. Each stage yields more information about the car's properties than the one before. At about 1 year of age, he will show his understanding of the toy's function by running its wheels along the floor.
3. Hide a favorite object under a cloth while the baby is watching.	When the infant takes the cloth away, discuss how this demonstrates her beginning understanding of object permanence, the knowledge that objects continue to exist even when the baby cannot see them. This discovery adds to her knowledge that the world has some consistency and dependability to it. Infants are beginning to have a mental representation of the object which explains why they can search and find the hidden toy now when they could not do it at 6 months of age. Compare this ability to understand object permanence with person permanence. Discuss how separation anxiety and protest when the mother leaves the room demonstrates that the baby now has a mental symbol of her mother and the discrepancy between that symbol and her not being there evokes crying and protest in an attempt to get the mother to return.
4. Engage the child in reaching for a pen which is extended to him.	The pediatric clinician can again demonstrate improved visual–motor functioning. The infant will shape his fingers midway through the reach, depending on the placement of the pen. This again is a reflection of neuromaturational development and greater efficiency of the visual-motor process.

(continued)

Table 3-2. (Continued)

12 months (1 year) of age

Maneuver	Comment
1. Again offer the extended pen to the child.	Starting at about 12 months of age, stranger anxiety often prevents the child from reaching toward a stranger.
2. Give the baby a pop-up toy or busy-box to play with.	Discuss the strategies that the child uses to figure out how to get the toy to perform. The baby who uses various schemes such as banging, shaking, and poking has developed more ways to use objects and to extract meaning from objects. This broadens her cognitive understanding of how the world works. Use these exploratory schemes for discovering causality as a teachable moment in response to the classic complaint of most parents that 1-year-olds are "into everything." Emphasize that while this can be annoying to parents and cause for safety concerns, it is the toddler's way of learning about the objects in his environment. Discuss ways to amuse busy toddlers while the parents cook, eat, and go about their normal routines.
3. The child's autonomy and stranger anxiety can be seen when the child tries to fend off the physical examination.	This presents an opportunity to discuss with parents the child's temperament, level of persistence and intensity, and autonomy regarding everyday activities.

15 months of age

Maneuver	Comment
1. In many cases the pediatric clinician need not do anything to provoke an example of the child's growing autonomy. Most children scream as soon as they get into the room with strangers.	The pediatric clinician can model *how* to anticipate and limit the baby's stranger anxiety *by* slowly approaching the child using his or her voice as a distraction technique. If that approach is unsuccessful, the pediatric clinician can point to his or her own disappointment and how other family members or friends who see the child infrequently may feel rejected by the child.
2. Give the child a toy telephone and see whether he can demonstrate functional use by putting the phone to his ear. Ask him to let a doll talk on the phone.	Discuss the child's ability to represent the use of a toy phone on a doll. This stage of cognitive development signals the beginning of symbolic representation, when the child can use one object to represent another object that is not present. Children at this age can demonstrate the functional use of cars, dolls, and care-giving activities such as feeding, and can imitate house-work such as vacuuming and washing dishes.

18 months of age

Maneuver	Comment
1. Give the child a container and blocks.	Note the seemingly endless delight that toddlers have in dumping and filling. There is a sense of satisfaction and fulfillment to the activity. There is also a cognitive component. Toddlers are learning about the properties of objects in space, about completing a task (when the bucket is full), and about a parent's reaction to the toddler's goal of filling and dumping. This also gives the pediatric clinician the opportunity to talk about throwing objects and offer suggestions for how to handle limit setting with young toddlers.

(continued)

Table 3-2. (*Continued*)

24 months (2 years) of age	
Maneuver	Comment
1. Give the child a book.	Talk about the child's attempts at exploring the book-turning pages, looking at all the pictures. Does the child bring the book to the parents to show them or ask them to read it? This activity also offers the opportunity to talk about the importance of reading aloud to young children and the concept of dialogic reading—or asking the child open-ended questions (see Chapter 7). Comment on "joint attention," ways to support the child's attention, and following the child's lead in storytelling.

30 months of age	
Maneuver	Comment
1. Demonstrate the child's receptive language skills by asking the child to complete two- and three-step commands.	Watching their child perform these tasks correctly can be particularly important for parents who are worried about their child's language development. Demonstrating the sophistication with which the child can follow directions often calms the fears of a parent who is worried about a child who is not talking as well as his age mates.

36 months (3 years) of age	
Maneuver	Comment
1. Use a ball to introduce simple games.	While playing ballgames with the child, point out the child's ability to take turns, understand reciprocity, keep the ball within the physical limits set by the game (between your legs and his), and kick it forward.

Adapted from Zuckerman B, Parker S. Teachable moments: assessment as intervention. *Contemp Pediatrics* 103–118, 1997.

    c. The **18- to 24-month period** is marked by struggles over control, by limit testing, and by the toddler's ability to get herself into serious trouble as she climbs too high or runs away too quickly from a parent. The physical examination and immunizations usually produce enough negative responses from the toddler to bring these issues to the surface. Since clinician and parent have both observed these behaviors, they create yet another TM, giving the clinician insight into how the parents understand the behavior and how they respond to it. It is important at moments like these to:
- *Empathize* with the parents. They need assurance that their child's behavior is normal, as is their frustration and embarrassment or anger at their child
- *Explain* that a toddler's autonomy struggles often feel like the child is "refusing to listen"
- *Model* verbal and behavioral strategies to help the child cope with the experience of being in the office, for example, demonstrating for the parents the importance of setting safe limits for the child while trying to avoid unnecessary power struggles regarding parental control, that is, "I know that you like jumping off high places, but jumping off the exam table is not safe"
- *Help* the child feel like she has mastered a stressful situation by commenting on her attempts at control: "I know it was hard for you, but you did a good job when I looked in your ears." Instead of the child feeling like a failure and the parents feeling embarrassed or angry or both, the family can feel that you understood and accepted their reactions and that you still like their child and respect their parenting efforts

B. Using history taking as a teachable moment.
    1. Evocative questions during history taking, especially in the first year of life, can create special TM. Such questions might include asking about the parents' own upbringing, the "ghosts/angels in the nursery" that influence their child-rearing practices, and their feelings about themselves as parents (see Chapter 10). Eliciting a family history of depression and alcoholism may help parents understand the impact

of these factors on their parenting and their fears about their child's (and their own) vulnerability to these or other mental health problems.

2. Questions about the **child's behavior and development** give parents a chance to discuss concerns in these areas. Especially useful in the early years are questions about the child's temperamental characteristics, developmental milestones, behavioral and family issues, and how the parents feel about these issues.

3. A dialogue about **parental disagreements** is another example of a potential TM during history taking. Asking how a family handles anger or resolves disputes often leads to a discussion of these issues and their impact on child behavior and development. The clinician might say that children benefit when they see their parents come to a peaceful conclusion after an argument, or point out that conflicts are an opportunity to teach children about frustration, anger, and disagreements without fear of the loss of love.

4. **Clinical judgment** is always required to distinguish when it is appropriate to expand and when to narrow the content of the discussion. Also, it is helpful to remember that while some parents find it helpful to discuss their feelings, others experience personal questions as intrusive. Sensing when not to intrude on the parents' privacy is as important as knowing what, how, and when to probe.

5. Finally, clinicians should be aware that TM also occur when children who are old enough to understand are asked directly about their health and behavior. Asking 3-year-olds whether they brush their teeth or eat their vegetables conveys the message that they have a responsibility to take good care of their bodies. The opportunity should not be missed.

C. Using the physical examination as a teachable moment.

1. The physical examination provides the pediatric clinician with a window into the child's behavior and development. One can comment how *this* child at *this* age responds to the examination, compared to her behavior at an earlier age. As the pediatric clinician performs the examination, he should narrate a running commentary about the findings: "Heart sounds great—good, strong heart! Lungs are clear . . . No sign of bronchitis. Ears have a little bit of fluid—do you think she is hearing okay?" This running narrative serves, first and foremost, to reassure mothers and fathers that their child is healthy. In this regard, one should avoid ambiguous statements such as: "Well, she doesn't sound too bad or I can't find anything wrong." Such equivocation does little to reassure and may set the anxious parent's mind racing.

2. The examination also serves as a natural springboard to elicit more information or concerns from the observing parent. Neutral, nonjudgmental comments about the child's behavior (e.g., "He certainly is a busy guy, isn't he?") may trigger a host of parental concerns, elicited all the more easily by focusing ostensibly on the child's physical examination and not the parental feelings.

3. Finally, the physical examination is a wonderful opportunity for the pediatric clinician to reframe the child's behavior in order to enhance parent–child interactions. One's demeanor toward the child serves as a model for the parent. Certainly, the physical examination must be approached with respect for the child and sensitivity to issues of power and control. For example, the obstreperous toddler who resists examination offers the opportunity to discuss the child's attempts at autonomy, individuation, and his understandable desire to maintain control of his body. The child who cries but then consoles himself sets the stage for a discussion of his coping skills.

BIBLIOGRAPHY

For clinicians

Parker S, Zuckerman B. Therapeutic aspects of the assessment process. In Meisels S, Shonkoff J (eds), *Handbook of Early Childhood Intervention*. New York: Cambridge University Press, 1990, pp. 350–371.

Zuckerman B. Family history: a special opportunity for psychosocial intervention. *Pediatrics* 87:740, 1991.

Zuckerman B, Parker S. Teachable moments: assessment as intervention. *Contemp Pediatrics* 103–118, 1997.

Web sites for clinicians

http://www.pediatriccareonline.org/pco/ub/view/Bright-Futures-Pocket-Guide/135503/5/core_concepts

http://www.pediatricsinpractice.org/new/teaching_center/curricular_mod_education.asp

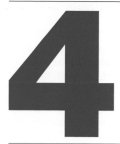

Anticipatory Guidance in Well Child Care Visits in the First 3 Years: The Touchpoints™ Model of Development

Joshua Sparrow
T. Berry Brazelton

I. **What is a Touchpoint?**
A. **Touchpoints are predictable developmental crises.** Each developmental spurt is preceded by a temporary regression. These regressions often consist of sleep disruptions, food refusal, increased crying, clinging, and seeking physical contact, or temper tantrums. When young children become disorganized, parents become disorganized too. The succession of Touchpoints in development is like a map that can be anticipated by both parents and clinicians. This helps prevent parental overreactions that may inadvertently reinforce regressive behaviors and lead to more serious developmental deviations, for example, in the areas of sleep, feeding, toilet training, and behavioral control. **Thirteen Touchpoints** have been noted through the first 3 years, beginning in pregnancy. They involve caregiving themes that matter to parents (e.g., feeding, sleep, discipline, toilet training), rather than traditional, static milestones. The child's negotiation of these Touchpoints can be seen as a source of satisfaction and encouragement, as well as a source of stress, for the family.
B. **Anticipatory guidance: observing child behavior to strengthen the clinician–parent relationship.** Parents find it reassuring that bursts and regressions in development are to be expected. This represents a shift in thinking for parents who, without this information, might misunderstand their child's behavior as pathological and question their own caregiving efficacy. In the face of these regressions, they wonder what they are doing wrong. Pediatric clinicians can share their observations of a child's behavior in the office when they offer anticipatory guidance about each touchpoint at every routine healthcare maintenance visit. This new knowledge, and the respectful, supportive relationship within which it is offered, will help parents feel less alone and more confident in themselves and in their child. For example:
1. **4 months.** Clinicians can predict that there will soon be a burst in cognitive awareness of the environment. It will be difficult to feed the baby. He will stop eating to look around and listen to every stimulus. This distractibility, if witnessed in the office, is well worth observing with parents (Chapter 3). To parents' dismay, he will begin to awaken again at night. What is going on? A greater capacity for visual accommodation that now allows him to focus on objects several feet away expands his awareness of his environment. No longer is the face of the parent who feeds him the sole point of interest for him. When parents understand this temporary regression in the area of feeding as a natural precursor to the exciting changes that follows, they will be less likely to feel that the infant's loss of interest in the bottle or breast represents a failure in their ability to nurture him. A simple, practical tip to share with parents to handle this challenge is that dimming the lights will reduce visual distractions during feedings.
2. **9 months.** Clinicians can expect a sequence of behaviors during the office visit that offers opportunities for developmental assessment, relationship building, and anticipatory guidance.
a. When the infant, held aloft in a parent's arms, first crosses the threshold of the doctor's office, she is likely to quickly glance at the clinician's face, begin to whimper, and turn to the parent for reassurance. This is evidence of the infant's growing capacity for social referencing—interpreting facial expressions. If the parent smiles encouragingly, the baby will begin to relax. If the parent looks wary, the baby will become more upset. The clinician can normalize stranger anxiety as a time when difficult behavior accompanies a new developmental step: the abilities to distinguish strangers and decipher facial expressions are consolidating. Parents may be embarrassed about the infant's unsociable behavior. But clinicians can admire the fact that the baby knows whom she cannot yet trust and that she can turn to parents for reassurance and reliable information about people and situations she does not yet understand. This is also a subtle way of signaling to parents

that their nonverbal communication can reassure the infant about the clinical encounter.

    b. Once the baby begins to relax, she may start to explore the new environment. Using her index finger, she will point at something, which she wants to find out about, a new accomplishment in both symbolic thinking and expressive communication that can be shared with parents. She may demonstrate new fine motor dexterity with her pincer grasp (apposition of thumb and index finger), reaching for the otoscope and other office equipment—another touchpoint in which a new developmental capacity brings new challenges. This provides a rapid assessment of infants' fine motor development and parents' ability to manage challenging behaviors. The clinician can comment positively on the new abilities, empathize with the new challenges for keeping the baby safe now, and join in problem solving to keep small objects out of reach that might choke her if she tries to swallow them.

    c. After the infant has made herself at home with her fine motor mastery of the new setting, she is likely to start demonstrating new gross motor skills next—scooting, cruising, and crawling. This is another new developmental step that will disorganize the whole family. The infant's behavior in the office provides an opportunity to observe her motor development as well as her parent's reaction and ability to manage the challenges of new mobility. The onset of mobility requires a new round of baby-proofing at home and, in the office, is another opportunity for shared observation and discovery: "She gets into everything now! What strategies have you discovered to help keep her out of trouble?" Parents are much more responsive to such discussions when they are directly tied to the baby's on-the-spot behaviors and offered in the context of a partnership, rather than teaching.

    d. Anticipatory guidance about the next touchpoint: expect the baby to be fussier and more easily frustrated until her drive to take her first step finally leads to success. Starting several weeks before, she is likely to start waking up at night every 3 to 4 hours. Parents may find her standing in her crib, gripping the rails, unable to get herself back down. She is so focused on motor development that she just cannot stop at night. Infants at this age spend more time in light sleep than at any other point in childhood. This temporary sleep cycle change may be necessary for motor learning and memory in preparation for walking. Parents may not be thrilled to learn this, but will be relieved that this regression is in the service of development, and should be temporary, provided that they limit their interactions with the infant when she awakens.

C. In premature infants, Touchpoints may be more anxiously awaited and may occur somewhat later. They will be even more important as opportunities for supporting parents who are vigilant for signs of possible long-term effects of prematurity.

D. Atypically developing children's Touchpoints may in some instances occur at different times or have different features from those of typically developing children. It is preferable to carefully observe, understand, and respect each child's behavior for evidence of developmental disorganization and reorganization rather than to make unhelpful comparative judgments.

II. The Touchpoints Model: a paradigm shift for clinical practice.

A. A paradigm shift positions clinicians to help parents handle temporary behavioral disorganization and the vulnerability it stirs up (Fig. 4-1). Pediatric clinicians are trained to look for failures, and parents sense this. The focus on problems leaves parents wary and defensive. When we start with their strengths, they are far more likely to reveal their vulnerabilities. Although many professionals endorse this paradigm shift, it is more difficult to interact with families accordingly. We are so well trained in our medical search for impairments that we can "fix," that it can be difficult to acknowledge parents' expertise, and look for opportunities to support their mastery.

B. Professionals can use the **guiding principles of the Touchpoints** Model as a framework for each encounter with families (Table 4-1). Several **guiding assumptions about parents** form the core of Touchpoints' practice (Table 4-2). Perhaps the most important for the clinician to keep in mind is that *parents are the experts on their child's behavior.* Together, professionals and parents can discover themes that recur and strategies to negotiate upcoming challenges.

C. Professionals are encouraged to offer anticipatory guidance in the form of a dialogue about how parents will feel and react in the face of predictable challenges to come. This is, in part, based on how they have dealt with related issues in the past.

D. Advice can be effective but only when requested and offered in the context of a relationship based on respect. Clinicians can also ask permission: "Would you like some advice?"

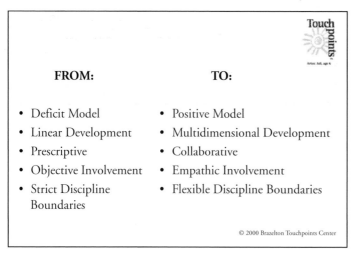

Figure 4-1. A Paradigm Shift.

This rapid maneuver changes the field in which advice is proposed and received and increases the likelihood that it will be acted upon.

Questions that presuppose parental expertise (e.g., "What have you found helps your baby to settle at night?") set the stage for professionals to add suggestions to parents' wisdom.

III. **Systems theory (Fig. 4-2) defines clinicians' interactions with families: each member of the caregiving system is in balance with each other member.**

   A. If a clinician wants to participate in the system's success, she or he must become an equal member of the system. Touchpoints' guiding principles and parent assumptions can be used to re-equilibrate power imbalances within clinician–family interactions.

   B. If there is a stress on the system, each member must adjust to the stress. As a result, stress becomes an opportunity for learning.

   C. As a member of the caregiving system, the professional must learn to understand and value the culture, religion, and beliefs of the other members. Understanding a different culture is a lesson in humility, for the more we learn, the more we realize how much escapes us. Such a stance, which empowers the families we work with to transform us, is a far cry from one that assumes the superiority of science and that may result in talking down patients, in giving instructions that may be incompatible with their values.

   D. To join the caregiving system and help sustain its equilibrium, clinicians may find it helpful to greet families with an initial positive observation of the infant or child's behavior, for example, evidence of temperament or stage of development. Other meaningful behaviors to be shared with parents are those that offer evidence of a child's own satisfaction in a new accomplishment. When a child succeeds at a developmental task, he expresses his satisfaction as if to say: "I did it!"—a powerful observation to share with parents. This inner feedback cycle (Fig. 4-3) is self-reinforcing, mobilizing new energy for the next developmental achievement. This cycle, coupled with the parent's reinforcing behaviors (the external feedback cycle), fuels the processes of development driven by the maturation of the central nervous system. Clinicians can share their observations of these two cycles and encourage parents to enjoy them, if they do not already: "You look so thrilled to see your little girl stack that second block on the first—and so does she!"

Table 4-1. The guiding principles of the Touchpoints Model

Value and understand the relationship between you and the parent
Use the behavior of the child as your language
Value passion wherever you find it
Focus on the parent–child relationship
Look for opportunities to support mastery
Recognize the beliefs and biases that you bring to the interaction
Be willing to discuss matters that go beyond your traditional role

Table 4-2. Touchpoints parent assumptions

The parent is the expert on his or her child
All parents have strengths
All parents want to do well by their child
All parents have something critical to share at each developmental stage
All parents have ambivalent feelings
Parenting is a process built on trial and error

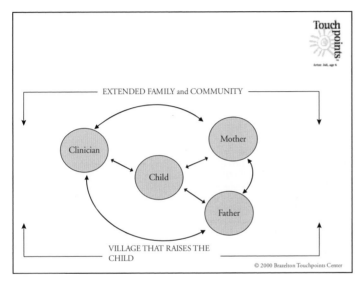

Figure 4-2. A Systems Approach to Using Touchpoints with Children and Families.

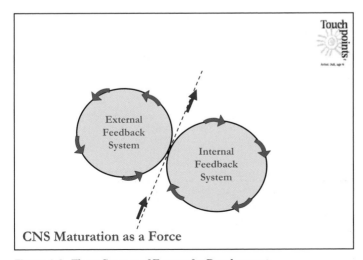

Figure 4-3. Three Sources of Energy for Development.

E. Child behaviors that are meaningful for clinicians to share with parents emphasize the child's strengths and the parents' major contributions to the child's development. As a result, parents are more likely to openly participate in history taking and sharing concerns. Each visit can strengthen the parent–clinician working relationship, as parents come to trust that, along with their strengths, their vulnerabilities will be respected and valued.

F. The trust of parents is also more readily won when clinicians demonstrate their understanding of and sensitivity to the predictable developmental needs of their child. For example, when the clinician respects a 9-month-old's stranger anxiety by postponing further attempts to engage her until the infant initiates a bid for engagement, the clinician has demonstrated her expertise in child behavior. She has also shown her capacity to care for a child more powerfully than by simply saying "I care."

IV. **Touchpoints: a relational model of development.** Each touchpoint stresses the parent–child relationship. The openness to guidance and support during these developmental crises creates an opportunity for clinicians to deepen their relationships with family. The predictable stresses of a child's developmental surges are matched by parents' passionate desire to do well by the child. As clinicians join parents in their urge to foster the child's optimal development, each contact becomes rewarding to the parents as well as to clinicians.

BIBLIOGRAPHY

Brazelton TB. Soapbox: how to help parents of young children: the Touchpoints Model. *Clin Child Psychol Psychiatry.* 3(3):481–483, 1998.

Brazelton TB, Sparrow JD. *Touchpoints Birth to Three: Your Child's Emotional and Behavioral Development* (2nd ed), Cambridge, MA: Da Capo Press, 2006.

Sparrow JD, Brazelton TB. A developmental approach to the prevention of common behavioral problems. In McInerny TK, Adam HM, Campbell DE, et al. (eds), *American Academy of Pediatrics Textbook of Pediatric Care* (1st ed), Elk Grove Village, IL: American Academy of Pediatrics, 2008.

van de Rijt-Plooij H, Plooij F. Infantile regressions: Disorganization and the onset of transition periods. *J Reprod Infant Psychol* 10:129–149, 1992.

Web site for professionals

http://www.touchpoints.org/

5

Difficult Encounters with Parents

Barbara Korsch

I. **Description of the problem.** No honest clinician in pediatrics can claim to love all patients all of the time or to communicate well with everyone who appears in the practice. There are certain names on the day's schedule that make the clinician's heart sink and feel fatigued in advance.

II. **Factors in difficult encounters.** The situations that trigger negative emotions are not the same for every clinician. It is of fundamental importance for each clinician to develop awareness and insight into his or her own individual sensitivities and idiosyncrasies to minimize counterproductive encounters and to develop strategies for assuring his or her own well-being.

   A. **The clinician–parent relationship.** It is too easy to blame the parent: "The mother was a poor historian" or "She was ignorant, opinionated, and uncooperative." Unflattering labels are often used to take the onus and the blame off the clinician. If it were entirely the parent's "fault" that the medical encounter was difficult, there would be no way of mending the relationship. It is more productive for the clinician to realize that a ruptured relationship usually involves both sides. Knowledge, critical self-awareness, and an explicit focus of interest on the communication process and where it went wrong are helpful in this regard.

   B. **Ambiguity.** Clinicians are trained to solve problems and finish tasks. They want diseases that can be named (labeling is one approach to mastery) and symptoms that can be cured. Yet patients' problems often defy simple solutions. A common reason for difficult encounters lies in the clinician's (or parents') discomfort with this ambiguity. Patients with symptoms that do not point to a known disease entity are annoying and frustrating.

   C. **The overanxious parent.** In pediatrics, the parent who recites the child's complaints in an overanxious and overemotional manner is judged the equivalent of the hypochondriac in adult practice. He or she is equally unpopular and frequently given short shrift, although sympathetic listening to the concerns might reveal significant issues underlying the emotionality. Concluding that "it is the parent who is the problem" and not the child, too often does not lead to problem recognition, empathy, and sympathetic treatment.

   D. **Slow treatment response.** Just as clinicians thrive on the instant gratification of a patient's getting well quickly, so too are they annoyed by patients who do not respond to treatment. Blaming the patient for a poor response to treatment (even unconsciously) impedes the collaboration with the family. The clinician needs to join the family and patient in facing their common disappointments: " I know you had hoped to see him better by now. So did I. But we will have to be patient a little longer. We do know we are on the right track."

   E. **Clinician limitations.** All clinicians encounter certain issues, which lead them to communicate less effectively because of special sensitivities. There may be something in the parent's personality or in the presenting illness of the child that touches a sensitive nerve in the clinician. This often leads to overidentification, which interferes with accurate empathy. It is crucial that the physician develops enough awareness of these special vulnerabilities so that they do not interfere with optimal patient care "—physician knows thyself."

      1. A frequent barrier to effective communication lies in the clinician's difficulty in accepting his or her own limitations. A parent who "shops" for medical care; who quotes other authorities ("When the child next door had the same thing, the doctor gave him antibiotics and he was fine the next day"); who reads independently and forms strong opinions ("I read on the Internet that new medicine A is really more effective"); who challenges directly ("How many children have you raised doctor?" or "How many kids with this condition have you treated?" or "How long have you been in practice?")— these are all unpopular parents. The reason, often, is that the health professional needs to feel that parents will accept *only his or her* authority. The idea that a parent might inquire elsewhere, quote information or misinformation from the Internet,

and that there are other valid (and sometimes better) ideas may seem unacceptable. But such paternalism is unjustified in all respects, especially in a therapeutic alliance between clinician and patient's family.

2. Failure to accept personal limitations in knowledge and competence may lead the clinician to perceive patients as difficult. A simple, "You know, I have not really seen this particular combination of signs and symptoms before. I would like you to see Dr. X who has more experience in this line," may be an effective approach that relieves clinician stress and parental anxiety.

F. **Cultural differences.** The clinician's lack of knowledge about cultural factors that may provoke certain kinds of patient symptoms or behavior can also lead to irritation and impatience. For instance, resistance on the part of certain Latino families to have their daughter's perineum inspected might be interpreted as ignorance and resistance. The informed clinician understands that the mother's reluctance is not a personal reaction but is based on the cultural belief that privacy must be protected in young girls at all costs. There are also differences in cultures of medical care and it is increasingly important for the clinician to assess the families' ideas concerning complementary or alternative medical practices and to include these in the joint decision making.

1. Cultural sensitivities pose special challenges in our Western culture. We take pride in our nonpatronizing approaches, with patients and clinician working as partners, and on maximum information sharing and joint decision making. There are problems in applying this approach with all patients in all situations. Yet even in our community, there are instances where patients do not wish to be informed and desire their clinician to make important decisions for them.

2. In many other societies, communication about health and illness is handled much less openly. This is true within families where relatives protect family members from information, and also applies in the clinician–patient relationship. Being informed about fatal illness and bad prognosis may be considered harmful to the patient. These patients' belief systems need to be explored and respected by the clinician, even when his own preferences are different. Over time an agreement may be achieved, but the relationship and trust can be damaged by insensitive insistence that our approach be used.

3. Decision making is especially difficult for those patients who have been taught not to challenge their clinicians or to ask questions. They may suffer when pressured to decide, for fear of angering the doctor, and also because they do not have the necessary knowledge.

4. Another cultural barrier with which everyone is struggling has to do with language, and as the population gets more heterogeneous increased skills in using interpreters and overcoming language barriers will be needed.

G. **Patient perceptions.** Encounters will become difficult when family perception and the doctor's idea of the nature of the severity of the problem are different.

1. "No Come Nada." Often mothers perceive it as a serious medical problems when the child does not eat as much of or the kind of food as they feel he needs. Whereas it seems the doctor at the sight of a bouncy rosy-cheeked child on an examination table, and a normal growth curve, does not take the problem seriously. Hence the endless "no come nada" cases, which exasperate the pediatrician and frustrate anxious mothers.

2. Vaccine refusal. As new vaccines are developed, or when more information regarding alleged ill effects of immunization is publicized by the media, families become anxious and come to believe that the effects of immunizations are more harmful than beneficial. Here again empathetic listening is more helpful than judgmental responses. Allowing the mother to mention a few of her specific concerns will be necessary to get her to be receptive to the clinicians' recommendations.

H. **Ambiguous boundaries.** Some parents are unwilling to assume any responsibility, thus putting everything onto the clinician's shoulders. ("Can you tell my daughter to stand up straight or she will make her back crooked"? or "Oh! doctor, tell me what to do! You have got to help me"!) Having once become trapped in such a situation, the clinician will subsequently have to deal with a parent who continues to act helpless and expects him or her to solve every problem. This is a no-win situation with inevitable disappointment for the family. Instead, the clinician needs to support and mobilize the parents' resources and to help the family take ownership of their problems. Recognizing and setting clear boundaries about what the clinician is (and is not) able to do and establishing reasonable expectations for parent–patient responsibility is one of the essential principles of avoiding counterproductive clinician–parent communication.

I. **Judgmental attitudes.** Besides the need for power, authority, success, and the wish to please, other attributes of the clinician constrain open communication. Some clinicians do not like fat children; others overreact to lack of cleanliness. Ways of dressing, sexual orientation, or mannerisms may trigger emotional reactions in clinicians of which they are not even aware.

J. Overidentification. Certain diagnoses (such as developmental disability, leukemia, and visual impairment) may arouse feelings based on the clinician's personal experiences that negatively color the encounter. Overidentification, which is also a lack of boundary setting, is as counterproductive to the therapeutic alliance as is a lack of empathy.

K. Systems problems. Another barrier to good clinician–patient relationships lies in systems problems: lack of time; difficulty in obtaining relevant data; excess waiting time for families, which angers them even before they begin the encounter; pressures imposed by quality control and utilization review committees; fear of litigation; and the many other irritants in the healthcare system. When clinicians themselves feel abused by the system and helpless to overcome certain obstacles to optimal care, they are likely to transfer their frustrations to colleagues, families, and patients. Acknowledgment of the pressures for all involved and allowing mutual expression of frustration will often clear the air and lead to better cooperation (e.g., "I can understand that it annoys you that you are not seeing the same doctor today. It is difficult for me too because we could work things out better if I had all the information at hand. In the meantime, let us do the best we can.").

L. Time constraints. Especially in busy practices, patients who take a lot of time are very irritating. Clearly, there are patients who suffer from such extreme psychosocial or emotional problems that they do not fit into the constraints of regular medical practice. Patients who arrive without appointments, bring in two children, or ask for advice for other family members need to be redirected with appropriate boundaries and limit setting. It will save the clinician's time and frustration to learn to detect the truly pathologic personalities as early as possible so their care can be appropriately shared with mental health professionals or outside community agencies.

Instances of this type, however, are far less frequent than are those in which extra time is needed due to ineffective communication and the failure to recognize communication breakdown. When in the course of an encounter, the clinician feels annoyed and impatient, repeating the same message with the sense that it is not getting across (e.g., "What you need is just a regular bedtime routine" to a mother who is struggling to survive in a chaotic and overwhelming family situation), he or she needs to consider: What is going wrong? Why am I angry? Why does this parent act so aggressively? Is there another approach that I could try? What can I learn from this difficult encounter that could help this family or parent?

III. Dealing with difficult encounters.

A. Address the problem. Acknowledging that it is the *encounter* and not the parent that is difficult is the most important step. A number of techniques can be helpful.

1. Confront the parent: *"You seem angry. Can you tell more about why?"*
2. Acknowledge the difficulty: *"I am having a problem here. I feel we are talking at cross-purposes. Let us see whether we can get off to a better start. What I really need to hear from you right now is . . . ."*
3. Use the common concern over the child: *"Let us watch him walk together. Perhaps we will observe the things that concern you about him, and then we can discuss plans."*
4. Offer a concrete sign of wanting to help. For instance, if a parent is anxious about a sibling who will be getting out of school, allowing her to call a neighbor on the office telephone may turn things around. An extra diaper from the office supply or a quarter for the parking meter may make the point that the clinician does indeed want to help.

B. Expand the system. After setting boundaries for what can appropriately be dealt with, it may be time to expand the system.

1. Include other family members: "Could you get your husband to come in or telephone me so we can include his ideas in our planning?"
2. Call on other members of the healthcare team, depending on the urgency and the main focus of the problem.
3. Look to the community—not necessarily to a health professional but perhaps to the family's clergy or other religious adviser. Sometimes the grandparent becomes a key figure.

C. Give it time. Many things cannot be dealt with on a single visit, and if the task cannot be completed to the parent's or the clinician's satisfaction, both will be frustrated. But if the clinician is able to deal at least partially with the problem and can explicitly defer some of the other concerns to a later occasion, harmony can be restored toward the end of the visit. Solutions may also be more likely after a certain amount of reflection and time has passed. Frequently, the parents who annoy the clinician the most are those who require the most prompt follow-up.

BIBLIOGRAPHY

Asnes AG, Shenoy A. The difficult pediatric encounter: insights and strategies for the pediatric practitioner. *Pediatr Rev* 29:e35–e41, 2008. doi:10.1542/10.1542/pir.29-6-e35.

Korsch BM. Do you know these patients? High risk pediatric encounters. *Pediatr Rev* 10:100–105, 1988

Korsch BM, Gozzi EK, Francis V. Gaps in doctor-patient communication. I. Doctor-patient interaction and patient satisfaction. *Pediatrics* 42:855–871, 1968.

Miller R, Rollnick S. *Motivational Interviewing.* New York, NY: The Guilford Press, 1991.

Prochaska JO, DiClemente CC. Transtheoretical therapy: toward a more integrative model of change. *Psychotherapy* 20:161–173, 1982.

Quill TE. Recognizing and adjusting to barriers in doctor-patient communication. *Ann Intern Med* 111:51–57, 1989.

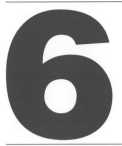

Helping Families Deal with Bad News

Richard D. Goldstein
Maria Trozzi

I. **Issues in delivering bad news.** The task of sharing bad news is among a clinician's most solemn responsibilities and a special human encounter. In addition to competently understanding the medical facts to be shared, it demands presence and authenticity on the part of the clinician. Balancing blunt honesty with encouragement and, fundamentally, some hope, requires a high level of practice. Clinicians can struggle with finding this balance, and often enter these conversations with discomfort and feelings of incomplete preparation.

   A. **What is bad news?** Sharing bad news involves complex medical communication during critical life events. In every area of medicine, there are times when bad news must be communicated. In pediatrics, bad news can be the diagnosis of a serious chronic illness, a significant developmental disability, or a fatal disease. But bad news is not simply a function of the severity of the disease process. It also refers to the impact of the shared information on the recipients' sense of quality and meaning in life, their expectations, and their goals.

   B. **More than a communication of facts.** Cassell has written that "the imperative to tell the truth seems an insufficient guide to what you should tell patients." A more complete perspective requires that the sharing of information reduce uncertainty, provide a basis for action, and strengthen the patient–clinician relationship. This becomes possible when the clinician looks beyond stating facts and prognosis and attempts to appreciate how the receiver of the information will understand the matters in focus. This patient-centered approach involves attempting to grasp how the new reality and options might seem to the patient and family and helping them with first steps in its integration. Information and the way it is conveyed itself can be an important therapeutic tool with direct implications for later management.

   Studies document long-lasting consequences of poorly or negatively perceived disclosure affecting the patient–doctor alliance and a parent's understanding of the clinician's attitudes toward their child. Conversely, successfully conveyed bad news can establish helpful themes and foci for the parents to use in their efforts to clarify the goals of their child's care.

   C. **The clinician's role.** Research has found that clinicians generally project a limited set of personae in communicating bad news. They have been described as the inexperienced messenger, the emotionally burdened, the rough and ready, the benevolent but tactless, the distanced doctor, and the empathic professional. Although each approach can be effective, empathic professionals may be the best because they are able to share bad news in an understanding way that affirms hope and a committed relationship with the patient.

   It is important for the clinician to understand his or her personal feelings before attempting to communicate bad news. Understanding that these apprehensions exist and working to minimize their impact helps increase the potential for meaningful communication. It is not uncommon for a clinician's apprehensions to be based upon fear. Commonly expressed fears include the fear of being at fault and blamed, the fear of unleashing a disagreeable reaction, or the fear of not knowing all the answers during a critical conversation. Many clinicians feel that the skills involved in this communication are untaught or unknown and worry about performing at the level the situation demands. Clinicians may also experience a personal discomfort with illness and death, which can exhibit itself as a discomfort with hopelessness.

   Minimizing clinician-based impediments to communication is not simply a matter of acting in the way the clinician believes the recipient desires, but rather one of assuring that this communication does not undermine a parent or dissolve hope. It is important to reinforce the goals the family have for their child. Most of the time, there will be opportunities for further refinements in the future and the sharing of news is the beginning of the process.

D. Difficulties with prognosis. Clinicians should be wary of prognosis. Studies investigating prognosis have found that clinicians are accurate only 20% of the time and tend to be overly optimistic. Although studies have shown that more experienced clinicians tend to have less error, there is also a correlation between the length of a relationship with a patient and a lowered likelihood that the prognosis will be correct. Despite this tendency toward error on the part of clinicians, patients nonetheless seek a clear disclosure of information. They interpret hidden or minimal information as their doctor withholding frightening information. Patients who receive more elements of prognostic disclosure are more likely to report communication-related hope, even when the likelihood of cure is low. To help balance the hazards of sharing prognosis is to tell parents how their child's clinical treatment condition will be monitored over time.

II. The process of delivering bad news. Different circumstances present different constraints. It would be simplistic and inaccurate to portray the successful giving of bad news as following a formula. It relies not only on technique, but also on experience and instinct. There are, however, certain helpful keys to a successful encounter.

A. Tell the family as soon as possible and in person. Studies of parents' reactions to bad news about their children have demonstrated that most families would prefer to be told as soon as the healthcare provider suspects there is a problem. Sensitive clinicians must feel comfortable sharing available information, even if it is incomplete or uncertain as long as the clinician spells out the steps and duration of time to obtain a firm diagnosis. Critical conversations are best not conducted on the telephone. Planning an in person meeting, when possible, also will allow the family time to make sure the right people are in attendance.

B. Prepare a roadmap. Preparation for the sharing of bad news begins with an understanding of the facts and the clinician's emotional response to them. But the communication of those facts should be organized and well-paced. This is improved when some thought has been given to the manageable number of points that the family can hear. In encounters that promise to be emotionally overwhelming, parents are often unable to understand more than a very limited number of bits of information. Before entering into this conversation, it is helpful to rehearse what language and terminology will be used, consciously trying to avoid medical terminology, and what, if any, crucial decision must be made right then, and what the next step will be. Clinicians should conceive of a way to talk about the problem that is accurate while not relying on too much medical terminology.

C. Prepare a space. When circumstances permit, critical information should be shared in a private and safe environment. Ideally, this is a room free of distractions or interruptions. Except in cases of older children and adolescents who should be involved, this is best done away from the bedside for hospitalized patients or at an arranged time for outpatients. The key decision makers should be present, generally parents and guardians. Some thought should be given to seating arrangements, assuring that the people giving and those receiving the news are proximate. The numbers of healthcare personnel and family members should be restricted to the minimum necessary to assure a less distracted and more emotionally attentive interaction. Support staff, for example, social work or clergy, should be included when possible. The room should be supplied with tissues.

D. Make the space feel secure. The requirement for being culturally competent cannot be overstated. All who will share bad news must be mindful of the cultural implications of language, whether spoken or through body language. The name of the child and the parents should be known before the conversation begins as well as how they would prefer to be addressed. Allow for all participants to come in and be seated before beginning. If possible, beepers and phones should be silenced. Once the door closes, every effort should be made for all involved to remain in the room until the interaction concludes. Everyone in the room should introduce themselves. It must be clear that the family has the clinician's undivided and unrushed attention.

Attention to body language can be helpful. Sitting at the same level, facing the parents and establishing eye contact promotes directness and connection, provided it does not seem threatening. It is just as important to read the body cues of the receivers, respecting their defenses and looking for opportunities to reassuringly meet their gaze.

E. Diagnose the recipients of information. Different parents have different needs for information and details. The success of the encounter relies in part on understanding those needs and addressing them appropriately. As the meeting begins and an agenda is set out, a helpful opening can be asking parents what they understand of the situation and what they want to know. As they speak, the appropriate level of detail with which to speak may be deduced to inform the clinician's sharing of medical information. The terminology they use can be employed, and their priorities can be reflected in the shape of the ensuing discussion.

F. Communicate for them. Receiving bad news represents a major life event to a family. Part of that experience is certain to be a high degree of emotion. That emotion will predictably influence the encounter and may cloud the communication.

Speak about essential facts in small aliquots and wait for their questions to elaborate on details. Watch for their saturation point and stop the flow of words when it is sensed. Acknowledge all parent responses. It is powerful to absolve parents of responsibility for misfortunes if that is possible. When appropriate, let them know that this is only the first of many discussions and be clear about what is required of them at this point.

When the answer to a parent's question is unclear, it is important to distinguish between responses that cannot be answered due to the clinician's knowledge (e.g., "I don't know the answer to that question, but I will help you find out") and responses to questions that are essentially unanswerable (e.g., "It is difficult to say what your child will be like 5 years from now"). In the latter case, it is helpful to explain why the question cannot be answered, and how the illness will be monitored over time to help answer the question.

G. Monitor and maneuver through emotional density. The emotions experienced during the sharing of bad news are an essential part of the communication. The manner of communication can be shaped by communicating the central issue and then pausing. Silence will invite response. A response with affect reflects fuller communication than one that asks only for clinical details. Regardless of the response, focus on it and address it, while keeping in mind the roadmap.

The clinician must model permission to express emotions during the exchange. There are technical aspects to show that feeling is permitted to be a part of the exchange of information. Draw it out with silence, with affirmation followed by a pause, or with body cues. The common desire to soothe distress with reassurance should be controlled as it can sometimes cut off the development of the parent's perspective, although this should not be done without feeling. Nonetheless, feelings expressed deserve an empathic response.

Parents often have concerns related to the impact of the situation on siblings. When conditions permit, it can be helpful to explore whether they have concerns about disclosure to siblings or worries about their coping. It is productive to explore this area with them, affirming its importance.

Some parents have complained about hearing the phrase "I'm sorry" too much from health professionals. While they appreciate the sympathy, and it is important to express it, they want to know, for example, that although the situation is dire everything is being done so that it does not hurt their child, or that although there is great uncertainty, strong efforts will be made to understand as much as possible and work toward their expressed goals of care. Fundamentally, parents want to know that their clinician is a strong, committed advocate who will focus his or her efforts and intellect on promoting what is in the best interest of their child.

H. Answer their questions. It is important to ask parents if they have any questions and answer them. Parents are sometimes too overwhelmed to know what, if anything, to ask. If they feel unable to ask questions, it can be helpful to ask them to summarize what they have heard. As they do so, the clinician may need to gently shift their focus to essential concerns or, sympathetically, reiterate basic facts.

I. Finish in alliance. When it is clear that the essential points have been communicated, that there is a sense of how they are managing the information, and critical and timely decisions have been made, it is time to end the meeting. The last words generally belong to the clinician and can have a lingering impact. One useful sequence is to offer an empathic statement for the situation they find themselves balanced by a pledge to work toward their expressed goals of care. Any decisions made should be reiterated, available supports reviewed, and the timing of the next occasion to meet should be stated. The meeting can be adjourned if there are no further questions.

BIBLIOGRAPHY

Buckman R. Breaking bad news: why is it still so difficult? *BMJ* 288:1597–1599, 1984.

Cassell EJ. *Talking with Patients, Vol 2: Clinical Technique.* Cambridge, MA: MIT Press, 1985, pp. 148–193.

Carr J. Six weeks to twenty-one years old: a longitudinal study of children with Down's syndrome and their families. Third Jack Tizard Memorial Lecture. *J Child Psychol Psychiatry* 29:407–431, 1988.

Christakis NA, Lamont EB. Extent and determinants of error in doctor's prognoses in terminally ill patients: prospective cohort study. *BMJ* 320:469–472, 2000.

Fallowfield L, Jenkins V. Communicating sad, bad, and difficult news in medicine. *Lancet* 363:312–319, 2004.

Friedrichsen MJ, Strang PM, Carlsson ME. Breaking bad news in the transition from curative to palliative cancer care: patient's view of the doctor giving the information. *Supportive Care Cancer* 8:472–478, 2000.

Mack JW, Wolfe J, Cook EF, et al. Hope and prognostic disclosure. *J Clin Oncol* 25:5636–5642, 2007.

Miller SZ, Schmidt HJ. The habit of humanism: a framework for making humanistic care a reflexive clinical skill. *Acad Med* 74:800–803, 1999.

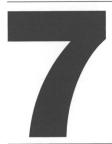

Promoting Early Literacy

Perri Klass

I. **Description of the problem.** Children who grow up without being read to and with little exposure to books and to printed language during the first 5 years of life are at a greatly increased risk for reading failure and general school failure. They are likely to reach the age of school entry with poorer language skills, poorer school readiness, and poorer motivation. Coming from print-poor environments, such children may be unskilled in handling books, lacking positive associations with books as sources of pleasure and information. Children who are not able to develop reading skills on grade level in first grade are at increased risk to continue through elementary school and even high school reading below grade level, which puts them at risk for school failure and its concomitant risks, from low self-esteem to dropping out.

II. **Epidemiology.** Approximately one-third of the U.S. children enter school without the requisite language preparation to learn to read on schedule. Reading difficulties in the early years of school may reflect the child's school entry skills, as well as language issues and learning disabilities. When reading skills are tested in the fourth grade, approximately one-third of the children in the United States cannot read on grade level. Low socioeconomic status and poor parental literacy skills significantly increase children's risk of reading problems.

III. **Etiology/contributing factors.** There are many reasons why children may not be read to or may grow up in print-poor environments.
   - Parents who were not themselves read to as children may not understand the importance of reading aloud especially to very young children.
   - Parents who have limited literacy skills may not be in the habit of using written language (newspapers, magazines, books, written messages) to convey or receive information.
   - Adults who struggled in school, or who still struggle with written language, may look on reading aloud as a difficult task, or a reminder of failure and defeat.
   - Families may be under significant time stress, lack resources to buy books, or live in areas where appropriate children's books are not easily available.
   - Non–English-speaking parents may not have books available in their languages, may be intimidated by books in English, or may deliberately refrain from reading (or even speaking) to their children in their native language in the hope that the children will grow up speaking English.
   - Parents who are themselves educated may not be directly caring for their own young children, or may feel unsure about what books and reading techniques are suitable for infants and toddlers.
   - Families in the 21st century are faced with many competing modes of "entertaining" young children, including television, video, and electronic media.
   - These same electronic alternatives are available to parents and may work against "face time" with young children or "family time" centered around books.

IV. **Which families need literacy promotion?** Literacy promotion in pediatric primary care should be offered to all families, regardless of socioeconomic status and parents' educational level. Special attention should be paid to families whose economic circumstances or educational background make reading aloud more challenging for parents or place their children at additional risk, to parents who have not completed high school, to parents whose English language skills are limited, to adolescent parents, and to families under extreme social and/or financial stress. Since one goal of reading aloud is to link books with pleasure in the child's mind, literacy promotion should take place on a highly positive note, encouraging parents to help their children learn and achieve, and recommending an experience, which both parent and child are likely to enjoy.

   A. **History.** *How are your child's language skills? Do you read aloud to your child? What books do your children enjoy? Are books a part of your daily routine with your child? Does anyone in the family have a library card?* Ask children directly: *What is your favorite book?*

B. Identifying families at risk. It is important to try and identify parents who may be at increased risk and may need extra help because they themselves have limited literacy skills. Their children are at risk for reading difficulties and school problems, and these families may also be at additional health risk because of the parent's limited ability to understand other written materials, including prescriptions, handouts, and pamphlets (Chapter 97). Asking about parental literacy level may feel uncomfortable and intrusive, and it may be easiest to ask for objective information (i.e., how far a parent went in school) as a routine part of patient intake; asking all parents for this information also removes the risks of making assumptions about literacy level. One study has shown that the number of children's books in the home can be a good indicator of parental literacy level, with parents who claim less than 10 children's books in the home are more likely to perform poorly on a test of health literacy. For families of concern, a more detailed family history, such as a parent history of learning problems or school retention, may offer important information for counseling parents and screening children.

V. Management: literacy promotion in primary care.

A. A model for effective literacy promotion. Reach Out and Read (ROR) was founded in 1989 by pediatric clinicians and early childhood educators. ROR advocates a three-component model of literacy promotion in pediatric primary care.

1. Primary care providers are trained to counsel parents about books and reading aloud at the health supervision visit.
2. Providers give each child a new, age-appropriate children's book at every health supervision visit from 6 to 60 months, so that the child acquires a home library of 9 to 10 books by school entry age.
3. Literacy-rich waiting rooms reinforce the message with displays about reading aloud, family literacy, libraries; with gently used books that children can take home; and, whenever possible, with volunteers in the waiting room who read aloud to children and thereby model reading-aloud techniques for parents are an option for some practices.
   In multiple published studies, ROR has been shown to result in significantly higher rates of parents reading to children, significantly more positive attitudes toward books and reading on the part of parents and children, and significantly improved receptive and expressive language skills in high-risk children as young as 18 months.

B. Anticipatory guidance. Anticipatory guidance offered to parents around literacy should be

1. Brief and age appropriate.
   a. Parents need to understand what to expect from young children with respect to books and reading (e.g., that it is normal for a 6-month-old immediately to put a board book in his mouth or that a 2-year-old may not sit still for an entire story).
   b. Encourage age-appropriate dialogue, as in asking a toddler to name a picture or asking a 4-year-old to tell you what he thinks will happen next.
2. Linked to other issues of behavior and development discussed in the health supervision visit.
   a. Discuss reading at bedtime in the context of discussing sleep issues and bedtime routines.
   b. Offer suggestions for how to incorporate books into other aspects of the child's routines.
   c. Encourage parents who are looking at childcare and preschool programs to look for situations where books are available and reading aloud is built into the schedule.
   d. When talking about watching television or videos or electronic games and young children, offer reading aloud as an alternative entertainment.
   e. Discuss the importance of reading aloud in the context of language exposure and acquisition for infants and toddlers.
   f. Discuss the relationship of reading aloud and school readiness for preschoolers.
   g. Introduce the concept of "dialogic reading." Dialogic reading is a style of book sharing in which parents encourage toddlers and preschool-aged children to comment on pictures and the story, to engage the child and promote a conversation about the book or story.
3. Positive and reinforcing for the parents.
   a. Give parents positive feedback if they are already reading.
   b. Emphasize the importance of the parent's voice in the child's development.
   c. Encourage physical contact between parent and child, cuddling, "face time," all of which will make the books and reading more desirable and important to a young child.

    d. Present reading with the child as something that should be fun; acknowledge the parent's wish to see the child learn and succeed.

    e. Encourage bilingual and non–English-speaking parents to read in whatever language is most comfortable; acknowledge the importance of storytelling and oral traditions.

C. Using books in the examination room.

  1. If books are available to be given to the child at the visit

    • Bring the book early in the visit.

    • Offer the book to the child and observe the child's behavior with the book while you speak with the parent.

    • Use the book as part of your observation of the child's developmental skills.

D. Choosing age-appropriate books for children.

  1. For **6–12 months of age**, choose small board books, with pictures of faces and only a few words per page.

  2. For **1–2 years of age,** choose board books with pictures of familiar objects, family life, and animals; choose simple stories and books with rhyme and repetition.

  3. Some 2-year-olds still need board books; many can handle paper pages, and enjoy books with more complex stories; rhyme and repetition remain important.

  4. For **3–5 years of age,** it is often helpful to offer the child a choice of books. Fantasy stories are popular, as are funny stories and family stories; also consider alphabet books and counting books.

E. Books as developmental observation tools.

  1. Observe fine motor development as child handles book, looking for pincer grasp in turning pages and pointing with one finger (at 9 months of age), for increasing skill in handling paper pages (by 2 years of age).

  2. Assess speech and language as child responds to book: infants should vocalize, 1- to 2-year-olds should label with single words, and older children may be asked to name objects or colors.

  3. Discuss child's language with parents in the context of the book: by 15–18 months, children begin filling in words at the ends of familiar sentences; by 2 years, they can "read" familiar books to themselves or their stuffed animals.

  4. Assess parent–child interaction and whether parent is able to pick up child's cues, answer child's questions, and respond to child's interests.

  5. At the 4- or 5-year-old visit, use the book as a tool to look at the child's school readiness skills, asking the child to name colors, count objects, identify letters on the page, and describe what is happening in illustrations.

VI. Clinical pearls and pitfalls.

  • Be sure to have the book in the room during the visit and not to use it as a "give-away" (like a sticker or a lollipop) at the end of the visit.

  • Model simple dialogic book-reading strategies in the examination room—pointing at pictures and naming them with infants and toddlers ("That's a baby, where's the baby's nose?"), asking more complicated questions with older children ("What do you think will happen if he gives that cookie to the mouse?").

  • Compliment parents when children take pleasure in the books, or manifest book-handling skills ("He (or she) really seems to like books—that's because you read to him (or her) at home.")

  • If there are any concerns about the parent's own literacy skills, encourage the parent to enjoy the book with the child without emphasizing the word "read," by talking about looking at books together, naming the pictures, and telling a story.

  • Be prepared to offer referrals to adult and/or family literacy programs to parents who express a desire to improve their own literacy skills.

  • With non–English-speaking families, it is of course very helpful to have books available in the appropriate language; but when this is not possible, parents should be encouraged to look at pictures and discuss books with their children, even when they cannot read the words.

  • Older siblings can be encouraged to read aloud to younger children.

  • Do not let this become a drill, or a way of pressuring children to read early. Reading aloud should be about enjoying books together. Older children will certainly begin to pick up information about print and letters, and parents can encourage this, but hearing a story should not be a test!

  • Help parents understand the link between a younger child who enjoys being read to—in part, because it means parental attention and "face time"—and an older child who likes books and feels eager and ready to learn to read.

BIBLIOGRAPHY

For parents

Web sites

http://www.reachoutandread.org/parents/
http://www.readingrockets.org/
http://www.bankstreet.edu/literacyguide/main.html

Books

Lipson ER. *The New York Times Parent's Guide to the Best Books for Children* (3rd ed), New York: Three Rivers Press, 2000.
National Research Council. *Starting Out Right: A Guide to Promoting Children's Reading Success.* Washington, DC: National Academy Press, 1999.
Silvey A. *Everything I Know I Learned From A Children's Book.* New York: Roaring Book Press, 2009.
Trelease J. *The Read-Aloud Handbook* (6th ed), New York: Penguin, 2006.

For professionals

Duursma E, Augustyn M, Zuckerman B. Reading aloud to children: the evidence. *Arch Dis Child* 93(7):554–557, 2008.
High PC, LaGasse L, Becker S, et al. Literacy promotion in primary care pediatrics: can we make a difference? *Pediatrics* 104:927–934, 2000.
Klass P, Dreyer BP, Mendelsohn AL. Reach Out and Read: literacy promotion in pediatric primary care. *Adv Pediatr* 56:11, 2009.
Mendelsohn AL, Mogilner LN, Dreyer BP, et al. The impact of a clinic-based literacy intervention on language development in inner-city preschool children. *Pediatrics* 107:130–134, 2001.
National Research Council. *Preventing Reading Difficulties in Young Children.* Washington, DC: National Academy Press, 1998.

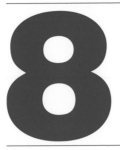

A Family Systems Approach to Pediatric Care

Carol Hubbard
William Lord Coleman

I. **Description of the issue.** Pediatric clinicians know well the impact that family function has on children. Behavioral, emotional, or physical complaints in a child may be a manifestation of underlying distress in the family system. Just as children are affected by their families' well-being, children's own health and behavioral issues can, in turn, disrupt the family balance, may make parents feel frustrated or powerless, and strain marriages and other relationships. In 2002, the American Academy of Pediatrics (AAP) Task Force on the Family summarized a large body of research about families, concluding that children's physical and emotional health and cognitive and social functioning are strongly influenced by how their families function, and that there is much pediatric clinicians can do to nurture and support families. In this and other policy statements, the AAP has suggested that pediatric clinicians assess family relationships, health and behaviors, screen and refer parents for physical and emotional problems when needed, and practice "family-centered care," on the basis of collaboration with families and recognition of their strengths, an important component of an effective medical home. Professionals who treat children are uniquely positioned to positively impact family functioning, as they may be the only ones in regular contact with the family during the early years of a child's life.

A. **The pediatric clinician's attitude toward families.** Sometimes pediatric clinicians may label challenging families as "dysfunctional," "resistant," and "noncompliant." Instead, viewing family members as "multistressed" and identifying their strengths can enable clinicians to be more supportive and empathetic. Thinking of family members as separate from the constraints or problems in their lives allows the clinician to view the "problem as the problem, rather than the family as the problem"—an approach known as "externalization." The clinician can become more aware of the family's strengths and resources by getting to know about the family outside the context of the problem. Remaining respectfully curious and interested in a family, and believing that it has the capacity to grow and change, builds a collaborative relationship and gives a sense of hope to both the family and the clinician.

B. **The importance of language.** By listening carefully to the words family members use and the "stories" or narratives they tell to explain their experiences, pediatric clinicians can learn much about their attitudes and values. Ambiguous or emotionally laden terms should be clarified (e.g., what a father means when he says "pops" his son when he misbehaves). Respectfully clarifying language is especially important when working with families from different cultures. By listening carefully and using the family's own words and phrases, the clinician can more effectively communicate with them. In addition, making the extra effort to learn and use family members' names (rather than the generic "Mom" or "Dad"), in addition to the child's name, powerfully conveys the clinician's interest in the whole family.

II. **Assessing and addressing problems within a family context**

A. **How family issues present.** Parental or family medical and/or social–emotional health issues and other stressors should be explored in the initial family history and/or while providing ongoing care for a child. Some parents/caregivers may be open in discussing broader family issues and seeking guidance, but others may not perceive such issues as falling in the province of the pediatric clinician. The clinician should be aware of clues or "red flags" that raise the suspicion of underlying family stress (Table 8-1).

B. **Shifting the focus from the child to the family unit.** Techniques that can help to explore a problem within a family context include the following:

1. Showing empathy for parents by acknowledging the impact of the child's problem on the family: *"This must be a challenge for you all to deal with as a family. How are you handling it?"* An opportunity for such a comment can occur when parents use the term "we" to refer to the people affected by the child's issues.

2. Asking directly *"Who are all the people affected by your child's medical (or developmental or behavioral) issue?"*

35

Table 8-1. "Red Flags" for potential family factors in a child's presentation

1. An ambiguous chief complaint or reason for the visit
2. Recurrent, multiple, or chronic complaints without an obvious medical explanation
3. Lack of improvement of symptoms with standard therapy
4. Sudden unexplained changes in a child's behavior or health
5. Unusual parental concern or anxiety about a child
6. Concerning parental behavior and affect (anger, hopelessness) in the office
7. Obvious conflict or estrangement between family members
8. Conflicting or very different parenting styles
9. A major family transition or crisis

   3. Soliciting family members' opinions about the source of the difficulties, *"What do you think is going on?"* and inviting them to work together with you to address the problem.

C. Gathering family information. Information gathering can sometimes jump start the therapeutic process toward better family functioning by encouraging family members to think about the issues involved. History taking also provides an opportunity for the clinician to comment on a family's strengths and past efforts to address problems. Key areas to consider are found in Table 8-2. It may take more than one visit to obtain a detailed family history, or family information may unfold over time as a pediatric clinician cares for a child and his or her relationship with the family grows. Further techniques for understanding a family include.

   1. Eliciting family narratives. Family stories or narratives develop over time to explain past behavior, events, or illness, and are shaped by family members' perceptions, emotions, and selective memories of past events. Subsequent events are often interpreted in light of the preexisting story or interpretation and may perpetuate the problem

Table 8-2. Gathering family information

Family structure and relationships	Who is considered part of the family? Strength of the parent's relationship? Sibling relationships? Who is in charge and makes decisions ("the Executive")? Who provides emotional support? Appropriateness of boundaries between the members and generations
Family/parenting style	Cohesive versus disengaged and distant? Adaptable versus rigid? How is affection demonstrated?
Communication style	Can difficult subjects be discussed?
Sources of stress on the family	Internal or external stressors? Recent crises or transitions: deaths, births, children leaving home, divorce, illness in family members, substance abuse, domestic violence? Is the home perceived as a safe place?
Background	Ethnicity and culture Religion Education level Parent's upbringing and families of origin (and how their own parenting has been shaped by their experiences)
Environmental factors	Socioeconomic level Employment Neighborhood School Peer relationships Community agency involvement Sources of support outside the family

or perception, for example, the "self-fulfilling prophecy." A child, for example, may be labeled "bad" or the "black sheep of the family," and much of their behavior interpreted with that bias. The clinician can listen for such themes and guide family members to remember other details (exceptions to the dominant narrative) that might support a different "story," one with a more positive slant.

2. **Circular questions.** This useful technique involves asking one family member about the perceptions of another. Examples include asking a child *"How do you think your mother feels when you and your sister argue?"* or asking a parent *"What do you imagine your spouse thinks about your son's illness?"* Circular questions can be used with several family members present to encourage dialogue and understanding of each other's points of view, or with one person at a time to learn more about their relationships with other family members.

3. **Scaling questions.** Asking a patient to rate severity of pain on a scale of 1–10 may be familiar to clinicians. Similarly, family members can be asked to rate the magnitude of a situation (e.g., level of stress or alternatively the hopefulness or coping ability in the household), a behavior (e.g., child's opposition or cooperation), or their own feelings (e.g., enjoyment of time at home). Each family member should rate the same issue. This allows sharing of their perspectives and discussion of differences in their responses, which can help to move toward problem solving. A powerful follow-up question is to ask *"What could happen (or what would be different) to make that number just a bit better"* (e.g., to increase from a four to a five) thus encouraging discussion leading to cooperative solution building.

4. **Family drawings.** If a child is present she can be asked to *"Draw your family doing something."* The child's perceptions may provide information about the family structure and dynamics. The drawings can be reviewed with parents, opening more opportunity for discussion.

5. **Positive feedback.** Liberal use of compliments, supportive statements, and positive feedback reminds the family of previous success, reinforces positive behaviors, and instills hope. They are appropriate at any time during the evaluation or management stages of family encounters and are one way the clinician can reinforce positive parenting techniques. A *positive reframe* of a negative perception often serves to change the family narrative in a way that facilitates solution building.

D. **Maintaining a focus on solutions.** Clinicians trained in the biomedical model are accustomed to focusing on problems, spending considerable time with patients discussing the problems in detail. When working on a family issue in a busy office setting, it is often more productive to move quickly to discussing solutions after the clinician has an understanding of the situation. Using scaling questions and asking what would change to make the rating better, or simply asking what would be different if things were better, can help family members to think more about solutions and less about problems. The pediatric clinician can help the family to come up with goals that are mutually agreed upon, realistic, and achievable. The goals should be defined as a desirable new behavior or situation, not simply the absence of an old problem. Successfully making small changes is energizing for a family and gives them renewed hope. Bringing a family together as a group to work together with the clinician to "co-construct" solutions is a first step in effecting positive change.

III. **Meeting with the family.** There are times when it is useful to gather the family together, to learn more about a child's issues, to provide them with information (e.g., about a new diagnosis), or to brainstorm about a problem. Simply letting parents know that they are welcome to bring significant family members or support-givers to the child's appointments can lead to opportunities for group discussion. A family meeting is more effective when the affected family members are present, particularly the family decision maker or "executive." Ideally this person should attend at least one meeting for the clinician to form an alliance with them. A meeting may allow the clinician to meet previously "hidden" but important members. It can be informative to ask which family members are absent, what they would think about the topics being discussed, and if they could attend another meeting. A positive, supportive tone, with emphasis on past family successes and on realistic expectations will motivate family members to work together. The meeting will be more productive if focused on goals and solution building rather than lengthy descriptions of the problem. A suggested format for a family interview is given in Table 8-3.

IV. **When to refer.** Referral to a mental health or other professional is appropriate when the pediatric clinician's work with a family has not ameliorated the problems or when family issues are uncovered that are outside the clinician's ability or comfort level (e.g., substance abuse or domestic violence). Other factors to consider in deciding on referral include the severity and acuity of the problem and any associated protective or risk factors.

Table 8-3. Steps in convening a family meeting

1. **Contact the family to arrange the meeting.** Have them write down their questions in advance. Encourage participation of the affected members and include members perceived as authority figures.
2. **Before the meeting, formulate your thoughts, questions, and hypotheses about what family factors may be contributing to the problem.**
3. **Find a place to meet with adequate seating for all participants** (a conference room or after-hours waiting room).
4. **Greeting and seating:** Perform introductions and explain the purpose of the meeting.
5. **Social or warm-up time:** If appropriate, ask demographic information about each person (e.g., their connection with the group). Identify the authority figures or spokespersons. Try to match your communication style (e.g., warm, reserved, joking) to the family's.
6. **Problem identification/information sharing:** Briefly introduce the issues to be discussed. Then ask each person to describe the problem. Encourage them to be specific and to describe behavior and feelings. Direct communication between members is facilitated and blaming discouraged. Attempts are made to engage all members.
7. **Goal definition:** Past attempts at solutions are discussed, emphasizing successes. Be positive and encouraging about the group's strengths and the possibility of progress. Assist the family in defining what they would like to see change. Goals should be specific, positive, and realistic.
8. **Homework assignment:** Suggest specific, small, achievable tasks to be done by individual family members before the next meeting to move the group closer to the goal.

BIBLIOGRAPHY

Web sites

www.healthychildren.org, family life section

Books and articles

Allmond BW, Tanner JL. *The Family is the Patient* (2nd ed), Philadelphia: Lippincott Williams & Wilkins, 1999.

American Academy of Pediatrics Institute for Family-Centered Care. Policy statement: family-centered care and the pediatrician's role. *Pediatrics* 112:691–696, 2003.

American Academy of Pediatrics. Family pediatrics: report of the Task Force on the Family. *Pediatrics* 111:1541–1571, 2003.

Coleman W. Family-focused pediatrics: a primary care family systems approach to psychosocial problems. *Curr Probl Pediatr Adolesc Health Care* 32:255–314, 2002.

Coleman WL. *Family-Focused Behavioral Pediatrics: Clinical Techniques for Primary Care.* Philadelphia: Lippincott Williams & Wilkins, 2001.

Freedman J, Combs G. *Narrative Therapy: The Social Construction of Preferred Realities.* New York: W.W. Norton & Company, Inc., 1996, p. 47

Madsen W. *Collaborative Therapy With Multi-Stressed Families.* New York: Guilford Press, 1999, pp. 1–3, 167.

McDaniel S, Campbell TL, Seaburn DB. *Family-Oriented Primary Care.* New York: Springer-Verlag, 1990.

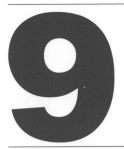

Using Difficult Child Behavior in the Examination Room to Help Parents

Gregory F. Hayden
Barry Zuckerman
Marilyn Augustyn

I. **The importance.** A range of positive and negative parent and child behavior happens in examination rooms. Children are uncertain and stressed; parents may feel under pressure in the spotlight. Under these circumstances, some children will impulsively climb furniture, whine and yell at mother, or display other problematic behaviors that elicit anger, frustration, or excessive concern in the parent.

II. **The child's perspective.** This is a special moment for children. They may be upset or anxious for a variety of understandable reasons. Maybe they got up earlier than usual, breakfast was rushed or even omitted in the hurry, maybe the bus was late, maybe finding a parking space was difficult, maybe the wait in the waiting room was long. These previsit issues are coupled with recollections of what happened to him the last time he was in this room—maybe immunizations, maybe a finger stick or venipuncture, or maybe a forced and painful ear examination. Doubtless, the examination room offers many interesting possibilities for exploration—a door with a knob, drawers with handles, a wastebasket, a sharps disposal unit, a sink with running water and a paper towel dispenser, boxes of latex gloves that make interesting balloons, and much more. Although children do not want to get into trouble as their mother is preoccupied talking with the doctor, some children will engage in a behavior for their own amusement or need at the same time, with the plan in some cases to get the mother's attention.

III. **The parent's perspective.** This is also a difficult moment for the parent, especially if she has other important or acute stresses at home or work. Many thoughts and emotions may fly through her head as she tries to concentrate on what you are saying about fluoride and the temperature of her hot water heater. Maybe she felt embarrassed last visit because her child was very uncooperative. When he now misbehaves while you are in the examination room, she is unsure what to do. At some level she is aware that her threats ("Stop that or else...") do not seem to work very well. Spanking seems sometimes to work, but she does not think you would approve. A bribe is another possibility ("Behave and I'll take you to...on the way home."). Anything she does, however, will call the behavior to your attention and she is hoping that you are either too preoccupied to notice or too hurried to talk to her about it.

IV. **The clinician's perspective.** When your patient misbehaves you have to decide whether or not to intervene and, if so, you do not want to offend the child's parent nor do you want the child to hurt himself and you want to decrease the noise level in the office and return focus to your history taking, physical examination, and anticipatory guidance.

V. **Potential responses**
   A. Wait for the parent to respond.
   B. Observe the parent's approach and effectiveness.
   C. If the parent does not respond or is ineffective in controlling the child's behavior, model setting limits.
   D. Skip the remainder of the routine anticipatory guidance and intervene in the moment by eliciting information and providing advice.
   Possible interventions include the Coleman's "5 Rs"
   1. Reassurance (acknowledge the mother's emotional distress, e.g., "You probably find this type of behavior really challenging at times...")
   2. Recipes (offer advice, generic wisdom; discuss time-out or model an actual time-out in the examination room)
   3. Readings (books, pamphlets, and Web sites about behavior and discipline)
   4. Rx's (e.g., begin attention deficit/hyperactivity disorder (ADHD) work-up with eventual treatment if further testing suggests this diagnosis)
   5. Referral (e.g., to a mental health clinician for evaluation and guidance if behavior problems have been severe and frequent)

VI. Obtaining more history

  A. *Why do you think your child is behaving this way today? Does he or she act like this at home? Does he or she behave the same way with other adults (other parent/grandparent, teacher, etc.)? Does this behavior bother you?*

  B. *What do you do at home? Does it work? Do you sometimes feel overwhelmed?*

  C. *Would you like some help with this? What kind? Would you be willing to talk to a child psychologist (or other professional) about this?*

VII. Clinical pearls

  A. Cultural sensitivity. It is critically important to recognize cultural differences between your own values and the family's values. Opening with a question such as, "Is this behavior OK with you?" may give you a small window into the family's expectations. Respect to parents and other authority figures (like doctors) is important in many cultures, and parents will often respond with speed and directness at signs of disrespect.

  B. Make a note about this episode in the chart so the next time you see the parent you can ask him or her about ongoing occurrences and whether any interventions have been helpful.

  C. If the parent hits the child in front of you, it is important to acknowledge what just happened. Ignoring it will implicitly tell the parent it is "OK." You can respond that your office is a "no hitting" zone followed by a discussion about what a child learns by being spanked: hitting is OK. Children love to imitate, especially people whom they love and respect. Spanking demonstrates that it is all right for people to hit people, and especially for big people to hit little people, and stronger people to hit weaker people.

  D. Tell the parent that spanking a child when angry makes it very difficult to maintain control and the child could be injured. It also teaches the child to hit when frustrated or angry. As the child's clinician, you need to ensure his or her safety. If the spanking seems excessive (e.g., hitting with an object) or has resulted in injuries (e.g., bruises or welts), tell the parent that you will need to involve protective services for a more thorough investigation of the home. Acknowledge that you know the parents love the child and reassure them that you will support them through the process but that for the child's safety, an investigation needs to occur. Never contact protective services without telling the family or your chances to maintain the relationship will be severed.

BIBLIOGRAPHY

Howard BJ. Advising parents on discipline: what works. *Pediatrics* 98:809–814, 1996.

Howard BJ. Discipline in early childhood. *Pediatr Clin North Am* 38:1351–1369, 1991.

Ivey CL. Effective discipline: gain without pain. *Contemp Pediatr* 8:108–113, 1991.

Stein MT, Coleman WL, Epstein RM. "We've tried everything and nothing works": family-centered pediatrics and clinical problem-solving. *J Dev Behav Pediatr* 22 (2 Suppl):S55–S60, 2001.

Wissow LS. What clinicians want to know about teaching families new disciplinary tools. *Pediatrics* 98:815–817, 1996.

Wissow LS, Roter D. Toward effective discussion of discipline and corporal punishment during primary care visits: findings from studies of doctor-patient interaction. *Pediatrics* 94:587–593, 1994.

10

Promoting Parental Self-Understanding

Barry Zuckerman
Pamela M. Zuckerman

I. Description of the problem. Adults are challenged when they become parents first. The tasks are novel and often cause concerns, anxieties, and fears. New parents must also address previously unexplored values and attitudes now brought to the fore by the birth of their baby. New day-to-day activities and routines, new problems needing solutions, and normal struggles and uncertainties can elicit heightened emotional responses from parents.

Mundane and minor matters can elicit worry (e.g., parents' great anxiety when their infant has not had a bowel movement in 2 days). More serious and threatening experiences also cause internal upset (e.g., a mother's feelings of exhaustion and being literally consumed by her ever-hungry new infant; a father's dismay at his wife's physical and at times emotional unavailability as she completely focuses on the new infant).

In addition to these universal early experiences, parents know that ahead of them are the even more challenging tasks and risks of child rearing.

- How will they protect the child from their own occasional frustration, anger, or irritability?
- How will they avoid being overindulgent and also set limits that are not too harsh or arbitrary?
- How will they balance providing praise appropriately and correcting unwanted behaviors effectively without being either too strict or overly permissive?

II. Process of self-understanding. The pediatric clinician's input around child development information and child-rearing strategies is often inadequate to help parents negotiate the myriad feelings and the complex tasks involved in successful parenting. One thing in which parents really need to be successful is to develop an understanding and insight into their own past, especially their relationship to their own parents, and also to understand their own patterns of behavior. Self-understanding for parents develops over time through review of their past upbringing through remembering, retelling, reflecting on, and perhaps reinterpreting past events. This process is catalyzed and assisted through ongoing conversations with spouse, relatives, friends, and other parents and professionals.

Without adequate self-understanding, problems can arise for parents when experiences, attitudes, and fears arising from their own upbringing, cause them to respond inconsistently or behave inappropriately toward their child. And when parents do direct excessive anger, withdrawal, sarcasm, harsh criticism, or rigid orders toward their child, it can be upsetting, confusing, and ultimately damaging for the child. To short circuit inappropriate responses to their child, parents need to be aware of the origins of their attitudes and behaviors. Again, this is achieved through reflection and self-exploration.

Pediatric clinicians can foster self-understanding in parents by asking key questions at critical times and then listening to the answers. Questions that are particularly important address parents' attitudes and values, especially as they relate to their own childhood and how their parents raised them. Growing up in a family that is overly strict or harsh or lacks emotional warmth can program children to recreate the same family style when they become parents. But when parents have reviewed their own upbringing thoughtfully, have considered which aspects were positive and which were not, and have decided how they would like to raise their own children, research shows they are much less likely to repeat maladaptive patterns learned in the past.

A. Questions for self-understanding. There are a number of simple, straightforward questions pediatricians can ask that will help parents begin to look at their own personal stories and make connections between their current experiences being a parent now and their past experiences as a child growing up.

General themes to be addressed include experiences of love, nurturing, separation, care when distressed, times of feeling threatened, and experiences of loss. Other related topics, which may also be helpful, include experiences of being disciplined, the presence of siblings, and changes in the relationship with the parents during adolescence and adulthood. Parents can be relieved when they gain insight into the connections between difficult events in their past and unexpected eruptions in their present life with their

Table 10-1. Questions for parental self-reflection

These questions can be asked over the course of many visits over many years.

Do you plan to raise your child like your mother and father raised you? What was your parents' philosophy in raising children? What was it about it that you liked? What was it about it that you did not like?

How did you get along with your parents? How did the relationship evolve throughout your youth and up until the present time?

How did your relationship with your mother and father differ and how were they similar? Can you describe three characteristics of your childhood relationship to each of your parents? Why did you choose these adjectives? Are there ways in which you try to be like, or try not to be like, either of your parents?

Do you recall your earliest separations from your parents? What was it like? Did you ever have prolonged separations from your parents?

What kind of discipline did your parent use? Did your mother or father differ? What impact did that have on your childhood, and how do you feel it affects your role as a parent now?

Did you ever feel rejected or threatened by your parents? Were there other experiences you had that felt overwhelming or traumatizing in your life, during childhood or beyond? Do any of these experiences still feel very much alive? Do they continue to influence your life?

Did anyone significant in your life die during your childhood or later in life? What was that like for you at the time, and how does that loss affect you now?

How did your parents communicate with you when you were happy and excited? Did they join with you in your enthusiasm? When you were distressed or unhappy as a child, what would happen? Did your father and mother respond differently to you during these emotional times? How?

Was there anyone else besides your parents in your childhood who took care of you? What was that relationship like for you? What happened to those individuals? What is it like for you when you let others take care of your child now?

If you had difficult times during your childhood, were there positive relationships in or outside of your home that you could depend on during those times? How do you feel those connections benefited you then, and how might they help you now?

How have your childhood experiences influenced your relationships with others as an adult? How has your childhood shaped the ways in which you relate to your children?

Adapted from Siegel DJ, Kaetzel M. *Parenting from the Inside Out.* New York: Putnam Books, 2003.

children. When these connections are made and parents gain insight into some of the underpinnings of their own behavior, parents are often then able to let go of some struggles or rigidity they are involved in with their children.

The pediatric clinician can begin with gentle questions (Table 10-1) to open the door, to invite parents to remember, to retell, and to rethink the emotional meanings of their past lives in context with their new role as a mother or as a father. Because the pediatric clinician is a trusted professional, the parents can tolerate and respond thoughtfully to these personal questions. The pediatric clinician need not ask all these questions at one visit and should consider this as an ongoing conversation that may vary in need and intensity at different stages in the child's development or parents' life circumstances.

  B. **New use of family history.** Family history is traditionally used to identify risk for genetically loaded diseases. Routine family history can be expanded to highlight two common parental health problems affecting children: depression (3% of adult men and 9% of adult women) and alcoholism (12% of adults).

Beyond the potential genetic risk, these disorders convey risk through multigenerational parenting dysfunctions and role modeling starting with grandparents during the childhood of the parents. When the parents were younger, their depressed or alcoholic parents may have difficulty with emotional regulation and availability to their children, and they may be unable to set consistent limits and are reflected in poignant stories of adult children of alcoholics, whose descriptions of difficulties with self-esteem, nurturing, and relationships suggest problems originating in their childhood. Some alcoholic parents physically and sexually abuse their children. These stories demonstrate how the adult child of an alcoholic may become a dysfunctional parent even though he or she is not alcoholic. Although not yet clearly defined, the parenting of adult children of depressed parents may also be impaired even if they are not depressed. Pediatricians obtaining a family history should therefore ask about the presence of either of these problems in the child's grandparents. If a grandparent suffered from either of these problems, a pediatrician should then ask the following questions:

1. Since it runs in families, do the parents or their siblings have any similar problems?
2. If yes, are they being treated?
3. If no, do they think their childhood experiences affect their parenting? For example, are they overprotective, overly strict, or have trouble showing emotions?

This type of discussion with the pediatrician provides the parents with an opportunity to become aware of their parents' influence on their own parenting. If there is not a significant problem at that time, identification of the problem in the family provides the opportunity for parents to talk about their childhood experiences, and their concerns regarding their own feelings and their ability to nurture, support, and promote the self-esteem of their own children. The pediatrician should continue to bear this history in mind; sometimes issues will arise during specific stages of the child's development such as adolescence, and a parent may develop depression or alcoholism throughout the time.

While asking specific listed questions or family history, the clinician needs to spend a little time to listen to the parent's responses. However, you do not have to listen indefinitely or hear it all at once, nor do you have to respond with explanations or advice immediately. If necessary, the appropriate "referral" is to a spouse, friends, or selected family members. The professional can say something like, "It sounds like you have many memories and feelings. I would encourage you to talk to your spouse, sister, or friends about them to give you insight into what you want to do and don't do as a parent."

Outside the pediatric office setting, the issues can be explored in greater depth and complexity in the parents' circle of friends and family, and with other therapeutic professionals if appropriate or desired. Spouses and friends can assist parents in continuing the process of insightful exploration, "making sense" of a parent's personal history with supportive, empathic, emotionally directed conversations.

Both science and clinical experience tell us that parents' self-understanding can greatly enhance their ability to be good parents and to foster their children's optimal development. The pediatric clinician's role is to raise the issues and support the process of parental self-understanding through reflection and discussion with others. A continuity of care setting allows questions and the unfolding answers and their clarification and import to occur over time.

BIBLIOGRAPHY

For parents

Siegel DJ, Hartzel M. *Parenting from the Inside Out.* New York: Penguin Putnam, 2003.

For professionals

Fraiberg S, Adelson E, Shapiro V. The Nursery. *J Am Acad Child Psychiatry* 14:387–421, 1975.

Mav M. Attachment: overview with implications for clinical work. In Goldberg S, Muir R, Kerr J (eds), *Attachment Theory: Social, Developmental, and Clinical Perspectives.* Hillsdale, NJ: Analytic Press, 1995, pp. 407–474.

Zuckerman B. Family history: a special opportunity for psychosocial intervention. *Pediatrics* 87(5):740–741, 1991.

Zuckerman B, Zuckerman P, Siegel DJ. Promoting self-understanding in parents—for the great good of your patients. *Contemp Pediatr* 22(4):77–90, 2005.

11

Behavioral Screening

Terry Stancin
Ellen C. Perrin

I. **Description of the problem.** Regular surveillance and periodic screening for behavioral problems in pediatric settings is important because effective child intervention techniques result in a more positive impact on behavioral problems if children are identified and referred for appropriate services early. Studies in primary care settings have shown that close to 25% of children have significant behavioral problems, yet pediatric clinicians fail to identify many of them, and refer successfully only a minority of children to mental health professionals for further evaluation and treatment.

Effective monitoring consists of regular *surveillance*, characterized by repeated observations over time, and periodic *screening* using validated instruments at regular intervals. In the context of routine pediatric care, surveillance of a child's emotional and behavioral health status should be a part of every health supervision visit, and screening is recommended at specified visits. Further evaluation may be performed by pediatric clinicians or may be deferred to a mental health consultant.

II. **Selection and utilization of behavioral screening instruments.** Most surveillance and screening methods available for behavioral problems rely on caregiver report, often via questionnaires or rating scales. Standardized surveillance and screening instruments allow comparisons to normative standards, analogous to showing parents a child's weight on a standardized growth chart. Most can be administered in advance of clinical encounters and scored easily by clerical staff, and thus are efficient and inexpensive methods for collecting information. As electronic methods of administering and scoring such questionnaires become more widespread and accepted, the efficiency and utility of their use will increase further. Rating scales can be an excellent way to collect and compare the opinions of multiple observers as well, especially teachers.

The use of standardized screening instruments and other systematic procedures have been shown to increase identification of child behavior problems in primary care settings. Monitoring of behavioral/emotional status using standardized instruments should occur within the context of a clinical evaluation of every child, combining information from the checklist with the history, direct observation, physical examination, and diagnostic tests. Formal screening procedures should be psychometrically sound, acceptable to parents, accurate, cost effective, and fit into the practice setting.

If a concern is identified on regular surveillance (or as part of a periodic schedule), an appropriate next step would be a "first-stage" screening instrument. These are generally brief parent questionnaires, standardized to identify children in need of further evaluation. Additional clarity will be obtained from a "second-stage" screening instrument, administered by the pediatrician or a mental health consultant, and often available in formats for completion by multiple observers.

A. **Selection of instruments depends on the particular goals of screening but should take into consideration the following factors:**
  - Ages of the children to be screened
  - Informants (parent, teacher, and child)
  - Characteristics of available screening tools (sensitivity, specificity, acceptability, efficiency, and cost)
  - Impact of procedures on practice (e.g., training and supervision of staff responsible for implementation and maintenance of screening procedures)
  - Cost and reimbursement issues
  - Procedures for further evaluation and interventions of children who screen positive
  - Mental health resources available
  - Possible adverse consequences of screening

  Table 11-1 contains a list of some behavioral screening instruments that have been recommended because of their acceptable psychometric characteristics and utility in primary care settings. Comparative studies are just emerging, which will assist with decisions about selecting one method over others.

Table 11-1. Selected behavioral surveillance and screening methods

Title of instrument	Screening focus	Informant*	Ages (years)	Time (minutes)	Comments
Surveillance					
Bright Futures Tool and Resource Kit http://brightfutures.aap.org	Forms for different screening purposes	Parent	0–21+	Varies by form	Tool kit of various forms and screens to accompany Bright Futures recommendations for developmental and behavioral surveillance and screening.
Parents' Evaluation of Developmental Status (PEDS) www.pedstest.com	Developmental and behavioral concerns	Parent	0–8	5	Questions prompt parents to observe and describe concerns.
First-Stage Screening					
Ages and Stages Questionnaire— Social Emotional (SE) http://www.agesandstages.com	Social and emotional behavior	Parent	0.5–5	10–15	Eight questionnaires for different ages. Can be used alone or in conjunction with ASQ-3. English and Spanish.
Brief Infant–Toddler Social-Emotional Assessment Scale (BITSEA) http://www.pearsonassessments.com	Emotional competencies and problems of infants and toddlers	Parent	1–4	15	Developmentally and clinically sensitive.
Pediatric Symptom Checklist (PSC) http://www2.massgeneral.org/ allpsych/psc/psc_home.htm	General psychological functioning	Parent	4–16	<5	Specifically designed for use in pediatric settings to screen for psychosocial dysfunction. Cutoffs, but no standard scores. Can be downloaded and used free of charge.
Strengths and Difficulties Questionnaire (SDQ) http://www.sdqinfo.com	General behavioral functioning	Parent, teacher, adolescents	3–16	5	Twenty-five items of positive and negative attributes. Scores interpretable as normal, borderline or abnormal. Free in public domain. Available in many languages.

(continued)

Table 11-1. (Continued)

Title of instrument	Screening focus	Informant*	Ages (years)	Time (minutes)	Comments
Second-stage screening					
Behavior Assessment System for Children (BASC-2) http://psychcorp.pearsonassessments.com	Multidimensional behavioral screening and assessment	Parent, teacher, and child self-report formats	2–22	10–20	Broad-based measure of pathology. Provides a profile of internalizing and externalizing problems, other problems (atypicality, withdrawal); and adaptive skills. Standard T-scores provide norm-based comparisons by age and gender. Validity check included. Norms available by age and gender. Computer scoring recommended.
Child Behavior Checklists (CBCL, TRF, YSR) http://www.aseba.org/	Multidimensional behavioral screening and assessment	Parent, teacher, and child self-report formats	1½–Adult	20	Broad-based measure of pathology. Provides a profile of internalizing and externalizing problems. Standard T-scores provide norm-based comparisons by age and gender, with DSM-compatible scales. Spanish versions available. Computer scoring or Internet administration recommended.
Infant-Toddler Social-Emotional Assessment Scale (ITSEA) http://www.pearsonassessments.com	Emotional competencies and problems of infants and toddlers	Parent	1–4	30	Extension of BITSEA. 17 subscales address four domains; focus on strengths and weaknesses. Developmentally and clinically sensitive. English and Spanish. Computer scoring available.

*Parent = parent or a primary caregiver.
Portions adapted from Perrin E, Stancin T. A continuing dilemma: whether and how to screen for concerns about children's behavior in primary care settings. *Pediatr Rev* 23: 264–282, 2002 and from Stancin T, Aylward GP. Screening instruments: behavioral and developmental. In Ollendick T, Schroeder C (eds). *Encyclopedia of Pediatric and Child Psychology*. New York: Kluwer Academic/Plenum publishers, 2003, pp. 574–577. Test author information available upon request and at most test Web sites.

B. Incorporating behavioral instruments into practice. Tools intended for regular surveillance are generally short and appropriate to administer routinely to all children in a setting such as the pediatric clinician's waiting room.

1. The "first-stage" screening measures focus on broad concerns such as general psychosocial dysfunction, disruptive behavior, and family functioning, and can be completed and scored in less than 10 minutes. Examples include instruments such as the Ages and Stages-SE and the Brief Infant–Toddler Social-Emotional Assessment Scale (BITSEA) for young children, and the Pediatric Symptom Checklist (PSC) for children older than 4 years.

2. A longer, "second-stage" screening instrument may follow positive results of a first-stage screening, or whenever a clinician suspects or has identified a problem, to obtain more detailed information about the nature and severity of behavioral concerns. These more detailed assessments can be obtained using the Child Behavior Checklist (CBCL), the Behavioral Assessment Scale for Children (BASC-2), and the Infant–Toddler Social-Emotional Assessment Scale (ITSEA), all of which tend to be multidimensional in focus and have normative standards by which to evaluate the nature and severity of problems.

C. Cautions regarding the use of standardized questionnaires:
- Interpretation of results must take into account the fact that any caregiver's perceptions are subject to biases. Procedures that rely on parent report may yield false negative results when the parent does not perceive behaviors as problematic. Use of multiple informants is ideal.
- Screening procedures carry costs for implementation (e.g., purchase of materials, implementation costs, scoring, and subsequent care).
- New administrative demands are placed on office staff to administer questionnaires properly. Training, supervision, and expertise are necessary to ensure proper scoring and valid interpretation of results. To properly interpret results, the clinician must be familiar with and understand the meaning of a test's psychometric properties and norms.
- Screening is intended to identify those in need of further evaluation and assessment, not to provide a diagnosis. Because of the complexities described above, pediatric clinicians should seek consultation from a knowledgeable pediatric psychologist when selecting and incorporating formal rating scales into practice.

D. Beyond screening. Most pediatric clinicians will benefit from help with the *management* of children with behavioral problems even more than with their *identification. Screening for any condition presupposes a system in place for following up appropriately when a problem is identified.* Communication between mental health professionals and primary care clinicians is often cumbersome and frequently inadequate. Therefore, a collaborative relationship with one or more mental health professionals in the community is advisable. New models of collaborative care and improved payment mechanisms are urgently needed to create a fully responsive system for regular and comprehensive child health supervision and care.

BIBLIOGRAPHY

Dobrez D, Lo Sasso A, Holl J, et al. Estimating the costs of developmental and behavioral screening of preschool children in general pediatric practice. *Pediatrics* 108:913–922, 2001.

Glascoe FP, Dworkin PH. Surveillance and screening for development and behavior. In Wolraich ML, Drotar D, Dworkin PH, et al. (eds), *Developmental and Behavioral Pediatrics: Evidence and Practice.* Philadelphia, PA: Elsevier/Mosby, 2008, pp. 130–144.

Perrin E, Stancin T.A continuing dilemma: whether and how to screen for concerns about children's behavior in primary care settings. *Pediatr Rev* 23:264–282, 2002.

Sheldrick RS, Perrin EC. Surveillance of children's behavior and development: practical solutions for primary care. *J Dev Behav Pediatr* 30:151–153, 2009.

Stancin T, Aylward GP. Screening instruments: behavioral and developmental. In Ollendick T, Schroeder C (eds), *Encyclopedia of Pediatric and Child Psychology.* New York: Kluwer Academic/Plenum Publishers, 2003, pp. 574–577.

Vogels AGC, Crone MR, Hoekstra F, et al. Comparing three short questionnaires to detect psychosocial dysfunction among primary school children: a randomized method. *BMC Public Health* 9:489, 2009 [Epub ahead of print].

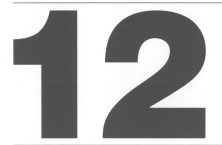

Developmental and Academic Surveillance and Screening

Kevin P. Marks
Frances Page Glascoe

I. **The problem of underdetection.** Most children with developmental and behavioral problems have subtle symptoms that are not readily apparent in the absence of measurement. Because few medical professionals use standardized screening tests routinely, 70%–80% of children with disabilities are not detected prior to school entrance and vital opportunities for early intervention are missed. As few as 2 years of early intervention prior to school entrance increases the likelihood of high school graduation, employment, and independent living and reduces the rates of teen pregnancy, criminal activity, and violent crime.

II. **Pearls.** Timely early detection relies upon frequent, periodic screening where measures are promptly scored and interpreted, ideally before the visit begins. Frequent, periodic screening is important because developmental–behavioral problems tend to worsen over time, especially when a history exists of adverse psychosocial risk factors such as poverty, exposure to domestic violence, parental mood disorders, parental substance abuse, negative approaches to parenting, child abuse/ neglect, etc. When an efficient clinic system is in place, developmental–behavioral screening does not necessarily lengthen the well-child visit and yet it simultaneously raises the quality of care with a parent-centered approach.

The optimal tools for identifying developmental and behavioral problems in primary care are those that

- Have proven levels of accuracy (at least 70%–80% of children with and without problems should be detected correctly) and have been properly standardized and validated on a large, national, general (not referred) sample of children.
- Are feasible in a primary care setting and rely on information from parents. Parent-report screens take little time to administer (because parents can complete them in waiting or examination rooms). Parents, regardless of their level of education or parenting experience, are equally able to provide predictive information about their children. For non–English-speaking parents, many screens are published in multiple languages.
- Offer both evidence-based surveillance as well as screening, and they are easy to use because pediatric clinician need not elicit skills directly from children who may be fearful, uncooperative, sick, or asleep.

III. **Pitfalls.** While surveillance (meaning clinical observation and judgment) is important, the informal methods typically deployed are associated with limited identification rates. Non-standardized, non-validated checklists lack definable scoring/referral criteria and many include items that are far too easy for the age levels given. Checklists lack any proof of accuracy.

IV. **Tools.** Several good quality measures relying on information from parents are presented in Table 12-1. Several of these can be administered directly to children by clinicians who prefer this approach. Other alternatives to direct measurement are to (a) send such parents home with a copy of parent-report screen and ask that he or she complete it with other caregivers or (b) refer for screening through the public schools or through child find services through the Individuals with Disabilities Education Act (see list of referral resources below to locate them for every state and region).

V. **Making it work in primary care.** There are many approaches to organizing pediatric settings so that developmental and behavioral problems can be easily detected and addressed while also maintaining patient flow and office efficiency. Table 12-1 is a list of such methods and Web sites for specific tools often have useful information on how to apply them in busy practices. In settings where there are healthcare providers, such professionals can and should document carefully both medical history and physical examination findings to determine whether organic conditions are contributory. The physical examination should include attention to growth parameters, head shape and circumference, facial and other body dysmorphology, eye findings (e.g., cataracts in various inborn errors of metabolism), vascular markings, and signs of neurocutaneous disorders (e.g., café-au-lait spots in neurofibromatosis, hypopigmented macules in tuberous sclerosis), muscle strength, tone, presence of abnormal reflexes, and disturbance of movement.

Table 12-1. Parent-report, standardized, validated, and accurate developmental–behavioral screens

Screens for primary care—general screens					
Parent-report developmental and/or behavioral screens	Age range	Description	Scoring	Accuracy	Administration time and cost
Parents' Evaluations of Developmental Status (PEDS). (2006) Ellsworth & Vandermeer Press, Ltd. 1013 Austin Court, Nolensville, TN 37135 Phone: 615-776-4121; fax: 615-776-4119 http://www.pedstest.com ($30.00) See electronic options below. **Training options:** downloadable slide shows with notes, case examples, and handouts, Web site discussion list (covering all screens), short videos coming soon) some live training.	Birth to 8 years	10 questions eliciting parents' concerns in English, Spanish, Vietnamese, and many other languages. Written at the 4th–5th grade level. Determines when to refer, provide a second screen, provide patient education, or monitor development, behavior/emotional, and academic progress. Provides longitudinal surveillance and triage.	Identifies children as low, moderate, or high risk for various kinds of disabilities and delays	Sensitivity 74%–79%; Specificity 70%–80% across age levels.	About 2 min (if interview needed) **Print materials** ~$.31 **Admin.** ~$.88 Total = ~$1.19
Ages and Stages Questionnaire-3 (3rd ed., 2009). Paul H. Brookes Publishing, Inc., P.O. Box 10624, Baltimore, MD 21285 Phone: 1-800-638-3775). ($249) http://www.pbrookes.com/ See electronic options below. **Training options:** purchasable videos, case examples, and live training.	1–66 months	Parents-report, elicits children's developmental skills in 5 domains with 30 items and 6–7 overall questions using an age-appropriate form for each well visit. Reading level varies across items from 4th to 5th grade. Proven feasible for office use with an option to complete at home (ideally before the visit). Online and mail-out approaches are used for child find programs. In English, Spanish, French, Korean, and others.	Straightforward (refer/no-refer) cutoff scores, along with a near cutoff monitoring zone per age interval.	Sensitivity (overall 86%), 82.5%–89.2% across all age intervals; Specificity (overall 85%), 77.9%–92.1% across all age intervals.	10–20 min (dependent upon whether the ASQ-3 is completed in a clinic, at home, or by direct interview) **Materials** ~$.40 **Admin.** ~$4.20 Total = ~$4.60

(continued)

Table 12-1. (*Continued*)

Screens for primary care—general screens

Parent-report developmental and/or behavioral screens	Age range	Description	Scoring	Accuracy	Administration time and cost
PEDS: Developmental Milestones (Screening Version) Ellsworth & Vandermeer Press, Ltd. 1013 Austin Court, Nolensville, TN 37135 Phone: 615-776-4121; fax: 615-776-4119 http://www.pedstest.com ($275.00). Electronic options coming soon. **Training Options:** 2-min movie on Web site, plus slide shows with notes, case examples, handouts, some live training, and a discussion list.	0–8 years	PEDS-DM consists of 6–8 items at each age level (spanning the well visit schedule). Each item taps a different domain (fine/gross motor; self-help, academics, expressive/receptive language, social-emotional). Items are administered by parents or professionals. Forms are laminated and marked with a grease pencil. It can be used to complement PEDS or stand alone. Written at the 2nd grade level. A longitudinal score form tracks performance. Supplemental measures are included (see descriptions below): the M-CHAT, Family Psychosocial Screen, Pictorial PSC-17, the SWILS, the Vanderbilt ADHD scale, and the Brigance Parent–Child Interactions Scale. In English and Spanish.	Cutoffs tied to performance above and below the 16th percentile for each item and its domain. On the assessment level, age equivalent scores are produced and enable users to compute percentage of delays.	Sensitivity 75%–87%; Specificity 71%–88% to performance in each domain. Sensitivity 70%–94%; Specificity 77%–93% across age intervals	About 3–5 min Materials ~$.02 Admin. ~$1.00 Total ~$1.02

Narrow-band screens for primary care (*for psychosocial risk, mental health, and autism spectrum disorder. These are valuable adjuncts in primary care and elsewhere but should not be used as the sole measure of developmental–behavioral status*)

Ages & Stages Questionnaires: Social-Emotional (ASQ:SE) Paul H. Brookes, Publishers, P.O. Box 10624, Baltimore, MD 21285 Phone: 1-800-638-3775). ($149) http://www.pbrookes.com/ **Training options:** live training, training video	3–65 months	Parent-report tool designed to complement the ASQ, the ASQ:SE consists of 8 intervals with 22–36 items per age interval (4–5 page questionnaire). Items focus on self-regulation, compliance, communication, adaptive functioning, autonomy, affect, and interaction with people. Items are based on parental recall and do not ask parents to elicit developmental skills so quicker to complete than the ASQ.	Single (above or below) cutoff score indicating when a referral is needed	Sensitivity 71%–85%; Specificity 90%–98% in detecting children with social-emotional delays/a need for an early intervention and/or mental health referral	10–15 min Materials ~$.40 Admin. ~$4.20 Total = ~ $4.40

Brief-Infant–Toddler Social-Emotional Assessment (BITSEA); Harcourt Assessment, Inc, 19500 Bulverde Road, San Antonio, TX 78259 Phone: 1–800–211–8378 ($105.00) http://pearsonassess.com/ **Training options:** none	12–36 months	42-item parent-report measure for identifying social-emotional/behavioral. Problems and delays in competence. Items were drawn from the assessment level measure, the ITSEA. Written at the 4th–6th grade level. Available in Spanish, French, Dutch, and Hebrew. Has a CD-ROM for ease of scoring.	Cut-points based on child age and sex show presence or absence of problems and competence.	Sensitivity 80%–85%; specificity 75%–80% in detecting children with social-emotional problems and in need of an early intervention and/or mental health referral.	5–7 min Materials ~$1.15 Admin. ~$.88 Total ~$2.03
Modified Checklist for Autism in Toddlers (M-CHAT) (1999). Free download including follow-up interview at http://www. mchatscreen.com Included in the PEDS:DM. See electronic records options below. **Training options:** none	16–30 months	Parent report of 23 questions modified for American usage at 4th–6th grade reading level. Available in multiple languages. Screens for Autism Spectrum Disorder (ASD). Downloadable scoring template and .xls file for automated scoring. Requires a follow-up interview (also downloadable in English and Spanish, in response to problematic performance). M-CHAT Follow-up Interview is designed to reduce false positive M-CHAT results and reduce the number of expensive comprehensive ASD diagnostic evaluations	Cutoff based on 2 of 3 critical items or any 3 from the 23-item "yes or no" checklist. Clarifies ASD concerns with failed M-CHAT items	Initial study demonstrated sensitivity at 90%; specificity at 99%. Note: a revised 7-item M-CHAT is under development. Subsequent studies recommended that a failed M-CHAT (6%–10% of children at 18 and 24 months) should lead to an in-office, standardized "M-CHAT Follow-up Interview."	About 5 min (excluding the M-CHAT Follow-up Interview) Print Materials ~$.10 Admin. ~$.88 Total = ~$.98

SCREENS FOR OLDER CHILDREN (these screens focus on academic skills and mental health, including ADHD screening and are brief enough for primary care).

Safety Word Inventory and Literacy Screener (SWILS). Glascoe FP, Clinical Pediatrics, 2002. Items courtesy of Curriculum Associates, Inc. The SWILS can be freely downloaded at: http://www. pedstest.com/ and is included in the PEDS:DM. **Training Options:** none	6–14 years	Children are asked to read 29 common safety words (e.g., High Voltage, Wait, Poison) aloud. The number of correctly read words is compared to a cutoff score. Results predict performance in math, written language, and a range of reading skills. Test content may serve as a springboard to injury prevention counseling.	Single cutoff (refer/ no-refer) score indicating the need for a referral	78%–84% sensitivity and specificity across all ages	About 7 min (if interview needed) **Materials ~$.30 Admin. ~$2.38** Total = ~$2.68

(continued)

Table 12-1. (Continued)

Screens for primary care—general screens

Parent-report developmental and/or behavioral screens	Age range	Description	Scoring	Accuracy	Administration time and cost
Pediatric Symptom Checklist (PSC): Jellinek MS, Murphy JM, Robinson J, et al. Screens school age children for academic and psychosocial dysfunction. Research studies and downloads at: http://www2.massgeneral.org/allpsych/psc/psc_home.htm or http://www.brightfutures.org/mentalhealth/pdf/professionals/ped_sympton_chklst.pdf Pictorial PSC (PPSC, is more effective with Spanish-speaking and low-SES families) can be downloaded at www.dbpeds.org and is also included in the PEDS:DM. **Training Options:** none	PSC age range is 4–16 years. PPSC age range is 4–16 years.	Parent-report, 35 short statements of problem behaviors including both externalizing (conduct) and internalizing (depression, anxiety, adjustment, etc.). Ratings of never, sometimes or often are assigned a value of 0, 1, or 2. For children 4–5 years old, referral cutoff score is 24 or higher; 6–10 years old, 28 or higher; 11–16 years old, the (Youth Report) Y-PSC referral cutoff score is 30 or higher. Factor scores identify attentional, internalizing, and externalizing problems. Factor scoring is freely downloadable at: http://www.pedstest.com/links/resources.html	Single cutoff (refer/ no-refer) score	All but one study showed high sensitivity (80%–95%) but somewhat scattered specificity (68%–100%).	About 7 min (if interview needed) Materials ~$.10 Admin. ~$2.38 Total = ~$2.48

Electronic Records Options for Screening with Quality tools

Company	Training/Support options	Description and Pricing
CHADIS (http://www.chadis.com/) PEDS, ASQ, M-CHAT, and other measures online for touch screen, tablet PCs, keyboards, telephony, and parent portal methods. Spanish language version coming soon.	Downloadable guides, live training at exhibits, and other training services on request.	CHADIS also includes decision support for a large range of other measures, both diagnostic and parent/family focused, such as the Vanderbilt ADHD Diagnostic Rating Scale, and various parental depression inventories. CHADIS offers integration with existing EHRs. works with a range of equipment/applications, and automatically generates reports. Pricing is ~$2.00 per use.
Press/Forepath.org (www.pedstest.com) PEDS, M-CHAT online for keyboard and tablet PCs. (PEDS:DM, Spanish language and other translations coming—June, 2009)	Slide shows, Web site FAQs, e-mail support, online videos, discussion list	This site offers PEDS and the Modified Checklist in Toddlers for applications including tablet PCs, keyboards (allowing for actual comments from parents). Offers a parent portal (wherein families do not see the results), etc. Scoring is automated as are summary reports for parents, referral letters when needed, and ICD-9/procedure codes. In English and Spanish (with other languages coming soon along with the PEDS:DM). Integration with electronic records is available as is data export and aggregate views of records. $1.00–$2.00 per use (depending on volume).

Patient Tools (www.patienttools.com or http://pediatrics.patienttools.com/why-pediatrics.asp) (PEDS, M-CHAT, ASQ, ASQ:SE, PSC and others measures online for tablet PCs)	Webcasts/webinars, live support by phone, e-mail	Patient tools offers the ASQ, ASQ:SE, M-CHAT, PEDS, PSC, the Vanderbilt ADHD Scales, and a wide range of behavioral/mental health measures for adolescents and adults. A parent portal approach is available via Survey Tablets. Equipment including docking stations is rented, lease-purchased, or purchased ($74.00–$1320) after which $58.00 per month is the ongoing cost of hosting, data storage, telephone technical, installation support. Copyrighted measures are licensed from their publishers and incur per use fees. From www.pedstest.com (above) at $1.00–$2.00 per use depending on volume.
Brookes Publishing (www.agesandstages.com/) (ASQ via CD-ROM installed on keyboard computers, web-based scoring service coming in June 2008)	Live training, online training, purchasable training videos, e-mail LISTSERV	ASQ on a CD-ROM enables users to click answers and receive an automated score. The software offers aggregation of results, report writing templates, and progress tracking.
Curriculum Associates (www.cainc.com) (Brigance Screens-II online for keyboards. English only but with Spanish-language score/administration forms)	Live training, online training, e-mail, and phone support, customer suggestion box	This service, web-based or via CD-ROM, provides clickable datasheets, which automatically calculate scores including age equivalents, quotients, progress indicators, at-risk cutoff scores quotients, etc. Aggregated reports are available through the online service. $3.00–$5.00 per use, depending on volume.
Riverside Publishing (http://www.riverpub.com/) for Battelle Developmental Inventory along with the screening version (BDIST-II) online via keyboards, and/or CD-ROM	Web site FAQs, e-mail support, live workshops, webcasts/webinars	Scoring services include report writing, all via web-based services. The Web site indicates a version for Personal Digital Assistants (PDAs), but this will be phased out shortly. In English and Spanish. Pricing, ~$765 per year

When screening test results are problematic, referrals should begin with IDEA services. This allows intervention to commence even while children typically need to wait for medical specialty examinations, autism-focused clinics, etc. It may seem odd to refer for treatment before a diagnosis is finalized, but with young children (who are those who benefit most from early intervention), eligibility criteria are generally only a percentage of delay, and do not require specific nosology. Clinicians do not need to confirm a diagnosis before referring.

BIBLIOGRAPHY

For parents

Patient education

American Academy of Child and Adolescent Psychiatry: facts for families has numerous handouts that can be downloaded for free. Written in multiple languages, they address such topics as divorce, disaster recovery, and how to choose a psychiatrist (www.aacap.org).
British Columbia Council for Families has articles, online questionnaires, and links to resources on a variety of parenting and family topics. Carries individual and bulk copies of books and brochures on such topics as adolescence, marriage, family cohesion, and child development, as well as a parenting program. Nobody's Perfect (www.bccf.bc.ca/).
Children and Youth Health is from the South Australian Department of Human Services, this site has extremely rich information for parents on a huge range of psychosocial issues for teens and young children. Diapers are "nappies" and ear infections are "glue ear," but other than that, the depth and quality of parenting advice is unparalleled (www.cyh.sa.gov.au).
Kids' Health is promulgated by the Nemours Foundation, this site has excellent information on health and safety, emotional and social development, and positive parenting, focused on teens and younger children (www.kidshealth.org/).
Early Childhood Connections has sections for parents and professionals interested in developmental and behavioral issues in early childhood. It houses parent information sheets (Adobe Reader is required) in various languages including Arabic, Bosnian, Chinese, Croatian, Somali, Spanish, Turkish, Vietnamese, and English (www.rch.org.au/ecconnections).

Referral and disability resources

Exceptional Parent (P.O. Box 3000 Dept. EP, Denville, NJ 07834, 1-800-562-1973). Published monthly, this journal also produces an annual resource issue that lists Web site, phone numbers, and addresses of organizations devoted to specific disabilities and conditions, parent-to-parent programs, mental health resources, parent training, and information services, etc. (http://www.eparent.com).
First Signs includes information on early detection and treatment of autism (www.firstsigns.org).
American Academy of Pediatrics: Find a Pediatrician to locate general as well as developmental-behavioral, neurodevelopmental, and other subspecialty pediatricians (www.aap.org/referral).

For professionals

The American Academy of Pediatrics' Section on Developmental and Behavioral Pediatrics Home Page has a Web site with information on typical and atypical child development, current information on reimbursement, and coding, updates on quality tools, etc. (http://www.dbpeds.org/)
National Early Childhood Technical Assistance System has a Web site listing all the coordinators for 0–3 and preschool programs, state by state. These individuals have complete lists of early intervention programs. The site provides phone numbers, e-mail, and street addresses (www.nectac.org).
American Academy of Pediatrics Medical Home provides support for a "model of delivering primary care that is accessible, continuous, comprehensive, family-centered, coordinated, compassionate, and culturally effective (www.medicalhomeinfo.org).
Glascoe FP, LaRosa A. Developmental screening and surveillance. *Pediatrics-Up-To-Date.* http://www.uptodate.com.
American Academy of Pediatrics Council on Children with Disabilities, Section on Developmental Behavioral Pediatrics, Bright Futures Steering Committee, Medical Home Initiatives for Children with Special Needs Project Advisory Committee. Identifying infants and young children with developmental disorders in the medical home: an algorithm for developmental surveillance and screening. *Pediatrics* 118(1):405–420, 2006. doi:10.1542/peds.2006–1231.

Wolraich ML (ed.). *Disorders of Development and Learning: A Practical Guide to Assessment and Management* (3rd ed), Chicago: Mosby-Year Book, Inc., 2002.

2009 MMWR recommendations for blood lead screening of medicaid-eligible children aged 1–5 years: an updated approach to targeting a group at high risk. Available at: www.cdc.gov/mmwr/preview/mmwrhtml/rr5809a1.htm?s_cid = rr5809a1_e.

For guidance in conducting a pediatric neurodevelopmental examination, the following online video is helpful: http://library.med.utah.edu/pedineurologicexam/html/home_exam.html.

ABCD Screening Academy (http://abcd.nashpforums.org/).

Harvard's implementation research Web site (http://www.developmentalscreening.org).

13

Screening for Social–Emotional and Behavior Delays in Early Childhood

Margaret J. Briggs-Gowan
Leandra Godoy
Alice S. Carter

I. **Introduction.** According to the National Survey of Children's Health, 11.3% of children in the United States are affected by emotional, behavioral, or developmental conditions, based on parental report. Across all ages of childhood, as many as one in five children are estimated to have mental health problems. Social–emotional and behavioral problems that first emerge in the early childhood (by 5 years of age) often persist within early childhood and are predictive of mental health problems in elementary school. However, many young children do not receive needed mental health services. Lack of attention likely prolongs and exacerbates children's difficulties and contributes to increased parent and family stress. Pediatric clinicians are increasingly essential to the early identification and referral for children with social–emotional/behavioral problems. Clinicians must balance identifying mental health problems with competing medical and developmental demands that are inherent to routine healthcare maintenance. Screening, which relies on the use of an assessment tool, is considered by many to be a necessary supplement to developmental surveillance.

II. **Goals and benefits of screening.** The general goal of developmental/behavioral screening is to identify children who may be experiencing delays or difficulties in a particular developmental domain (e.g., language, cognition, social–emotional). A primary goal of screening is to identify children from a large pool who may be at elevated risk in a relatively quick and cost-effective manner. Once identified, practitioners employing multigated or multistage screening can follow up with children whose scores fall within the "at-risk" range with a longer measure or clinical interview to obtain more detailed information about the specific nature of the child's difficulties and to help in referral or treatment planning. Screening is particularly important in early childhood because some young children have limited contact with formal childcare or preschool settings. These children are unlikely to come into contact with childcare or educational professionals who may help to identify delays.

III. **Considerations for early childhood**
   A. **Behaviorally specific tools.** Screening tools that inquire about specific behaviors help to establish whether the level of behavioral problems reported by a parent is higher than that normally expected for the child's age. This is especially important for parents of young children, as they often have difficulty determining when difficult child behavior crosses the boundary between normative and atypical and warrants worry or concern. Many parents who report high levels of behavioral problems do not endorse feeling worried or concerned about these issues.
   B. Tools that assess both **behavioral problems and competencies** offer a balanced view not only of problem areas, but also of areas of strength for the child. This information can help to guide decisions about next steps for follow-up assessment and referral.
   C. **Cognitive and language delays** may increase the young child's risk for social–emotional/ behavioral problems. Thus, social–emotional screening should be considered when delays in these other domains are evident.
   D. **Importance of multiple informants.** Young children can behave very differently in different contexts or settings. Screeners that have forms for both parents and childcare/preschool teachers can offer important insight into similarities and dissimilarities in how children behave in the family/home context compared with that in the childcare setting.
   E. **Access to follow-up care.** A common barrier to screening is the limited capacity of the current mental health system to manage referrals for young children. Identifying and building referral relationships with agencies and service providers in the region to facilitate referrals is an important step to support the successful implementation of screening.

IV. **Choosing a screening tool.** Several screening tools that focus on social–emotional/ behavioral problems and are appropriate for use with young children, aged 0–5 years, are presented in Table 13-1. The screening tools presented in this table meet most or all of the following criteria:

Table 13-1. Social–emotional/behavioral problem screeners for early childhood

	Ages and Stages Questionnaires Social–Emotional (ASQ-SE) www.brookespublishing.com	BASC-2 Behavioral and Emotional Screening System (BASC-2 BESS) Preschool Form www.pearsonassessments.com	Brief Infant–Toddler Social & Emotional Assessment (BITSEA) www.pearsonassessments.com	Devereux Early Childhood Assessment (DECA) www.devereux.org	Devereux Early Childhood Assessment for Infants and Toddlers (DECA I/T) www.devereux.org	Eyberg Child Behavior Inventory (ECBI) Sutter-Eyberg Student Behavior Inventory-Revised (SESBI-R) http://www3.parinc.com
Age range	6–65 months	3–5 years	1–3 years	2–5 years	4 weeks to 3 years	2–16 years
Respondent Forms	Parent	Parent Childcare/teacher	Parent Childcare/teacher	Parent Childcare/teacher	Parent Childcare/teacher	Parent Childcare/teacher
Number of items	22–36 items	25–30 items	42 items	33–37 items	33–36 items	36–38 items
Completion time	10–15 minutes	5–10 minutes	7–10 minutes	10 minutes	5–10 minutes	5–10 minutes
Validity	Acceptable	Acceptable	Acceptable	Acceptable	Generally acceptable	Acceptable
Description of item content	Self-regulation Compliance Communication Adaptive Autonomy Affect Interaction with people Problem	Behavioral Emotional Adaptive skills	Internalizing Externalizing Dysregulation Competence Social relatedness Atypical	Problem behaviors Initiative Self-control Attachment	Initiative Attachment/ relationships Self-regulation	Behavior problems
Scores	Problem	Problem	Problem Competence	Total protective factors, behavioral concerns	Total protective factors	Total intensity score, total problem score

57

- Screening tool is in checklist format and is written at a sixth grade reading level (or lower);
- Parents can complete the screener independently in 10 minutes or less;
- Available in English and Spanish;
- Acceptable reliability and validity;
- Cut scores are based on large standardization samples.

It may be beneficial to follow at-risk screening results with a clinical interview or more lengthy measure. Several norm-referenced tools, which are appropriate for such second-stage screening with acceptable reliability and validity, are provided below:

- **Behavior Assessment Scale for Children (BASC-2 Preschool)** measures behavior problems and adaptive skills for children aged 2–5 years. (Available at: www.pearsonassessments.com)
- **Child Behavior Checklist (CBCL/1.5–5)** is a checklist which measures emotional and behavioral problems in children aged 1.5–5 years. (Available at www.ASEBA.org)
- **Devereux Early Childhood Assessment Clinical Form (DECA-C)** is a checklist measure appropriate for parents or other primary caregivers of children aged 2–5 years. (Available at http://www.devereux.org)
- **Infant–Toddler Social & Emotional Assessment (ITSEA)**, a checklist measure for profiling social-emotional/behavioral problems and competencies in 1- to 3-year-old children, is available at http://www.pearsonassessments.com.
- **Preschool and Kindergarten Behavior Scales (PKBS-2)**, a checklist measure of problem behaviors and social skills in 3- to 6-year-olds, is available at http://www.proedinc.com.
- **Social Skills Improvement System (SSIS)**, a checklist measure of social skills, behavior problems, and academic competence in children aged 3–18 years, is available at: www.pearsonassessments.com.

V. **Sociocultural issues.** Social–emotional/behavioral health screening is best implemented with an understanding of the sociocultural issues that play a role in the process. Culture-specific values and norms influence parents' expectations for child behavior including whether and when they expect particular behaviors or skills to emerge. Sociocultural factors also influence parents' intentions for raising their children and the opportunities and encouragement they provide. Unfortunately, most screeners (including those in Table 13-1) have not been normed within specific cultural groups. In addition, during the translation from one language to another some items may lose their intended meaning because population-specific behavioral and linguistic issues may be overlooked. Clinicians should therefore be mindful of sociocultural and linguistic issues when interpreting screening results.

BIBLIOGRAPHY

American Academy of Pediatrics. Committee on Psychosocial Aspects of Child and Family Health and Task Force on Mental Health. Policy statement—the future of pediatrics: mental health competencies for pediatric primary care. *Pediatrics* 124(1):410–421, 2009.

American Academy of Pediatrics . Committee on Children with Disabilities. Developmental surveillance and screening of infants and young children. *Pediatrics* 108(1):192–196, 2001.

Carter AS, Briggs-Gowan MJ, Davis NO. Assessment of young children's social-emotional development and psychopathology: recent advances and recommendations for practice. *J Child Psychol Psychiatry* 45(1):109–134, 2004.

Christensen M, Emde R, Fleming C. Cultural perspectives for assessing infants and young children. In Delcarmen-Wiggins R, Carter A (eds), *Handbook of Infant, Toddler and Preschool Mental Health Assessment.* New York, NY: Oxford University Press, 2004, pp. 7–23.

Web resources

The American Academy of Pediatrics (AAP). National Center for Medical Home Implementation Web site (http://www.medicalhomeinfo.org/index.html) has information related to surveillance and screening for providers (http://www.medicalhomeinfo.org/Screening/DevProvider.html) and families (http://www.medicalhomeinfo.org/Screening/DevFamily.html).

The Center for Disease Control Web site has a section on developmental screening for healthcare providers (http://www.cdc.gov/ncbddd/child/screen_provider.htm).

The Developmental-Behavioral Pediatrics division of the American Academy of Pediatrics Web site has a section dedicated to screening (http://dbpeds.org/screening/).

The Bright Futures Web site has information and resources about prevention, early detection and the Medical Home (http://brightfutures.aap.org/index.html).

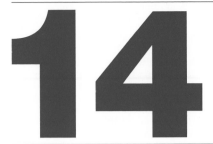

Behavioral Management: Theory and Practice

Edward R. Christophersen
Sarah S. Nyp

Traditional behavioral management techniques can be very useful to the primary care clinician. This chapter describes the concepts and techniques that parents can routinely use in interacting with their children.

I. Techniques to teach or improve behaviors.

A. Time-In and verbal praise.

1. *Time-In* refers to brief, nonverbal, physical contact provided to a child when a parent notices that the child is displaying appropriate or acceptable behavior. Examples include a pat on the back or a tussle of the hair. Time-In can be described to parents as a two-handed approach. One hand is on the child. The other hand is over the parent's mouth. This description illustrates to parents the importance of providing physical contact as an encouragement to the child to continue the current behavior. The nonverbal nature of the communication decreases the chances of distracting the child from the behavior. If a child is sitting quietly while working on puzzles with her sibling and her mother "interrupts" the appropriate play and interaction by providing a verbal comment, even verbal praise, the child is less likely to continue the activity. The physical contact of Time-In provides the child with knowledge that the behavior was noticed, without distracting the child from the acceptable activity. Parents should be encouraged and educated to provide their children with Time-In whenever their children are engaging in acceptable behavior. They should not wait for "good behavior."

2. *Verbal praise* is provided when a child has done something "good." The best time to use verbal praise is during natural breaks in an activity. For example, when a child is engaged in a coloring activity, the parent should provide lots of brief, nonverbal, physical contact (time-in). Once the child has finished coloring or stops coloring to show it to a parent, verbal praise is appropriate.

   Advantages. Time-in and verbal praise encourage children to continue to engage in acceptable behaviors. When applied correctly, these techniques take no additional parent time and do not distract children.

B. Incidental learning.

Children learn behaviors by being around individuals who engage in those behaviors. This is called *incidental learning*. For example, if both parents smoke cigarettes, their child is significantly more likely to become a smoker than if neither parent smokes. A surprising number and variety of children's behaviors appear to have been learned incidentally, including language, gestures, and anger management strategies.

Advantages and disadvantages. Incidental learning can be achieved without any additional effort on the part of the parents. They need only be aware that such learning occurs naturally and be cognizant of incidental learning during the time they spend with their children. The negative side is that children also learn behaviors the parents never intended for them to learn (e.g., swearing).

C. Modeling.

1. Two basic modeling techniques exist: live and video recordings. Most modeling procedures work best if the model is approximately the same age as the target child. For example, a 6-year-old boy who has previously had his teeth cleaned by a dentist and who behaved appropriately during the procedure could be observed live or on video recordings while being examined. A second child who observes the dental procedures being performed on this model can learn both what to expect of dental procedures and how to react to those procedures.

   Advantages and disadvantages. Children are more likely to believe what they see a peer doing than what their parents *tell* them, particularly if the two messages are contradictory (e.g., one a verbal message that the child should relax, and the other the anxiety that a child feels in the dental chair). However, modeling can teach maladaptive behaviors as well as adaptive behaviors. For example, if a child is observing a peer model in the dentist's office and the peer model becomes very upset, the target child will probably have a more difficult time when it is his turn for the procedure.

D. Reinforcement. No other topic in the behavioral literature has been more misunderstood than reinforcement. An item or activity can be said to have reinforcing properties for an individual child if and only if that child has previously worked to obtain access to that item or activity.

1. *Choosing rewards.* Under the right circumstances, reinforcement, by definition, will work with virtually any age group and with many different behaviors. However, no item or activity can be accurately described as a reinforcer unless and until it has produced a change in behavior. For example, although candy is reinforcing for the vast majority of children, it cannot be referred to as a reinforcer until it has been demonstrated that the child will either work to obtain the candy or stop a behavior that prevents him from receiving it.

   Principles of reinforcement, or the manner in which the reinforcer is made accessible to a child, are extremely important.

   a. **Small rewards offered frequently are better than large rewards offered infrequently.** A physical hug offered several times during a household chore will usually be more effective than a big reward at the end of the chore. Small rewards during the chore and a reward at the end will also work nicely.

   b. **Repetition, with feedback, enhances a child's learning.** A child will learn more from performing the same task repeatedly, with help from his parent, than from performing it once. Although parents will often expect their child to perform a task correctly the first time, the child will actually learn the task better if he has many opportunities to practice. For example, a child who helps one of his parents to do the laundry several times each week for 2 years will probably be able to do the laundry for the rest of his life.

   c. Making the choice to participate in acceptable behavior is a learning process. Children learn more quickly and retain the learning better if they are **relaxed while they are learning.** While helping children to acquire the skills to make appropriate choices can be very frustrating, the parent who becomes angry or impatient only exacerbates the situation. Similarly, an upset child does not learn as rapidly or as permanently as a calm child. Parents should be reminded that children learn a significant amount about what behaviors are "appropriate" by watching how their parents respond when presented with frustrating or otherwise challenging situations.

   d. **Warnings only make behavior worse.** Although parents have a natural tendency to warn their children, it is far more effective to discipline the child (provide a consequence) for not performing the task after the first time the request is ignored and then give the child another opportunity to fulfill the command, rather than frequent warnings that the tasks must be done. In fact, children who receive warnings prior to consequences, often learn that they may continue to disobey their parents several times before they will either be forced to complete the request or receive a consequence. This "planned ignoring" on the part of the child often becomes increasingly frustrating to the parent.

   e. **A behavior must already be learned before it can be reinforced.** If the child does not know how to perform the expected behavior, offering a reward, in lieu of teaching the child how to perform the behavior, is ineffective. For example, if a child has never tied his own shoes, offering him a new bicycle if he ties his shoes is not likely to be effective.

   Advantages and disadvantages. Reinforcing items and activities frequently can become part of normal, everyday life without substantial planning on the parents' part. Examples may include 10 minutes of one-on-one time playing catch with a parent or an extra story at bedtime. It should also be noted that reinforcing items and activities may sometimes be inadvertent. For example, when a parent waits until their child has been crying for several minutes in the morning, the parent may be reinforcing that child for crying. If the same parent had picked their child up BEFORE he started crying, however, he would be reinforcing the child for playing quietly in his crib instead of waiting until he was crying.

   In addition, the child's behavior may return to its prereinforcement level as soon as the reinforcers are no longer available. For example, in research on the use of reinforcers for automobile seat belt use, many children stopped wearing their seat belts as soon as the reinforcers were no longer available. Procedures that have been shown to be successful in maintaining desired behaviors after reinforcement ceases include gradually making the reinforcer available less often (e.g., on the average, every second behavior is reinforced, then every third behavior, then every fourth behavior). Once a behavior becomes habitual, the individual will engage in it whether it is reinforced or not.

E. Conditioned reinforcers. Many items and activities that have no intrinsic reinforcing properties can take on reinforcing properties. Money, for example, is not usually a reinforcer to a small child. When the child learns what he can purchase with money, it begins to take on reinforcing properties. As another example, to a distressed child in the middle of the night, even the sound of the bedroom door opening can take on reinforcing properties, as the child associates the sound of the door opening with receiving attention from a caregiver.

Advantages. Conditioned reinforcers are usually more readily available than the actual reinforcer, and most children will work just as hard for a conditioned reinforcer as they will for the actual one. Conditioned reinforcers, such as money, also have the advantage that they can be traded for a wide variety of items or activities as the child's tastes and preferences change.

F. The token economy. Conditioned reinforcers work best if there is a consistent method of exchange. In the case of money, the exchange system is already in place, and the money becomes a "token" of what can be purchased. Entire "token economies" have been devised as treatment programs for children from age 4 years to adulthood. The term token economy refers to the organized manner in which tokens are gained and lost, as well as what can be purchased with them. The success or failure of a token economy depends almost entirely on how it is implemented and on how many reinforcing activities are realistically available to the individual who must earn, lose, and spend tokens. The mere use of tokens does not make a token economy.

Token economies are most effective when they are used as motivational systems to encourage children to engage in socially appropriate behaviors. Three different types of token economies are widely used with common behavioral problems:

1. A **simple exchange system** provides a means of keeping track of the child's appropriate and inappropriate behaviors. A list of behaviors can be posted on the door of the refrigerator. As the child completes assigned or volunteered tasks or chores, he marks these on the "positive side" of the exchange chart. Similarly, as the child engages in inappropriate behaviors, he marks these on the "negative side." When the child wants a special privilege or activity, there must be more positive marks than negative marks to "afford" the special privilege. The simple exchange system is appropriate for children aged 5–12 years.

2. Under **chip systems,** the child earns a token, such as a poker chip, for positive behaviors. Each time poker chips are earned, the parent acknowledges the child's appropriate behavior while offering chips. The child is then expected to take the chips from the parent's hand, look the parent in the eye, and say, "thank you." In this way, the child not only receives the tokens for the appropriate behavior, but also practices appropriate social behaviors. Similarly, when the child engages in a behavior that loses chips, he is expected to hand the chips to the parent politely and may receive one chip back for "taking the fine so nicely." The chip system is useful for children aged 3–7 years.

3. The **point system** is similar to the chip system but can be much more sophisticated. Points can be used to motivate children and teenagers to practice the behaviors they are lacking, such as taking feedback well and sharing their feelings appropriately. Each time they engage in these types of behaviors, they earn points that can be used to purchase items and activities they want. The point system is useful for children aged 6–16 years.

G. Fading. Fading refers to changing something gradually instead of abruptly changing it. For example

- For a toddler who is drinking too much juice, a cup can be provided with juice, which is gradually diluted from 100% juice to 90% juice:10% water, then 80% juice:20% water, and so on, until the toddler is drinking pure water from the cup.
- Raising training wheels on a bicycle 1/8 in. every 2 weeks until they are about 3 inches off the ground and no longer necessary.
- Changing a child's bedtime 15 minutes each night at daylight savings time instead of abruptly changing it the entire hour in one night.
- Teaching a child how to swallow pills by starting out with very small cake sprinkles to wash down with a favorite beverage, then moving to slightly larger pieces of candy. Typically using six to eight steps (sizes) is very effective.

Advantages and disadvantages. Fading often helps to avoid confrontations with a child. It can be used to accomplish something without incident that otherwise may have been difficult to accomplish. The disadvantage of fading is that parents have to spend more time than they would if their child could abruptly make the desired changes.

II. **Procedures to decrease or discourage behaviors.**

A. **Time-Out.** Probably the most frequently recommended disciplinary technique is time-out. As initially used, time-out was actually referred to as "time-out from positive reinforcement." Over the past three decades or so the term has been shortened to "time-out," and, in doing so, the idea of removing a pleasant interaction has been ignored or forgotten. Time-in and time-out are effective from the age below 1 year to early adolescence. **It is very important for parents to realize that in absence of good "time-in," there really is no such thing as "time-out."** There is often confusion regarding how long a time-out should last. This question can be answered by discussing with parents the purpose of time-out. The purpose is two-fold. The first is to stop the undesired behavior (noncompliance, tantrum, etc.). The second is to encourage the development of self-quieting (calming) skills. Once a child is able to sit silently with quiet hands and feet, the child has accomplished both of these goals.

The following variables have the most impact on the effectiveness of time-out:
- It must be presented immediately after an inappropriate behavior.
- It must be presented every time the inappropriate behavior occurs.
- The time-out must remove or make unavailable an otherwise pleasant state of affairs (i.e., time-in), in most cases ALL interaction with the parent must cease.
- The time-out should not be considered "over" or "finished" until the child has quieted down.
- All warnings about using time-out should be carried out.
- The child should be completely ignored during the time-out, regardless of how outrageous the behavior might become. One study demonstrated that time-out becomes more effective when the time-in is "enriched" (more fun, more enjoyable) and becomes less effective when the time-in is "impoverished."

Advantages. Time-in and time-out provide parents with an effective alternative to nagging, yelling, or spanking. Their consistent use also encourages children to develop self-quieting skills (a child's ability to calm himself without the assistance of a parent). It encourages these skills because the parents are modeling the ability to cope with an unpleasant situation and because the child is learning how to cope with feelings he experiences when he does not like something his parents have done.

B. **Extinction.** Extinction is defined as the withdrawal of all attention after a child engages in undesirable behaviors. One of the most common example of extinction is not paying attention to a child's whining. When used properly, extinction involves completely ignoring a child's whining.

A major problem with using extinction is an initial sharp increase in the child's inappropriate behavior, called an *extinction burst*. For example, when a child is ignored during a temper tantrum or when whining, these behaviors usually increase in intensity and duration at first, perhaps discouraging the parents from continuing the extinction procedure. If the parents continue with the extinction procedure, however, the change in the child's behavior will usually be forthcoming.

Although extinction procedures are often successful, parents may not be able to tolerate the technique. Several modifications have been made to make extinction techniques more acceptable to parents. For example, the "day correction of bedtime problems technique" involves teaching the parents to use extinction for whining and fussing during the day. The parents then gain confidence in their ability to use it properly, and the child learns that the parents will follow through with the use of extinction once they start it. Only after the parents and the child are familiar with the use of extinction during the day are the parents encouraged to use it at bedtime. The day correction technique is actually more effective than using extinction only at bedtime.

Advantages and disadvantages. Extinction procedures have been effective with many different childhood problems. The time necessary to educate parents on the use of these procedures is reasonable, given the constraints of primary care practices. The main disadvantage is the extinction burst and the parents' inability to tolerate their child's initial distress at being ignored.

C. **Planned ignoring.** The parents gradually ignore their child's behavior for longer and longer periods of time (as opposed to introducing complete extinction abruptly). Planned ignoring may result in less of an extinction burst, but it takes longer to be effective. Probably the most common use of planned ignoring is for bedtime resistance.

D. **Spanking.** With spanking, caregivers can vent their own frustration at the same time they are discouraging a child from engaging in the behavior that resulted in the spanking. In addition, spanking will often produce an immediate decrease in the child's behavior.

Advantages and disadvantages. Spanking can teach a child that hitting is an acceptable way to express frustration or anger. The child, after being spanked, is likely to avoid or try to escape from the caregiver who administered the spanking. To maintain its effect, the magnitude of spanking often must increase over time (harder spanking). This may lead to injury or abuse. Spanking can also result in other discipline methods losing their effectiveness. Thus, a child who is frequently spanked at home is less likely to be responsive to the use of extinction at daycare. Since time-in and time-out can produce virtually the same effects as spanking but without the side effects, spanking should not be recommended for parents.

E. **Job grounding.** This is a form of grounding whereby the child has control over how long the grounding is in effect. When a child has broken a major rule (e.g., gone to a shopping center by bike without telling parents), he is "grounded." The child loses all privileges (including television, telephone, having a friend over, playing with games, snacks and desserts) until he has completed one job properly. The jobs, which can each be written on a 3″ × 5″ card, should be agreed upon by both parent and child during a quiet, peaceful time, should not be one of the child's typical household chores, and should take 5–10 minutes to complete (washing the windows of the family car, picking up pet waste from the yard). The child, upon being grounded, is asked to pick from a stack of cards that are held face down by the parent. Once the job is chosen, the child is restricted from all activities, with the exception of family meals and homework, until the job is completed. The parents are instructed to refrain from nagging, prodding, and reminding. As soon as the child has completed the job (most jobs should take only 5–10 minutes to complete and be tasks that the child has done many times before), he is "off grounding." Job grounding differs from traditional time-based grounding in that the child determines how long the grounding lasts and, under most circumstances, the child has the option of getting the job done without missing valued social activities.

Advantages and disadvantages. Job grounding is usually effective, it lets the child practice a job that he probably did not want to do in the first place, and it gives him the opportunity to avoid losing a valued activity. The disadvantage is that if the child has no planned activities, he may stall on completing the job until some external motivation is present.

F. **Habit reversal.** Habit-reversal procedures were developed for use with habit disorders and motor or vocal tics. Habit-reversal training requires a level of cognition not reached before a mental age of about 4–5 years.
  1. Components of habit reversal are the following:
     - Increase your child's awareness of the habit on a daily basis.
     - Keeping track of how often the habit occurs is the only way that the parent and child can tell when progress is being made.
     - On a daily basis, the child should look into a mirror while performing the habit on purpose.
     - Parents help the child to become aware of how his body moves and what muscles are being used when he performs the habit.
     - The child identifies each time he engages in the habit by either raising his hand when the habit occurs, or by stating something like, "that was one," when the habit occurs.
     - If parents see the habit occur but the child does not appear to be aware that it occurred, parents use a prearranged signal, gesture, or expression to help make the child aware.
     - Self-monitoring: The child can record each occurrence of the habit on a 3 × 5 card.
     - Competing response should be practiced daily.
     - Have the child practice his competing response in the mirror. This helps the child become comfortable with the response and assures him that the competing response is not noticeable socially. For example, a child who is blinking his eyes excessively can practice blinking his eyes very gently and the child who is pulling his hair can practice holding his thumbs on the waist of his pants.
     - The child is encouraged to use the competing response when he feels the urge to engage in the habit or in situations where the child has a history of engaging in the habit.
     - The child is encouraged to use the competing response for 1 minute following the occurrence of the habit.
     - Stress anxiety reduction procedures (all should be practiced daily).
       - Progressive muscle relaxation training
       - Visual imagery
       - Breathing exercises

2. Parent Involvement
- **Feedback.** Parents work with the child to increase awareness of his habit by helping him identify the habit when it occurs.
- **Support and encouragement.** Parents encourage their child to use the competing response and praise the child for doing so. Parents also praise any noted decrease in rates of the habits.

Although many children and adolescents will notice a decrease in their habit within a couple of days, the greatest change from using these habit-reversal procedures occurs during the second and third month.

Advantages and disadvantages. Habit-reversal training is effective and has no physical side effects. The overall reduction in habit disorders and tics is also far greater with this technique than with medication. The disadvantage is the time it takes to teach and monitor, as well as the time it takes to reduce the habit disorder (usually days).

G. Positive practice is the procedure of having a child practice an appropriate behavior after each inappropriate behavior. For example, when a previously toilet trained child wets his pants, he is required to practice "going to the bathroom" 10 times; five times from the place where the accident was discovered and five times from such alternative sites as the front yard, the backyard, the kitchen, and the bedroom. When used correctly, with no nagging or unpleasant behavior on the part of the caregivers, positive practice can produce dramatic results.

Advantages and disadvantages. Positive practice gives a child many opportunities to practice appropriate behaviors. This technique is typically effective quickly. The disadvantages include the length of time necessary to implement the practice, as well as the fact that the practice should be done immediately after the inappropriate behavior, which is not always convenient.

H. Practice, Praise, Point Out, and Prompt. Several of these procedures can be combined into a very effective teaching tool. For example, when a child's interruption is a problem, they can be taught an alternative to interrupting. Encourage the parents to practice having their child gently place her hand on the parent's forearm, and the parent immediately place his or her hand on the child's hand and ask her what they would like to say. This should be practiced daily with a reward for practicing. The parents should "point out" to their child when the parents wait instead of interrupting, or when a character in a book is seen to be waiting. The parents can also "prompt" their child to place her hand, for example, on Daddy's arm when she wants to get his attention. This strategy combines incidental learning, modeling, reinforcement, and praise.

III. General remarks and conclusions.
- Although the term "behavior management" frequently has been used to refer to coercive action taken in an effort to discourage a child from engaging in inappropriate behavior, many positive alternatives are available. Generally, the emphasis should be on teaching children appropriate behaviors, rather than concentrating on reducing inappropriate behaviors.
- The single most important consideration in implementing such behavior management strategies is taking a history that can help to identify precisely what strategy should be offered to the caregiver and how to offer that strategy. The clinician now has a variety of evidence-based behavior management strategies available for dealing with situations encountered in the provision of care to typically developing children with minor behavior problems.
- As with many of the "medical interventions" offered to parents from the clinician, the use of written handouts summarizing the treatment recommendations can be very helpful to the parent who is trying to follow the clinician's recommendations.

BIBLIOGRAPHY

For parents

Christophersen ER. *Little People: Guidelines for Commonsense Child Rearing* (4th ed), Shawnee Mission, KS: Overland Press, 1998.
Christophersen ER, Mortweet SL. *Parenting that Works: Building Skills that Last a Lifetime.* Washington, DC: American Psychological Association, 2003.
Schmitt BD. *Your Child's Health* (2nd ed), New York: Bantam Books, 1991.

Web sites

http://www.patienteducation.com/
http://www.disciplinehelp.com/

For professionals

Christophersen ER. *Pediatric Compliance: A Guide for the Primary Care Physician.* New York: Plenum, 1994.

Christophersen ER, Mortweet SL. *Treatments that Work with Children: Empirically Supported Strategies for Managing Childhood Problems.* Washington, DC: American Psychological Association, 2001.

Mortweet SL, Christophersen ER. Coping skills for the angry/impatient/clamorous child: a home and office practicum. *Contemp Pediatr* 21(6):43–55, 2004.

Schmitt BD (ed). *Pediatric Advisor.* Englewood, CO: Clinical Reference Systems. Computer software, 2003.

Schriver MD, Allen KD. *Working with Parents of Noncompliant Children: A Guide to Evidence-Based Parent Training for Practitioners and Students.* Washington, DC: American Psychological Association, 2008. http://www.aap.org/ConnectedKids/.

15

Coping with Stressful Life Events/Transitions

Maria Trozzi
Richard D. Goldstein

I. **Description of the problem.** Families facing transition and major life events ranging from disclosure by a parent of major illness or divorce, to the death of a loved one including a pet, to moving. Telling a child that her sibling has Down syndrome or a major disability can be an event recalled through a lifetime. At its root, change is hard. Multiple changes challenge the best of families. Oftentimes, the change impacts both the parents and the child. The parent's capacity to face the stressor, model good coping skills, and provide anticipatory guidance for his/her child is critical to the child's adjustment. As important, each successful adjustment is a positive predictor of the child's next adjustment.

II. **Factors that influence successful adaptation**
   A. **Child/family history of stressors.** The platform from which a family adjusts to an acute stressor may be rocky or smooth. The family challenged historically with multiple, or ongoing, or chronic stressors such as poverty, domestic violence, or addictions, faces a more difficult adjustment to a new, acute stressor. For the child who has faced multiple losses, changes, and disruptions in her caregivers, any new stressor can be magnified.
   B. **Temperament.** The child's temperament is a factor in how she/he faces a stressor. In fact, the child's temperament sometimes influences whether an event is interpreted as stressful. For the shy, slowly adapting 3-year-old child, a birthday party in a bowling alley may challenge all his coping skills and may overwhelm him. For a child whose temperament is easy going, and/or whose history includes visits to a bowling alley with older siblings, this birthday party is joyfully anticipated and presents challenges easily faced.
   C. **Developmental age/regrieving.** The lens with which a child understands the stressor or anticipated transition is informed by his developmental stage. That is, his cognitive capacity will change as he develops and the *meaning* he gives to the stressor will significantly change. His developmentally based awkward/confusing understanding will determine his experience and ability to adjust successfully.

   For example, the 6-year-old child facing the birth of his first sibling will understand the event differently than a 2-year-old. Competitiveness for the caregiver's attention, meaning given to the new family constellation, meaning of the very definition of family, and the effect this birth has on his daily routine both inside and outside his home are all considerations for older siblings. However, the 2-year-old's capacity to understand a new sibling's appearance in his family, his ability to express feelings meaningfully, not just rotely, as well as his experiencing of this newest family member differ significantly from an older child.

   For many children, this stressor is considered "normative"; that is, most children face the birth of a sibling and are able to successfully adapt to the challenges inherent to "sharing" the primary caregiver. On the other hand, the death of a parent, divorce, and the diagnosis of a sibling with a significant special need are considered "nonnormative" stressors. These or any stressors that can be construed as a loss will be revisited by the child at each new developmental stage and will be regrieved.

   For instance, the 4-year-old child, whose 2-year-old brother is diagnosed with autism, has a very limited understanding of the impact of this stressor. She can observe and experience stress and grief as it manifests itself within the family unit; she can accompany her brother to therapies and even engage in them herself as his "helper"; she can react to his behavioral differences. As this older sister grows, she will make *new meaning* of her brother's disability, and how it affects her. At 9 or 10 years of age, it would be normal for her to feel embarrassed by his behaviors at times when she has friends visit at home. For this reason, she may avoid bringing friends home. As a senior in high school, she may feel guilt and relief as she leaves the family home to become a college student. At each stage of her development, she will regrieve this loss as it affects her and her family.

   D. **Culture.** Socioeconomic, ethnic, religious, and cultural differences matter when assessing the impact on what constitutes a stressor or the presumed magnitude on a child's adjustment. A family's religious beliefs and ideology are often the protective factors that affect the stressor's impact on the parent and the child.

Also, as the child faces the stressor, the contextual meaning is affected by the "normalization" of the stressor; the absence or prevalence of the "event" should be regarded within this cultural context to assess the magnitude of the stressor as it impacts the child. For 3–8-year-olds in Africa, going to a funeral is normative but not for most children acculturated in the United States. Getting braces or birth control at 16 years may be viewed more as a "right of passage" for some adolescents than a stressor. On the other hand, adjusting to an extended family member's move into a child's bedroom for the foreseeable future, facing a parent's arrest and anticipating his prison term, and losing one's home due to financial hardship are even more stressful if the child also has to face the additional stress of feeling isolated from other children's experiences.

III. General principles of management

A. Parents need to face it first. No matter what the stressor on the family, the parents need to face it first. A parent's capacity to face the stressor and demonstrate equipoise has a significant impact on the outcome of the child's adjustment. Crisis theory reminds us that re-establishing equilibrium after the onset of a stressor is primarily dependent on how well the adult models appropriate coping skills.

For example, in the immediate aftermath of Hurricane Katrina, millions of television viewers watched families being temporarily sheltered in New Orleans Superdome. In many cases, parents and family members lay on cots as children played near them. Each adult caregiver's emotional capacity to face her tragic and painful circumstances and to demonstrate parental competence, emotional safety, and guidance were critical to her child's emotional adjustment to this significant stressor.

B. Scaffold; do not overprotect. No parent wants her children to suffer ever. All parents want to protect their child from harm, pain, and grief. It is counterintuitive to allow children to confront the stressor head on. Parents need to "buffer" children by titrating amounts of stress so the child can develop new coping skills to master this new stressor and not become overwhelmed.

In fact, when a child feels sad or mad, which is often the case when she faces a transition, anticipating and allowing for those normal feelings is useful. A child experiencing separation brings up feelings of helplessness, grief, sadness, and confusion in parents as they watch their child struggle with dependence and autonomy. Understanding that the coping skills the child accrues in the process of separating, the pride when she feels successful, and the permission to experience a full range of appropriate feelings set a stage for future successes during transitions to a new classroom, a new school, etc.

Shielding the child from difficult information like a grandparent's life-threatening illness and hospitalization, and continuing on as though nothing were amiss, may feel protective but of course, the child feels the stress in the household and often the isolation from being outside this family emergency. In many situations, he worries that the situation is even worse than it is since no one talks about it.

As the child struggles to understand changes in people's routines, new feelings, new experiences, and overt manifestations of stress at home, he needs to be reassured that his parents can continue to care for him, that he is safe, and that these worries are temporary. In the face of a new or difficult experience, pediatric clinicians should use their guidance on the following principles:

- Name it; name that which the child witnesses or experiences.
- Use language that is developmentally appropriate.
- Check in with the child to assess his meaning.
- Clarify as the situation changes.
- Give permission to the child to ask questions.
- Provide reassurance.

Children benefit from the important adults in their life to assure them that they are capable. "I know you'll be okay." "You'll do a great job." "I wouldn't ask you to face something that I didn't think you could." "We'll face this together. I'm always here to help." These reassuring statements boost the child's confidence to face the unknown territory ahead. *Tell* them do not *ask* them because they will deny it.

C. Stress the importance of continuing and reinforcing routines. The predictability of routines such as mealtimes, bedtimes, pacing of the day, etc. creates a safety net for children when they are facing normative changes and difficult stressors. This is not the time for well-meaning helpfulness such as long evenings out, missed bedtimes, introducing new foods, new routines, and unnecessary changes. Less is more.

D. Advise parents to check in with the child. It is important not to pathologize the child's response to a stressor or transition. In many cases, the child's emotional response is a *normal one when facing an abnormal event.* What is important is to check in with your child. In a private moment, simply ask her how she is doing: "I want to check in with you about how you're doing with the divorce.... with grandpa living with us.... with your sister leaving for college?" This is not a time for fixing it; it is a time for listening and acknowledging the feelings. It is important to not trivialize the child's experience of the event, or her feelings. If the child says, "I'm OK" parents should acknowledge his being "okay" for now and might use a strategy called the "third person plural" to normalize some feelings that the child may have; e.g., "Some kids of your age would worry about .... ." or "Often, kids fight with their older siblings right before they leave for college because it's easier to leave 'mad' than 'sad'. What do you think?"

E. **Help identify ways the child shows stress.** Look to the child's historical response to stress. Sleeping and eating disturbances, temporary regressive behaviors, such as thumb sucking or bedwetting, and tantrums are typical in younger children. Moodiness, more sibling fighting, and irritability are more common in older children.

Parents should be aware that some older children might try to protect the parent(s) they deem vulnerable. Look for signs of their demonstrating hypermaturity and adultified behaviors (being the "good" one, more responsible, more mature, the peacemaker). There can be far reaching sequelae when parents unintentionally promote their child's self-esteem in this way. This is particularly true for children whose parents are mentally ill, facing addictions, and parenting a child with severe special needs.

IV. **Specific management for stressful situations.** A few common stressful situations are named below with some brief guidelines for pediatric clinicians to ask parents to consider.

A. **When a grandparent is very sick.** The following guidelines will help parents navigate through this difficult time and create an opportunity to promote their child's mastery of copying skills. Specifically, it is important to

1. **Describe in simple terms the declining health of a grandparent.** Every visible change or alteration in arrangements requires a clear, simple explanation.

2. **Prepare the child for visits to the hospitalized grandparent.** Children, even very young children, can benefit from visiting their grandparents in the hospital *if* they are prepared for what they will see, hear, and experience.

3. **Find other teachable moments from the children's friends or neighbors' experiences.** This helps to normalize this inevitable teachable moment. Point out how the families return to normal routines after a grandparent's death.

4. **Prepare the child for his grandparent's imminent death.** Although it seems counterintuitive, the best way to protect your child's emotional health is by sharing information with him that will affect him.

5. **Tell the child in clear terms what death means.** For example "When Nana dies, her body will stop working completely, for always." Avoid euphemisms that can confuse; for example, "We lost Nana," or "Nana passed."

6. **Encourage them to find ways for the child to help as a grandparent's health declines or is hospitalized.** This is critical. Even very young children like to be involved in helping. It makes them feel an important part of the caring and giving process.

7. **Discuss with parents how they can model their own authentic grief to your children.** Children learn from observing the important adults in their life during these difficult times. It is fine to express emotions in front of your child as long as there is an explanation of the feeling; sad or angry or exhausted and the assurance that the parent is still available to care for the child.

8. **Encourage the parent to look for cues that the child is affected by the illness or death of his grandparent.** The child is watching and listening and learning from them when they are talking on the phone or to others at the hospital. The information he overhears can be confusing, frightening, or overwhelming.

9. **Be careful not to overload the child with information.** Children will let you know what they need to know, how much, and when if you listen to them.

10. **Parents do not need to be perfect.** They are being called upon to be a son or daughter, a sibling, a caregiver, and a parent all at once in the most stressful of life's events.

B. **Welcoming a new sibling.** If a spouse were to ask his partner to enthusiastically welcome a second permanent partner into the marriage, one quickly understands the feelings stirred up when a parent expects her first -born child to welcome a new baby sibling! Adaptation is a process that is repeated with each new major developmental milestone.

1. **Advise parents to be prepared for ambivalence.** Both parents and children may have ambivalent feelings when considering the new baby. Making emotional room

for the new routines; initial exhaustion; and displaced feelings of guilt, jealousy, and abandonment can be challenging, particularly if parents are not prepared for them.

2. **Advise parents to find special alone time.** Making a "special alone" time weekly for each of the older children when they are coping with the additional new sibling is worth the energy. It need not be a large quantity of time but just between parent and child, if possible, away from the new baby. Talking about the anticipated special time is part of the solution.

C. **Transitions to childcare/school/college.** Each transition from the initial family unit to daycare, kindergarten, middle school, high school, and college enlarges the child's sphere of influence, the parents' impact on the child's development, and is often positively anticipated for the excitement inherent in each transition.

   1. **Normalize feelings of grief for the parent at each transition.** Although these transitions are inherent to a child's development, they represent a loss of control (Who can ever care for her the way I do? Will she know me when I return at the end of the day?)

   2. **The parent needs to prepare himself/herself first for the feelings that are a normal part of facing "the unknown".** With each successful transition, the child (and the parent) builds a sense of mastery coping with and managing fears about the unknown. Recognizing that separation and adaptation are processes that are accomplished incrementally is essential. Baby steps.

D. **Being a typical sibling.** As adults, many typical siblings of children with disabilities will confess to ambivalent feelings toward their parents and the affected sibling at different periods of their childhood.

   Remind the parent that the child is often expressing normal feelings to abnormal situations. Frequent hospitalizations of the affected sibling, special caregivers entering and exiting their household, different expectations of the typical sibling, and periods of embarrassment are but a few of the situations that can exacerbate feelings, whether they express them or not, of frustration, jealousy, guilt, and loneliness in the typical sibling.

   The parent also may have his/her own feelings of guilt about not having time or emotional energy for the typical child in the family, and expecting too much from them during times of acute stress. Whenever possible, finding regular time with the typical child without their sibling benefits both the child and the parent.

E. **Financial hardships.** Teaching children about money, its value, and its management is a developmental process that is often overlooked within the family. From the time children are as young as 3 years, and at each subsequent developmental stage, understanding money, its power, and meaning within the family and the community is valuable as one tool for decision making.

   Regardless of the family's socioeconomic status, the family may be forced to face financial hardships that affect the child. Although no one would ever invite this stressor, there are hidden *opportunities* for the child. When facing a financial hardship, encourage parents to consider the following tasks:

   1. Reassure the child that although financial changes may impact the family on some levels, they, the parents, are in charge and will always keep the family safe.

   2. Be concrete about the changes that are to happen; telling a child that, "we have to tighten our belts," do not explain to the child what will be the same and what will be different.

   3. Projecting blame on a family member for the financial hardship should be avoided. Many preadolescents and adolescents benefit from frank discussions about why a family vacation has to be "down-sized" or why a new pair of jeans or the latest cell phone is not possible at this time. This may lead them to consider ways in which they can contribute the family's well being, by babysitting or doing lawn work. Losing a home, moving in with relatives, or becoming homeless, even temporarily, challenges the best coping skills in families. Parents should be reminded of the child's critical need to feel safe. The parent's very presence, especially emotional availability, can create a safe haven for a child when his familiar home is no longer his.

BIBLIOGRAPHY

Levetown M. Communicating with children and families: from everyday interactions to skill in conveying distressing information. *Pediatrics* 121:e1441–e1460, 2008.

Masten A, Best K, Garmezy N. *Resilience and Development: Contributions from the Study of Children Who Overcome Adversity*. University of Minnesota.

Shonkoff JP, Jarman FC, Kohlenberg TM. Family transitions, crises, and adaptations. *Curr Probl Pediatr* 17(9):507–553, 1987.

For parents

Trozzi M, Massimini K. *Talking with Children about Loss*. New York: Putnam-Penguin, 1999.
Youngs BB. *Stress and Your Child: Helping Kids Cope with the Strains and Pressures of Life*. New York: Fawcett Columbine, 1995.

Web sites

www. childcareaware.org/dailyparent.
www.zerotothree.org.
Center on the Social and Emotional Foundations for Early Learning. www.csefel.uiuc.edu/.
www.naeyc.org.
www.cyfernet.org.
www.siblingsupport.org.

16

Managing Behavior in Primary Care

Barbara Howard

I. **Description of the problem.** Behavioral and emotional issues comprise an estimated 25%–50% of all pediatric problems raised by parents. Pediatric primary care clinicians are in an ideal position to deal with such concerns: they are well known to the family, generally respected, viewed as supportive by both parent and child, and already know much about the child and the family. In addition, the office setting is seen as friendly, nonstigmatizing territory.

II. **Identifying problems.**

A. **Open-ended questions.** The first requirement for addressing behavioral problems is their identification. This is not always easy because children rarely ask for help and the parents may not realize that the clinician has either the interest or the expertise to help. Discussing behavior and development at each visit, using screening questionnaires, and educating oneself to have practical advice will all encourage parents to discuss psychosocial concerns. Open-ended questions (ones that cannot be answered by one word), such as "How are things going?" allow the parent and child to express their own agenda for the visit. For children aged 3 years and older, an interview of the child first can convey their centrality to the visit and elicits their point of view before they have heard (and potentially clammed up from) parental complaints. In other families, the clinician may need to ask specifically about *behavior at home, at school, or in day care.* Another approach that broadens the agenda is to ask routinely, "What is the hardest part of taking care of an X-month-old?"

B. **Observations in the office.** Observations of behavior in the office and waiting room can be revealing. Toys in the examination room are an invaluable way to observe the child's behavior and development (as well as to enhance the enjoyment of the visit). These observations can then be used to start the discussion (e.g., "I noticed that he is very active. How is that for you at home?"). Such comments should be asked in a nonjudgmental way so that the parents' response can reveal if they view the behavior as problematic. The clinician's own feelings and intuitions about the child and family should be compared with parental and child reports and used to raise questions or to formulate clinical hypotheses about the child's behavior. Asking the child to draw a person and relate a story about that boy or girl or a Family Kinetic Drawing ("Everyone in your family doing something.") can be very informative about the child's perceptions as well as about their cognitive and fine motor skills.

C. **Screening questionnaires.** Questionnaires can be a valuable time saver and tool for identifying behavioral problems and adding to office documentation. Validated screening tools are now recommended as standard care as informal methods have low sensitivity (see Chapter 12).

D. **Collecting additional information.** The next task is to collect additional information by questions, observations, direct physical examination or testing, and usually requesting information from other sources such as notes from childcare or school report cards (see Chapter 67). Depending on the acuity of the problem and time available, this may be deferred to a scheduled follow-up visit.

III. **Managing behavioral problems.**

A. **Defining the problem and setting goals.** The first step to successful problem resolution occurs during the initial discussion in defining the problem. After initial open-ended questions, it is crucial to elicit details about the onset and attempted solutions, as well as times when the problem was not present to look for relevant causal factors. A survey of the areas of daily functioning (including bedtime, meals, toileting, peer interaction, separation abilities, family relationships, and school adjustment) is all needed to detect patterns that suggest areas of weakness or dysfunctional management.

It is important for the clinician to summarize the parent's (or his or her own if the parent has none) concerns to demonstrate that their worries have been heard. The clinician should formulate and explain his or her clinical hypotheses about the underlying child, family, and environmental factors contributing to the child's behavior. The problem should be discussed nonjudgmentally and reframed in a positive light and in terms of new specific desired behaviors rather than the ending of a behavior (e.g., "You would like him to listen to instructions [rather than to not act up]").

The initial discussion should set the stage for treatment by clarifying the problem, setting a positive tone, engaging other family members by determining how it affects them, and not blaming or insulting the child (who may be listening).

The next step is to convey some *hope and confidence* that a solution is possible and *collaboratively design an initial plan* or "homework" that addresses relevant goals for behavior change. It is important to guide family members in selecting homework tasks that apply to the family dynamic that seems causative, include tasks for each family member that are doable and measurable, and are of a scope that is not overwhelming but also not trivial. Additional diagnostic information comes from seeing how the family acted on this advice when they come for a follow-up.

B. **Levels of intervention in primary care.** There are different levels of behavior management suitable for different practitioners depending on their amount of interest, skill, time available for this work, and acceptability as advisors to the family.

1. **Education.** The simplest level of behavioral intervention is caregiver's education. This usually entails informing the family about what the behavior may mean to the child, what behavior is normal for age, how temperament may be involved, and how behaviors may be reinforced, for example, by attention. This level of intervention should also include teaching families how to set up the environment to reduce the child's frustration and stress and how the caregivers should model how to manage emotions themselves, for example, through self control, verbalizing feelings, or walking away.

2. **Advice.** The second level of intervention involves all of the above plus giving specific advice for the problem behavior. Obtaining details about a specific incident's antecedents (what happened before the problem behavior, the behavior itself (what the child did), and the consequences (both feelings and actions for the child and the parent)) is essential and will generally reveal patterns of family interaction. Often children act up at times when they are being asked to make a transition to a new activity or other repeated situations such as the morning rush. In other cases, the meaning of the behavior is revealed such as opposition sparking when parents argue. Clarifying these patterns may be all that is needed for a family to solve the problem for themselves. Further coaching may be needed on how to anticipate these scenarios and how to verbalize about, praise, and give marks or points for even small improvements in emotion control or flexibility.

3. **Dealing with underlying issues.** Higher-level interventions involve dealing with underlying issues in the child, adult, family interaction, or the environment. To successfully work on this level, the clinician needs to understand and make hypotheses based on a transactional model that takes into account mutual influences among these factors.

   a. **Child issues.** Child issues that result in frustration such as functional weaknesses in motor skills, language, emotional regulation, or attentional control may need further evaluation. Treatment for weaknesses can be advised including such things as special education support, adopting bypass strategies, therapy for strengthening skills, reducing demands, and medication.

   The behavior itself or the situations eliciting the problem may have meaning to the child that must be addressed directly or symbolically. Clinicians may efficiently hypothesize these meanings on the basis of an understanding of developmental stages and commonly associated family issues, for example, sibling jealousy that emerges when infants begin to crawl and get into the other's toys. Other ways of determining the meaning of a behavior include asking directly, "What does it make you think when he does that?" or telling the child or family "Any kid who ... (e.g., wonders if a divorce is his fault might act up to see if his parents still care)" while watching the person's emotions. Sometimes the meaning can be inferred from a reaction to "homework" that addresses the issue, for example, infantilizing activities during special time for the child who seems to act up due to seeking more nurturance.

   There are common patterns of family dynamics associated with child behavior problems at different ages. For example, young children may be out of control when a laissez-faire style has resulted from a reaction against a parent's own history of being punished harshly as a child. Sleeping problems in a child may result when there is marital discord causing ambivalence about the parents sleeping together.

Biting may occur when parents cannot agree on whether or not to use corporal punishment. School underachievement may occur when a sibling is glorified for academics. Promiscuity may signal incest or sexual abuse. Substance abuse may result from depression. After gathering data for a hypothesis about meaning the clinician shares this with the child and/or family and works both to help the family members clarify and communicate their feelings and to establish new adaptive ways of interacting that are no longer based on reactions to these issues but fill the needs of all parties.

  b. **Parent issues.** It may become clear after simple advice has failed that interfering parent issues need to be addressed such as the parent viewing the child as special or vulnerable, inability to tolerate angry emotions from the child due to their own past exposure to violence, inability to prevent interfering with the other parent's management, covert satisfaction in a child's misbehavior, or lack of energy or motivation to do the hard work of behavior management.

    Eliciting past experiences that are reawakened during child management is often the key. Engaging cooperation from all relevant adults is always helpful and may be essential. When the adult understands how their own issue is affecting the child's behavior they are better able to change their interaction patterns. Writing down the costs and benefits to maintaining the interaction patterns is a useful intervention as is done in motivational interviewing. Referral for further individual work or therapy for the adult may also be needed.

  c. **Interactional issues.** A parent with reasonable overall parenting skills may still be susceptible to maladaptive practices with an individual child. This may be due to a mismatch in temperament with the child, an unreasonable expectation given to this child's attributes, or a change in circumstances or different energy from other periods of parenting for providing adequate attention to the child's positive behaviors. Education and clarification may be sufficient, but providing alternative nurturers for the child is sometimes the only solution.

  d. **Environmental issues.** It is not unusual for a child's behavior to be due to outside conditions especially with the current culture of extensive time in childcare. Toxins such as lead, poor-quality care by others, and models or stress from observing dysfunctional adult behaviors should all be considered when kindly, reasonable parents are unable to resolve child behavior in a previously well-adjusted child. The mediating factors may also be sleep debt, hunger, sibling, or peer influence or abuse. These factors often occur in combination with the above so that all need to be addressed.

C. **Special "problem visits."** Once a problem has been identified, one or more visits of longer duration than usual are generally needed. To arrange an effective "problem visit," the vitally important people in the child's life should be invited to attend, if possible. Boyfriends, neighbors, or babysitters, for example, may be crucial to the solution of the problem if parents give consent for them to attend.

  1. **Visit duration.** Frequently, a longer (e.g., one-half to 1 hour) problem visit can be scheduled at the beginning or the end of the workday, when no sick children are waiting to be seen and telephone calls can be postponed. (It is often advantageous to schedule the problem visit at the beginning of the day, when clinician energy is high). Sometimes the most delicate or powerful issue is not raised until the last moments of the visit in a "parting shot." Such important statements at the end of the hour need to be acknowledged with appropriate empathy, recorded in the chart, and promised as first agenda items at the next visit (which may need to be scheduled sooner, depending on the information revealed).

    Another problem occurs when families or key family members arrive late for an appointment. This may be an important statement of that person's ambivalence about the issues being discussed. The emotional difficulty can be acknowledged directly and with empathy, but the visit should be kept on schedule.

  2. **Space considerations.** Many offices lack an examination room large enough to seat all the family members. A conference room or even the waiting room may better serve and can be private enough before or after regular office hours.

  3. **Documentation of the visit.** Since details of the session are critical to understanding and managing the problem and documenting complexity for billing, the clinician should leave adequate time to write down the salient aspects of the visit. Note taking is possible during the session for some clinicians, but should be interrupted when it interferes with the therapeutic alliance with the family and the patient.

  4. **Billing for the visit.** It is important that the extended problem visit be adequately billed with a higher level of care usually based on time spent. Patients should be informed

of the fee *before* the first extended visit. Offering to accept payment over time may decrease the burden of the extra fee for some families. Third-party reimbursement may be available depending on the diagnosis, the clinician's experience and training, and state insurance regulations. Clinicians generally cannot refer their own patients to themselves and record the visit as a consultation. Experience suggests that most patients *are* willing to pay for counseling if they are able. Many of the barriers to adequate billing are in the mind of the clinician, who is insecure about whether she or he really has something valuable to offer.

D. **Expanding counseling skills.** Books, journals, lectures, videotapes of master therapists, workshops, courses, and fellowships in behavior and development, child psychiatry, or family therapy are available to help clinicians strengthen their behavioral counseling skills. The ultimate method, however, is through experience. For example, working as cotherapists with a more experienced clinician in the session with the family is a very valuable format. Case discussions with another clinician or in a group provides support and often helps clarify the family's and clinician's emotional reactions, as well as providing input into the content and process of management. This process is called *supervision* and can be either direct (another professional attends the counseling session or observes through a one-way mirror) or indirect (the other professional reviews cases later from audiotape, videotape, verbatim process notes, standard notes, or recall, and makes suggestions to be incorporated into future patient visits). The Bureau of Maternal and Child Health has funded a number of Collaborative Office Rounds demonstration projects to provide such case discussion for groups of 8 to 10 practicing pediatric clinicians, or a similar group can be assembled with an agreement to pay the supervisor for their time.

E. **Communicating with schools.** Some behavioral problems are situationally specific and occur only in school or day care. In such cases, it is useful to obtain an objective description of the problem from the school. Have parents sign a note of consent for two-way communication at the first visit that can be faxed to the other relevant sites. A behavioral questionnaire can be sent to the teacher via the child, mail, fax, or an online system or a written note requested. Ideally, direct telephone contact between clinician and teacher is the most revealing. (It is easiest to reach teachers at 7:30 A.M. or noon.) Teachers are generally very grateful for the clinician's interest and can be extremely helpful in providing more information about the family and the child. A single clinician visit to a school to meet one child's teachers, principal, and guidance counselors can facilitate communication for years to come about many children.

F. **Making effective referrals.** One of the most important (and underrated) skills of the primary care clinician lies in making effective referrals. An estimated 68% of mental health referrals made for children are unsuccessful because the family has been poorly prepared, important members do not perceive the problem as significant or treatment as valuable, the family has negative perceptions of mental health professionals, or there is a poor fit between the specialist's therapeutic style and the family's or child's expectations.

1. **Help the family to identify their distress.** The first steps in making an effective referral are to ensure that each member of the family feels that his or her voice has been heard and to identify the distress that will motivate the family and child to accept counseling. It is always better for a clinician to refer the family for a problem that bothers *them*, even if it is not the one that appears primary to the clinician (e.g., a referral for the child's truancy rather than the father's alcoholism). The therapist taking on the case may need to do further work before the family is able to face the central issue.

2. **Discuss issues in a constructive way.** Behavioral and family issues should be discussed in nonjudgmental terms, citing their strengths and using issues from the family's current (rather than past) situation to suggest further work. In the case of a separation from an abusive spouse, for example, one might say, "It took so much courage to make this break that I can see that you really want what is best for your son. Now you can focus on improving your relationship with him and seeing him as a different kind of male from your ex-husband."

3. **Find the appropriate referral.** The next step in making an effective referral is to identify an appropriate consultant for the family. The clinician should inquire about the family's past experiences with counseling and demystify the process of counseling (e.g., by pointing out that therapy is just like the talking that has been going on in the exploratory sessions).

It is helpful to have ready the names and telephone numbers of several therapists who are available and have interest and skills in the type of problem at hand. This takes some preparation in getting to know the counseling style of a cadre of therapists: for example, what kinds of cases they prefer; whether they practice cognitive behavioral therapy, family therapy, or psychodynamic therapy; and whether they offer groups. Determine their fees and accepted insurance and how best to exchange information with them.

Consider introductory face-to-face meetings with local therapists. This provides some basis for discussing the therapists with families and will facilitate future communications between physician and therapist. The clinician should ideally provide the family and patient with details about the therapists so that they can make an informed choice. The gender of the therapist is not usually central to the success of treatment, although some family members may have a strong preference, which should be respected. The relationship of the family with this professional is vital to the treatment, so they should be actively involved in the initial referral. In addition, they should be told that they can always change counselors, should the need arise. This is important so that their problems do not go unresolved simply because of an initial mismatch.

4. **Follow-up.** Finally, it is important for the family to know that the primary care clinician will stay involved and will continue to manage other problems as before. This reassures them that they are not being rejected, especially if they have revealed information about themselves that could be perceived as undesirable. The clinician should be clear in defining exactly what problems will be handled by which professional, obtain written consent to communicate, and stay in touch with the referral therapist to assist or back up the therapist's plans and to facilitate ongoing communication with the family.

G. **Alternative counseling strategies in the office.**
   1. **Groups for families.** Group sessions for a number of families concerning common behavioral problems (e.g., temper tantrums, toilet training, discipline issues, choosing a day care provider, homework strategies) can be an effective way to address those issues and to provide parents with a support system of other parents in similar circumstances. Other groups can be made available for parents of children with a specific problem, such as attention deficit/hyperactivity disorder, oppositional defiant disorder, or developmental disabilities. Local branches of national diagnosis-specific organizations may already offer these or may arrange them when sufficient interest is shown. It has been shown that noncategorical groups, for example, for parents of children with a variety of chronic illnesses, can be as effective as diagnosis-specific groups. One-time sessions may be arranged to deal with crises, such as a publicized suicide, disaster, abuse in a local childcare center, or death of a public figure. For families, the existence of others with similar problems can be a tremendous relief in itself.

   These groups can be led by a primary care clinician in the practice or by an outside consultant, or co-led by both. They may be offered in the office or elsewhere, sponsored by the practice, or simply made known to patients in the practice. It is important to remember that the needs of the individual child or family are frequently not entirely met by these groups, so the leaders must carefully monitor the participants and ensure that supplemental support, guidance, or management is available if needed.
   2. **Group checkups.** There are some advantages to offering health supervision visits in groups. By seeing eight 6-month-old babies together over 1 hour, the clinician can spend much more time providing teaching, anticipatory guidance, and discussion of behavioral issues. It is important to also offer some private time for each family; however, as there may be issues that they do not care to share in a group.
   3. **Call hour.** Many offices have a designated call-in hour for health and behavior questions conducted by either the physician or an experienced nurse or nurse practitioner. Although telephone consultations have obvious major disadvantages, when supervised carefully they can be part of a spectrum of office services for dealing with behavioral problems and help motivate families for behavior counseling if the call line information alone does not suffice.
   4. **Housing other professional disciplines within the practice.** Many practices are choosing to provide office space for specialists from other disciplines to deal with specific behavioral and emotional problems. In private practices, the specialist may receive the space free, share in the costs and income of the group, set lower fees for patients from the practice, be paid a salary by the group, or be a totally independent contractor renting space and billing independently. The practice benefits by having a known, trusted, and readily available person to whom to refer their patients. The entire practice can be strengthened by the comprehensive care that ends up being delivered within its walls.

BIBLIOGRAPHY

Allmond BW, Tanner JL, Gofman HF. *The Family Is the Patient.* Baltimore: Williams & Wilkins, 1999.

Coleman WL. Family-focused pediatrics: solution-oriented techniques for behavioral problems. *Contemp Pediatr* 14:121–134, 1997.

Coleman WL, Howard BJ. Family-focused behavioral pediatrics: clinical techniques for primary care. *Pediatr Rev* 16:448–455, 1995.

McDaniel S, Campbell TL, Seaburn DB. *Family-Oriented Primary Care: A Manual for Medical Providers.* New York: Springer-Verlag, 1990.

Shepard SA, Dickstein S. Preventive intervention for early childhood behavioral problems: an ecological perspective. *Child Adolesc Psychiatr Clin N Am* 18(3):687–706, 2009.

17

Pain

Neil L. Schechter
William T. Zempsky

I. **Definition and background.** Pain is defined by the International Association for the Study of Pain as "an unpleasant sensory and emotional experience associated with actual or potential tissue damage or described in terms of such damage." This definition implies that pain has two components—a neurophysiologically determined sensation that results from stimulation of nociceptors and the interpretation of that stimulus, which is impacted by a host of genetic, personality, cognitive, developmental, experiential, and emotional factors. These may magnify or dampen the amount of pain and suffering that the stimulus causes to the individual. Recent research suggests that previous repeated exposure to painful stimuli, for example, can significantly alter nociceptive processing. Current understanding of pain, therefore, implies that because of individual biological and experiential variation there is no set amount of pain "allowable" for a given injury or illness and, therefore, care must be individualized for each child. This section will focus on acute pain; chronic pain problems such as headache and functional abdominal pain are reviewed elsewhere in Chapters 21 and 49.

Historically, pain has been undertreated in children for a variety of complex reasons. Difficulties with pain assessment in children, social attitudes, and ethical and financial constraints on research diminished interest and allowed for the persistence of myths ("infants do not feel pain") that denigrated the importance of treatment. There has been an outpouring of research in the last 20 years, however, and it is now clearly established that by the end of the second trimester, fetuses have in place the anatomical and chemical capabilities to experience discomfort. Preterm and newborn infants may, in fact, be hyperalgesic because they have the same number of nociceptors in a smaller surface area and because they lack descending modulation of pain through psychological means.

Inadequate pain management clearly has short- and long-term negative consequences. Untreated pain may inhibit immune function, induce stress hormone release, increase blood pressure, inhibit healing due to immobility, and decrease the pain threshold, which subsequently results in hyperalgesia and allodynia. Inadequately addressed pain in young and school-aged children with illness causes unnecessary suffering; worries about procedure pain during routine healthcare maintenance can dominate the encounter reducing the value and enjoyment of the visit for the child and the clinician. For many children with chronic conditions, inadequately treated procedure pain is the worst part of their illness, often worse than the disease itself and creates anxiety about subsequent medical encounters.

II. **Diagnosis.** Adequate assessment is the cornerstone of pain treatment and the individual's self-report of his/her discomfort is the gold standard for assessment. Pain assessment typically focuses on measures of pain intensity. In adults and children older than 8 years, the visual analogue scale that quantifies pain intensity from 0 to 10 is traditionally used. Because of developmental immaturity in children aged 3–8 years, modification of the visual analogue scale is necessary. Color scales, cartoon faces, manipulatives such as poker chips representing pieces of hurt, and photographs of children in discomfort have all been used as modified visual analogue scales. Of those available, the Faces Pain Scale-Revised is the most commonly used and has the strongest psychometric properties. For children younger than 3 years who typically cannot seriate, physiologic parameters (increased heart rate, increased respiratory rate, decreased SaO_2) and behavioral measures such as facial expression, body position, and crying have all been used as nonspecific indicators of pain. Attempts have been made to cluster together these parameters into clinically usable scales (examples of these include the FLACC, CHEOPS, and OBSR). Scales for term infants (N-PASS) and preterm infants (PIPP) have also been developed as well as for children with significant developmental disabilities (Non-communicating Children's Pain Checklist—NCCPC-R). When an intervention occurs to address an elevated pain intensity rating, a repeat assessment should typically occur within an hour to ascertain the efficacy of the intervention. Pain intensity rating scales are often inappropriate for children with chronic pain who should not be queried repeatedly about their level of discomfort. Functional scales such as the FDI and the CALI should be considered for that population.

III. Treatment.

A. General principles. The primary goal of treatment of children with acute pain is to make him or her as comfortable as possible, recognizing that it may not be possible to eliminate all discomfort. There needs to be a balance between pain relief and the side effects associated with treatment. A number of general principles have emerged, however.

   1. It should be generally assumed that whatever hurts an adult will hurt a child and appropriate pain relief should be planned.

   2. A preventative approach is key. Where pain is predictable, it makes much more sense to prevent pain from occurring than to ablate it once it has occurred. This suggests that around-the-clock dosing as compared with PRN dosing is preferable.

   3. Pharmacologic, cognitive-behavioral, and physical approaches should be considered for all pain problems.

   4. Nonnoxious routes of administration should be used, avoiding intramuscular, rectal, or intranasal routes if possible.

   5. Needle sticks are extremely troubling for children and wherever possible, needle pain should be addressed. This typically involves adequate preparation, parental involvement, technical variables (such as site selection, needle length, and position), distraction, and if possible local anesthetics when procedures are nonemergent.

   6. Prolonged pain may lead to sleep problems and immobilization and both of these problems can increase pain. Both should be considered when addressing pain.

B. Behavioral/cognitive/approaches. These nonpharmacologic approaches vary, depending on the type of pain and the age of the child. In situations where limited pain may be magnified by anxiety, they may be the only approach necessary. In general, however, they are used in conjunction with pharmacologic approaches.

   1. Parental presence and demeanor. Parental presence during painful procedures and parental involvement in treatment decisions often has a significant impact on pain the child experiences. During procedures, parents can function as a "coach," stroking, soothing, or talking to the child. They can be instructed in age-appropriate pain relieving techniques. In general, when parents can be included in treatment decisions, they feel less anxious and less helpless and their security is often transmitted to the child and pain is reduced. Research has shown children whose parents are overly apologetic or overly solicitous report more pain and display more pain behaviors than children whose parents are matter of fact and resolute.

   2. Preparation. Knowledge about the pain and its expected time course also reduces anxiety about it, which has the effect of decreasing pain. Discussion about illness and procedures clearly improves coping. Preparation for procedures should include a description of how the child will feel as well as a more detailed description of what will happen. When preparing a child for a painful procedure, the timing of the preparation should be determined by the child's developmental age and temperamental style. In general, the younger the child, the closer the preparation to the procedure.

   3. Visual imagery/distraction/hypnosis. These techniques help children cope with painful illnesses or painful procedures by focusing their attention away from their discomfort and promoting relaxation. Approaches in this category include breathing techniques, blowing on pin-wheels, blowing bubbles, being told stories, reading books, and imagining a more pleasant, desirable place through guided imagery. Hypnosis actively involves the child in a fantasy and uses suggestion to reframe the experience.

C. Physical approaches. Massage, heat, cold, pressure, and vibration in the form of transcutaneous electrical nerve stimulation all work by flooding the nervous system with nonnoxious stimuli, thereby decreasing the impact of the painful stimulus. The immobilization that often accompanies illness or surgery can result in increased pain. Therefore, physical therapy is often a beneficial modality to reduce both acute and chronic pain.

D. Pharmacologic approaches. A number of categories of pharmacologic agents are helpful in pain relief. They may have direct pain-relieving properties, anxiety-reducing properties, or potentiate analgesia.

   1. Local anesthetics. A number of local anesthetics are presently available, which should be used during pain associated with needle insertion or other painful procedures involving the skin.

   • **Eutectic mixture of local anesthetics (EMLA),** a topically administered combination of lidocaine and prilocaine, is extremely effective for venous cannulation, phlebotomy, and reservoir access, and has some efficacy on the pain associated with injections as well. EMLA requires approximately 1 hour to work, and provides 2–4 mm of anesthesia.

Table 17-1. Dosing data for Acetaminophen and NSAIDs

Drug	Usual adult dose	Usual pediatric dose	Comments
Oral NSAIDs			
Acetaminophen (paracetamol)	650–1000 mg q 4 hr	10–20 mg/kg q 4 hr	Acetaminophen lacks the peripheral anti-inflammatory activity of other NSAIDs
Ibuprofen	400–600 mg q 4–6 hr	6–10 mg/kg q 6–8 hr	Available as several brand names and as generic; also available as oral suspension
Naproxen	500 mg initial dose followed by 250 mg q 6–8 hr	5 mg/kg q 12 hr	Also available as oral liquid
Celecoxib	100–200 mg q 12 hr	For patients <2 yr of age, not approved. For patients ≥10 kg to ≤25 kg, 50 mg q 12 hr. For patients >25 kg 100 mg q 12 hr	COX-2 inhibitor may cause less bleeding and gastritis

- **LMX4, another topical cream,** is 4% lidocaine encapsulated by liposomes, which allow for transdermal delivery. It is available without prescription and works in approximately 30 minutes.
- **Lidocaine** can also be injected almost painlessly if it is buffered with sodium bicarbonate and injected slowly with a small needle.
- Topical refrigerants or **vapocoolant sprays** produce immediate anesthesia for a few seconds and may reduce injection or immunization pain.

2. **Drugs for Mild to Moderate Pain.**
   a. **Acetaminophen and nonsteroidal anti-inflammatory drugs (NSAIDs) (Table 17-1).** These categories of drugs act peripherally and inhibit cyclooxygenase, which has a role in prostaglandin synthesis. All of the drugs in this category have a "ceiling" effect, beyond which no further analgesia is achieved.
      - **Acetaminophen,** the most commonly used drug in this category, provides analgesia but has no anti-inflammatory effect.
      - Unfortunately, all available over-the-counter **NSAIDs,** which have anti-inflammatory activity, also have associated bleeding and gastrointestinal side effects. These agents are preferable to acetaminophen for pain, which may be associated with inflammation such as the pain of otitis media, pharyngitis, and muscular aches.
      - **COX-2 inhibitors,** were developed to reduce the side effects often associated with NSAIDs and initially held great promise. Unfortunately, they have been associated with increased cardiovascular events in older adults and except for celecoxib have been removed from the market.

3. **Drugs for moderate to severe pain.** Opioids (Table 17-2) are the drugs of choice for moderate to severe pain. There are known predictable side effects associated with these drugs, such as constipation, respiratory depression, and itching, and these should be anticipated. Although diversion and abuse of these drugs for illicit purposes exists, concerns about addiction, which have hampered the legitimate medical use of these drugs in the past, should not prevent the provision of adequate pain relief.
   - Although still a popular choice for mild moderate pain, **codeine** use is problematic given that 10%–15% of persons cannot metabolize codeine into morphine, which is required for its action.
   - Oral agents such as **oxycodone, hydrocodone,** and **oxymorphone** are alternatives, which are effective for pain. When these drugs are used in fixed drug preparation with an NSAID (i.e., acetaminophen/codeine (Tylenol #3), acetaminophen and oxycodone (Tylox, Percocet)), care should be taken to avoid excessive NSAID ingestion.

Table 17-2. Dosing data for opioid analgesics

Drug	Equianalgesic parenteral dose	Equianalgesic oral dose	Recommended adult dose[1] parenteral	Recommended adult dose[2] oral	Recommended pediatric dose parenteral	Recommended pediatric dose oral
Morphine	10 mg	30 mg	10 mg q 3–4 hr	30 mg q 3– hr	0.1 mg/kg. q 3–4 hr	0.3 mg/kg. q 3–4 hr
Codeine	130 mg	200 mg	Not recommended	30–60 mg q 4 hr	Not recommended	0.5–1 mg/kg. q 3–4 hr
Hydromophone	1.5 mg	7.5 mg	1 mg q 3–4 hr	2–4 mg q 3–4 hr	0.02 mg/kg. q 3–4 hr	0.04–.08 mg/kg. q 3–4 hr
Oxycodone	Not available	30 mg	Not available	5–10 mg q 3–4 hr	Not available	0.2 mg/kg. q 3–4 hr
Methadone	10 mg	20 mg	5–8 mg q 4 hr	5–10 mg 3–4 hr	0.1 mg/kg. q 6–8 hr	0.1–0.2 mg/kg. q 6–8 hr
Tramadol				50–100 mg q 6 hr		

[1] Doses refer to children older than 6 months.
[2] Greater than 50 kg.

- **Tramadol** is an analgesic that has the features of both a mu agonist and a selective serotonin reuptake inhibitor (SSRI) and is efficacious for both acute and chronic pain. It typically causes less sedation than traditional opioids.
- For severe pain, **morphine** remains the drug of choice. It can be administered through a number of routes and its pharmacokinetics are well-established in children. These agents can be used safely in children but should be used with caution in a carefully monitored setting in infants.
- For severe pain that persists, **long-acting opioids** (morphine (MSContin), oxycodone (OxyContin), morphine sulfate (Kadian)) are available but should only be prescribed for chronic pain, not acute unstable pain. When using a long-acting opioid, a short-acting opioid should always be prescribed simultaneously for breakthrough pain.
- **Methadone** has recently gained favor as opioid for chronic pain given its unique activity as an N-methyl-D-aspartic acid antagonist.

4. **Adjunctive drugs.** Drugs in this category include anticonvulsants (**pregabalin** and **gabapentin**) and antidepressants (**amitriptyline** and **duloxetine**), which have efficacy against the pain of nerve injury and neuropathic pain. This type of pain, which is often opioid resistant has unique characteristics and is often described as burning, shooting, or electric. Treatment of comorbid anxiety should be considered using medications such as **benzodiazipines** and SSRIs. Management of sleep disorders using **melatonin, amitriptyline, trazodone,** or **zolpidem** may also be necessary.

IV. **Summary.** Most acute pain problems are treatable using relatively simple, safe approaches. A small percent of cases will require regional or other anesthetic approaches. A systematic approach to assessment is the cornerstone of adequate treatment. Unless pain is documented, it cannot be adequately treated nor can the success of interventions be monitored. Multimodal treatment (pharmacologic, cognitive-behavioral, and physical approaches) is essential in any comprehensive plan for pain relief.

BIBLIOGRAPHY

Books and Journals

Berde CB, Sethna NF. Analgesics for the treatment of pain in children. *N Engl J Med* 347:1094–1103, 2002.

McGrath PJ, Walco GA, Turk DC, et al. Core outcome domains and measures for pediatric acute and chronic/recurrent pain clinical trials: PedIMMPACT recommendations. *J Pain* 9:771–783, 2008.

Schechter NL, Berde CB, Yaster M. *Pain in Infants, Children, and Adolescents* (2nd ed), Philadelphia: Lippincott Williams & Wilkins, 2003.

Eccleston C, Palermo TM, Williams ACDC, et al. Psychological therapies for the management of chronic and recurrent pain in children and adolescents. *Cochrane Database Syst Rev* (1), 2003. Art. No.:CD003968.

Web sites

Pediatric pain Web site available at www.dal.ca/~pedpain Dalhousie University supports a superb Web site that serves as a clearinghouse of pediatric pain information for children, families, and clinicians. They also sponsor a list serve on pediatric pain for clinicians.

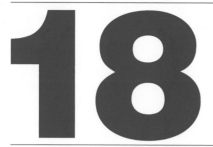

Early Childhood Development in Low- and Middle-Income Countries

Ilgi Ozturk Ertem

I. Description of the problem.

   A. The importance of early childhood development (ECD) and developmental risks or difficulties that begin during early childhood are increasingly recognized as important contributors to childhood morbidity in low- and middle-income (LAMI) countries. Although prevention of childhood mortality remains the focus in such countries, many countries are looking to promote ECD via healthcare delivery systems. Universal principles for the promotion of ECD in LAMI countries are multidimensional:

   - **Optimal development is the basic right of the child.** All but two countries have ratified the United Nations Convention of the Rights of the Child. The convention has brought increased awareness around the globe that regardless of place of residence, an environment that promotes his/her full developmental potential is a basic right of the child.

   - **Development during early childhood has economic implications for nations.** Research on cost-benefit analyses has emphasized that return for investment per human capital is highest during early childhood compared with any other period in the life cycle.

   - **Research has made it possible to better understand the links between physical health and psychosocial development.** The biomedical model that has dominated the approach to healthcare delivery in LAMI countries has limited attention to psychosocial and developmental issues. Recent research emphasizes that causes of poor health (e.g., malnutrition) also affect child development and that causes of poor development (e.g., unresponsive caring environments) also have an impact on health. The Lancet series entitled "Child Development in Developing Countries" has drawn attention to the need for the promotion of ECD in LAMI countries. International organizations such as the World Health Organization (WHO) and the United Nations Children's Fund (UNICEF) have shown increased appreciation that when healthcare delivery includes a developmental context, there are beneficial effects on survival, physical health, and development.

   - **Healthcare systems are often the only existing infrastructures reaching young children.** Research in Western countries has shown that professionals can support child development during pediatric healthcare encounters. Healthcare encounters are often the only opportunity available for professionals in LAMI countries to positively influence caregivers of young children.

   B. Risks to ECD are multiple in LAMI countries. Figure 18-1 describes a life cycle approach to developmental risk factors in LAMI countries, broken out further below.

   - **Little information on child development may reach families**. Young children may not be regarded as receptive to interaction and may not be given opportunities for exploration and play. Gender inequalities may place women at higher risk for difficulties in caring for themselves and in providing developmentally appropriate care to their young children.

   - **Maternal depression** in LAMI countries is at least as prevalent and has all the consequences that are present for children and families in Western cultures. Furthermore, recent research has shown that in LAMI countries, young children of depressed mothers have higher rates of low-birth weight and life-threatening disease such as diarrhea and other infections compared with children of mothers who are not depressed.

   - Because of displacement in war zones or moves into urban life, **the support of extended family may be lost.** As women increasingly join the work force without appropriate childcare facilities, they may need to leave their young children in the care of other children or alone in homes and shelters.

   - **Far fewer encounters with healthcare providers** take place in LAMI countries, and these are typically not for routine healthcare maintenance but during acute illness.

   - **Healthcare professionals may not be equipped with information on developmental or psychosocial issues.** Mental health professionals may not exist or are very

PRECONCEPTION	PRENATAL/ PERINATAL	NEWBORN	INFANCY/ EARLY CHILDHOOD
			Lack of appropriate child care
			Child health problems/chronic illness
			Inadequacies in nurturing and stimulating qualities of the caregiving environment
Problems/deficiencies in maternal health and nutrition	Maternal mortality Perinatal asphyxia Low birth weight Prematurity	Inadequate caregiver– newborn relationship and interactions	Iron deficiency
Inadequate birth interval	Perinatal complications/ infections	Neonatal infections/ complications	Iodine deficiency
Unintended pregnancy	Congenital/chromosomal abnormalities	Developmental/sensory impairments	Malnutrition and micronutrient deficiencies
Parental consanguinity			

EXPOSURE TO ENVIRONMENTAL TOXINS ⟶

PROBLEMS IN CAREGIVER PHYSICAL AND MENTAL HEALTH ⟶

DEFICIENCIES IN THE SOCIAL AND ECONOMIC ENVIRONMENT ⟶

nutrition, safe housing, environmental hygiene, living-wage jobs, gender equality, caregiver education, child care, preschool opportunities and schools, access to public and private goods and services, access to healthcare and trained healthcare providers, exposure to violence/war.

Figure 18-1. Life cycle Approach to Developmental Risk Factors.

few in number and multidisciplinary teams typically may not exist. Existing professionals and healthcare systems may view support to the development of young children as a luxury that is not relevant to healthcare.

C. **Strengths and protective factors that foster resilience during early childhood in LAMI countries.** Risks, strengths, and resilience coexist even in the most deprived populations. As risks to optimal development differ within populations, reasons for resilience may also differ.
   • The primary role of the mother in caring for her young child, the slow pace of daily life, the presence of fathers and extended family, and the "whole village" that circle and nurture the child may be important protective factors for a young child's development.
   • Substance abuse by women, a major risk in Western populations, is less common in most LAMI countries.
   • Healthcare professionals are often highly regarded in the community exerting significant influence on behavior.
   • Systems that high-income countries spend large funds to install, for example, home visiting for the delivery of primary care, healthcare stations that are regarded as part of communities, may be already in place in LAMI countries.

D. Strategies to promote ECD in LAMI countries. The promotion of ECD does not require expensive equipment, or expensive and lengthy training programs. When existing strengths within local resources are identified, the remaining challenge then involves increasing motivation to place emphasis on promoting ECD:

- **Develop locally owned sustainable interventions.** Interventions resembling episodic relief work do little to ameliorate problems in the long run. A thorough understanding of the magnitude of problems and strengths within communities is needed to ensure a match between interventions and what the population needs, what it can achieve and sustain. It is by building local capacity that a sustainable approach can be developed. Particularly, academic centers in LAMI countries can be supported to transmit knowledge flow from other countries, develop culturally appropriate and innovative interventions, and test their effectiveness.

- **Assess theoretical construct.** Culturally appropriate interventions that reflect "state-of-the-art" teachings on child development are needed. ECD may be a new concept in LAMI countries and may be dominated by outdated theories and models. For example, outdated models that have been adopted from Western cultures may result in the removal of children physically or conceptually from the context of their relationships and environments when attempting to promote their development. Such old models may focus on the neurodevelopmental milestones of the child, child-centered screening, procedures and interventions that do not foster relationships with caregivers. These models are not likely to provide benefit. Practices based on such beliefs and models need to be identified and changed.

- Current theories that place **caregiver–child interactions at the center of promoting child development,** interventions that enable relationships and partnerships with caretakers, that allow nonthreatening, supportive environments within healthcare delivery, and interventions that regard young children as active participants in the process would be most effective.

- **Adopt a comprehensive approach.** As risks to development are multiple, so must interventions be comprehensive. It will not be enough to enhance the play skills of malnourished children who may also have untreated infections. Similarly, it will not be a sufficient boost to brain development if these children are fed and given medications only. Health professionals must take all components of health and psychosocial care into account together.

- **Assess and increase motivation and training of healthcare staff.** The following questions can assess the backgrounds and motivation of healthcare staff: Is up-to-date information on child development a part of preservice or in-service training? What are the knowledge, skills, and attitudes of healthcare clinicians related to monitoring and supporting ECD? How can healthcare clinicians be motivated to take on another and new agenda?

- **Identify minimum standards.** When identified in each community and setting, key elements that promote child development may prove to be easy to institute, inexpensive, and cost-effective. For example, in hospital settings the hospitalization of children and adults on separate wards, hospital accompaniment of children by caregivers at all times, home made toys at the bedside, and trained healthcare workers who discuss the child's development with the caregiver may be low-cost interventions that can promote ECD.

- **Support continuity of care.** Continuity of healthcare clinician may not be emphasized in LAMI countries. Receiving healthcare from one clinician works to promote child development in two directions: it enhances families' experience through better healthcare worker–family communication, and it enhances healthcare workers' experience through opportunities for natural observations of child and family development.

- **Adopt an opportunistic approach.** Incorporating the promotion of child development into community programs, family planning, safe motherhood, obstetric care, delivery, postpartum care, immunizations, nutrition counseling, ill child ambulatory care, and hospitalizations are examples of opportunistic approaches.

- **Involve men as well as women.** The role of fathers, extended family, male leaders in community, and policy makers should not be overlooked and may have more impact in LAMI countries than recognized in the Western world.

- **Attend urgently to specific problems.** Children affected by war, displacement, the HIV/AIDS pandemic, natural disasters, developmental disorders, orphanage care, abuse, neglect, and exploitation deserve specific attention and comprehensive care throughout the world.

- **Work for peace and equality throughout the world.** In all of our efforts to better child health and development, we must remember that these depend most on peace and equal distribution of resources throughout the world.

II. Examples of interventions.

   A. WHO/UNICEF Care for Child Development Intervention (CCDI), developed by the WHO Department of Child and Adolescent Health and Development and UNICEF, uses the window of opportunity that arises when the child comes in contact with the healthcare system. The CCDI is a standardized interview, which assesses how the caretaker plays with and communicates with the child. Observations and intervention strategies offered to parents during the interview include listening to caregivers and giving specific reinforcement for ways they support their child's development; observing for positive interactions between infants and caregivers during the healthcare visit; using basic home made toys to facilitate interactions; pointing out responses of the infant and the role of the caregiver in eliciting these responses; and providing ideas for age-appropriate stimulation. Healthcare workers then explore with the child's caregiver the potential for such interactions in the home; discuss obstacles that caregivers may face to help the child develop; and ways they can overcome these obstacles. The intervention can be delivered anywhere and adds approximately 10 minutes to the health visit. The training period is approximately 1.5 days. Training materials, comprising of workbooks and videotape for facilitators and trainees have been tested in the field and have been revised by the WHO and UNICEF to be used globally.

   B. Training of healthcare professionals: an example from Turkey. Over two decades, Ankara University School of Medicine Developmental-Behavioral Pediatrics (DBP) Unit has been collaborating with the Turkish Ministry of Health, the WHO, and UNICEF, to develop training programs for healthcare clinicians on ECD. As a result of these collaborations, training programs have been developed for healthcare clinicians at different levels: 1) 3-day course for primary healthcare providers (general practitioners, nurses, midwives); 2) 5-day course for pediatricians who will be providing healthcare and follow-up of high-risk children; 3) 2-month training program for teams that will be founding DBP units at pediatric training hospitals; and 4) 2-year program in training subspecialist pediatricians in DBP. The content of the training programs includes concepts and theories of ECD starting from pregnancy to preschool years, risks to optimal development, ways to decrease risks, preventing developmental delay, common psychosocial problems, techniques for developmental monitoring and for supporting child development, early identification of children with developmental delay, services for children with developmental difficulties, and community resources available for early intervention and rehabilitation. All training methods are interactive, experiential, and problem based. Materials comprise a book in Turkish on developmental–behavioral pediatrics, DVDs with slides presentations, local video recordings of children and caregivers demonstrating typical development, and case scenarios for developmental difficulties. All of the programs have started and are intended to go to scale in Turkey. We find that the topic of ECD has an enchanting effect. When introduced in a form that is appropriate to the context of their ongoing work, healthcare professionals are highly motivated to take on as their mission the promotion of ECD.

   C. Training of community workers: example from India. The Ummeed Child Development Center in Mumbai, India, conducts a Child Development Aide (CDA) Training Program: This program trains community workers from not-for-profit organizations (NPOs) and schools, serving low-income populations in India. The NPOs include governmental and nongovernmental organizations, which provide community-based rehabilitation and early childhood education in slums, orphanages, and maternal and child healthcare programs. Ummeed aims to create resources within these organizations with direct access to children at risk for and with developmental disabilities. A CDA is trained to promote normal development, educate the local population regarding prevention of disabilities, identify children "at risk" and with special needs, and carry out simple interventions in various areas of development and education. The curriculum is based on the transactional model of child development and family-centered approaches. The training program is full time, for 6 months with an additional 1-year mentorship program onsite.

BIBLIOGRAPHY

Ertem IO, Pekcici EB, Gok CG, et al. Addressing early childhood development in primary health care: experience from a middle-income country. *J Dev Behav Pediatr* 30:319–326, 2009.

Ertem IO, Dogan DG, Gok CG, et al. A guide for monitoring child development in low- and middle-income countries. *Pediatrics* 121:e581–e589, 2008.

Ertem IO, Atay G, Bingoler BE, et al. Promoting child development at sick-child visits: a controlled trial. *Pediatrics* 118:e124–e131, 2006.

Grantham-McGregor S, Cheung YB, Cueto S, et al. International Child Development Steering Group. Developmental potential in the first 5 years for children in developing countries. *Lancet* 369:60–70, 2007.

Maulik PK, Darmstadt GL. Childhood disability in low- and middle-income countries: overview of screening, prevention, services, legislation, and epidemiology. *Pediatrics* 120(Suppl 1):S1–S55, 2007.

Richter LM. Poverty, underdevelopment and infant mental health. *J Paediatr Child Health* 39: 243–248, 2003.

Web sites

Ummeed Child Development Center, Mumbai, India: http://www.ummeed.org/index.asp

World Bank Toolkit Examining ECD in Low Income Countries: http://www.siteresources. worldbank.org/Examining_ECD_Toolkit_FULL.pdf

19

Self-Regulation Therapy

Karen Olness

I. **Background and introduction.** Training in self-regulation can prove useful for pediatric clinicians and for the children and adolescents they serve. Training in self-regulation techniques provides a sense of mastery and coping abilities for children. Controlled studies have increasingly provided evidence for the effectiveness of such training in conditions such as prevention of juvenile migraine and irritable bowel syndrome and anxiety associated with medical or dental procedures. Early training in self-regulation can extinguish negative conditioned physiological responses such as tachycardia or hyperventilation and thereby avoid more complex adult problems. The average child can learn self-regulation techniques quickly, and initial training requires only a few office visits.

A. **Definitions.**

1. **Hypnotherapy** refers to focusing attention on specific mental images for therapeutic purposes. It often, but not always, involves relaxation. Children, for example, may be physically active when practicing self-hypnosis. All hypnosis is, in fact, self-hypnosis although the term hetero-hypnosis is used to refer to the training period when the child is being taught self-hypnosis. Pediatric clinicians who teach self-hypnosis to children must consider each child's interests, learning styles, and imagery preferences.

2. **Imagery.** This term is often used for training in self-regulation. It is important that teachers of imagery recognize that mental imagery preferences vary among individuals. Although most children are skilled in visual imagery, many prefer to focus on auditory, kinesthetic, or taste/olfactory imagery.

3. **Biofeedback** provides visual or auditory evidence of physiological changes. A bathroom scale and a blood pressure monitor, for example, are biofeedback devices. Many child appealing small biofeedback devices have been developed, which provide feedback of peripheral temperature, galvanic skin resistance, heart rate, heart rate variability, and/or muscle responses. Neurofeedback requires larger equipment. In order to effect changes in physiological responses, children and adolescents are taught self-hypnosis strategies such as favorite place imagery or kinesthetic imagery or progressive relaxation.

II. **Self-regulation in pediatric care.**

A. **Applications.** The pediatric clinician may recommend training in a self-regulation method as primary or adjunct treatment for a number of problems (Table 19-1). These include habit problems such as hair pulling, thumb sucking, or nail biting; chronic illnesses including asthma, hemophilia, diabetes, cancer, or migraine; performance anxiety including sports, examinations, musical performance, and speaking; and enuresis, warts, conditioned fears and anxieties, sleep problems, pain associated with procedures, chronic pain, and attention deficit disorders. The addition of biofeedback to training in self-hypnosis makes the training more interesting for many children and helps them to understand that by changing their thinking, they can control body responses.

B. **Principles of self-regulation treatment.**

1. Assess the **presenting problem** to rule out causes that may require other types of treatment such as enuresis associated with constipation or a urinary tract infection.

2. Assess the interest of the child and his or her **willingness to practice self-regulation techniques.** If the problem is of primary concern to the parent, rather than the child, the child may not wish to invest the requisite practice time.

3. Determine the **child's interest, likes, dislikes, fears, and learning patterns** to choose an approach that is likely to be appealing and practical.

4. Because practice is the job of the child, not the parents, **teach the child without the presence of parents in most cases.** Parents may be present during the initial part of the interview. The pediatric clinician might say, in the presence of both the child and parent, *"Your mother is not allowed to remind you to practice. On the way home*

Table 19-1. Applications of self-regulation in pediatrics

Pain management
    Acute (procedures in office or emergency room)
    Chronic (sickle cell disease, hemophilia, recurrent headaches, etc.)

Habit problems
    Thumb sucking
    Hair pulling
    Simple tics
    Enuresis
    Habit cough

Reduction of anxiety in chronic conditions
    Malignancies
    Hemophilia
    Sickle cell disease
    Lupus erythematosus
    Tourette's syndrome
    Diabetes
    Cyclic vomiting

Improved performance
    Sports
    Drama
    Music
    Exams

Control of conditions involving autonomic dysregulation
    Raynaud's phenomenon
    Reflex sympathetic dystrophy
    Dyshidrosis
    Conditioned hyperventilation
    Conditioned dysphagia

Prevention
    Migraine
    Anxiety

Other
    Insomnia
    Parasomnias
    Warts
    Disfluencies
    Conditioned hives
    Fears (e.g., flying)
    Eating problems

---

the two of you can discuss a way to remind yourself to practice, for example, a sign on your bedroom door."
5. Be certain that the child **understands something about the mechanism of the problem.** This can be achieved by simple drawings and concrete language (e.g., diagramming the urinary tract or a pain pathway). The pediatric clinician can ask the child to make his or her own drawing.
6. Emphasize your **role as a coach or a teacher.** You cannot force the child to practice. The child decides if and when he or she will do the practice.
7. Communicate in a way that increases the **child's sense of coping and mastery.** Provide the child some choices. For example, say to a child with cancer, "You've done well with your biofeedback practice. You can decide whether to practice in the morning or afternoon or evening and, when you're ready, you can show your mom or dad how you do it."

Table 19-2. Organizations providing training

American Society of Clinical Hypnosis
140 N. Bloomingdale Road
Bloomingdale, IL 60108-1017
Phone: 630-980-4740
www.asch.net

Association for Applied Psychophysiology and Biofeedback
10200 West 44th Avenue, #304
Wheat Ridge, CO 80033-2840
Phone: 303-422-8436

Society for Clinical and Experimental Hypnosis
Massachusetts School of Professional Psychology
221 Rivermoor Street
Boston, MA 02132
www.sceh.us

8. Encourage the child to think about **how life will be different when he or she no longer has the problem.** What would be different? What is the desired outcome? A child who has no mental picture of the benefits may not be ready to practice a self-regulation method.

9. Plan with the child some **system to record progress,** such as a calendar or sticker chart. It is important to record not only symptoms and severity but also the frequency of practice.

C. Self-regulation training.

1. **Imagery.** Self-regulation involves directing a child's imagination to focus his attention, at which time the child can give herself or himself instructions to regulate or control a sensation, physiological function or action. The teacher or coach suggests imaginary involvement that is appealing. For example, a child can imagine riding a bicycle to a favorite place and can inform the teacher when he or she arrives and is ready to give himself or herself a specific instruction or suggestion. Most children enjoy being offered such control.

2. **Control.** Not only is it therapeutically sound to provide a child control in a training sessions but this also aids in determining if the child is interested in resolving a habit or performance problem. For example, if the child does not reach the favorite place (in the above example), this may mean that he or she is not motivated to change or has not understood what is being taught or perhaps did not enjoy the imagined bike riding. The use of "canned" instructions removes the child's ability to choose and is contraindicated.

3. **Therapeutic suggestions** should be consistent with the child's wishes and previous explanations. The pediatric clinician and child should have agreed on the purpose of the visit and should be very clear about what the child wishes to achieve. Suggestions should be concrete and refer to language used in earlier explanations and drawings. For example, *"When you're ready, you can tell your bladder to send a message to your brain to wake you up when the bladder is full. Tell your brain to wake you up completely and send a message to your legs to get out of bed and walk to the toilet."*

4. **Audiotaping training sessions** and giving a CD or DVD to a child is helpful to some. It is important to emphasize that the CD is for help in the first practice days but that the goal is for the child to do the practice on his or her own in the way he or she prefers.

5. **Access to the pediatric clinician.** Because parents should not be the reminders or reinforcers, the child must be able to ask the teacher about the practice, when necessary. After the initial visits for training, scheduled telephone or e-mail follow-up may be helpful to children.

6. **Early training for children with chronic diseases.** It is more efficient and effective to train young children with chronic diseases (such as hemophilia or sickle cell disease) in self-regulation soon after the diagnosis. Children who develop conditioned anxiety, nausea, and other symptoms associated with procedures can also benefit from self-regulation training, but, in general, much more training time is required.

D. Anticipatory guidance. Clinicians may choose to include the teaching of self-regulation techniques in their anticipatory guidance. For example, preschoolers can be encouraged to use their imaginations during physical examinations. They can be asked, *"Where would* *you like to be now?"* If the child says, "At home" or "At the playground" the response is *"Good. Pretend you're there right now. Tell me what you are doing."* This type of interaction can be repeated at each visit and is likely to be remembered by the child if he or she comes in later for a procedure. For younger children who must undergo procedures, nurses, clinic assistants, and parents can be instructed in holding techniques that give a child a sense of control (e.g., sitting upright on a nurse's lap). Keeping a supply of pop-up books, headphones, CDs with appropriate music or stories, or bubbles provide excellent distracters that mitigate the distress of procedures. The simple suggestion that a child pretends he or she is blowing out birthday candles will make it easier to tolerate procedures.

Regardless of whether the pediatric clinician decides to study this area by taking formal training workshops, he or she can practice using everyday language in a way that is encouraging and inspires confidence. For example, during a visit for a minor injury, the clinician may say, *"When you go home, what's the first thing you will do?"* This gives the child the expectation that the procedure will end and he will go home and all will be well. Or saying, *"Your blood looks strong and healthy"* is a powerful positive message for most young children.

III. **Training for the professional.** Basic training workshops in biofeedback and hypnosis are available through several professional organizations (Table 19-2). After taking basic training, clinicians who wish to teach self-hypnosis or biofeedback to children and adolescents should take specialty workshops taught by healthcare professionals who are experienced in working with children. These workshops should be at least 20–24 hours and include at least 6 hours of supervised practice of techniques.

After taking this training, the pediatric clinician should seek a mentor who can be available via phone and e-mail to provide guidance and support. Fortunately, most children learn easily and benefit from the experience; this is encouraging to the novice clinician-teacher. The learner should also attend follow-up workshops, watch videotapes of other teachers, and read basic textbooks and journals sponsored by professional societies. There are board examinations in both biofeedback and hypnosis. Finally, the pediatric clinician who is developing these skills should learn and benefit from practicing biofeedback and hypnosis for himself or herself. This provides valuable lifelong benefits.

BIBLIOGRAPHY

For parents

Culbert T, Kajander R. *Be the Boss of Your Pain [Book and Kit].* Minneapolis, MN: Freespirit Publishing, 2007.

Culbert T, Kajander R. *Be the Boss of Your Stress [Book and Kit].* Minneapolis, MN: Freespirit Publishing, 2007.

Kuttner L. *No Fears, No Tears.* Canadian Cancer Society. *No Fears No Tears 13 Years Later.* Canadian Cancer Society, 955 West Broadway, Vancouver BC. V5Z 3 × 8. Canada. Films available at www.fanlight.com.

Thomson L. *Harry the Hypno-potamus: Metaphorical Tales for the Treatment of Children.* Norwalk, CT: Crown House, 2005. www.crownhouse.co.uk.

For professionals

Barabasz AF, Olness K, Boland R, et al. *Medical Hypnosis Primer: clinical and research evidence.* New York: Routledge, 2009. www.routledgementalhealth.com.

Culbert T, Olness K. *Integrative Pediatrics.* New York: Oxford, 2009.

Olness K, Kohen DP. *Hypnosis and Hypnotherapy for Children* (3rd ed), New York: Guilford, 1996.

20 Psychopharmacology

Elizabeth Harstad
Alison Schonwald

I. **Description of the Problem.** The use of psychopharmacologic agents in children most commonly occurs in the treatment of attention-deficit/hyperactivity disorder (ADHD)/impulse control problems, mood and anxiety symptoms, and psychosis. Although many studies demonstrate highly effective and safe treatment of pediatric ADHD, data for efficacy with most other symptom complexes is less compelling. Because of the paucity of research on children, most use of medications for non–ADHD symptoms remains "off label." In the United States, 20% of children and adolescents have a diagnosable mental health disorder that requires intervention or monitoring and interferes with daily functioning. Primary care providers currently assume all mental healthcare for the majority of affected children. With the increased recognition of childhood psychiatric disorders, ease of obtaining information on the Internet, and ongoing marketing of psychotropic medications, the need for primary care providers to stay current with treatment options remains clinically imperative.

II. **Epidemiology.**
   - Mental health disorders affect up to 20% of U.S. children and adolescents.
   - ADHD affects 3%–9% of U.S. children.
   - Depression affects up to 3% of children and 8% of adolescents.
   - Anxiety disorders affect up to 15% of those younger than 18 years.
   - By some estimates, bipolar disorder affects close to 1 million children and adolescents in the United States at any given time. Several studies have reported that more than 80% of children who have early-onset bipolar disorder will meet full criteria for ADHD.

III. **Deciding to treat with medication.** Determining that a child's presentation indicates the need for psychopharmacology requires
   - Identification of target symptoms.
   - Review of appropriate home and school supports and interventions.
   - Degree to which symptoms causes functional impairment.
   - Informed consent.

   These decisions can be complicated by difficulties in clearly diagnosing the pediatric population, as well as concerns about potential long-term effects of psychotropics on brain development. Children with depression, anxiety, severe aggression, or psychotic thinking should work with a therapist, who can help identify contributing stressors, and teach the child strategies to cope better with tension, worries, fears, and negative thoughts. For many, however, individual psychotherapy will be augmented by psychopharmacological intervention. When medication is deemed necessary, it is helpful to use validated rating scales to monitor progress. Examples of such scales are the Clinical Global Impression Scale, Aberrant Behavior Checklist, Self-Report for Childhood Anxiety Related Emotional Disorder (SCARED), and Multidimensional Anxiety Scale for Children (MASC). See bibliography for information regarding these tools.

IV. **Medical and philosophical controversies.** In the past several decades, clinicians have had to extrapolate the findings from adult psychopharmacology to children, and only recently have research studies become available to document the efficacy and safety of these medications in children. Many of the medications used have potentially serious side effects, which must be weighed against the adverse effects of not treating difficult or dangerous behaviors with medication. With the increasing prevalence of mental health disorders recognized in children, there is more and more of a need to understand and provide effective and safe treatment. Debate remains over which clinicians are best suited to oversee both behavioral and medication management and, in some areas, a paucity of clinicians limits options.

V. **History: key clinical questions.**
   - *"What are your greatest concerns at this time? How impairing are these behaviors or feelings?"* Medication may be helpful to the child whose depression, anxiety, or aggression prevents adequate learning, participation in the classroom, or social success. Setting realistic expectations to improve sleep, brighten affect, or improve school behavior comes from clear discussion of what the problems are and how the medication will help.

Table 20-1. Selective serotonin reuptake inhibitors (SSRIs)

Brand name (generic name)	Age and approved indications	Off-label clinical indications	Metabolism	Preparation	Start dose per day (mg)	Target dose per day (mg)
Celexa® (citalopram)	No pediatric approval	Depression, anxiety, OCD	Weak IID6, IIIA4, IIC19	10, 20, 40 mg 10 mg/5 mL	5–10	10–60
Lexapro® (escitalopram)	≥12 yr: depression	Anxiety	Weak IID6, IIIA4, IIC19	5, 10, 20 mg 5 mg/5 mL	1.25–5	2.5–20
Luvox® (fluvoxamine)	≥8 yr: OCD	Depression, anxiety	IA2, IIIA3–4, IIC19	25, 50, 100 mg; 100, 150 mg ER	12.5–25	25–300
Paxil® (paroxetine)	No pediatric approval; not recommended for depression under 18 yr	Anxiety, OCD	IID6, IIIA4	10, 20, 30, 40 mg; 12.5, 25, 37.5 mg CR 10 mg/5 mL	5–10	10–60
Prozac® (fluoxetine)	≥8 yr: depression ≥7 yr: OCD	Anxiety	IID6, IIIA3–4, IIC19	10, 20, 40 mg 20 mg/5 mL	2.5–10	5–20 MDD 20–60 OCD
Zoloft® (sertraline)	≥6 yr: OCD	Depression, anxiety	Weak IID6, IIC19	25, 50, 100 mg 20 mg/mL	12.5–50	25–200

MDD, major depressive disorder; OCD, obsessive compulsive disorder; ER, extended release; CR, controlled release.

Table 20-2. Atypical and tricyclic antidepressants

Brand name (generic name)	Age and approved pediatric indications	Off-label clinical indications	Metabolism	Preparation	Start dose per day	Target dose per day
Atypical antidepressants						
Buspar® (buspirone)	No pediatric approval	Anxiety, depression	IIIa4	5, 10, 15, 30 mg	2.5 mg	20–60 mg divided tid
Desyrel® (trazodone)	No pediatric approval	Sedation, anxiety	IIIa4/5	50, 100, 150, 300 mg	25 mg	25–150 mg qhs
Effexor® (venlafaxine)	Over 18 yr; not recommended for depression under 18 yr	Depression, anxiety, ADHD	IId6, IIIa4	25, 37.5, 50, 75, 100 mg; 37.5, 75, 150 mg ER	37.5 mg XR	37.5–225 mg XR
Remeron® (mirtazapine)	No pediatric approval	Insomnia, depression, anxiety, weight loss	IId6, IA2, IIIa4	15, 30, 45 mg	15 mg qhs	15–45 mg
Wellbutrin® (bupropion)	No pediatric approval	Depression, ADHD	IIb6, IIIa4	75, 100 mg; 100, 150, 200, 300 mg ER	50 mg SR	50–200 SR bid, 150–450 XL qd
Tricyclic antidepressants						
Anafranil® (clomipramine)	Over 10 yr for OCD	ADHD	IId6, Ia2, IIa4/5	25, 50, 75 mg	25 mg	Up to 200 mg (2–5 mg/kg)
Norpramin® (desipramine)	No pediatric approval	ADHD, chronic pain	IId6	10, 25, 50, 75, 100, 150 mg	10–25 mg	100–200 mg (2–5 mg/kg)
Pamelor® (nortriptyline)	No pediatric approval	ADHD	IId6	10, 25, 50, 75 mg 10 mg/5 mL	10–25 mg	0.5–4 mg/kg, plasma level 50–175 ng/mL
Tofranil® (imipramine)	Childhood enuresis in children older than 5 yr	ADHD, depression	IId6, IIc9, 11c18/19, IIa4/5	10, 25, 50, 75, 100, 125, 150 mg	10–25 mg	75 mg

OCD, obsessive compulsive disorder; ADHD, attention deficit/hyperactivity disorder; ER, extended release.

Table 20-3. Atypical and tricyclic antidepressant side effects

Medication	Notable side effects	Management considerations
Buspar® (buspirone)	Dizziness, drowsiness, headache, nausea, vomiting	Use with caution in patients with renal of hepatic disease
Desyrel® (trazodone)	Sedation, priapism	Use for insomnia
Effexor® (venlafaxine)	Sustained hypertension	Avoid in patients with high BP
Remeron® (mirtazapine)	Sedation, increased appetite, rare agranulocytosis	Use for insomnia and poor appetite, consider monitoring CBC count
Wellbutrin® (bupropion)	Weight loss, tics, activation, lower seizure threshold	Avoid in patients with bulimia or anorexia, uncontrolled seizures, risk for seizures
All tricyclics	Increases PR, QRS, QTc; tremor, sedation, dry mouth, constipation, blurry vision, dizzy	Monitor vital signs, plasma levels and EKG; do not provide more than 1 week supply to patients at risk for overdose

QTc, corrected QT; CBC, complete blood cell; BP, blood pressure; EKG, electrocardiograph.

- *"What interventions or medications have been tried in the past?"* Confirming that therapeutic and behavioral support has been appropriately offered is often the first step. Positive and negative responses to different medications and doses might give information for the decision of what medications to consider or avoid.
VI. **Treatment.** Dosing in children is often not established. Although taking the adult dose and dividing it by 75 yields an approximate mg/kg/day dosing target, this could underestimate the dose required. It is important to consult the package insert and the clinical trial literature for more specific dosing guidelines. When dosing guidelines for psychiatric indications are not available, there may be some guidance from the dosing for other indications.
   A. **Selective serotonin reuptake inhibitors (SSRIs).** SSRIs are often chosen to treat depression and anxiety in children and adolescents. A newer formulation in this group includes escitalopram, an S-enantiomer of citalopram (Table 20-1). This group of medications requires no laboratory monitoring, and most come in liquid and pill forms. Side effects are usually minimal; however, there is a risk of manic activation and suicidal ideation, which families must closely monitor. The Food and Drug Administration (FDA) black box warning regarding the increased risk of suicide must be discussed and weighed against the adverse effects and possible risk of suicide associated with untreated depression. The SSRIs are not as toxic in overdose as tricyclic antidepressants. SSRIs generally require several weeks to reach full efficacy and should be weaned over weeks to minimize withdrawal symptoms. Cytochrome P450 interactions are common with fluoxetine, fluvoxamine, and paroxetine. Common medications with which they can interact include dextromethorphan, theophylline, phenytoin, tricyclic antidepressants, and atomoxetine.
   B. **Atypical and tricyclic antidepressants.** Several antidepressants that work via mechanisms other than selective serotonin reuptake inhibition are also widely used, though few are approved in the pediatric population (Table 20-2). Several atypical antidepressants have side effect profiles that must be carefully considered when prescribing (Table 20-3).
   C. **Antiepileptics and mood stabilizers.** This group of medications has played an increasing role in treating childhood bipolar and impulse/aggression disorders (Table 20-4). They are often well tolerated but may require combined pharmacotherapy and sometimes blood tests for monitoring (Table 20-5). Many interact with commonly used medications, such as antidepressants.
   D. **Atypical neuroleptics.** With less risk for extrapyramidal side effects than the first generation of antipsychotics, atypical neuroleptics are used with increasing frequency in children with psychosis, bipolar and disruptive behavior disorders, tic disorders, and autism (Table 20-6). However, they can have significant short- and long-term side effects, and only modest data indicate efficacy and safety. The only medications with FDA approval in children are risperidone and aripiprazole. Risperidone, olanzapine, and quetiapine are linked to weight gain, and possibly to diabetes and hyperglycemia. Electrocardiograph (EKG) changes are seen most prominently with ziprasidone, and prolactin elevation most prominently with risperidone. Clozapine (Clozaril) has significant risk of agranulocytosis, and is associated with seizures and myocarditis; it is rarely prescribed

Table 20-4. Antiepileptics and mood stabilizers

Brand name (generic)	Age and approved pediatric indications	Off-label clinical indications	Metabolism	Preparation	Start dose per day	Target dose per day or plasma level
Depakote® (divalproex sodium)	≥10 yr: epilepsy	Manic episode, mixed mania, behavioral disorders, prophylaxis of major depression	Glucuronidation, mitochondrial oxidation	125 mg sprinkles: 125, 250, 500 mg tabs; 250, 500 mg ER	10–15 mg/kg divided tid, or qd with ER	Plasma level 50–125 mg/mL
Keppra® (levetiracetam)	≥4 yr: seizures	Bipolar disorder	Not extensively metabolized	250, 500, 750, 1000 mg tabs; 500, 750 mg ER tabs; 100 mg/mL solution	5–10 mg/kg/day divided bid or tid	60 mg/kg/day
Klonopin® (clonazepam)	Panic disorder over 18 yr, seizure disorders in children	Anxiety with insomnia	IIIa, nitro-reduction in liver then excreted in urine	0.5, 1, 2 mg tabs: 0.125, 0.25, 0.5, 1, 2 mg wafers	0.01–0.03 mg/kg divided bid–tid	0.02–0.2 mg/kg
Lamictal® (lamotrigine)	Adjunct for partial seizures in children, bipolar disorder in adults	Mood stabilization, depression	Glucuronidation	25, 100, 150, 200 mg tabs; 2, 5, 25 mg chewable; 25, 50, 100, 200 mg ER; 25, 50, 100, 200 mg orally disintegrating tabs	Dosing depends on weight, age, and concomitant medications	Consult package insert for titration schedules
Lithium® (lithium carbonate)	≥12 yr: Bipolar disorder	Explosive or extreme aggression, major depression with predictors of bipolar disorder	100% bioavailability, mostly excreted by kidneys	150, 300, 600 mg caps, 300, 450 mg ER tabs; 8 mEq/5 mL,	Dose by weight	Plasma level 0.6–1.2 mEq/L
Neurontin® (gabapentin)	Adjunct for partial seizures in children older than 3 yr	Anxiety, posttraumatic stress disorder	Not metabolized	100, 300, 400 mg caps; 600, 800 mg tabs; 250 mg/ 5 mL solution	100–300 mg divided tid	400–2400 mg divided tid
Tegretol® (carbamazepine)	Childhood epilepsy	Mania, intermittent explosive disorder, rage	IIIa4	100 mg chewable; 200 mg tab; 100, 200, 400 mg ER tabs; 100 mg/5 mL suspension	7–10 mg/kg	Plasma level 8–12 mcg/mL
Topamax® (topiramate)	Partial onset seizures, or primary generalized tonic-clonic seizures and Lennox–Gastaut syndrome in children older than 2 yr	Mood stabilization	Not extensively metabolized	25, 50, 100, 200 mg tabs: 15, 25 mg sprinkles	1–3 mg/kg or 25–50 mg/day	5–9 mg/kg up to 200–400 mg
Trileptal® (oxcarbazepine)	Childhood epilepsy	Mania, intermittent explosive disorder, rage	Reduced by cytosolic liver enzymes, IIC19, IIIA4/5	150, 300, 600 mg tabs; 300 mg/5 mL suspension	8–10 mg/kg, up to 600 mg divided bid	Target dose based on weight

ER, extended release.

Table 20-5. Side effects of antiepileptics and mood stabilizers

Medication	Side effects	Management considerations
Depakote® **(divalproex sodium)**	Nausea, vomiting, pancreatitis, hepatitis, weight gain, thrombocytopenia, tremor, rash	Baseline CBC count, LFTs, BUN/Cr, EKG, follow up CBC count, LFTs, plasma level; take with meals
Keppra® **(levetiracetam)**	Drowsiness, aggression, irritability, leukopenia, neutropenia	Serum creatinine, BUN, CBC count
Klonopin® **(clonazepam)**	Headache, drowsiness, ataxia, dizziness, confusion, hepatic dysfunction, paradoxical CNS stimulation can occur	Monitor CBC count, LFTs; tolerance may develop; risk of dependence increases with duration of treatment and in those with prior history of drug or alcohol abuse
Lamictal® **(lamotrigine)**	Rash, nausea, vomiting, dizziness, ataxia, drowsiness, headaches	Monitor CBC count; discontinue if rash appears at any time given concern for SJS or TEN
Lithium® **(lithium carbonate)**	Weight gain, kidney and thyroid dysfunction; low therapeutic index	Baseline EKG, baseline and follow up thyroid and kidney function, plasma level q 1–3 mo
Neurontin® **(gabapentin)**	Disinhibition in 10%–15%	Few medication interactions, no serum monitoring
Tegretol® **(carbamazepine)**	Neutropenia, agranulocytosis, hepatitis, rash, sedation	Baseline CBC count, LFTs, TSH, EKG and follow-up CBC count, LFTs, plasma level; consider HLA-B*1502 genotype screening in patients of Asian descent prior to initiating medication as it increases risk of SJS and/or TEN
Topamax® **(topiramate)**	Weight loss	May be used to minimize weight gain
Trileptal® **(oxcarbazepine)**	Sedation, dizziness, headache, nausea, impaired concentration	Consider monitoring sodium levels; many CNS effects are dose related

CBC, complete blood cell; LFTs, liver function tests; TSH, thyroid stimulating hormone; EKG, electrocardiograph; BUN/Cr, blood urea nitrogen/creatinine; SJS, Stevens–Johnson syndrome; TEN, toxic epidermal necrolysis; CNS, central nervous system.

for children. Regular monitoring, including blood work, is recommended for all atypical neuroleptics (Table 20-7). Patients should be monitored routinely for abnormal involuntary movements; the Abnormal Involuntary Movement Scale (AIMS, see Bibliography section) is often useful. Weight should be documented prior to treatment, at 1, 2, and 3 months, and then at quarterly intervals; practitioners should consider switching to a different antipsychotic agent for weight gain ≥5% of the initial weight or other metabolic derangements. Atypical neuroleptics may interact with antidepressants and antiepileptics.

VII. Clinical pearls and pitfalls.
- "Start Low, Go Slow": Start at the lowest possible dose and increase slowly. Children may respond to a lower dose of medication than an adult needs and may have more side effects as the dose increases.
- Consider the rest of the picture: If the medication "stops working" or seems to have new side effects, ask if there are other contributors to the child's presentation, such as classroom changes, stressors at home, concomitant illness, new medications, or puberty.
- Choose medications with side effects in mind: For children who have trouble sleeping you may opt for a sedating drug, while in overweight children you may avoid medications that tend to cause weight gain.
- Read the newspapers and the journals: Pediatric psychopharmacology is a hot topic in the media, where parents often learn both valid and invalid information. New medications and new potential side effects of older medications are often well publicized, so keep on top of the field to provide top care.

Table 20-6. Atypical neuroleptics

Brand name (generic)	FDA approval in children	Off-label clinical indications	Metabolism	Preparation	Start dose per day	Target dose per day
Abilify® (aripiprazole)	≥13 yr: Schizophrenia; ≥10 yr: Bipolar	Psychosis, manic, and aggressive symptoms	IId6, IIIa4	2, 5, 10, 15, 20, 30 mg; 10, 15 mg disintegrating tab; 1 mg/mL	2–5 mg	10–30 mg/day
Clozaril® (clozapine)	No pediatric approval	Severe psychosis not responsive to other neuroleptics	Ia2, IId6, IIIa4, IIA6, IIC9, IIC19	25, 100 mg tabs	12.5 mg	up to 300 mg/day
Geodon® (ziprasidone)	No pediatric approval	Psychosis, manic, and aggressive symptoms, Tourette's syndrome	IIIa4, Ia2, IID6	20, 40, 60, 80 mg caps	20 mg bid	1–3 mg/kg up to 160 mg divided bid
Risperdal® (risperidone)	Irritability in autism; ≥13 yr: schizophrenia; ≥10 yr: bipolar	Psychosis, manic, and aggressive symptoms	IId6, IIIA4	0.25, 0.5, 1, 2, 3, 4 mg tabs; 0.5, 1, 2, 3, 4 mg orally disintegrating tabs; 1 mg/mL suspension; Long Acting form via injection	0.125–0.5 mg bid	0.5–6 mg divided bid–tid
Seroquel® (quetiapine)	No pediatric approval	Psychosis, manic, and aggressive symptoms	IIIa4, IID6	25, 50, 100, 200, 300, 400 mg tabs; 50, 150, 200, 300, 400 mg ER tabs	12.5–25 mg	25–600 mg divided bid
Zyprexa® (olanzapine)	No pediatric approval	Psychosis, manic, and aggressive symptoms	Ia2, IIIa4, IID6, IIC9	2.5, 5, 7.5, 10, 15, 20 mg tabs; 5, 10, 15, 20 mg orally disintegrating tabs	1.25–2.5 mg	2.5–20 mg divided qd–tid

ER, extended release.

Table 20-7. Monitoring parameters for atypical neuroleptics

Timeline—Months

Baseline	1	2	3	6	9	12	Ongoing
BMI	BMI	BMI	BMI	BMI	BMI	BMI	BMI (Q 3 MOS)
Blood pressure and pulse			Blood pressure and pulse	Blood pressure and pulse	Blood pressure and pulse	Blood pressure and pulse	Blood pressure and pulse (Q 3 MOS)
Neuromotor signs and symptoms			Neuromotor signs and symptoms	Neuromotor signs and symptoms	Neuromotor signs and symptoms	Neuromotor signs and symptoms	Neuromotor signs and symptoms (Q 3 MOS)
Fasting blood glucose and lipids			Fasting blood glucose and lipids		Fasting blood glucose and lipids		Fasting blood glucose and lipids (Q 6 MOS)
Electrolytes, full blood count[1], renal and liver function						Electrolytes, full blood count[1], renal and liver function	Electrolytes, full blood count[1], renal and liver function (Q 12 MOS)
Consider EKG[2]							
Consider prolactin[3]							

[1] Clozapine may require more frequent evaluation of complete blood cell count with differential.
[2] An **EKG** should be checked for patients on ziprasidone or clozapine at baseline, and if taking ziprasidone, during titration and at maximum dose.
[3] Morning **prolactin** should be checked at baseline if abnormal sexual signs or symptoms are present or at any time in which they appear.

BIBLIOGRAPHY

For parents

American Psychiatric Association and American Academy of Child and Adolescent Psychiatry. "Parents Med Guide: The Use of Medication in Treating Childhood and Adolescent Depression: Information for Patients and Families." Available at: www.parentsmedguide.org/pmg_depression. html

For professionals

Bostic JQ, Prince J, Frazier J, et al. "Pediatric Psychopharmacology Update." Available at: http://www.psychiatrictimes.com/p030988.html

Dulcan M (ed). *Helping Parents, Youth, and Teachers Understand Medications for Behavioral and Emotional Problems*. Arlington, VA: American Psychiatric Publishing, Inc, 2007.

Kutcher SP. (ed). *Practical Child and Adolescent Psychopharmacology*. New York: Cambridge University Press, 2002.

The Abnormal Movement Scale (AIMS) is available at: http://www.cqaimh.org/pdf/tool_aims.pdf

Information regarding access to many monitoring and/or screening scales can be found at: www.schoolpsychiatry.org

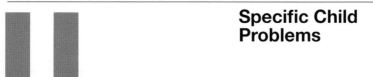

Specific Child Problems

21

Abdominal Pain

Claudio Morera

I. Description of the problem.
A. Definition.
Chronic abdominal pain (CAP) is episodic or continuous abdominal pain for at least 2 months. It might or might not interfere with daily functioning. **Recurrent abdominal pain** (RAP) is a clinical description and not a diagnosis. To avoid confusion from initial descriptions of the problem, it is better called **CAP** and it can be organic abdominal pain and **functional abdominal pain** (FAP).

B. Epidemiology.
- CAP can be 2%–4% of all pediatric visits.
- Weekly abdominal pain is reported in 13% of middle school and 17% of high school students.
- FAP prevalence in pediatric gastroenterology, using very strict criteria, has been reported in 7.5%.

C. Etiology.
1. **Organic abdominal pain.** Although the list of possible etiologies is large, only 10%–25% of children presenting with CAP have an identifiable organic etiology. **Table 21-1 shows a list of disorders that can present as CAP that can mimic FAP.**
2. **FAP.** FAP is the main cause of CAP in the pediatric age group. It used to be an exclusion diagnosis; currently diagnostic criteria have been developed that allows a positive diagnosis. A combined interaction of altered gastrointestinal (GI) motility, visceral perception, and psychological factors is the main pathophysiologic mechanism. The biopsychosocial model provides the conceptual basis to FAP, including such potential etiologies as genetics, postinfectious, certain foods like sorbitol and other carbohydrates, psychological stress, school stress, other anxiety, etc. The concept of health and disease as well as coping skills also may play a role. Parents of patients with FAP have more GI complaints, anxiety, and somatization. Their understanding and acceptance of the biopsychosocial concept is associated with recovery.

II. Making the diagnosis of FAP.
The main purpose is to establish the diagnosis of FAP, which was an exclusion diagnosis, but clinical diagnostic criteria have been developed to make a positive diagnosis of FAP with minimal workup (Rome III Criteria, Table 21-2)

A. Signs and symptoms.
The abdominal pain is typically periumbilical, lasts 30–60 minutes, and occurs during the day (rarely awakening the child from sleep). It might or might not be associated with alterations in daily functioning. In most cases, the pain pattern cannot differentiate organic from functional, but the presence of red flags (Table 21-3) has a high positive predictive value for organic disease.

If there is some loss of daily functioning and additional somatic symptoms (headaches, limb pain, or difficulty sleeping), FAP syndrome is present.

B. Differential diagnosis.
The initial differentiation is between organic and FAP. Other functional bowel disorders associated with pain should also be considered, that is, irritable bowel syndrome, abdominal migraine, functional dyspepsia, etc.

C. History: key clinical questions.
1. *"When did the abdominal pain begin? How often does it occur? Where does it hurt? Has the child locate the area by pointing with one finger?"* Establish origin point in time (at least 2 months), frequency (at least once a week), and localization.
2. *"Has there been weight loss?"* Investigation of red flags.
3. *"How is the stooling pattern?"* Constipation or diarrhea must be investigated as a potential red flag as well as other functional GI disorder like irritable bowel syndrome.
4. [To both parent and child] *"What do you think is going on? What do you do when the pain starts or to control it? How does it interfere with daily functioning, school missing, etc? Are there similar symptoms or other functional disorders in family members?"* It is important to start with open questions and let both parents and patient elaborate. We need to determine how much the symptoms impair functioning, what is the reward system in the family, what behaviors are reinforced (health or disease), what are

Table 21-1. Organic abdominal pain that can mimic functional

- Carbohydrate malabsorption
- Parasitic (Giardia)
- IBD
- Constipation
- Allergic enteropathy
- Celiac disease
- Antibiotic-associated diarrhea
- Peptic ulcer
- GERD
- Eosinophilic esophagitis
- Crohn's disease
- Cholelithiasis
- Pancreatitis

IBD, inflammatory bowel disease; GERD, gastroesophageal reflux disease.

the fears and prior experiences with chronic pains. The objective is to understand the family concept of health and disease, their understanding of the biopsychosocial concept of disease, coping skills, and presence of anxiety, depression or somatization in the family as well as in the child

D. **Behavioral observations.** Observe parent–child interaction (is the patient allowed to answer questions, is he or she treated as if he or she was younger, etc?) and reaction to pain complaints. Observe developmental state of the patient as well as body posture, dressing, etc.

E. **Physical examination.** A complete physical examination is essential. Any area not examined at this time should be clearly noted so it can be examined in the future.

F. **Laboratory evaluation.** If the history and physical examination suggest a specific etiology, appropriate tests should be ordered. Otherwise, the initial laboratory evaluation should be quite limited and is oriented to rule out most organic conditions (Table 21-4).

III. **Management.**

A. **Objectives.** Identify and treat organic diseases producing CAP, decrease pain, and modulate the impact of chronic pain in daily functioning. These are met by a thorough clinical evaluation and the establishment of a clear management and treatment plan with realistic expectations with the patient and the family.

B. **Initial treatment strategies.**

1. **Education.** On the initial evaluation, the clinician should explain that most children will not have an identifiable organic etiology for their pain and will fulfill the criteria for FAP. The clinician should explain that the objective of the initial visits is to find organic disease, if present, and to manage the symptoms with available interventions. Explain the interaction between GI motility, enhanced sensation, and psychological factors including anxiety. It is important to explain that FAP is better understood using a biopsychosocial model. Close to 75% of children whose parents understood and accepted the psychological component improved their symptoms.

2. **Medication.** In most patients the initial visit is enough to establish a positive diagnosis of FAP, to order a minimal workup plan, and to design a management plan.

   Famotidine: In a double-blind placebo-controlled trial in patients with FAP and dyspeptic symptoms using famotidine (H2 blocker) at 0.5 mg/kg twice a day 68% of patients in the treatment group improved versus 12% in the placebo group.

   Migraine medication: (See Chapter 49) For patients with FAP and diagnosis of abdominal migraine.

Table 21-2. Diagnostic criteria for childhood functional abdominal pain

Criteria fulfilled at least once per week for at least 2 months before diagnosis
Must include all the following:

- Episodic or continuous abdominal pain.
- Insufficient criteria for other functional gastrointestinal disorders.
- No evidence of an inflammatory, anatomic, metabolic, or neoplastic process that explains the subject's symptoms.
- If some loss of daily functioning and additional somatic symptoms (headaches, limb pain, or difficulty sleeping) functional abdominal pain syndrome is present.

Table 21-3. Red flags

- Involuntary weight loss
- Decreased linear growth
- Pubertal delay
- Significant vomiting
- GI blood loss
- Chronic diarrhea
- Anemia
- Persistent pain in right upper abdomen or right lower abdomen
- Nocturnal pain. Pain awakening the child at night
- Dysphagia
- Arthritis
- Perianal disease
- Unexplained fever
- Dysuria
- Inflammation signs (elevated ESR, elevated CRP, etc)
- Family history of inflammatory bowel disease or peptic ulcer disease

ESR, erythrocyte sedimentation rate; CRP, C-reactive protein

3. **Diet.**
   Fiber: The evidence supporting the use of fiber to treat FAP is weak and inconclusive. On the other hand, it is an inexpensive intervention that might benefit some patients. The recommended dose of daily intake is the age in years after 2 years of age plus 5–10 g. Adult recommended dose is 30 g/day. It can be provided through diet or by adding extra fiber supplements.

   Lactose: There is inconclusive evidence that a lactose-free diet decreases symptoms in children with FAP. Two studies have compared lactose-free diet with lactose-containing diet. There were no differences in rate of recovery or increased pain in lactose digesters versus lactose non-digesters. Lactose intolerance and FAP seem to be two different entities.

4. **Behavioral interventions.** There have been several trials of cognitive-behavioral therapy and they provide evidence that it may be useful in improving pain and disability. Programs include reinforcement of well behavior, distraction, cognitive coping skills training like self-efficacy statements, self-induced relaxation, and self-administration of rewards. The training is directed to both patients and parents. Adding behavioral intervention to the use of fiber has been shown to offer better results to fiber alone.

5. **Parents' role.** As stated before, caretakers play a key role in the management of pediatric FAP. Cognitive-behavioral interventions are reinforced by the parents so it is essential that they understand and accept the psychological component of FAP to improve outcome. Also they report the presence of red flag symptoms and should be instructed to recognize and report them to the clinician.

C. **Back-up strategies.** Since the pain of FAP can persist even after initial interventions, it is essential for the clinician to remain vigilant for an etiologic cause and not to be discouraged. Support and reinforcement of the functional nature of the condition is vital. We are aiming for care and control rather than cure, using a similar approach of coping as it is used for other chronic conditions. It is also important to understand that failing

Table 21-4. Initial workup

Complete physical examination—including rectal examination, examination of spine, and neurologic examination

Initial laboratory examination
    Urinalysis (culture in females)
    CBC count, erythrocyte sedimentation rate (ESR), and C-reactive protein (CRP)
    Liver and kidney profiles
    Stool for ova and parasites

Lactose breath test (if suggested by history and physical)

Abdominal ultrasound (if suggested by history and physical)

CBC, complete blood cell.

to find an organic cause or failure of control with initial management does not mean that FAP is not the diagnosis. Do not transmit your uncertainty to the patient by escalating diagnostic tests; rather refer to a specialist *"not because I don't know what you have but to have specialized management."*

IV. Clinical pearls and pitfalls.
- There is no substitute for a complete and thorough initial history and physical examination. Unnecessary laboratory and radiologic tests often lead parents to believe that there is an organic etiology for the abdominal pain. Clinical criteria and minimal negative initial workup (Table 21-4) are enough to diagnose FAP.
- Explain to the child that abdominal pain is common in children of their age and that the pain does not mean that there is something wrong.
- It is important for parents to understand that the pain is a product of a combination of physiological and psychological stressors with no one more important than the other.
- Keep close follow up. Initially, monthly visits and more frequent phone follow-up calls are advisable. It reinforces the idea that you are not ignoring the pain and also help coaching the behavioral interventions.
- Do not discourage second opinions or referral to specialist if a family is uncomfortable with your evaluation of their child's abdominal pain. Offer options of specialists, which you consider have a reasonable approach to FAP and discourage "doctor shopping."
- If FAP syndrome is present (FAP with other somatic symptoms, see Table 21-2) refer the child to a specialist (gastroenterologist or mental health professional) who has an expertise in the management of these conditions.

BIBLIOGRAPHY

Chogle A, Saps M. Environmental factors of abdominal pain. *Pediatr Ann* 38:396–400, 2009.

Crushell E, Rowland M, Doherty M, et al. Importance of parental conceptual model of illness in severe recurrent abdominal pain. *Pediatrics* 112:1368–1372, 2003.

DiLorenzo C, Coletti R, Lehmann H, et al. American Academy of Pediatrics Subcommittee on Chronic Abdominal Pain and NASPGHAN Committee on Abdominal Pain. Clinical report. Chronic abdominal pain in children: a clinical report of the American Academy of Pediatrics and the North American Society for Pediatric Gastroenterology, Hepatology and Nutrition. *J Pediatr Gastroenterol Nutr* 40:245–248, 2005.

DiLorenzo C, Coletti R, Lehmann H, et al. American Academy of Pediatrics Subcommittee on Chronic Abdominal Pain and NASPGHAN Committee on Abdominal Pain. Technical report. Chronic abdominal pain in children: a technical report of the American Academy of Pediatrics and the North American Society for Pediatric Gastroenterology, Hepatology and Nutrition. *J Pediatr Gastroenterol Nutr* 40:249–261, 2005.

Huertas-Ceballos AA, Logan S, Bennett C, et al. Pharmacological interventions for recurrent abdominal pain (RAP) and irritable bowel syndrome (IBS) in childhood. *Cochrane Database Syst Rev* (1), 2008. Art. No.: CD003017. DOI: 10.1002/14651858. CD003017.pub2.

Huertas-Ceballos AA, Logan S, Bennett C, et al. Psychosocial interventions for recurrent abdominal pain (RAP) and irritable bowel syndrome (IBS) in childhood. *Cochrane Database Syst Rev* (1), 2008. Art. No.: CD003014. DOI: 10.1002/14651858. CD003014.pub2.

Rasquin A, DiLorenzo C, Forbes D, et al. Childhood functional gastrointestinal disorders: child/adolescent. *Gastroenterology* 130:1527–1537, 2006.

Weydert J, Ball T, Davis M. Systematic review of treatments for recurrent abdominal pain. *Pediatrics* 111:e1–e11, 2003.

For parents

Web sites

International Foundation for Functional gastrointestinal Disorders IFFGD: http://www.iffgd. org/site/gi-disorders/kids-teens

22

Anorexia Nervosa and Bulimia Nervosa

Angela S. Guarda
Alain Joffe

I. **Description of the problem.** Anorexia nervosa and bulimia are clinical syndromes belonging to a spectrum of conditions best understood as disorders of dieting behavior. The two key characteristics common to both diagnoses are (1) **morbid fear of fatness** coupled with (2) a **disturbance in eating habits** comprising one or more behaviors concerned with the consumption or disposal of ingested calories. These behaviors include restricting intake, binge eating, excessive exercise, self-induced vomiting, and/or laxative/diuretic/diet pill abuse. The main distinction between anorexia nervosa and bulimia is ultimately weight, with anorexia being defined by underweight.

- Patients with anorexia nervosa have a body weight that is at least 15% below ideal body weight or fail to gain the amount of weight normally expected during the pubertal growth spurt. The term anorexia nervosa is a misnomer, since it implies lack of appetite, which is not a symptom of this condition. Although patients may deny hunger in their attempts to rationalize their dieting behavior, they are constantly preoccupied with thoughts about food and weight. Hypothalamic amenorrhea is also a prominent finding and a consequence of starvation. The applicability of this criterion to younger adolescents who may have not yet achieved menarche or who normally have irregular periods is problematic. Recent data suggest that the presence or absence of amenorrhea does not correlate with severity or prognosis and is not a useful diagnostic criterion. Besides restricting calories and exercising excessively, a subset of anorectics also binge and may vomit or abuse laxatives and diuretics. This purging anorectic subgroup tends to have a worse prognosis and is at higher risk of morbidity.
- All patients with bulimia nervosa engage in binge eating, characterized by the ingestion over a 2-hour period of an amount of food that is distinctly greater than the amount most individuals would consume under similar circumstances. These binge eating episodes are accompanied by feelings of guilt and lack of control. Patients with bulimia nervosa are further subdivided according to whether or not they purge in an attempt to prevent weight gain. Purging behaviors include self-induced vomiting or use of laxatives, diuretics, or enemas. Patients with bulimia who do not purge alternate periods of bingeing with severe dietary restriction and/or excessive exercise.

A. **Epidemiology.**
- It is estimated that up to 1% of young females may have anorexia nervosa. Adolescent onset between the ages of 12–18 years is found in 50% of cases.
- Approximately 2%–3% of late adolescent and young adult females meet psychiatric diagnostic criteria for bulimia nervosa, with age of onset (approximately 18 years) being slightly older than that for anorexia. A brief period of anorexia nervosa often precedes the onset of bulimia and bingeing behavior with associated weight gain.
- Males account for at least 10% of individuals with eating disorders.
- Both disorders are seen across all racial, ethnic, and socioeconomic groups. Overall, however, higher rates of eating disorders characterized by restricting and low weight are seen in Caucasian women and higher rates of bingeing and high weight are seen amongst African American women.

B. **Genetics.**
1. The concordance rate for anorexia nervosa among monozygotic twins is 55% (vs. 7% for dizygotic pairs), suggesting a genetic basis for this syndrome. First-degree relatives of probands are eight times more likely to develop anorexia than are first-degree relatives of healthy controls. The heritability of anorexia nervosa is estimated to be 33%–84%.
2. The concordance rate for monozygotic twins with bulimia (22.9%) is higher than that for dizygotic pairs (8.7%). The heritability of bulimia nervosa is estimated to be 28%–83%. This is high for a psychiatric condition and indicates that individual genetic vulnerability to an eating disorder is a significant predisposing factor.

C. **Etiology.** There is no single cause for an eating disorder. Factors that may precipitate its onset or contribute to sustaining an eating disorder are the following:

1. **Sociocultural.** Our society places a high premium on being thin, especially for women. Thinness is often equated, implicitly or explicitly, with success, attractiveness, and self-control. Not surprisingly, women in professions in which thinness is prized, such as models or ballet dancers, have higher rates of eating disorders.

2. **Physiologic.** During female puberty, there is a widening of the hips and increased deposition of adipose tissue. These normal changes run counter to pervasive socio-cultural pressures for thinness that target female adolescents. This may lead to a preoccupation with weight and a dissatisfaction with one's emerging body shape. The preponderance of affected females versus males also suggests that the estrogenic hormonal milieu may play a role in the onset of eating disorders.

   Patients with anorexia nervosa and/or bulimia nervosa have been shown to have multiple metabolic, hormonal, and neurotransmitter abnormalities. However, most of the abnormalities result from starvation or from the purging behaviors associated with eating disorders, thereby precluding a straightforward cause and effect relationship from being established. Some of these secondary abnormalities, however, for example, delayed gastric emptying or preoccupation with food secondary to starvation, are believed to contribute to sustaining the disordered eating behavior.

3. **Developmental.** Predisposing adolescents to the development of eating disorders are such temperamental or personality factors as being introverted, perfectionist, self-critical, or eager to please. Patients who primarily restrict calories tend to be risk-avoidant. In contrast, those who binge and purge may be self-injurious or display impulsive behaviors such as substance abuse, sexual promiscuity, and shoplifting.

   Adolescence is a time of great physiological, psychological, and sociocultural change. Adapting to a markedly changed body, developing a personal and sexual identity, and separation from parents are all important developmental tasks. At this time, adolescents who are otherwise vulnerable to the development of an eating disorder are particularly sensitive to comments about being too fat and to media images that portray thinness as the ideal of beauty, sexual attractiveness, and selfcontrol.

4. **Familial.** Families of patients with eating disorders have been characterized as either hostile and chaotic or overly enmeshed and rigid. However, ongoing research indicates that many characteristics associated with families of patients with eating disorder are also typical of families of chronically ill children, suggesting that these patterns of interaction are a consequence rather than a cause of the illness.

II. **Making the diagnosis.**

A. **Signs and symptoms.** Young women rarely disclose an eating disorder to their primary care clinician. Just as patients with anorexia deny hunger as they pursue the ideal body shape, so too will they ignore or cover up various manifestations of their illness. They may wear bulky clothing in an attempt to hide their weight loss, deny fear of fatness, or be quite secretive about their bingeing, vomiting, or abuse of laxatives or diuretics. Hence, the clinician must maintain a high index of suspicion and gently but firmly pursue the diagnosis when symptoms suggest or are consistent with an eating disorder.

The signs and symptoms associated with eating disorders are highlighted in Table 22-1. What is apparent on physical examination is a function of whether the patient is starving herself to the point of being significantly underweight and/or whether she uses purging techniques to control her weight. Girls who develop anorexia nervosa prior to the onset of or early in puberty will present with failure to gain the weight normally expected with physical maturation or with delayed onset of secondary sexual characteristics or primary amenorrhea.

B. **Differential diagnosis.** In developing a differential diagnosis, clinicians should remember that patients with illnesses whose signs and symptoms are similar to anorexia nervosa and bulimia generally indicate discomfort with these manifestations and do not have a persistent and overriding concern with body shape and weight. While they may, initially, be pleased with a limited amount of unexpected weight loss, they become alarmed as their weight continues to fall. They do not exclusively limit fat and calories and concerns about weight and body shape do not preoccupy them to the exclusion of all else. Diseases that can mimic these disorders are listed in Table 22-2. A thorough history that addresses all aspects of an adolescent's life (HEADSS: Homelife, Education, Activities/Affect (e.g., mood), Drug use, Sexuality/sexual behaviors, and Suicidal thoughts/actions), a careful physical examination and perhaps a few screening laboratory tests (such as an erythrocyte sedimentation rate (ESR), stool for occult blood, and thyroid-stimulating hormone (TSH)) are generally sufficient to exclude these diagnoses.

Table 22-1. Signs and symptoms of eating disorders

	Associated with starvation	Associated with purging
General	Hyperactivity or lethargy Irritability Sleep problems Dizziness, confusion Syncope Hypothermia	Dizziness, syncope Confusion
Skin	Subcutaneous fat loss Dry, brittle hair or loss of hair Lanugo hair on torso or face Yellow skin	Ulcerations, scars, or calluses on back of hand over knuckles Perioral acne
Oral		Dental caries Enamel erosion or discoloration of teeth (lingual surface) Parotid gland hypertrophy
Cardiovascular	Hypotension Bradycardia	Arrhythmias
Gastrointestinal	Constipation Decreased bowel sounds	Epigastric tenderness Gastroesophageal reflux Abdominal distension Ileus
Neuromuscular	Muscle weakness/wasting	Muscle weakness, paresthesias
Extremities	Decreased deep tendon reflexes cold, mottled hands and feet	Decreased deep tendon reflexes
Genitourinary	Thin, pale, dry, atrophic vaginal mucosa, amenorrhea, low libido	Edema of feet
Musculoskeletal	Osteopenia/fractures	

Note: Patients who are malnourished and engaged in purging behaviors will display signs and symptoms from both columns.

    C. History: key clinical questions. Clinicians should focus their questions in the following areas:
- weight and dietary history
- extreme concerns about being fat and dissatisfaction with body shape
- methods used to lose weight or prevent weight gain, including exercise patterns and details of bingeing and purging episodes
- symptoms of a concomitant affective disorder
- use of drugs and alcohol.

Table 22-2. Differential diagnosis of eating disorders

CNS	Hypothalamic disorders (e.g., brain tumor)
Endocrine	Addison's disease
	Diabetes mellitus
	Hyperthyroidism
Gastrointestinal inflammatory bowel disease	Achalasia Malabsorption syndromes (celiac disease)
Immunologic	Systemic lupus erythematosus
Gynecologic	Pregnancy
Psychiatric	Depression Thought disorders
Miscellaneous	Any detected malignancy Drug abuse (e.g., amphetamines, alcohol)

CNS, central nervous system.

1. **How do you feel about your current weight? What would you like to weigh?** Begins to elicit information about fear of fatness and body shape dissatisfaction (e.g., feeling fat or wanting to lose "just a few more pounds" even when the teenager appears emaciated).

2. **What is the most and least you have ever weighed since puberty began and how old were you at each of those times?** (For prepubertal girls: what is the least/most you have weighed in the last few years?) Establishes baseline measurements and reflects degree of weight loss. Updating of growth charts is essential.

3. **Tell me what you ate for breakfast, lunch, dinner, and snacks yesterday and was this a typical day for you?** Establishes caloric intake, meal patterns, and food preferences and helps indicate distorted thoughts about food or restriction of food repertoire to low-calorie, low-fat choices. Information must be obtained in great detail (e.g., what was on the sandwich? how much of it was eaten?).

4. **Tell me about your exercise routine. How many hours do you spend exercising in the average week? Have you increased the amount of exercise you do lately?** Patients with eating disorders will often exercise intensely as a way to increase caloric expenditure and/or to compensate for binge eating episodes. Information about the specific types and duration of exercise should be elicited. Solitary aerobic exercise is often favored over team sports.

5. **How often do you weigh yourself?** Frequencies greater than once daily indicate an overpreoccupation with body weight.

6. **How would you generally describe your mood—happy, sad, down, etc.? How did you feel last year?** Depression is commonly associated with eating disorders, either as a primary or secondary phenomenon since starvation induces a syndrome of depression. Screening questions about sleep problems; decreased concentration; fatigue; loss of interest in usual activities; frequent crying; and feelings of self-blame, guilt, or suicidal behavior should be covered.

7. **Which of the following have you used to control your weight: laxatives/enemas, water pills (diuretics), diet pills?** These represent commonly used weight loss methods. Any positive answers should be followed up with questions about frequency of use and amounts used.

8. **How often do you binge eat? Tell me exactly what you ate during your last binge?** A true binge includes consumption of large quantities of food, often several thousand or more calories. In contrast, some young women mistakenly interpret eating a few cookies or an ice cream sundae as a binge. During a binge episode, food is usually consumed quickly and while alone.

9. **How do you feel before and after you binge? Are there situations or feelings that trigger binge episodes?** Binge eating typically is associated with feelings of lack of control, self-deprecating thoughts, and guilt. Binges are often triggered by specific feelings such as being disappointed, feeling criticized, lonely, or bored.

10. **How often do you vomit after a binge episode? Do you need to gag yourself to vomit?** These questions elicit details of the binge/purge cycle. Some patients with bulimia have lost their gag reflex and may be able to spontaneously vomit or regurgitate food at will.

D. **Behavioral observations.** While eliciting the history, it is important to note the patient's general affect and willingness to answer questions directly. Patients with eating disorders often minimize their symptoms. They typically show little concern for a degree of weight loss that others would find alarming and are ambivalent about entering treatment. The interviewer should note the quality of interactions between patient and family, such as who answers questions and how family members regard each other. It is often helpful to initially interview the adolescent alone to build rapport and trust and later to obtain a collateral history from parents without the patient in the room.

E. **Physical examination.** Key aspects of the physical examination are noted in Table 22-1. Severely anorectic patients with a greater degree of weight loss will display more of these features, especially if they also binge and purge. Conversely, patients with bulimia alone may display few physical findings and be of normal weight or above. Patients must be undressed completely (except for a gown and underpants) to accurately assess their physical condition. Examination of the breasts and external genitalia (pubic hair development, testicular size) to assess sexual maturity rating should also be performed; a pelvic examination may also be indicated for adolescents who are sexually active.

F. **Tests.** Patients with severe anorexia nervosa or bulimia are likely to have several abnormal laboratory test results, but it is not essential to identify all of them. Table 22-3 includes the most commonly noted abnormalities that can help to confirm or eliminate the diagnosis or identify potentially life-threatening conditions. However, in the presence

Table 22-3. Laboratory values in eating disorders

Hematologic	Anemia (mild)
	Leukopenia
	Thrombocytopenia
Endocrine	Follicle-stimulating hormone/luteinizing hormone: low/low normal
	Thyroxine/thyroid-stimulating hormone: low/low normal
	Elevated cortisol (in starvation)
GI	SGOT/SGPT normal or elevated
	Salivary amylase increased (in vomiting)
Renal	BUN normal or elevated
	Urine pH >7
	Urine-specific gravity normal or elevated (may also be very low in anorectic patients who drink excessive water).
Metabolic	Metabolic alkalosis
	Decreased Na^+, K^+, Cl^-
	Ca^{++} normal or low
	Mg^{++}, PO_4 normal or low
	Increased CO_2
ECG	Low voltage
	Bradycardia
	Depressed T waves
	Prolonged QTc interval

GI, gastrointestinal tract; SGOT, serum glutamic oxaloacetic transaminase; SGPT, serum glutamic pyruvic transaminase; BUN, blood urea nitrogen; ECG, electrocardiogram.

of the classic syndrome of anorexia nervosa or of bulimia marked by fear of fatness and dieting behavior, an exhaustive diagnostic workup is generally not indicated. Gastrointestinal complaints are common among such patients and almost always remit with behavioral treatment.

III. Management

A. Primary goals.
Restoration of weight is the primary goal in the treatment of patients with anorexia nervosa. Until this goal is achieved, patients may not benefit from other therapeutic modalities as a result of the intense preoccupation with food and weight and depressive symptoms sustained by their starved state. For patients with bingeing and purging behaviors, normalization of eating behavior and cognitive behavioral therapy including maintenance of a food log and identification of triggers for bingeing are initial goals. Other goals for patients with eating disorders include the following:

- education about nutrition based on the food pyramid and eating three regular meals daily
- improvement in personal, social, and family functioning
- correction of medical complications
- treatment of comorbid psychiatric conditions (e.g., depression, anxiety disorders, drug and alcohol abuse)
- parent training. Empirical evidence suggests that family therapy aimed at training parents to refeed their child and help him or her to block his or her eating disorder behavior is more effective than individual treatment.

B. Treatment.
Management of a young woman with an eating disorder depends on a number of factors: the stage of the illness at which the patient is diagnosed; the primary behaviors employed to control weight and their intensity; the clinician's assessment of the family dynamics and the level of support likely to be offered by her family; the presence of a concomitant affective disorder and/or substance abuse problem; and, finally, the skill level of the clinician in working with these patients. In general, younger patients with supportive families and recent onset of the eating disorder without significant comorbidity can be effectively managed by the primary care clinician on an outpatient basis.

The optimal outpatient treatment of most patients occurs with a multidisciplinary treatment team consisting of a pediatric clinician, nutritionist, mental health worker, and nurse. More complicated patients, those who fail to gain weight after 1–2 months of outpatient therapy or those with a long-standing eating disorder will likely require

Table 22-4. Indications for psychiatric hospitalization

Weight less than 60% of normal weight for height
Continued weight loss or failure to gain weight in anorexia nervosa or to decrease binge-purge behavior in bulimia following 2–3 months of outpatient treatment
Cardiovascular compromise
  Cardiac arrhythmias
    Bradycardia (slower than 40–50 bpm)
    QTc prolongation >500 ms
  Postural hypotension with presyncopal symptoms or systolic blood pressure less than 70 mm Hg
Hypothermia (<36°C)
Significant dehydration
Electrolyte disturbances (e.g., K⁺ <2.5 mEq/L, metabolic alkalosis)

Electrolyte disturbances (e.g., K^+ <2.5 mEq/L, metabolic alkalosis)
Severe psychiatric symptoms, e.g., comorbid depression or anxiety or substance abuse
Suicidal ideation or recurrent self-injurious behavior

admission to a specialty inpatient treatment program. Immediate hospitalization is necessary if any of the conditions in Table 22-4 are present.

The primary care clinician is ideally suited to serve as coordinator of the treatment process. Often, he/she has a long-standing relationship with the patient and her family and can explain the nature and severity of the illness. The clinician can also assume the role of monitoring weight gain and the potential medical complications of the illness (such as amenorrhea or hypokalemia).

1. **Weight gain.** Patients should be weighed weekly dressed in a gown and underpants only. They should urinate before being weighed since water loading is often used by patients to artificially raise their weight and can be detected by checking urine specific gravity. The goal should be a slow, steady gain of 1–2 pounds per week. The target weight should be the 50th percentile for the patient's height and pubertal development. Restoration of menses is a reliable indicator that an appropriate weight threshold has been achieved. Patients usually tolerate an initial caloric intake of 1500–2000 kcal/day, with increments of 500 kcal per week until the patient gains at least 1 pound per week. Weight gain usually occurs once the adolescent consumes 3000–4000 kcal/day; 1000 kcal of the total daily intake may need to be provided in a liquid supplement form, for example, as three 350 cal supplements daily between meals. It will be necessary for the clinician or nutritionist to be very specific about what kinds of foods the young woman will need to eat to reach her daily caloric requirements. Many young women with eating disorders have developed a list of "forbidden" foods and will need considerable firm, concrete instruction and support in changing their diet and in broadening their food repertoire. Parents should be instructed to select the menu during the early treatment phase. A family therapy approach developed in England at the Maudsley Hospital and adapted by Locke and Le Grange uses a highly prescriptive 20-session family therapy program to put parents in control of their son's or daughter's nutrition and exercise (sessions 1–10) and then gradually returns control to the adolescent (sessions 11–20).

2. Restrictions on activities and privileges are necessary for underweight patients, both as a means of assuring the child's safety and because patients are unlikely to gain weight if permitted to exercise. In most cases, no exercise should be permitted until the goal weight is achieved.

3. **Body image.** Much of the ongoing treatment will revolve around addressing the young woman's concerns about her body shape and fear of fatness. The clinician can review with her what happens to a young woman's body as she matures (e.g., the hips widen) and that these changes do not indicate that the patient is becoming fat. Many young women find it helpful to know that their peers are struggling with the same issues and that our society creates unreasonable expectations for them in terms of defining characteristics for physical attractiveness and success. Finally, it may help to remind patients and families that body image improves last and often lags behind normalization of eating behavior by 3–6 months, but that it will improve if the patient's behavior changes.

4. **Nutrition.** In conjunction with the nutritionist, the role of proper nutrition as critical to appropriate physiologic functioning should be stressed. Since many patients with eating disorders are concerned with athletics, it may be helpful to indicate that optimal

performance requires adequate intake of essential nutrients. Many adolescents (and their parents) have inaccurate information about the caloric content of various foods and the appropriate diet for a maturing adolescent. It is important to stress, for example, that a low calcium diet, coupled with a hypoestrogenic state, can lead to osteopenia that may be irreversible and that this complication occurs early, often within 6 months of the onset of amenorrhea. Many of the symptoms the patient experiences and finds distressful are due to physiologic alterations secondary to weight loss; clarifying this relationship will lend credence to the team's insistence on weight gain. The importance of choosing foods following the food pyramid guide should be stressed. Some fat should be consumed with each meal (in a society that emphasizes no-fat foods, teenagers may not be aware of the importance of some dietary fat to the body's normal functioning) and no diet, fat-free or sugarless products should be eaten until the target weight is achieved.

5. **Purging.** Teenagers may not be aware that self-induced vomiting or regular use of diuretics or laxatives primarily results in water weight loss rather than true weight loss yet can induce dehydration or a variety of life-threatening complications. The clinician should routinely ask if patients have used or are using any of these products or to what extent they are purging. Hypokalemia (serum K^+ <3.0 mEq/dL) suggests a patient is vomiting at least daily and is potentially life threatening. Most deaths in eating disorders arise from cardiac arrhythmias due to electrolyte imbalances.

6. Family dynamics and problems that contribute to the eating disorder must also be assessed. Treatment goals and expectations among team members and the family must be clear so that the patient, family members, and members of the treatment team are not pitted one against another. Again, the clinician can play a critical role in coordinating these treatment efforts and assuring that everyone is in agreement with treatment plans. Family therapy is an essential component of the treatment for eating disorders among adolescents and has been shown to be more effective than individual therapy alone.

7. Medications, such as the serotonergic reuptake inhibitors, have been found to be helpful in decreasing episodes of bingeing and purging in bulimia; however, no medication has been found to be useful in achieving weight gain among patients with anorexia. Serotonergic antidepressants may be helpful in patients with comorbid anxiety and depressive disorders but usually will not be effective unless the starved state is reversed. Hormonal treatment to induce or regulate menses has not been demonstrated to be effective in preventing osteopenia; furthermore, it eliminates an important marker for gauging the adequacy of weight gain and may falsely reassure a young woman that "everything is okay" while rendering her more anemic. Refeeding and weight gain will usually result in resumption of menses and halt bone loss.

BIBLIOGRAPHY

For parents and patients

American College Health Association. Eating disorders: what everyone should know. http://www.acha.org/

ETR Associates. "Eating disorders—what? why?", "Dieting—what's normal? what's not?", "Food and feelings," among others. 1-800-321-4407. www.etr.org. Geared towards teenagers and young adults.

The National Institute of Mental Health. Eating disorders. http://www.nimh.nih.gov/health/publications/eating-disorders/index.shtml

Katzman D, Pinhas L. *Help for Eating Disorders: A Parent's Guide to Symptoms, Causes, and Treatments.* Toronto, Canada: Robert Rose, 2005.

Locke J, Le Grange D. *Help Your Teenager Beat an Eating Disorder*. New York: The Guilford Press, 2004.

Eating Disorders. www.bulimia.com (includes a variety of resources for parents and also lists treatment centers in the United States and Canada).

National organizations

National Eating Disorders Association (NEDA). www.edap.org

Eating Disorders Coalition for Research, Policy and Action. http://www.anad.org/

National Association of Anorexia Nervosa and Associated Eating Disorders (ANAD). http://www.anad.org/

Maudsley Parents. A site for parents of eating disordered children, http://www.maudsleyparents.org/

Academy for Eating Disorders. http://www.aedweb.org/index.cfm; includes videos for parents http://www.aedweb.org/video/parents.cfm

For professionals

American Dietetic Association. Nutrition intervention in the treatment of anorexia nervosa, bulimia nervosa, and other eating disorders. *J Am Diet Assoc* 106(12):2073–2082, 2006.

American Psychiatric Association (APA). *Practice Guideline for the Treatment of Patients with Eating Disorders* (3rd ed). Washington, DC: American Psychiatric Association, 2006.

Calero-Elvira A, Krug I, Davis K, et al. Meta-analysis on drugs in people with eating disorders. *Eur Eat Disord Rev* 17:243–259, 2009.

Claudino AM, Hay P, Lima MS, et al. Antidepressants for anorexia nervosa. *Cochrane Database Syst Rev* (1):CD004365, 2006.

Golden NH, Katzman DK, Kreipe RE, et al. Eating disorders in adolescents: position paper of the Society for Adolescent Medicine. *J Adolesc Health* 33(6):496–503, 2003.

Le Grange D, Eisler I. Family interventions in adolescent anorexia nervosa. *Child Adolesc Psychiatr Clin N Am* 18:159–173, 2008.

Powers PS, Bruty H. Pharmacotherapy for eating disorders and obesity. *Child Adolesc Psychiatr Clin N Am* 18:175–187, 2008.

Rome ES, Ammerman S, Rosen DS, et al. Children and adolescents with eating disorders: the state of the art. *Pediatrics* 111(1):e98–e108, 2003.

Treasure J, Claudino AM, Zucker N. Eating disorders. *Lancet* 375:583–593, 2010. doi:10.1016/S0140-6736(09)61748-7

23 Anxiety Disorders

Marianne San Antonio
Nili E. Major

I. **Description of the problem.** Anxiety is commonly a normal part of child development. The occurrence of stranger anxiety in the first year of life is an early example of what is developmentally appropriate anxiety. Fears about monsters and the dark are common in preschool-aged children, whereas school-aged children typically worry about injury and natural events (e.g., storms). Older children and adolescents often have worries about school performance and social competence. Distinguishing among normal fears and worries, temperamental variations, and clinically significant anxiety may be challenging. However, anxiety disorders are common in the pediatric population, and efforts to identify these children should be made, as effective, evidence-based treatments are available. Anxiety disorders in children are characterized by excessive and developmentally inappropriate worry that significantly impairs the child's functioning. The context in which anxiety symptoms are produced primarily differentiates the specific anxiety disorders. Below are commonly encountered specific disorders. Other anxiety disorders such as post-traumatic stress disorder, specific phobias, and selective mutism are discussed elsewhere in this book.

A. **Anxiety disorders.**
   1. **Generalized anxiety disorder (GAD)** is characterized by chronic and excessive worry in a number of areas (e.g., schoolwork, social interactions, family, health/safety, world events) that is difficult to control.
   2. **Separation anxiety disorder (SAD)** refers to excessive and developmentally inappropriate distress experienced when separated from home or major attachment figures.
   3. **Social phobia** is characterized by feeling scared or uncomfortable in social and performance situations due to fear of embarrassment.
   4. **Obsessive compulsive disorder (OCD)** is defined by the presence of obsessions or compulsions that cause marked distress, are time consuming (occupy a child for more than 1 hour a day), or significantly interfere with the child's normal functioning.

B. **Epidemiology.** Anxiety disorders are among the most common psychiatric disorders affecting children and adolescents. The lifetime prevalence for having any anxiety disorder ranges from 6%–20% across several large-scale epidemiological studies. Anxiety disorders are typically more frequent in girls than in boys, with ratios of 2:1 to 3:1 by adolescence. Anxiety disorders may begin at any time, but more than 70% of adults diagnosed with an anxiety disorder report that their symptoms started in childhood. The average age of onset for specific anxiety disorders varies widely among studies. Likewise, the long-term course of anxiety disorders diagnosed in childhood is somewhat controversial. In general, the more severe and impairing the disorder, the more likely it is to persist. Despite the remission of some initial disorders, new anxiety disorders may emerge over time. Also, there is an increased risk for later development of other disorders, such as depression and substance abuse. Anxiety disorders are highly comorbid with other anxiety disorders, as well as with other psychiatric disorders, such as attention-deficit/hyperactivity disorder, depression, substance abuse, oppositional defiant disorder, learning disorders, and language disorders.
   1. **GAD.** Reported prevalence rates range from 3%–5%. GAD is often highly comorbid with depression, leading to some speculation as to whether they are truly distinct disorders. Children with comorbid depression often have a poorer prognosis and longer duration of symptoms.
   2. **SAD.** SAD is the only anxiety disorder considered to be specific to childhood, as its onset must occur prior to 18 years of age. Prevalence rates are estimated to be between 3% and 5%. Although SAD typically has the highest remission rate of all the anxiety disorders, it remains a risk factor for the later development of anxiety and depressive disorders.
   3. **Social phobia.** The rate of lifetime social phobia in a community sample of adolescents was found to be 1.6%. There is evidence that social phobia in adolescents is a unique risk factor for the development of subsequent substance dependence disorders.

4. **OCD.** Prevalence of OCD ranges from 1%–4% in children and adolescents. In childhood, OCD is more common in boys with a ratio of 3:2. This changes to a slight female predominance in adulthood. Tic disorders are a common comorbid condition in children with OCD.

C. **Etiology.**
   1. **Genetic.** Although there are no specifically identified genes in humans for anxiety disorders, children who have a first-degree relative with an anxiety disorder are more likely to develop one themselves. Based on twin studies, estimated genetic heritabilities are modest, falling in the range of 30%–40%. Current research is looking at candidate genes in mouse models and biochemical functioning in the amygdala as possible sources of these disorders.
   2. **Environmental.** Families can play a role in a child's development of an anxiety disorder by modeling anxious behaviors. Parents may reinforce a child's avoidant behaviors, thereby increasing their frequency. Parents who are overinvolved, controlling, or highly critical of their children may also contribute to anxiety in their children. Transitions and losses, such as moving, the death of a relative, or a parent who loses a job, can also trigger anxiety in children. It is important to keep in mind that anxiety in a child can be a red flag for significant stress or violence in the home.
   3. **Temperament.** Children with a temperamental style known as *behavioral inhibition* are at increased risk for the development of anxiety disorders, particularly social phobia. These children typically exhibit fearfulness and withdrawal when faced with new people and situations.

II. **Making the diagnosis.**
   A. **Signs and symptoms.** The various anxiety disorders discussed here often share commonalities in their presentations. Children will frequently report somatic complaints. Anger, irritability, and crying are often present when the child is confronted with the fearful stimuli and may be misconstrued as oppositional behavior. The anxiety symptoms interfere with the child's normal functioning in school, with friends, and in the home. Common clinical presentations of the individual anxiety disorders are presented below, along with specific information regarding *Diagnostic and Statistical Manual of Mental Disorders, Fourth Edition, Text Revision (DSM-IV-TR)* diagnostic criteria *(with special attention paid to differences in criteria that pertain to diagnosis in children).*
      1. **GAD.** Children with GAD have anxiety and worry about a wide range of topics that is difficult for them to control. They are often conforming perfectionists who constantly seek approval and reassurance. Anxieties may take different forms at different ages:
         - Preschool: imaginary creatures
         - 5–6 years: threats to physical well-being
         - 7–14 years: school performance, health, personal harm
         - Adolescent: social issues

         Symptoms must be present for at least 6 months. *In children, only one associated symptom listed in the DSM-IV-TR is required for diagnosis.*
      2. **SAD.** Children with SAD exhibit distress when faced with separation from major attachment figures. Parents often note that their children with SAD
         - Follow them around the house
         - Refuse to be alone to sleep or to use the bathroom
         - Often worry excessively about their parents' safety and health
         - Experience nightmares with themes of separation
         - When away from home, are extremely homesick and fear being lost
         - Refuse to go to school or to camp
         - Experience stomachaches and headaches on weekdays but not weekends

         According to *DSM-IV-TR* criteria, symptoms must be present for at least 4 weeks, and onset must be prior to 18 years of age. Although SAD is considered a childhood disorder, symptoms may be present in adults as well.
      3. **Social phobia.** Children with social phobia experience fear associated with social scrutiny in social settings such as classrooms, restaurants, and extracurricular activities. These children may have difficulty reading aloud or answering questions in class, initiating conversations, eating at restaurants, using public restrooms, and attending social events. The duration of symptoms must be at least 6 months. There are a number of clarifications in the *DSM-IV-TR* pertaining to making this diagnosis in children:
         - Children must have the ability to develop age appropriate friendships, and the anxiety must occur in peer settings as well as with adults.
         - The anxiety may be expressed by crying, tantrums, freezing, or shrinking from social situations.
         - Children do not need to recognize that the fear is excessive or unreasonable.

4. **OCD.** Children with OCD have obsessions (recurrent and intrusive thoughts, impulses or images that cause marked distress) and compulsions (repetitive behaviors or mental acts that the person feels driven to perform in response to an obsession) that take up large parts of their day and interfere with how they function both at home and at school. When these rituals are confronted or broken, tantrums frequently occur. *Children do not need to recognize that the obsessions and compulsions are excessive or unreasonable for the diagnosis to be made.*
   - Common **obsessions** seen in childhood are concerns about getting dirty or sharing germs, danger to self or family, and the need to keep things in a particular order.
   - Common **compulsions** include excessive hand washing, checking things (e.g., seeing if a door is locked), putting things in order, and counting things.
   - Diagnosis can be delayed as children may attempt to hide their symptoms for as long as possible, and parents may inadvertently compensate for their atypical behaviors. For example, parents may tolerate increasingly frequent bathroom breaks, not realizing that their children are using these times to compulsively wash their hands.
   - Children may come to medical attention because of sequelae from their ritualistic behaviors, such as eczematous changes from repeated hand washing or encopresis resulting from refusal to use public restrooms.
   - As with all of the anxiety disorders, it is necessary to distinguish developmentally appropriate behaviors (e.g., wearing a "lucky" cap for sporting events), which rarely interfere with the child's life, from more serious and impairing symptoms of OCD.

B. **Differential diagnosis.** Normal, developmentally appropriate anxiety should always be considered in the differential diagnosis.
   - **Psychiatric disorders.** A number of psychiatric disorders may present with symptoms similar to those seen in anxiety disorders and should be considered in the differential. These include the following:
     - *Attention-deficit/hyperactivity disorder*—restlessness, inattention
     - *Depression*—social withdrawal, sleep difficulty, somatic complaints, irritability
     - *Autism spectrum disorders*—social withdrawal/awkwardness, repetitive behaviors, adherence to routines
     - *Learning disabilities*—persistent worry about school, school avoidance
     - *Psychotic disorders*—restlessness, social withdrawal

     It is important to keep in mind that these disorders may often exist as comorbidities with an anxiety disorder. Likewise, it is important to assess for comorbid anxiety when considering any of these disorders as a primary diagnosis.
   - **Physical conditions and drug effects.** The clinician should consider physical conditions that may present with anxiety-like symptoms such as hyperthyroidism, asthma, migraines, seizure disorders, hypoglycemia, cardiac arrhythmias, pheochromocytoma, or central nervous system disorders. Substance use or withdrawal (cocaine, amphetamines, caffeine, alcohol, cannabis) may result in symptoms that mimic anxiety, as might side effects from prescription (stimulants, antipsychotics, steroids) and nonprescription (cold medicines, antihistamines, diet pills) medications.
   - **Psychosocial problems.** Children with symptoms of anxiety should always undergo a thorough assessment for possible psychosocial stressors including abuse, neglect, parental mental illness, and violence in the home.

C. **Key questions and useful questionnaires.** When assessing a child for the presence of an anxiety disorder, it is beneficial to obtain information from multiple sources (parents, child, teachers). Children may be more aware of their own symptoms and inner distress, whereas parents may be more perceptive of the impact the anxiety has on the child's functioning. A combination of directed interviewing and the use of standardized screening tools can be helpful in revealing types and sources of anxiety.

1. **Interview questions for children**
   - *What kinds of things do you worry about?*
   - *Do you think you worry more than other kids?*
   - *Does worrying about things get in the way of sleeping, going to school, or having friends?*
   - *For how long have these worries been bothering you?*
   - *Are you afraid that something bad will happen to your mom or dad?*
   - *Do you have nightmares about getting lost or kidnapped?*
   - *Are you scared around large groups of children, such as at birthday parties?*
   - *Are there thoughts you cannot get out of your head?*
   - *Are there things that you do repeatedly to make another worry go away?*

2. **Interview questions for parents**
   - *Would you describe your child as nervous or a worrier?*

- *What things does he worry about?*
- *How does your child's worry interfere with daily activities like school, friendships, or fun?*
- *Does anyone in the family have a history of anxiety or depression?*
- *Does your child have any difficulty falling asleep alone?*
- *Does your child complain of headaches and stomachaches on weekdays but not on weekends?*
- *Does your child worry that he or she will do something embarrassing in front of other people?*
- *Is your child afraid of meeting or talking to new people?*
- *Does your child have bad or silly thoughts or images that he or she cannot get out of his or her head?*
- *Does your child have certain habits or rituals that he or she performs over and over (e.g., washing hands, counting objects, checking the door is closed)?*

3. **Questionnaires.** There are two broad categories of questionnaires that clinicians can use to screen for anxiety disorders.
   - General behavioral/emotional screens assess for symptoms of a wide range of disorders. Some general screens that may be familiar to clinicians are the *Pediatric Symptom Checklist* (PSC), the *Behavior Assessment System for Children* (BASC), and the *NICHQ Vanderbilt Assessment Scale*.
   - Screening tools that specifically assess for symptoms of anxiety disorders are also available. Examples of anxiety specific screens are the *Screen for Child Anxiety Related Disorders* (SCARED) and the *Multidimensional Anxiety Scale for Children* (MASC). Both are available in parent and child (self-report) versions. More recently, scales have been developed to assess for anxiety in younger children, such as the *Spence Preschool Anxiety Scale*.

III. **Management.** For children with mild symptoms of anxiety and limited impairment in functioning, education, and guidance may be sufficient. For those with higher levels of symptomatology and impairment, a referral to a mental health specialist for psychotherapy, and possibly medication, should be initiated.

A. **Parent education and guidance.** The first step in management is to educate both parents and children about the disorder. The discussion should include information about the symptoms of the disorder, course, treatment options, risks of treatment, and consequences of not seeking treatment. Parents and children should be given concrete suggestions and techniques for how to deal with symptoms at home and at school. Parents should try to attend to their child's concerns and help them find names for their feelings. They can model positive coping styles and help children to prepare for anxiety-producing transitions by practicing new routines and exploring new environments. They should try not to let children restrict their daily activities because of their anxiety.

B. **Psychotherapy.**
   1. **Cognitive-behavioral therapy (CBT).** Substantial evidence exists supporting the use of CBT in the treatment of pediatric anxiety disorders. CBT is a time-limited, goal-directed therapy in which patients learn to react in a different way to situations that are anxiety producing. Children learn to manage their somatic symptoms, restructure how they think about anxiety-provoking situations, face their fears via exposure techniques, and make plans for what to do if anxiety returns. A widely utilized CBT protocol known as the Coping Cat Program consists of 14–18 sessions over 3–4 months. Given the significant role that parents and families may play in the development and maintenance of anxiety symptoms, parents are frequently involved in the CBT treatment process. There have been a number of studies that have shown added benefit when a parent component is added to child CBT, particularly if the parent is anxious herself.
   2. **Play therapy.** Play therapy may work well for young children as well as older children with language or cognitive impairments that may prevent them from participating in CBT. Therapists use toys such as animals, dolls, blocks, and puppets to help the child express their feelings and experiences through play. Most of the existing literature regarding the use of play therapy focuses on trauma-related anxiety disorders. Further studies are needed to evaluate the efficacy of play therapy in the treatment of pediatric anxiety disorders.
   3. **Group psychotherapy.** For children with social phobia, group therapy may help them to confront their fears and facilitate positive interaction with others in an accepting group of people with shared problems.

C. **Medication.** Selective serotonin reuptake inhibitors (SSRIs), such as sertraline, fluoxetine, and fluvoxamine are the first-line medications used in children with anxiety disorders. There is no evidence that a particular SSRI is more effective than another in treating pediatric anxiety disorders. It may take 4 weeks to see an effect; if no effect is seen at that time, consider slowly increasing the dose. If a child has been stable for at least a year, a trial off of medication can be attempted (best done during a low-stress period such as summer vacation) (see Chapter 20). Of note, in February 2004 the FDA issued a black box warning on the use of SSRIs in pediatric patients due to studies that showed a small increased risk of suicidal ideation and behavior in patients with depression taking these medications. This has not been studied specifically in patients with anxiety. It is particularly important to monitor closely for these symptoms in the first 4 weeks of treatment. A recent randomized, controlled trial conducted in children with SAD, GAD, and social phobia showed that both sertraline and CBT were equally effective in reducing symptoms of anxiety compared with placebo, while a combination of CBT and sertraline was superior to either therapy alone. Other medications used in the treatment of pediatric anxiety disorders include venlafaxine, tricyclic antidepressants, buspirone, and benzodiazepines. Limited studies of the safety and efficacy of these medications are available.

    D. **School.** An Individualized Education Plan (IEP) or 504 plan may be needed to help the student handle anxiety in school. The teacher may also need to be educated about the disorder, and provided with strategies for how to best help the child with anxiety in the classroom.

IV. Pearls and pitfalls.

- New or worsening anxiety in a child can be a red flag for violence, trauma or stress in the home or community. An assessment of environmental conditions is encouraged.
- When a child presents with chronic somatic symptoms, perform a mental health assessment early on in the medical work-up.
- Panic attacks may occur with any of the anxiety disorders discussed here. These should not be confused with panic disorder, which is rare in children.
- Parents identified as having possible mental illness should be strongly encouraged to seek evaluation and treatment. The likelihood that a child will respond to treatment increases when the parent is receiving needed treatment as well.
- Remember that children can have magical thinking. If a bad thing happens in their family or community, talk to them about it. Sometimes, children may develop significant anxiety by believing that these events were their own fault.

BIBLIOGRAPHY

For parents

Books

Dacey JS, Fiore LB. *Your Anxious Child: How Parents and Teachers Can Relieve Anxiety in Children*. San Francisco: Jossey-Bass, 2000.
Manassis K. *Keys to Parenting Your Anxious Child*. New York: Barron's Educational Series Inc., 1996.

Web sites

National Institute of Mental Health is a federal agency that researches mental and behavioral disorders. www.nimh.nih.gov
Anxiety Disorders Association of America is a nonprofit organization that provides information regarding anxiety. www.adaa.org

For professionals

Connoly SD, Bernstein GA. Practice parameter for the assessment and treatment of children and adolescents with anxiety disorders. *J Am Acad Child Adolesc Psychiatry* 46(2):267–283, 2007.
March JS, Morris TL (eds). *Anxiety Disorders in Children and Adolescents* (2nd ed), New York: The Guilford Press, 2004.
Sakolsky D, Birmaher B. Pediatric anxiety disorders: management in primary care. *Curr Opin Pediatr* 20(5):538–543, 2008.

Web sites

Web site listing various pediatric anxiety scales, some with links to downloadable PDF versions. www2.massgeneral.org/schoolpsychiatry/screeningtools_table.asp
PDF versions of SCARED parent and child scales. Parent version: http://www.wpic.pitt.edu/research/CARENET/CARE-NETPROVIDERS/PDFForms/ScaredParent-final.pdf. Child version: http://www.wpic.pitt.edu/research/CARENET/CARE-NETPROVIDERS/PDFForms/ScaredChild-final.pdf

24 Asperger Syndrome

Celine A. Saulnier
Fred R. Volkmar

I. **Description of the problem.** Asperger syndrome (AS) is a neurodevelopmental disorder characterized by **marked impairments in social interaction** with a **repertoire of restricted interests and activities** as seen in autism, yet *with relatively preserved cognitive and language functioning*. The restricted interests tend to include **intense, unusual, and highly circumscribed interests** that can be all encompassing. Although formal language skills are intact, **conversational skills and pragmatic language are quite idiosyncratic and impaired.** Motor clumsiness is an associated, but not diagnostic feature of AS.

A. **Epidemiology.** The prevalence of AS is about 2–3 cases/10,000. Consistent with higher functioning autism, AS is much more frequent in boys. There is no predilection for any racial, ethnic, or socioeconomic group. In the past, good verbal skills have probably led to the condition being underrecognized and incorrectly diagnosed.

B. **Familial transmission/genetics.** In his original report, Hans Asperger (1943) suggested that the disorder tended to run in families. The limited available data support this assumption with perhaps one-third of cases having a close family member with the condition or a significant social disability.

C. **Etiology/contributing factors.** Although a precise etiology has not yet been specified, the apparently strong genetic basis and the unusual pattern of development strongly suggest the operation of neurobiological factors in pathogenesis.

II. **Making the diagnosis.**

A. **Diagnostic features.** It has been suggested that the disorder begins during infancy or childhood with clinical features that include the following:

1. **Impaired reciprocal social interaction** (*at least two*).
   - Impaired use of nonverbal behaviors such as social gaze, communicative gestures, body posture, and facial expressions
   - Failure to develop age-appropriate peer relationships
   - Failure to seek others to share enjoyment, interests, and achievements
   - Lack of social and emotional reciprocity

2. **Restricted repertoire of activities and interests** (*at least one*).
   - Unusually intense circumscribed interests that are abnormal in intensity and focus
   - Rigid adherence to nonfunctional routines and rituals
   - Stereotyped repetitive motor mannerisms
   - Preoccupation with parts of objects

3. **Symptoms** cause clinically significant impairment across areas of functioning (e.g., social, educational, occupational, etc.).

4. **No history of delays** in the general development of syntactic language, with single words developing by the age of 2 years and communicative phrases developing by the age of 3 years.

5. **No significant delays or impairments** in cognitive functioning, age-appropriate self-help and adaptive daily living skills, and curiosity about the environment. More recent research has shown that adaptive communication and socialization skills can be quite impaired in many individuals with AS, despite nonimpaired verbal cognitive skills, that is, the child may have good vocabulary and syntax but fail to appreciate social conventions in a conversation.

B. **Clinical features.**

1. **Age of onset.** AS is typically recognized after the age of 3 years, when atypical social interaction skills and preoccupied interests become evident. If the symptoms are detected prior to the age of 3 years, then the profile of impairments should not meet the criteria for autism or another pervasive developmental disorder (i.e., there should be no delays in the development of formal language).

2. **Language and communication skills.** In AS there should be preservation in the development of formal language skills prior to the age of 3 years, and language may even

appear to be a lifeline for the child early on. However, difficulties will arise as the child matures, particularly in pragmatic language (i.e., in the functional and social use of language). Conversational skills tend to be limited to topics of interest and as a result, communicative exchanges become one-sided and circumstantial. A failure to use and respond to nonverbal cues, such as gestures, body posture, and facial expressions is also observed. The rate and volume of speech in AS is frequently atypical, which is consistent with autism.

3. **Socialization skills.** The early development of socialization skills in AS may initially appear preserved in that social intent is typically present. Impairments in social interaction become evident when the child attempts to negotiate interactions, as when engaging in conversation. Although the child may be aware of and interested in others, their social exchanges become verbose monologues on their topics of interest without any monitoring of the respective interests of their conversational partner. Thus, there is a lack of social and communicative reciprocity.

4. **Behavioral problems.** Individuals with AS are often accused of conduct problems that tend to result from a lack of social understanding, such as empathy and concern for others. During school years, for example, individuals with AS may engage in inappropriate or atypical behaviors that are perceived as behavior problems when in reality they are consequences of the disorder. Unfortunately, these individuals can then become the victim of rejection and/or ridicule from peers, placing them at risk for developing comorbid conditions such as anxiety and depression.

5. **Cognitive function.** According to the *Diagnostic and Statistical Manual of Mental Disorders, Fourth Edition, Text Revision (DSM-IV-TR)* diagnostic criteria, cognitive functioning in AS is at or above age level (i.e., $IQ > 70$). Although this may be the case for generalized IQ scores, the cognitive profiles in AS tend to be highly variable (as in autism), with significant impairments evident in some cognitive abilities. In contrast to individuals with autism whose visual-spatial skills tend to be a relative strength, individuals with AS typically have more facility with verbal information, particularly rote, factually based information. The cognitive profile in AS is often, but not always, indicative of a nonverbal learning disability, where (in part) verbal IQ scores are significantly greater than nonverbal IQ scores.

6. **Motor skills.** Individuals with AS have been described as having poor gross motor coordination, which is in contrast to the gross motor agility that is often observed in autism, particularly early on in development. In addition to motor clumsiness, individuals may also present with fine motor difficulties, including difficulties with fine motor speed and dexterity and graphomotor weaknesses.

7. **Changes over time.** Although the preservation of skills in the early development of AS suggests that the disorder is a "milder" form of autism, the manifestation of AS over the course of life actually presents numerous challenges. First, because of the preserved cognitive skills and often advanced formal language skills, a child with AS may erroneously be perceived as a "problem child" for acting in inappropriate and maladaptive ways, and their needs may be overlooked and underaddressed. Second, the perseverative interests and social naivete can result in rejection bullying from peers. This rejection, coupled with an awareness of not being accepted, places individuals with AS at great risk for developing anxiety and depression, which is often the case beginning in adolescence and young adulthood. This can also be the outcome if an individual with AS does not receive the appropriate social, educational, and vocational supports to successfully navigate through life. Finally, adaptive or "functional" communication and socialization skills can be significantly impaired in AS, with large discrepancies observed between adaptive abilities and cognitive prowess. Yet, if these individuals fail to present with academic challenges (which often they do not), then their adaptive deficits tend not to be acknowledged or addressed appropriately in intervention. As a result, many individuals with AS struggle to achieve levels of independence in adulthood.

C. **Differential diagnosis.**

1. **Autism,** a pervasive developmental disorder that is marked by impairments in communication that were apparent prior to 3 years of age in addition to the socialization impairments and restricted interests that are observed in AS.

2. **Schizoid personality disorder,** a pattern of social detachment and restricted range of emotional expression that typically begins in early adulthood and is present across contexts. A qualitative distinction between AS and schizoid personality disorder is that in AS, there appears to be an intent for social interaction and distress as a result of failure to engage, whereas in schizoid personality disorder the desire for interaction is not likely present.

3. **Nonverbal learning disability** is a neuropsychological profile marked by well-developed rote verbal abilities in the presence of poor pragmatic language, along with deficits in nonverbal problem-solving abilities, visual-spatial–organizational difficulties, and poor arithmetic and graphomotor skills. Deficits in social perception and judgment are the product of this neuropsychological profile, rather than the hallmark of the disability, as is the case in pervasive developmental disorders.
4. **Semantic pragmatic language disorder,** a profile of preserved syntactic and phonological skills in the presence of impaired semantic and pragmatic language skills.

D. **History: key clinical questions.**
1. *"Do you have any concerns regarding your child's socialization and play skills?"* Impairments in socialization are the hallmark features of AS, as in autism and other pervasive developmental disorders.
2. *"Did you have concerns regarding your child's language development before the age of 3 years?"* Since delays/impairments in the development of language are characteristic of autism, it is essential to inquire about early language development for the purpose of diagnostic differentiation between autism and AS.
3. *"When your child developed speech, did it appear to be formal in nature or precociously verbose?"* Language development in AS is often precocious, yet it can be pedantic or formal in nature (like "little professors").
4. *"Does your child have any unusual interests or preoccupations with certain topics? If so, to what extent do they interfere with the child's ability to engage in social exchanges?"* Assess the presence of and degree of intrusion of preoccupations.
5. *Are there times when your child simply does not respond to sounds?* Hearing loss and possible seizure activity should always be ruled out.
6. *"Does your child seem to be improving? If so, what appears to be helping?"* What works for one child may not work for another, even with the same diagnosis. Treatment plans must always be individualized.
7. *"How are you, your spouse, and other members of your family managing?"* Like autism, AS is a family problem. All members need support.

E. **Physical examination.** There are no characteristic abnormal findings with AS.
F. **Tests and additional evaluations.**
1. **Tests.** No specific medical evaluations are routinely indicated. Specific tests may be indicated on the basis of specifics of the case. As in all ASDs, high-resolution chromosomes and DNA for fragile X should be considered on all patients. If results of those tests are normal, further testing should be considered in a tiered approach, including comparative genomic hybridization/microarray analysis for submicroscopic duplications and deletions.
2. **Evaluations.** As in autism, all children with AS should have a comprehensive, transdisciplinary evaluation that includes assessments conducted by, for example, a developmental and behavioral pediatric clinician, child neurologist, child psychologist or child psychiatrist, and a speech-language pathologist. Evaluation by an occupational and/or physical therapist will often prove useful, as well.

III. **Management.**
A. **Educational/behavioral management.** The educational and therapeutic programming for children with AS should consist of the same intensive and comprehensive intervention developed for individuals with autism and should be customized to meet the needs of each individual on the basis of his/her profile of strengths and vulnerabilities. Programs should incorporate a range of intervention strategies to enhance skills across areas, including conversation and social interaction skills, academic functioning, motor control, psychological functioning, adaptive functioning, and behavioral management. Social skills interventions can range from teaching social scripts and social stories in one-to-one settings to working with peers, dyads, and small groups to facilitate, practice, and generalize learned strategies within naturalistic contexts. Conversational skills can be improved upon by enhancing awareness of speech volume, tone, and nonverbal gestures, as well as by teaching individuals with AS to inquire about the interests of their conversational partner, while restricting their desire to focus on their own topics of interest.

Similar to autism, children with AS tend to learn rote and concrete information with ease, whereas abstract concepts and complex information are more challenging to comprehend. Therefore, applied behavioral analysis techniques that involve breaking down concepts into basic, identifiable parts tend to be successful. Additional academic supports can include strategies to enhance the organization and interpretation of visual material, particularly, organizing sequential visual material. When verbal abilities are a relative strength, supplemental verbal and written supports should be provided to

enhance comprehension of visual information, which may differ from treatment of autism where the emphasis tends to be on using supplemental visual aids. Organizational and self-management strategies can include the use of daily planners/schedules such as handheld devices, smartphones, etc. In fact, many computer software programs are developing applications for such devices that offer explicit, visual, and user-friendly supports. Finally, a mental health clinician can serve to provide a supportive advocate for the child with AS with whom to problem solve challenging social and academic experiences.
   B. **Medications.** In school-aged children with AS attentional difficulties are often prominent and may respond, at least in part, to stimulant and similar medications. Adolescents and adults appear to be at increased risk for significant anxiety and depression. For individuals with depression and anxiety, SSRIs (selective serotonin reuptake inhibitors) are often utilized.
   C. **Support for families.** Support for the families of individuals with AS can include parent support groups, sibling support groups, family and educational advocates, and respite services.
IV. **Prognosis.** In general, the outcome in AS is apparently better than that in higher functioning autism (i.e., autism associated with IQ in the normal range). Many individuals with AS marry and have families; they may be somewhat socially isolated and are often attracted to occupations that minimize socialization requirements.

BIBLIOGRAPHY

For parents organizations

OASIS (Online Asperger Syndrome Information and Support). Web resources for parents on Asperger syndrome and related disorders. www.aspergersyndrome.org
Autism Society of America. Largest nonprofit organization on autism and pervasive developmental disorders. Provides a wealth of written materials, including newsletters, book lists, meeting schedules, and research updates. 8601 Georgia Avenue, Suite 503, Silver Spring, MD 20910, Phone: 301-565-0433, Fax: 301-565-0834. www.autism-society.org
Asperger Syndrome Education Network (ASPEN). Education, support, and advocacy network for individuals with AS and their families. 9 ASPEN Circle, Edison, NJ. 08820. Phone: 732-321-0880. www.aspennj.org

Books

Klass P, Costello F. *Quirky Kids: Understanding and Helping Your Child Who Doesn't Fit in – When to Worry and When Not to Worry*. New York: Ballantine Books, 2003.
Ozonoff S, Dawson G, McPartland J. *A Parent's Guide to Asperger Syndrome and High-Functioning Autism*. New York: The Guilford Press, 2002.
Powers M. *Asperger Syndrome and Your Child: A Parent's Guide*. New York: Harper Resource, 2002.
Stewart K. *Helping a Child with Nonverbal Learning Disability or Asperger Syndrome: A Parent's Guide*. Oakland, CA: New Harbinger Publications, Inc., 2002.

For professionals

Kamp-Becker I, Smidt J, Ghahreman M, et al. Categorical and dimensional structure of autism spectrum disorders: the nosologic validity of Asperger syndrome. *J Autism Dev Disord*. 2010 Jan 20. PMID: 20087640.
Klin A, Volkmar FR, Sparrow SS (eds). *Asperger Syndrome*. New York: The Guilford Press, 2000.

25 Attention-Deficit/ Hyperactivity Disorder

Steven Parker
L. Kari Hironaka

I. Description of the problem.

A. Attention-deficit/hyperactivity disorder (ADHD) is not a simple medical diagnosis. Rather, it is a behavioral syndrome, suspected when a cluster of suggestive behaviors are consistently observed by parents and other caregivers early in the child's life. **In young children,** these behaviors cause significant dysfunction in most of the important aspects of the child's experience: challenging relationships with parents and other caregivers, teachers and peers, as well as behavioral and discipline problems in multiple settings, including home, school, and childcare. **In the adolescent and adult,** ADHD may impair job performance, adult relationships, academic achievement, and be associated with increased legal difficulties, motor vehicle accidents, smoking, and substance abuse.

1. **The** *Diagnostic and Statistical Manual of Mental Disorders, Fourth Edition, Text Revision* **(DSM-IV-TR) diagnostic criteria for ADHD are found in Table 25-1.** The *DSM-IV-TR* differentiates three types of ADHD: predominantly inattentive, predominantly hyperactive-impulsive and combined type. Although meeting these criteria may not be necessary to make a diagnosis in all cases, these criteria represent an excellent list of the symptoms for the pediatric clinician to explore during the diagnostic process.

2. Aside from the "official" behaviors endorsed by the *DSM-IV-TR*, other issues commonly seen in children with ADHD may be even more important to their social, emotional, and academic well-being. These include the following:

   - **Emotional lability or immaturity** (other children call him "a baby"; when mood swings are extreme, especially with hyperirritable periods, a diagnosis of bipolar disorder may be considered)
   - **Resistance to environmental reinforcement** (much less responsive to positive or negative reinforcement, often rendering behavioral interventions less effective)
   - **Little sense of physical safety** (leading to increased accidents).
   - **Aggressive behaviors** (a major red flag with perhaps the most problematic long-term prognosis, often related to later aggressive behaviors and full-blown conduct disorder if not addressed).
   - **An oppositional stance to the world** (another major red flag, suggesting a suboptimal and negative response of the environment to the behavioral challenges, perhaps presaging a full-blown oppositional defiant disorder if not promptly addressed).
   - **Poor social skills** ("socially tone deaf") and poor peer relations (heartbreakingly few friends).
   - **Low self-esteem** (perhaps the most common damaging long-term outcome of all).

B. Epidemiology.

1. Prevalence studies yield confusing results, depending on the criteria and means for ascertainment. Probably the best estimate is 5%–10% of American school children have ADHD.

   - ADHD has been found worldwide, whenever it has been studied, with rates ranging from 3%–18%.
   - Higher rates are seen in children from low socioeconomic status, but it is unclear whether this represents a true increase or is the result of an environment with fewer resources to ameliorate the challenging behaviors.

2. Male to female ratio had been classically estimated at about 4–6:1. However, recent studies suggest a lower ratio, perhaps as low as 2:1. This is because the diagnostic criteria are oriented to the male presentation (with many externalizing behaviors) and may miss many females (who tend to be diagnosed at a later date, if at all, presenting with subtle attentional challenges in school and difficulties in their social relations).

C. Comorbidity of other diagnoses and ADHD is quite high, although it is often ambiguous whether a second diagnosis has been caused by the ADHD or is cause of behaviors that look like ADHD or coexists as a discrete but interacting true second diagnosis

Table 25-1. ADHD: *DSM-IV-TR* criteria

1. Six or more of the following symptoms of inattention (or both) have persisted for at least 6 months to a degree that is maladaptive and inconsistent with developmental level:

Inattention
a. Often fails to give close attention to details or makes careless mistakes in schoolwork, work, or other activities
b. Often has difficulty sustaining attention in tasks or play activities
c. Often does not seem to listen when spoken to directly
d. Often does not follow through on instructions and fails to finish schoolwork, chores, or duties in the workplace (not due to oppositional behavior or failure to understand instructions)
e. Often has difficulty organizing tasks and activities
f. Often avoids, dislikes, or is reluctant to engage in tasks that require sustained mental effort (such as homework)
g. Often loses things necessary for tasks or activities (toys, school assignments, pencils, books, or tools)
h. Is often easily distracted by extraneous stimuli
i. Is often forgetful in daily activities

Hyperactivity-impulsivity
2. Six or more of the following symptoms of hyperactivity-impulsivity have persisted for at least 6 months to a degree that is maladaptive and inconsistent with developmental level:

Hyperactivity
a. Often fidgets with hands or feet or squirms in seat
b. Often leaves seat in classroom or in other situations in which remaining seated is expected
c. Often runs about or climbs excessively in situations in which it is inappropriate (in adolescents or adults, may be limited to subjective feelings of restlessness)
d. Often has difficulty playing or engaging in leisure activities quietly
e. Is often "on the go" or often acts as if "driven by a motor"
f. Often talks excessively

Impulsivity
g. Often blurts out answers before questions have been completed
h. Often has difficulty awaiting turn
i. Often interrupts or intrudes on others (such as butting into conversations or games)

A. Some hyperactive, impulsive, or inattentive symptoms that caused impairment were present before the age of 7 years.
B. Some impairment from the symptoms is present in two or more settings (such as in school or work and at home).
C. There must be clear evidence of clinically significant impairment in social, academic, or occupational functioning.
D. The symptoms do not occur exclusively during the course of a pervasive developmental disorder, schizophrenia, or another psychotic disorder and are not better accounted for by another mental disorder (such as a mood, anxiety, dissociative, or personality disorder).

American Psychiatric Association, *Diagnostic and Statistical Manual of Mental Disorders* (4th ed) Text Revision, Washington, DC: American Psychiatric Association, 2000.
[a]For individuals (especially adolescents and adults) who currently have symptoms that no longer meet full criteria, "in partial remission" should be specified.

(Table 25-2). More than one of these additional syndromes can be (and often are) identified in the same child. Some estimate that comorbid diagnoses are the rule, not the exception, and can be found in 50%–75% of all children with ADHD.

    D. Etiology. ADHD likely has no single invariant cause, but likely represents the final common pathway for a host of neurological and environmental risks.

        1. Genetic factors. The concordance rate of ADHD in identical twins is strikingly high: 0.6–0.8. In addition, first- and second-degree relatives (parents, siblings, and grandparents) of children with ADHD have a much higher incidence of the disorder (20%–25%). Abnormal level of protein production by candidate dopamine-related genes (*D4, D2, DAT*) is being implicated in some. These and other genes are active subjects of intense research.

Table 25-2. Comorbid disorders

Comorbid disorders	% Range of prevalence from several studies
Specific developmental disorders (academic skills disorders, language and speech disorders, motor skills disorder)	20–60
Mild mental retardation	3–10
Oppositional defiant disorder	30–60
Conduct disorder	10–50
Anxiety disorders of childhood or adolescence (separation anxiety disorder, avoidant disorder, overanxious disorder)	10–30
Depressive disorder	5–35 (in adults)
Bipolar disorder	0–10 (15% of adults)
Tic disorders	5–30
Other neurologic disorders	<10
Posttraumatic stress disorder	Unknown

2. **Medical risks.** Intrauterine exposure to maternal smoking and alcohol use increase the risk of ADHD. Premature and low-birth weight infants also show a higher prevalence. Increased lead levels, carbon monoxide exposure, and various heavy metals (e.g., cadmium) have been implicated in some cases.
   a. **Differences in the brain.** Animal studies and the effects of psychoactive medications have led to speculations of altered neurotransmitter profiles and brain function in persons with ADHD. Recent positron emission tomography and functional magnetic resonance imaging studies suggest underactivity in parts of the cerebral cortex, especially the frontal lobes, perhaps leading to the challenges in executive function and self-regulation described in ADHD. Other areas, which have been implicated in studies as having altered function include the cerebellar vermis, cingulated gyrus, frontal-striatal connections, basal ganglia, and brain stem.
   b. **Environmental factors.** Environmental issues, such as parental psychopathology and low socioeconomic status, likely play more of a role in exacerbating (or at least not ameliorating) the behaviors of ADHD, rather than as a causal agent. A family environment that includes poor monitoring of behavior and a punitive approach to discipline, for example, may magnify the symptoms of ADHD.
E. **Theories of ADHD.** The most popular current theory of ADHD, posited by Russell Barkley, is that ADHD represents **a disorder of "executive function."** This implies dysfunction in the prefrontal lobes so that the child lacks the ability for *behavioral inhibition or self-regulation* of such executive functions as nonverbal working memory, speech internalization, affect, emotion, motivation, and arousal. Because of this relative inability to inhibit, the child lives pretty much only in the "now" and lacks the ability to modify or delay behavior in view of future consequences.
F. **Prognosis.**
   1. Symptoms persist in the majority of young adults and adults, but change in nature (hyperactivity replaced by feelings of restlessness).
   2. Higher incidence of problems is seen, such as antisocial behaviors (about 20%), substance abuse (15%), and other *DSM* diagnosis (about 35%).
      However, a recent meta-analysis suggests that the incidence of substance abuse in teens is less with those who were treated with stimulant medication.
   3. The majority do well, especially those who were not aggressive or oppositional, who have a high IQ, and come from high socioeconomic backgrounds.
II. **Making the diagnosis.** There is **no *sine qua non*** for the diagnosis of ADHD. Rather, the pediatric clinician must analyze and integrate the reports of characteristic behaviors by multiple observers, occurring in a variety of different settings, over an extended period of time. These behaviors are described as occurring with greater intensity and frequency than is typical for other children of the same development age and, most importantly, **are causing significant problems in the child's functioning and relationships in those settings.**
A. **History: key clinical questions.**
   1. *"Tell me about the behaviors that concern you? What, exactly does he do? Give me a specific example."* It is important to obtain specific examples to see if the behaviors sound truly more severe than other children at the same developmental level, or if

the parent has a low tolerance for a "normal," albeit temperamentally active and intense child.

2. *"Who else is concerned about these behaviors?"* Since children with true ADHD are problematic in most or all settings across time and space, if only the parent is concerned but other significant caregivers or teachers are not, one's index of suspicious should be raised of an etiology other than ADHD.

3. *"When did you first become concerned about these behaviors?"* Often the symptoms have been present for a long time before coming to your attention. Conversely, the abrupt onset of behavioral problems may suggest a stressful trigger and etiology.

4. *"Tell me about his attention span."* Remember that the ability to watch TV or play video games for an extended period does not necessarily connote a good attention span. As these require no input from the child, he may interact without really paying a lot of attention. Instead, ask for examples of *internally mediated attention*, that is, paying attention to less compelling, more boring activities that require sustained attention to be successful. Ask questions such as: *"Is he a daydreamer? Easily distracted? Does he have a hard time completing tasks? Does he have a hard time listening to instructions? Is he a poor listener?"*

5. *"Tell me about his activity level."* Some children are obviously extremely active. For others, fidgety and nonpurposeful activity may be more salient than gross motor hyperactivity. Ask: *"Does he seem to be in constant motion? Is he fidgety, even when quiet? Does he engage in dangerous activities without a sense of fear? Does he talk a lot?"*

6. *"Is he impulsive?" "Does he often act without thinking? Does he interrupt and butt in on others when they are doing something? Is he often remorseful after an impulsive act, saying, 'I'm sorry, I just couldn't help myself'?"*

7. *"Tell me about how he expresses his emotions? Does he seem angry or depressed or anxious or incredibly irritable sometimes?"* The search for another cause (e.g., depression, anxiety, bipolar disorder) or comorbidity begins with the initial history taking.

8. *"Does he get along with other kids? Have many friends?"* Most children with ADHD have poor social relationships, which is a significant cause of unhappiness and low self-esteem.

9. *"Tell me about how he is doing in school or day care?"* It is important to get a sense of the level of dysfunction and suffering these behaviors may be causing in all-important aspects of his world, including day care/preschool/school functioning.

10. *"Given all the problems you describe, how do you think they have affected his self-esteem?"* Since enhancing self-esteem may be the pediatric clinician's number one long-term goal, it is helpful to raise the issue early on, especially for parents who have never considered this question before.

11. *"How do you deal with these behaviors? What has worked and what has not?"* Often a child with ADHD has engendered many negative, ineffectual, and punitive responses by his parents. Especially because of their relative lack of response to positive and negative reinforcement, do not be too quick to blame the parents for inadequate limit-setting in a child for whom it requires heroic efforts to set consistent limits and who does not respond all that well to them anyway.

12. *"Why do you think these problems are occurring? What do others say is the cause?"* The parents' theories of causation are important to make explicit. Often they have a direct impact on their response (e.g., "He's just a bad boy and could behave better if he wanted" can lead to punitive and deprecating interactions). This question can also bring out parental disagreements that can affect later treatment ("His father says he's 'just a boy' and there is no problem, but I'm with him all day and I know better!").

B. **Office observations/evaluation.**

1. Many children with ADHD can contain themselves in the short time of the visit. They may be on their best behavior in order not to provoke the powerful pediatric clinician and because the setting is mostly one-on-one with few distractions. Such "good behavior" in the office should not be used to rule out ADHD, which is dependent on his behavior in the usual familiar settings.

2. On the other hand, if a child has many ADHD behaviors in the office, these may help to confirm the diagnosis when otherwise suspected, and perhaps even represents a level of symptomatology that is more pervasive and intense than a child who can contain himself in the office.

3. **Physical examination** is rarely revealing, except insofar as it allows a window into the child's behavior and affect during the examination. Look for any neurologic signs, mild dysmorphic features, and signs of autonomic disturbance that might suggest

Table 25-3. ADHD questionnaires

NICHQ Vanderbilt Assessment Scale
Free and downloadable from the **NICHQ ADHD Toolkit Web site** http://www.nichq.org/

Revised Conner's Questionnaire—Teacher and Parent Rating Scales
Perhaps the best validated and also includes if child meets *DSM-IV* criteria; is very focused on ADHD, with little information on comorbidities (however, is not free).

a medical or genetic diagnosis. Assessing for the so-called **soft neurological signs** is interesting, but cannot be used to confirm or disconfirm the diagnosis of ADHD. A complete cardiovascular examination, including blood pressure and heart rate, should also be performed.

C. **Diagnostic tests.** Aside from an ADHD questionnaire, other testing is rarely indicated unless suggested by the history and physical examination (e.g., laboratory tests assessing thyroid function, electroencephalography, or magnetic resonance imaging when unexpected neurological findings are prominent). Computer-based studies of sustained attention (e.g., the "continuous performance task") are neither reliable indicators of the diagnosis nor response to treatment. **Psychological and educational testing** can be illuminating if academic problems are significant to identify a comorbid learning disability or other learning challenge. Some clinicians refer *all* children with ADHD for such testing; others first treat the ADHD and then refer only those children for whom significant academic difficulties persist.

D. **Principles of the diagnostic process once ADHD is suspected.**
   1. **Do your homework!** It is rarely sufficient or acceptable to take a suggestive history from a parent, observe the child in the office, and make a definitive diagnosis. The suggestive behaviors must occur in all the child's significant environments.
   2. **Obtain a description and seek corroboration of the child's behaviors from caretakers in all settings in which he spends time.** Since interviews with these providers are impractical, use ADHD-specific questionnaires (see Table 25-3). Ask the mother and father and other caregivers in the home to complete the questionnaires, as well as all significant outside professionals and caretakers (babysitters, grandparents, teachers, preschool and Head Start providers, childcare providers).
   3. **Review the behavioral descriptions and integrate them with the history and your understanding of the child and family.** Remember that these descriptions are not diagnostic. *They merely state whether the behavioral descriptions are consistent with (but not necessarily due to) a diagnosis of ADHD.* Clinical judgment must be carefully applied to sort out such information.
      a. Look for consistency of the reported behaviors and whether they suggest ADHD in all settings. If that is the case, the diagnosis may be more clear-cut.
      b. Look for inconsistencies of the reported behaviors in different settings. Variable descriptions are more problematic to interpret.
         • For example, extreme behaviors described at home but not at school may imply stress and/or problematic relationships at home and not true ADHD.
         • Conversely, problematic behaviors seen only in school may imply a learning disability, scapegoating, etc. at school, and not true ADHD.
         • On the other hand, some parents are quite accepting of their child's inattentive, impulsive behaviors at home or do not challenge the child to exert sustained attention and may downplay those symptoms in a child with true ADHD.
   4. **Diagnostic certainty is impossible.** Especially in situations of problematic environmental characteristics (poor "goodness of fit" with parent or day care/school, lots of family stress, early adversities in home environment and community, etc.), it can be impossible to gauge if the ADHD-like behaviors are a cause of problematic parental interactions or an effect of environmental adversities.
      a. In such cases, ask yourself a key question "How much trouble is this child in? How much dysfunction and suffering in his life are these behaviors causing, regardless of the etiology?" If the answer is "to a significant degree," then a trial of medications may be warranted despite the diagnostic uncertainty. Conversely, a child who seems to be coping reasonably well in his world may not require such intervention at this time.
   5. **Be mindful of potential comorbidities.** Since ADHD can be associated with learning disabilities, depression, anxiety, posttraumatic stress disorder, developmental disability, an unrecognized genetic syndrome, language delays, etc. (Table 25-2), a diagnosis

of ADHD should never shut out the possibility that other challenges may be either causing the behaviors or co-occurring.

6. **Discuss with parents your judgment on the diagnosis.** It is always helpful to have asked parents to read about ADHD and state whether or not they think their child fits the criteria. The disagreements between clinician and parent can be made explicit and discussed.

   a. If a parent disagrees with your diagnosis, intervention efforts are likely to fail. Rather than try to browbeat them into acceptance, allow them time to learn more and see if things improve. *"We disagree on whether your child has ADHD. But he's your child and you have to make the final decision. Why don't you read some more about it, talk to parents with kids who have ADHD, and let's see if things improve. I think because your child is having such serious problems at school (and at home, with friends, etc.) that we really need to try to help him out. So far nothing has worked well and I'm concerned that, unless we treat him for ADHD, things are only going to get worse. We'll hold for now, but why don't I see you back in a month or so and we can discuss this further."*

   b. It is helpful to explain ADHD to parents with simple metaphors: *"Your child is like a fast car in which the accelerator is stuck down and the brakes don't work very well. One way or another we need to get the brakes to be more effective."*

   c. A diagnosis of ADHD is often helpful because it **takes the onus off the child:** *"I know his behaviors can be exasperating, but mostly he really can't help it. ADHD is caused by differences in the brain, not because he is a 'bad kid' or 'lazy'."* Without the understanding that *biological* factors lead to the child's behavior, his actions are often interpreted as willful and manipulative, and may provoke an angry response, which then aggravates the child's feelings of being misunderstood and picked on.

   d. Explain that ADHD is a **chronic condition** and is unlikely to go away on its own.

   e. Encourage the parents to read and learn as much as they can to best help their child.

III. Management.

A. **Primary goals.** The goals of all treatment for ADHD are to enhance the child's successful functioning in the domains that have been impaired and causing distress. These areas almost always include his academic or preschool functioning, family and peer relationships, and self-esteem.

B. **Information for the family.** Explain to the family the nature of ADHD and what is known about its treatment, specifically that medication treatment has been demonstrated to be, far and away, the most effective treatment in most children with ADHD. Have well-chosen handouts for parents at the ready in the office to give to them for later perusal.

C. **Medication treatment.**

1. **Fundamental rules of ADHD medication treatment** (some of which should also be explained to the parents.)

   • **All decisions are reversible**. Once a decision has been made either to treat or not to treat with medications, it can be changed as circumstances warrant.

   • **Obtain ongoing feedback regarding efficacy and side effects** from the parents and the same caretakers who provided the initial history. This often best done by the provider faxing a brief weekly report (such as the Clinical Attention Problem Scales (CAPS), which can be downloaded for free at: www.dbpeds.org) to the clinician in the initial stages of treatment and then bimonthly once a stable dose is achieved.

   • **If one medication does not work, try another.** If a child is a nonresponder to methylphenidate, 80% of the time he will respond to an amphetamine preparation. Likewise amphetamine nonresponders do respond to methylphenidate in 66% of cases.

   • Improvement should be gauged in areas such **as improved academic performance** (volume of work, efficiency, completion, accuracy) as well as **behavior in the classroom, improved self-esteem, decreased disruptive behaviors, improved relationships with parents, siblings, teachers, and peers; and enhanced safety.**

   • In general, one is looking for **a dramatic and clearly beneficial response to the medications.** Reports that maybe there *might* be some subtle or minor changes are not sufficient to view the trial as successful.

   • **Medications are usually the most important, but not the only treatment.** However, the improvement in the child's behavior often greatly enhances attempts at limit-setting, school expectations, etc.

- **Medications are effective in 70%–80% of children with ADHD.** However, the lack of a beneficial response does not necessarily mean that the diagnosis is incorrect.
- **Parental agreement with a medication trial is essential.** Some parents are understandably reluctant to give their child a psychoactive medication. They may have read or heard of frightening side effects and "don't want my child to become a zombie." The clinician should acknowledge and respect such concerns: *"I understand why you are concerned. I am too—I don't want to put a child on medications unless I really think it's necessary and safe to do so, which, in your child's case, I do. First off, if we start this, you will be in* **complete control.** *If your child is having side effects that worry you or if the medications don't seem to be helping, we'll stop or change the medicine. If it doesn't seem to be helping, we'll stop or change. Just because we start medications, doesn't mean we have to continue them if you or I are unsatisfied with their effects. Second, these medications have been around for a long time and are really very safe. If there are any side effects—and these are usually mild anyway— they go away when the medication is discontinued. Third, there is no question that medications are the most effective way to treat ADHD that we have. So, think about it. I'm not going to start medications unless you give the okay. If you decide against it now, we can reconsider it in the future if things don't improve for your child. But I suggest giving them a try and seeing how things go."*

2. **Pharmacologic agents.**
   a. **Stimulant medications** remain the first line of medication treatment for ADHD. These include the various preparations of methylphenidate and amphetamines. Table 25-4 contains information concerning their use. All can be effective, but some children may respond to only one. When problems arise with one drug or it is ineffective, another in this group should be tried.
      - **Cardiovascular risk factors and side effects.** Concerns regarding the cardiovascular safety of the stimulants, specifically—the risk of sudden cardiac death (SCD), have sparked controversy and received much recent attention in the academic literature. Although tragic, SCD is fortunately a very rare event in children. Statements by the American Academy of Pediatrics and the American Academy of Child and Adolescent Psychiatry conclude that there is currently no compelling evidence that the risk of SCD is higher in children receiving medications for ADHD than for the general population.
      - Stimulant medications are associated with mild increases in blood pressure (2–4 mm Hg systolic and 1–3 mm Hg diastolic) and heart rate (3–5 BPM). These changes are generally not clinically significant. However, there is at least a theoretical risk that children with underlying cardiac disease taking ADHD medications may be at increased risk for SCD and should be screened for SCD risk factors prior to the initiation of a trial of medications. Screening should include the following:
         - Patient history of syncope, dizziness, chest pain, palpitations, change in exercise tolerance or shortness of breath with exercise, high blood pressure, and/or history of cardiac disease.
         - Family history of sudden or unexplained death in person aged <35 years, cardiac arrhythmias, cardiomyopathy, QT syndrome, or Marfan syndrome.
         - Electrocardiograms are generally not recommended for healthy children without identifiable cardiovascular risk factors or cardiac disease.
         - Children with presenting cardiovascular risk factors or known cardiac disease should be referred to a pediatric cardiologist before ADHD medication is initiated.
   b. Currently, the second line of ADHD medications, when a stimulant trial proves ineffective due to intolerable side effects or dubious efficacy, is **atomoxetine**, which unlike stimulants is specific noradrenergic reuptake inhibitor. As such, it has no potential for abuse and is unscheduled, with the ability to write for refills.
      - There is a small increased risk of suicidal thinking associated with atomoxetine and the Food and Drug Administration (FDA) has added a boxed warning to the label. Although the risk is small, the pediatric clinician should discuss this risk with the patient and his/her family. Children should be monitored for the onset of suicidal ideation, particularly over the first few months of treatment (see Chapter 20).
   c. Third-line medications such as clonidine, guanfacine, and bupropion are least effective in improving ADHD symptoms and are often used in addition to a stimulant to address aggressive behaviors (clonidine, guanfacine) or depression (bupropion).

Table 25-4. Stimulant medication: dosage and techniques of administration[a]

Pharmacologic agent	Starting dose	Maximum dose (FDA)	Usual dosing
First line			
Short-acting			
Amphetamine and dextroamphetamine (Adderall)	2.5–5 mg q day (bid)	40 mg	bid–tid (duration 4–6 hr)
Dextroamphetamine (Dexedrine)	2.5–5 mg q day (bid)	40 mg	bid–tid (duration 4–6 hr)
Dexmethylphenidate (Focalin)	2.5 mg bid	20 mg	bid (duration 4–6 hr)
Methylphenidate (Ritalin or Methylin)	5 mg bid	60 mg	bid–tid (duration 3–4 hr)
Long-acting			
Dextroamphetamine sulfate (Adderall XR)	10 mg q day	30 mg	qd (duration 8–12 hr)
Methylphenidate (Concerta)	18 mg q day	72 mg	q AM (duration 12 hr)
Methylphenidate (Daytrana patch)	10 mg patch	30 mg	Up to 9 hr "wear time" (duration ~12 hr)
Dextroamphetamine (Dexedrine Spansule)	5–10 mg q day (bid)	40 mg	qd–bid (duration 6–8 hr)
Dexmethylphenidate hydrochloride (Focalin XR)	5 mg q day	30 mg	qd (duration 8–12 hr)
Methylphenidate (Metadate CD or Ritalin LA)	10–20 mg q AM	60 mg	qd (duration 8 hr)
Methylphenidate (Metadate ER and Methylin ER)	10 mg q day	60 mg	qd (duration 8 hr)
Lisdexamfetamine (Vyvanse)	20 mg q day	70 mg	qd (duration 13 hr)
Second line			
Atomoxetine (Strattera)	0.5 mg/kg/day × 4 days; then 1 mg/kg/day for 4 days; then 1.2 mg/kg/day	Less of 1.4 mg/kg/day or 100 mg	qd–bid (in AM if no drowsiness or HS if there is)—(duration 24 hr)

[a]Adapted from: Practice parameter for the assessment and treatment of children and adolescents with attention-deficit/hyperactivity disorder. *J Am Acad Child Adolesc Psychiatry* 46(7):894–921, 2007.

    d. Dosage. In general, a medication is started at the lowest dose and then gradually increased until the optimal response or intolerable side effects are seen. Dosages can generally be titrated up every 1–3 weeks. Side effects can usually be minimized by altering the dosage, timing, or form (short- or long-acting) of medication. Table 25-5 lists the common clinical question and side effects and how they can be managed.

- It is best to **start medications or any changes on the weekend** or any time the parents can be the first to witness the effects. They can then be instructed to call the clinician on Monday and relate any benefits or concerns.
- A follow-up visit should be scheduled within a month of initiating treatment to review side effects and overall progress.
- Throughout treatment, **height, weight, blood pressure, and heart rate should be monitored.** Although some children may experience some mild growth suppression of height and weight, these effects cease once medication is stopped thus warrant close follow-up.
- Once the appropriate dosage is established, it should be reevaluated and adjusted upward as tolerance develops or as the child's growth necessitates a larger dosage. Follow-up visits should be scheduled several times throughout the year

Table 25-5. Stimulant medication: common clinical questions and side effects and management strategies

Common clinical questions	Management strategies
Short-acting or long-acting?	In general, long-acting preparations (8–12 hr) are preferable, unless the cost is prohibitive or parental preference
Decreased appetite?	Administer medication with or shortly after meals. Offer high calorie foods when hungry
	Encourage eating after school and/or before bedtime
	When severe, institute short periods off medication on weekends
Difficulty falling asleep?	Try an 8 hr, rather than 12 hr preparation. On the other hand, if the child is restless and overactive at bedtime, may try a short-acting PM dose
	Add a mild hypnotic such as an antihistamine or clonidine prior to bedtime
Dazed and/or withdrawn behavior?	Reduce dosage or discontinue medication and try a different class
Gradual return of hyperactive behaviors?	Increase dosage. Be sure is not "rebound" behavior when blood levels are waning
Gradual onset of symptoms of depression during periods of effective medication dose?	Discontinue medication and try another class. Consider referral for treatment of depression
Development of tics that were not present prior to starting medication?	Discontinue medication and try another class

to ensure medication efficacy, monitor for side effects, and assess for the development of comorbidities.

- The decision to treat only on weekdays or only during the school year is best made in consultation with the parents. **Improved school performance is always a priority,** but when the child's symptoms seem to have a lesser impact on home and peer relationships, weekday use only may be acceptable and will help minimize growth effects. However, when the child's relationships at home and with peers is a source of great contention and suffering, taking the medications every day, including holidays and vacations, may be the best option.

  e. **Duration of treatment.** In general, treatment will need to be continued into and through adolescence (except in the 10%–20% of children with ADHD who may completely "outgrow" the problem). The decision to end treatment can be periodically tested via trials off medication during times of low stress.

3. **Multimodal treatments.** In addition to medication, several psychological and social treatments should be considered.

   a. **Parent training in behavioral management.** This treatment aims to teach parents how to set limits, provide incentives for appropriate behaviors, and minimize emotionally destructive responses. Training adults (either parents or teachers) in behavioral management skills often requires referral to a specialized program for parents of children with ADHD. For parents, treatment may be done in small groups, which have the advantage of providing support as well as training. The clinician should recognize that the goal of behavioral management therapy is improvement in the environment in which daily living takes place, not to change the child's fundamental nature.

   b. **Additional therapies** may be needed depending on the circumstances of the family and the child. Individual psychotherapy for the child with ADHD should be considered in cases of oppositional and aggressive behaviors, as well as to improve self-esteem. There is, however, no evidence that individual psychotherapy improves the child's ability to pay attention or reduces impulsiveness. As the child gets older and becomes more self-aware, however, psychotherapy may facilitate an understanding of how his own behavior affects others. **Family therapy** may be useful for families in which the relationships are stuck in negative responses and for whom the child's behavior has engendered other significant family issues or who need a specific focus in communication skills. **Social skills training** for the child can be helpful in improving peer relationships.

c. **Criteria for referral.** Most primary care clinicians will be involved in two aspects of treatment: (1) explaining the condition to the child and the family and (2) prescribing and following medication. The American Academy of Pediatrics (AAP) Guidelines on Diagnosis and Treatment of ADHD recommend that the diagnosis of children aged 6–12 years is appropriate in a primary care setting. Psychosocial treatments will be given by others, though the clinician should be familiar with each type of treatment and the goals of each treatment strategy. The clinician should develop resources for referral and establish ongoing communication with those resources. When the child fails to respond to stimulant medication or develops unacceptable side effects or the diagnosis remains ambiguous, referral to a specialist, such as a developmental–behavioral pediatrician or child psychiatrist, is indicated.

BIBLIOGRAPHY

For parents

A.D.D. Warehouse. A one-stop shopping site with books, videos, and other products to help children with ADHD and their families to understand and manage ADHD problems. Contains an excellent annotated bibliography. http://addwarehouse.com/shopsite_sc/store/html/index.html

CH.A.D.D. (Children and Adults with Attention Deficit Hyperactivity Disorders). A national organization with local chapters throughout the country. Provides support to families, formation regarding local laws and school policies and an avenue for advocacy. http://www.chadd.org/

For professionals

The American Academy of Child and Adolescent Psychiatry practice parameter for ADHD. http://www.aacap.org/page.ww?section=Practice+Parameters&name=Practice+Parameters

Pliszka S, AACAP Work Group on Quality Issues. Practice parameter for the assessment and treatment of children and adolescents with attention-deficit/hyperactivity disorder. *J Am Acad Child Adolesc Psychiatry* 46(7):894–921, 2007.

The American Academy of Pediatrics clinical practice guidelines for ADHD. Diagnosis. http://aappolicy.aappublications.org/cgi/content/full/pediatrics;105/5/1158

Treatment. http://aappolicy.aappublications.org/cgi/content/full/pediatrics;122/2/451

The American Academy of Pediatrics Policy Statement on cardiovascular monitoring of children on stimulant medications. http://aappolicy.aappublications.org/cgi/content/full/pediatrics;122/2/451

The Cincinnati Children's Hospital Evidence-Based Care Guidelines for ADHD—a very helpful evidence-based toolkit for the management of ADHD. http://www.cincinnatichildrens.org/svc/alpha/h/health-policy/ev-based/adhd.htm

Clinical Attention Problem Scale. Available from Developmental Behavioral Pediatrics Online. http://www.dbpeds.org/articles/detail.cfm?id=23

The NICHQ ADHD Toolkit. Contains very useful, free, downloadable information, handouts for parents, questionnaires, history forms, etc. Available at the National Initiative for Children's Healthcare Quality. http://www.nichq.org/login_req.html?returnpage=/toolkits_publications/index.html

Autism Spectrum Disorders

Elizabeth B. Caronna

I. **Description of the problem.** Autism is a heterogeneous neurodevelopmental disorder. It is defined clinically by characteristic behavioral impairments in
   - Reciprocal social interactions
   - Verbal and nonverbal communication
   - Range and nature of activities or interests

   The *Diagnostic and Statistical Manual of Mental Disorders, Fourth Edition, Text Revision* (*DSM-IV-TR*) uses the umbrella term pervasive developmental disorders (PDDs) to include several disorders, which appear to have different etiologies, including autistic disorder, Rett syndrome, childhood disintegrative disorder, Asperger syndrome, and pervasive developmental disorder-not otherwise specified (PDD-NOS). Recently, there has been increasing use of the term autism spectrum disorder (ASD) as a diagnosis for individuals who show less severe impairment than individuals who meet *DSM* criteria for autistic disorder. The autism spectrum includes PDD-NOS, atypical autism, high-functioning autism, and Asperger syndrome. This shift in nomenclature reflects the broader conceptualization of the disorder to include more individuals with milder symptoms. It is likely that this change will be reflected in the upcoming version of the *DSM*. (In this chapter, the term ASD is used to denote autistic disorder, PDD-NOS, and Asperger syndrome. Rett syndrome and childhood disintegrative disorder will not be discussed in detail here. Asperger syndrome is addressed in greater detail in another chapter.)

   A. **Epidemiology.** The prevalence of ASD is hotly debated. As recently as the 1980s, prevalence estimates were in the range of 0.5–1/1000. More recent estimates have suggested a prevalence of ASD in the United States (including autistic disorder, PDD-NOS, and Asperger syndrome) as high as 9/1000. The dramatic increase in rate of diagnosed cases may be attributed to several different factors, including changes in diagnostic criteria and the broader definition of ASD, variation in case finding methods and diagnostic substitution, increased public and professional awareness of the disorders leading to earlier diagnosis and treatment, and a possible true increase in the prevalence.

   Rates of ASD are significantly higher in males than in females (approximately four to five times as common in males). It is likely that there is no difference in actual prevalence of ASD based on race, ethnic background, or socioeconomic status although cases of ASD are often misidentified or identified late in disadvantaged groups.

   B. **Etiology/contributing factors.** Historically, autism was attributed to cold, distant parenting, widely known as the "refrigerator mother theory." The accumulation of evidence that the disorder had a neurological basis (frequency of associated seizures, obvious genetic links, and pathological abnormalities in the brain) made psychodynamic theories of etiology untenable. In the majority of cases, the etiology of ASD is idiopathic. Advanced maternal and paternal age has been found to be associated with increased rates. There are a small number of cases in which there is an underlying metabolic, infectious, or genetic disorder (such as untreated phenylketonuria, congenital cytomegalovirus or rubella, tuberous sclerosis, fragile X syndrome, CHARGE syndrome, neurofibromatosis, or Down syndrome).

   A genetic contribution to ASD is supported by high rates of recurrence of autism in families with one affected child (3%–7% or higher), 25%–35% recurrence risk if a second child has autism, and twin studies that show up to 70% concordance for autistic disorder and 90% concordance for ASD in monozygotic twins. As expected, lower concordance is seen in dizygotic twins (<3% for autistic disorder and 10%–30% for broader phenotype). ASD is assumed to be a polygenic disorder resulting from gene–environment interactions. Recent studies have focused on genome wide studies, identifying microduplications and deletions associated with autism on several autosomal chromosomes. Several studies have identified different genes coding for proteins involved in synaptic connectivity. There is a high rate (up to 10%) of fragile X syndrome in individuals with ASD. Notwithstanding rampant speculation in the lay press and on the Internet, possible environmental triggers of the disorder in genetically predisposed individuals have not yet been identified.

II. **Making the diagnosis.**
   A. **Signs and symptoms.**
      1. *DSM-IV-TR* **criteria for autistic disorder.** The criteria for diagnosis of **autistic disorder** according to *DSM-IV-TR* are outlined below. The presence of impairment must be judged compared with children of the same developmental level or mental age. The *DSM* requires at least six criteria be met from the following three groups of symptoms.
         a. **Qualitative impairment of reciprocal social interactions (*at least two*).**
            • Marked impairment in the use of multiple nonverbal behaviors such as eye-to-eye gaze, facial expression, body postures, and gestures to regulate social interaction
            • Failure to develop peer relationships appropriate to developmental level
            • A lack of spontaneous seeking to share enjoyment, interests, or achievements with other people (e.g., by a lack of showing, bringing, or pointing out objects of interest)
            • Lack of social or emotional reciprocity
         b. **Qualitative impairments in communication (*at least one*).**
            • Delay in, or total lack of, the development of spoken language (not accompanied by an attempt to compensate through alternative modes of communication such as gestures or mime)
            • In individuals with adequate speech, marked impairment in the ability to initiate or sustain a conversation with others
            • Stereotyped and repetitive use of language or idiosyncratic language
            • Lack of varied, spontaneous make-believe play or social imitative play appropriate to developmental level
         c. **Restricted, repetitive, and stereotyped patterns of behavior, interests, and activities (*at least one*).**
            • Encompassing preoccupation with one or more stereotyped and restricted patterns of interest that is abnormal either in intensity or focus
            • Apparently inflexible adherence to specific, nonfunctional routines or rituals
            • Stereotyped and repetitive motor mannerisms (e.g., hand or finger flapping or twisting, or complex whole body movements)
            • Persistent preoccupation with parts of objects
               In addition, delays must be present in at least one of the core areas (social interaction, social communication, or symbolic/imaginative play) by the age of 3 years. Although some children with ASD demonstrate true regression, it appears that most have atypical features in the first year of life that may not be clinically identified at the time.
      2. *DSM-IV-TR*: **PDD-NOS.** This category is used for severe and pervasive impairment in development of reciprocal social interaction associated with impairment in either verbal or nonverbal communication or with the presence of stereotyped behaviors, interests, and activities, but criteria are not met for autistic disorder. This includes atypical autism because of late age of presentation, atypical symptomatology, and/or subthreshold symptomatology.
      3. **Clinical features.** Each child on the autism spectrum has a unique presentation with various levels of impairment in each of the three core symptom areas. The atypical behaviors are notable for lack of flexibility in social communication, behaviors, and interactions. Common presentations in the often overlapping domains are outlined below.
         a. **Abnormal social interactions.** Deficits specific to ASD include lack of joint attention (ability to share interest with another using language, gestures, and eye gaze). Eye contact is usually decreased or not used to modulate social interactions. Children with ASD may range from being very withdrawn and appearing unaware of other people to having variable or odd interactions with others. Despite common misconceptions, they may be quite affectionate with caregivers and have normal attachment to them. They have difficulty establishing friendships with peers, ranging from being aloof to being overly intrusive. They may lack the ability to feel empathy or "put themselves in another's shoes."
         b. **Atypical communication.** Regression of language skills in the second year of life occurs in up to 30% of cases. Children on the spectrum who have meaningful language may demonstrate immediate and delayed echolalia, scripted speech (language heard on videos or in adult conversation), unusual prosody (monotone or singsong quality to speech), pronoun reversal (I/you) or speaking in third person,

and preservative speech. They do not spontaneously use gestures usually acquired by a child's first birthday, including pointing and waving.

c. **Restricted activities/play.** Children with ASD show little imaginative play. Often they engage in repetitive games or routines with toys (lining up, smelling, tapping). They may focus on sensory aspects of objects (spinning fans, flashing lights) or develop fascinations and obsessions with unusual objects (sprinkler systems, picture hooks, manhole covers). They often demand sameness in routines, placement of objects, or other rituals, and may become very agitated with any change. They may engage in repetitive hand or body movement (hand flapping, spinning, rocking) instead of meaningful play.

d. **Rote memory, nonverbal skills.** Children with ASD may have advanced "splinter skills," such as being able to decode words at a much higher level than expected (hyperlexia), although they rarely have commensurate reading comprehension. They may learn to count into the thousands, say the alphabet backwards, or be able to complete puzzles with the pieces upside down so that no pictures are showing; though they are not able to communicate their wants or needs to their parents.

e. **Sensory sensitivities.** Many children appear to be hyper- or hyposensitive to sensory experiences. They may, for example, cover their ears to loud noises, become distressed by textures of food or clothing, or be insensitive to painful stimuli.

f. **Comorbidities.** Many children with ASD have intellectual disability, although as diagnostic categorization of ASD has broadened, the rates are dropping below 50%. Children with intellectual disability are more likely to develop seizure disorders as well (approximately 30%). Many have symptoms of hyperactivity and inattention, anxiety, obsessive-compulsive behaviors, self-injurious behaviors, pica, or aggression. Sleep disorders, gastrointestinal and feeding disorders, and allergies are also common.

B. **Differential diagnosis.**
1. **Global developmental delay/intellectual disability.** Cognitive abilities may be difficult to assess in young, nonverbal child. Severe cognitive deficits may be associated with some of the repetitive behavioral manifestations of ASD.
2. **Developmental language disorder.** In the absence of significantly inhibited temperament or anxiety disorder, the child with developmental language disorder alone should demonstrate normal reciprocal social interactions and appropriate play for age.
3. **Hearing impairment.** Although not common, it is important to rule out sensory deficits as a cause of language and social delays.
4. **Landau–Kleffner syndrome.** Also known as acquired epileptic aphasia, this may cause regression of language and other delays and can be diagnosed by sleep-deprived electroencephalography (EEG).
5. **Rett syndrome.** Rett syndrome is a sporadic X-linked disorder in girls that shares some behavioral features with ASD. It is, however, a distinct disorder with a characteristic course including deceleration of head growth, stereotypic hand movements, and dementia. Many cases of Rett syndrome can be confirmed by genetic testing for the *MECP2* gene.
6. **Childhood disintegrative disorder.** Childhood disintegrative disorder is much rarer than ASD and is notable for apparently normal development followed by regression in at least two (and typically all) of the following areas: language, social skills, adaptive behavior, bowel and bladder control, play, or motor skills.
7. **Severe early deprivation/reactive attachment disorder.** Children who have experienced significant abuse and neglect may exhibit some of the symptoms of ASD.
8. **Anxiety disorders/obsessive compulsive disorder.** There is overlap between these disorders and ASD, although typically children with primary anxiety disorders have joint attention and reciprocal social relations that children with ASD lack.

C. **History.**
1. **Screening tools.** There is an increasing pressure from both parents and professionals for earlier identification of ASD so that treatment can begin before the age of 3 years. In 2006 and 2007, the American Academy of Pediatrics (AAP) outlined algorithms for routine screening and surveillance for developmental disorders including ASD as part of well-child care. The AAP recommended screening for ASD at 18 and 24 months, and suggested a list of possible screening tools. One commonly used screening tool is the Modified Checklist for Autism in Toddlers (MCHAT), which is free and easily administered and scored. However, the tool is limited by its low sensitivity (11%) in the absence of follow-up questions for "failed" items. Pediatric providers are advised to use a combination of screening tools and ongoing surveillance to identify children at risk for ASD.

Children identified as being at risk for ASD who "fail" routine screening or surveillance with questions below should be referred to a specialist experienced in evaluating children with ASD (developmental pediatric clinician, neurologist, psychologist, or psychiatrist).

2. **Key clinical questions.** When a concern of ASD is raised, the following questions (modified from the CHAT and MCHAT) are informative.
   - *Does your child respond to his name?"* Parents often report that they wonder if their child is deaf since he does not respond to voice, although he does turn to other sounds.
   - *"Does your child prefer to play alone than with others?"*
   - *"Does your child ever use her index finger to point and to show you something? Does your child ever bring a toy over to show you?"* These look at joint attention, which is impaired in ASD.
   - *"Does your child* (older than 18 months) *ever pretend when he is playing? (e.g., pretend to talk on the phone or feed a doll)."* Symbolic play is delayed or absent in ASD.
   - Red flags **of development that warrant further evaluation of possible ASD**.
     - No babbling by 9 months
     - No gesturing by 12 months
     - No single words by 16 months
     - No functional, nonecholalic two-word phrases by 24 months
     - **ANY loss of language or social skills at any age**
3. Family history of ASD and/or parental concern warrant further investigation including history and observation to determine whether the child requires an evaluation by a specialist in the field of ASD.

D. **Physical examination.** Most children with idiopathic ASD have unremarkable physical examinations. Some have isolated macrocephaly. Most have normal neurologic examinations and no motor abnormalities. Because of the association of tuberous sclerosis with ASD, a careful skin examination is required.

E. **Additional evaluations.** The medical workup of ASD should be guided by clues from the history and physical examination.
1. Formal audiologic evaluation and vision testing should be performed on all children.
2. Lead level should be tested if pica or social risk is present.
3. **Genetic testing.** High-resolution chromosomes and DNA for fragile X should be performed on all patients. If results of those tests are normal, further testing should be considered in a tiered approach, including comparative genomic hybridization/microarray analysis for submicroscopic duplications and deletions.
4. Repeat newborn screen, if not available or performed.
5. Consider EEG if clinical concern of seizures or significant regression (rule out Landau–Kleffner syndrome).
6. Consider magnetic resonance imaging if seizures or focal neurologic examination.
7. Consider genetics consultation if dysmorphisms or a family history of multiple cases of ASD is present. The genetics of ASD are an area of intense study and clinical recommendations are in rapid evolution.
8. Consider metabolic studies if history or physical examination is notable for hypotonia, regression, or decompensation with minor illness, or atypical presentation of ASD.

III. **Management.**
The foundation of treatment for ASD includes intensive educational intervention with individualized instruction aimed at ameliorating the core symptoms of ASD. *See Chapter 27, "Treatment and Medical Management of Children with Autism Spectrum Disorders" in this volume.*

IV. **Clinical pearls and pitfalls.**
   - ASD is very common, yet there is often a significant delay between when parents express concerns about their child's development and when the diagnosis of ASD is given. This may result in unnecessary delay of early intervention at the time when it is thought to have greatest impact. Parents' concerns about their child's development should be evaluated seriously and watchful waiting is not always appropriate in toddlers with language and social delays.
   - In the primary care office, clinicians should be sensitive to the needs of the child with ASD by speaking in a quiet voice and not pushing the child beyond his or her comfort level with eye contact or social interactions.
   - Clinicians should be alert to "hidden" medical conditions that can cause behavioral changes in nonverbal children with ASD (dental pain, constipation, etc). (This will be discussed in greater detail in Chapter 27.)

BIBLIOGRAPHY

Books

Grandin T. *Thinking in Pictures and Other Reports from My Life with Autism*. New York: Vintage Books, 1995. (A fascinating account by an accomplished woman with autism.)

Grinker R. *Unstrange Minds: Remapping the World of Autism*. New York: Basic Books, 2007. (Written by an anthropologist who is the father of a child with autism, this book offers both a review of many aspects of the science of autism, and interesting descriptions of the experience of autism in a variety of cultural contexts.)

Wiseman N. *Could It Be Autism? A Parent's Guide to First Signs and Next Steps*. New York: Broadway, 2006.

For professionals

Johnson C, Myers S, The Council on Children With Disabilities. Identification and evaluation of children with autism spectrum disorders. *Pediatrics* 120:1183–1215, 2007.

Schafer GB, Mendelsohn NJ, Professional Practice and Guidelines Committee. Clinical genetics evaluation in identifying the etiology of autism spectrum disorders. *Genet Med* 10:301–305, 2008.

Rice C, Principal Investigators. Prevalence of autism spectrum disorders-, autism and developmental disabilities monitoring network United States, 2006. MMWR 58(SS10):1–20, 2009.

Web sites

Autism Society of America. www.autism-society.org. Contains resources for parents in English and Spanish.

Autism Speaks. www.autismspeaks.org. Contains resources for parents in English and Spanish.

Centers for Disease and Prevention. http://cdc.gov/ncbddd/autism/index.html. Information for families and professionals about prevalence.

First Signs. www.firstsigns.org. Contains link to "Autism Video Glossary", a resource for parents and professionals about early signs of ASD, and free downloadable version of the MCHAT screening tool.

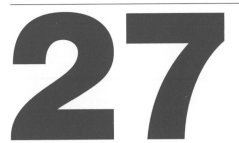

Complementary and Alternative Medicine in Autism Spectrum Disorders

Jodi Santosuosso
Eileen M. Costello
Elizabeth B. Caronna

I. **Description of the problem.** Complementary and alternative medicine (CAM) is commonly used for children with autism spectrum disorders (ASDs). These therapies can be extremely costly, few have been well studied with controlled trials, their placebo effect can be considerable, and many can be associated with significant risks. Parents of children with ASD are often frustrated by the failure of more traditional medical therapies to treat the core symptoms of ASD and the slow progress they see in response to well-accepted educational approaches, and for this reason, parents may turn to the promise of cure from nontraditional practitioners. Many parents of children with ASD utilize **both** widely accepted educational therapies and CAM. Thus primary care providers should routinely ask **all** parents of children with ASD about their use of CAM and be prepared to discuss treatments, data regarding efficacy or lack of efficacy (when available), and potential risks.

II. **Definition of CAM.** The National Center for Complementary and Alternative Medicine defines CAM as "a group of diverse medical and healthcare systems, practices, and products that are not presently considered to be part of conventional medicine," which includes mind–body interventions, biologically based practices, manipulative and body-based practices, and energy practices. Some treatments for ASD once considered "alternative" by healthcare providers are now so widely used that many now consider them conventional treatments. For example, sensory integration therapy for a variety of problem behaviors, and melatonin for sleep disturbances are now routinely recommended by many specialists in the field. (See Chapter 28 in this volume, "Treatments and Medical Management of Children with Autism Spectrum Disorders.") Similarly, many unproven treatments are ubiquitous in the lay press and on the Internet. Anecdotally, many parents have tried a restrictive diet even before their child has been formally diagnosed with ASD on the basis of recommendations from other parents or information from the Internet.

III. **Epidemiology and reasons cited for use of CAM therapies.** The most commonly used CAM treatments for ASD fall into two categories—biologically based practices and manipulative body-based practices. Up to three quarters of children with ASD may be treated with CAM; biologically based treatments are the most common, with higher rates of use in children with more severe symptoms of ASD. More than half of parents report that CAM treatments, including modified diets, vitamins/mineral and food supplements, are beneficial for their children with ASD, and many do not perceive risk associated with approaches that are promoted as being "natural." Unlike traditional educational or medical approaches, use of CAM gives parents more control over the therapy and, in some cases, promise of a cure. Despite considerable cost to families, as many of these therapies are "off label" and thus not covered by medical insurance, and risk of toxicity, many parents are eager to try unproven remedies that have been claimed to ameliorate symptoms of ASD.

IV. **Biologically based practices.** The controversy surrounding use of CAM for ASD is considerable and shows no sign of decreasing. The treatments discussed below are not meant to be an exhaustive list of all CAM used for children with ASD, but rather a list of several of the most commonly used treatments, an ever growing and evolving group of remedies not recommended by most medical practitioners.

A. **Gluten-free casein-free (GFCF) diet.** The elimination of the dietary proteins gluten (present in rye, wheat, and barley) and casein (present in dairy products) has been proposed as an effective treatment of ASD. True elimination of gluten and casein from the diet is difficult to implement and substitute foods can be expensive. The underlying theory is based on concerns about gastrointestinal problems (e.g., diarrhea) affecting digestion of proteins, food allergies, and abnormalities in gut permeability ("leaky gut" theory), allowing false opiate neuropeptides to cross the intestinal lining and enter the bloodstream, causing or exacerbating autistic behaviors. Although many parents report improvement in gastrointestinal problems on the GFCF diet, it cannot be recommended on the basis of available research data. Additional studies will be required to investigate whether there is a subset of children who do show true improvement of gastrointestinal symptoms or symptoms of ASD when on this elimination diet. Children on the GFCF diet should be monitored for nutritional deficiencies. (See Chapter 28 on Management of ASD.)

B. **Hyperbaric oxygen therapy (HBOT).** Used conventionally to treat carbon monoxide poisoning, HBOT has been recommended as a treatment of ASD on the basis of a theory that there is increased inflammation in the gut and brain and an aberrant response to oxidative stress in individuals with ASD. There are no randomized controlled trials (RCTs) to support the use of this therapy. Parents should be aware of the expense of time and money involved in this treatment and a risk of complications from high-pressure oxygen, including fire.

C. **Chelation.** The perception that heavy metal exposure, in particular mercury and lead, is related to increases in the diagnosis of ASD, has led to treatment through chelation, sometimes with industrial grade chemicals never designed to be used for medical use. Chemical chelation has evolved as an intervention despite the absence of data to support (1) the hypothesis that ASDs are related to heavy metals or (2) that chelation is safe or effective in this instance. Parents may ask their child's primary care provider to interpret results from nonstandard laboratory testing of blood, urine, stool, and hair for heavy metals. There has been one reported death of a child from hypocalcemia during a chelation treatment. Parents should be advised that chelation is not a proven treatment of autism, and is, in fact, potentially toxic.

D. **Intravenous immunoglobulin (IVIG).** IVIG has been used for the treatment of ASD on the basis of unproven theory of immune dysfunction/inflammation as a cause of autistic symptoms and small, uncontrolled studies that have claimed improvement in symptoms of ASD. The use of this therapy has not been supported by controlled studies, and the treatment carries the inherent risk of use of a pooled blood product. This is a costly, unproven treatment that presents considerable risk.

E. **Secretin.** First recommended in 1998 after a small study reported improved language and cognition in children administered with this gastrointestinal hormone during endoscopy, secretin has been extensively studied since. A review by the Cochrane group of 14 RCTs determined that no evidence exists that secretin is an effective treatment of ASD.

F. **Dietary supplements.**
   1. **Vitamins, minerals, and other supplements.** The use of dietary supplements, including high-dose vitamins, enzymes, antifungals, and probiotics, is well documented among families of children with ASD. Theories regarding deficiencies of nutrients or inability of the body to process their nutritional sources of nutrients are proposed as causes of symptoms of ASD, which are often held to be linked to gastrointestinal, allergic, or immune dysfunction that the supplements are purported to improve. Claims of powers of "detoxification" of some supplements are also given as reason for their use. Evidence from well-controlled, peer-reviewed studies is limited or not in existence to support the use of these various remedies.
   2. **Magnesium/vitamin B6.** Claims have been made that magnesium and vitamin B6 are useful in reducing autistic behaviors such as aggression and in improving eye contact and socialization. Insufficient data exist to support use of these supplements, and there is risk of sensory neuropathy from overdose of vitamin B6.
   3. **Dimethylglycine (DMG) and trimethylglycine (TMG).** DMG and TMG are thought to address behaviors purported to be related to immune dysfunction and are often used in conjunction with magnesium and vitamin B6 supplements. Anecdotal reports suggest that DMG and TMG can improve language, attention, and immune function in children with ASD. There are several small studies that do not demonstrate a positive effect and no studies supporting effectiveness of this intervention.
   4. **Amino acids.** Abnormal serotonin activity in the brains of individuals with ASD led to the approach to manipulate neurochemical activity through the use of amino acids, which are precursors to neurotransmitters. Common amino acid supplements include tryptophan, taurine, lysine, γ-aminobutyric acid, carnitine, and L-carnosine. L-carnosine is the only amino acid for which any data exist, in one small study of 31 peer-reviewed children who showed improvement over an 8-week trial of 800 mg daily. There are no peer-reviewed studies examining the effects of supplementation with the others.
   5. **Omega 3 fatty acids.** Studies have shown that children with ASD have decreased plasma levels of omega 3 fatty acids compared with typical children. The relevance of this finding is unclear as no clinical correlates were noted. One RCT in 13 autistic children with severe behavioral disturbance reported improvement in behaviors following a 6-week trial. This study has not been replicated. Side effects were limited to gastrointestinal discomfort, but there is a risk of environmental contamination of this nutritional supplement.

6. **Folate/glutathione.** Abnormal levels of antioxidants have been reported in children with autism, without clinic correlation, so the significance is unclear. Oxidative stress, which can result in neuronal injury, has been proposed as a possible etiology for the regression noted in up to one-third of children with autism. Folate and glutathione supplementation have been recommended to combat oxidative stress. Further research is required to assess the impact of folate supplementation.

G. **Probiotics, antifungals, and digestive enzymes.** These medications have been recommended on the basis of the unsupported theory that enteric yeast overgrowth due to antibiotic use or immune dysfunction triggered by vaccine administration causes gut wall inflammation, leading to increased permeability referred to as a "leaky gut," causing autistic symptomatology through release of "toxins" across the blood–brain barrier. There is no evidence-based data to support the use of probiotics or antifungals for the treatment of ASD.

H. **Body-based practices.**
1. **Auditory integration training (AIT).** Parents of children with ASD report high rates of auditory processing deficits. AIT purports to improve these deficits and to improve concentration through the use of headphones through which children listen to electronically modified voice, music, or sounds. Clinical trials thus far have not demonstrated effectiveness. The American Academy of Pediatrics considers AIT as an experimental therapy.
2. **Craniosacral massage.** Proponents of craniosacral therapy believe that gentle touch and manipulation of the skull and cervical spine will balance the cerebrospinal fluid and the membranes and tissues surrounding the spine and brain, thereby relieving stress and improving central nervous system function. There are no reported studies that evaluate this modality. Parents should be advised that the claims are biologically implausible and unlikely to be of any benefit.

I. **Vaccine refusal.** There is a common misperception that routine childhood vaccines have contributed to the increase in the prevalence of ASD. Theories of causal links between administration of the measles–mumps–rubella (MMR) vaccine or the vaccine preservative thimerosal and ASD have not been supported by numerous studies, and there is no peer-reviewed evidence to support such a relationship. The Institute of Medicine and the American Academy of Pediatrics have policy statements to this effect. Thimerosal was removed from routine immunizations in 1991, but distrust of vaccine safety is a frequent concern raised by parents in well-child visits, straining many relationships between pediatric clinicians and parents. Decreased rates of routine vaccination in the United Kingdom after the MMR-autism theory was first proposed resulted in increased rates of vaccine-preventable diseases. Parents who refuse vaccination should be counseled regarding these risks.

V. **Clinical pearls and pitfalls.**
- Primary care clinicians can help parents weigh the potential risks and benefits of CAM for ASD including the following:
- Rationale behind the treatment
- Financial cost
- Evidence of efficacy and/or toxicity
- Unproven claims of cure
- When parents chose to use CAM for ASD, pediatric clinicians should advise parents to
- Identify "target behaviors" of any intervention and keep data on those behaviors to assess possible improvement or deteriorations with treatment
- Use one treatment at a time to determine which treatment may be related to any behavioral changes
- Treatments proven to be ineffective, such as secretin, or dangerous, such as heavy metal chelation, should be warned against.
- Because the GFCF diet is among the most popular CAM interventions, primary care providers should identify clinical dietitians to whom to refer to assess for nutritional deficiencies associated with such diets.

BIBLIOGRAPHY

Web sites

Autism Watch. An interesting Web site offering a "scientific perspective on autism" updated by an individual physician. http://www.autism-watch.org/.
Cochrane Reviews. Includes several scientific reviews of treatments for ASD, including IV secretin, the GFCF diet, and vitamin B6/magnesium. http://www.cochrane.org/reviews/.

Books

Offit P. *Autism's False Prophets: Bad Science, Risky Medicine, and the Search for a Cure*. New York: Columbia University Press, 2008.

For professionals

Buie T, Campbell D, Fuchs GJ III et al. Evaluation, diagnosis, and treatment of gastrointestinal disorders in individuals with ASDs: a consensus report. *Pediatrics* 125:S1–S18, 2010.

Hanson E, Kalish LA, Bunce E, et al. Use of complementary and alternative medicine among children diagnosed with autism spectrum disorder. *J Autism Dev Disord* 37:628, 2007.

Heiger ML, England LJ, Molloy CA, et al. Reduced bone cortical thickness in boys with autism or autism spectrum disorders. *J Autism Dev Disord* 38:848–856, 2008.

Levy S, Hyman S. Complementary and alternative medicine treatments for children with autism spectrum disorders. *Child Adolesc Psychiatr Clin N Am* 17:803–820, 2008.

28 Treatment and Medical Management of Children with Autism Spectrum Disorders

Eileen M. Costello
Elizabeth B. Caronna

I. Description of the problem.

A. Treatment of core symptoms of autism spectrum disorders. Primary care providers are expected to help families make decisions about the management of a child with autism spectrum disorders (ASD). Because the spectrum is wide and includes a range of ability and disability, there is no one management strategy that works for all affected children. There is a growing body of research that supports the use of specific educational interventions as the foundation of therapy for ASD. However, individual children with ASD have variable responses to therapy, and there is regional variation in quality and quantity of available services. As a result, many families utilize a wide variety of therapies, both proven and unproven, in an attempt to treat both the core features of autism (deficits in verbal and nonverbal communication, impairment in social interactions, and restricted interests or repetitive behaviors) and the many associated difficulties commonly seen in children with ASD, such as deficits in sensory processing, sleep disturbance, gastrointestinal complaints, seizures, and anxiety or depression. (See Chapter 26 on Autism Spectrum Disorders and Chapter 24 on Asperger Syndrome in this volume for more information.) Pediatric providers should have a general familiarity with the strengths and limitations of both widely accepted and unconventional treatments for ASD and be able to steer parents toward evidence-based therapies available in the community whenever possible. (See as well Chapter 27 on Complementary and Alternative Medicine in Autism Spectrum Disorders in this volume.)

B. Medical and psychiatric comorbidities. The primary care provider should be alert to common medical comorbidities in ASD and for signs of medical symptoms that may be obscured by, or difficult to assess because of, the symptoms of ASD. For example, changes in behaviors of children with ASD (such as self-injury or aggression) may be attributed to worsening symptoms of ASD, causing an underlying medical disorder unrelated to ASD (such as gastroesophageal reflux or a dental abscess) to be missed. Challenges of history taking and detailed physical examination in the nonverbal or noncompliant child with ASD may compound this problem. Psychopharmacologic management, although not demonstrated to improve the **core** deficits in autism, can be helpful in managing some associated symptoms.

II. Educational interventions.

Intensive educational and behavioral programs have the best track record for improving outcomes of children with autism. As soon as a child is diagnosed with an ASD, immediate enrollment in an intensive educational or behavioral program is indicated. For children younger than 3 years, rapid referral for Early Intervention Services is crucial. Consensus statements from experts from both the educational/psychological and the medical fields recommend that Early Intervention should include active engagement of the child using a structured, consistent approach for a minimum of 25 hours per week, 12 months per year, with as much one-on-one engagement as possible. After the age of 3 years, services are typically provided through the public school system. Family training, in which parents learn to apply the educational and behavioral techniques in use during the school day, is a critical element of any program. Most research has focused on effectiveness of interventions with young children, but these interventions are also the foundation of instruction of older children, teens, and adults with ASD.

Three main types of educational interventions have been described. Each has unique components as well as components shared with the other two. Which therapy "works" for a child is determined by family preference, regional availability of qualified therapists, and the child's characteristics. With some children, there must be some "trial and error" before an effective individualized educational program is realized. Although no single therapy can be recommended above all others based on available evidence, it is clear that intensive services provided by skilled therapists with expertise in working with children with ASD are critical for success. The rate of progress depends on both the quality of the therapy provided and on the child's learning style and intellectual level. However, with appropriate instruction, all children with ASD can be expected to make demonstrable progress over time.

A. Applied behavioral analysis (ABA). ABA is a systematic and structured approach to instruction based on the science of behavior and learning which utilizes observation, data collection, and positive reinforcement to teach communication, academic, and social skills and to reduce problem behaviors. ABA can be used in both structured and naturalistic settings by skilled therapists, and programs such as Pivotal Response Training and Verbal Behavior Therapy also are grounded in the theories of ABA. Instruction based on ABA is widely used in preschool- and school-aged children, but the cost of one-on-one instruction of the intensity recommended in most studies can be prohibitively expensive. Coverage of the cost of these services through medical insurance and educational systems varies both by state and locally, but there are growing efforts by advocacy groups to mandate coverage of ABA and other therapies through medical insurance. ABA is the best studied of the educational approaches for ASD.

B. Structured teaching. The Treatment and Education of Autistic and related Communication-handicapped Children **(TEACCH)** program is the most prominent example of structured teaching for children with ASD. This method "structures" the physical environment and teaching techniques using visual supports and a predictable routine. The use of visual schedules fosters a predictable sequence of daily activities and structures activities. The emphasis of this method is on improving skills and modifying the environment to adapt to the learning preferences and needs of children with ASD.

C. Developmental approaches.

1. **Developmental, Individual Difference Relationship-based model (DIR).** The focus is on "Floortime" sessions of play of parent or therapist with the child to enhance relationships and foster emotional, social, and cognitive growth through developmentally appropriate play that taps the child's strengths. This therapy is directed at building "biologically based processing capacities" including auditory processing and language, motor planning and sequencing, visual-spatial processing, and sensory modulation.

2. **Relationship Development Intervention (RDI)** is designed to use positive reinforcement through a systematic, parent-based intervention to promote interactive behaviors that engage the child in a social relationship, first with an adult, and then with peers.

3. **Social Communication/Emotional Regulation/Transactional Supports (SCERTS).** The SCERTS model combines elements of the programs described above to promote social communication initiated by the child. It is typically used in classrooms and is well-suited to inclusive classroom settings.

D. Other interventions directed at specific aspects of ASD.

1. **Alternative Communication Strategies.** Many children with ASD have stronger visual than verbal reasoning abilities, so a variety of visual supports are commonly used in home and school settings. Alternative communication uses a range of simple to technologically advanced tools such as sign language, objects, photos, drawings, and computer-based technologies. It is most important for preverbal or nonverbal children.

2. **The Picture Exchange Communication System (PECS)** is in wide use. In this system, a child initiates a request by using a small picture of something he desires (such as a food or a toy) in exchange for the item. This system incorporates ABA and developmental principles and is effective with many children.

3. **Visual supports** such as the pictures or icons used in PECS can also be used in other ways, such as providing visual schedules, supporting vocabulary development, and for behavioral management strategies.

4. **Speech and language therapy.** The majority of children with ASD will require speech and language therapy to address their deficits in expressive and receptive language and social communication. Most children with ASD benefit from both individual and group speech and language therapy. There is evidence to support the use of **pragmatic language therapy,** which focuses on using language for social interaction, rather than the production of speech.

5. **Social skills training.** There is growing evidence to support that joint attention and symbolic play skills can be taught and that they will generalize to other settings. Joint attention is a precursor to social language development, and it is a focus of instruction in young and nonverbal children with ASD. Social skills training, designed to help children respond to social overtures of other children and adults, promote imitation of social behavior, and reduce stereotypes or other perseverative behaviors, can benefit children with ASD of all ages and level of disability. Formal social skills curricula and programs are often used in schools and may occur individually or in small groups of children with ASD or with typical peers.

6. **Occupational therapy.** Many children with ASD have difficulties with fine and gross motor skills that may be addressed through occupational therapy (OT). School-based OTs can help with classroom accommodations to promote social interaction, increased attention, and organization. **Sensory integration (SI)** therapy is a specialized type of OT designed to address the difficulties with processing sensory information that is common in ASD. Examples of SI include the use of swings to help with gravitational insecurity, brushing the skin to decrease sensory sensitivity, or the provision of sensations that the child seeks, such as deep pressure, to elicit or reinforce a desired behavior.

E. **The older child.** There is less research supporting programs designed to support older children and adolescents with ASD. Many of the educational approaches described above are used with school-aged children through adolescence, but often educational services designed specifically for children with ASD are harder to find outside of the early childhood period. In part, this is due to lack of empiric evidence for treatments for these older age groups. Older children are more likely to receive services designed to address their comorbid learning disability or cognitive impairment, rather than the social impairments specific to ASD.

The majority of children will require an individual education plan (IEP) throughout their schooling. Because of the range of behaviors and skills in affected children, some will require a substantially separate school program, whereas others can thrive in a regular educational setting with additional supports in place. Most students, even those with milder symptoms of ASD, will require support in social skills and academics. They may require significant academic accommodations, and many require aides to succeed in an inclusive educational setting. (See also Chapter 24 on Asperger Syndrome for more information about educational programs.)

Social reciprocity remains a concern for the majority of older children, and teens are at risk for loneliness, bullying, anxiety, and depression. Ironically, the children with milder symptoms of ASD and Asperger syndrome who are more likely to be educated in "mainstream" or inclusion settings are those most likely to be tormented by bullies because of their quirky behaviors. Their impairments in social communication, "reading" social cues, and lack of "street smarts" puts them at high risk, and primary care providers should ask specifically about bullying during clinical visits.

"Transition plans" are a part of an IEP for individuals approaching adulthood. A transition plan considers the student's strengths and potential for further education or a vocational career beyond high school. Students, parents, teachers, and professionals who have supported the family are involved in transition planning from the middle adolescent years.

Since sexual development progresses in a typical manner for teens with ASD, they may have the potential to find themselves in high-risk situations at school or in the community that they do not have the social skills to navigate. For older children and adolescents who have higher verbal and cognitive skills, the issue of disclosure of the diagnosis is also an issue that arises that must be addressed on an individual basis, and the primary care provider may be called upon by parents to offer guidance through this process.

III. **Medical management.** Most medical care for children with ASD is provided in the primary care setting, and children with ASD may require twice as much time per office visit than typically developing children. Time spent familiarizing the child with the office setting, instruments, and procedures will increase comfort, cooperation, and effectiveness of an office visit. Common challenging behaviors, especially in children with limited language, should prompt a thorough history and physical examination to eliminate an occult source of pain such as otitis, sinusitis, dental abscess, constipation, occult fracture, or esophagitis due to reflux.

A. **Medical comorbidities.**

1. **Sleep disturbance.** Sleep problems are common in children with ASD and include delayed sleep onset and nighttime wakening. Sleep problems increase stress on families and can negatively affect quality of life during waking hours. Evaluation for an underlying medical etiology such as gastroesophageal reflux or sleep apnea should be considered on the basis of the history and physical examination.

In addition to usual sleep hygiene practices, a variety of agents have been used to enhance sleep. Over-the-counter diphenhydramine can be tried in low dose to hasten sleep onset, though activation, rather than sedation, is common and may limit its usefulness. Evidence suggests that abnormal melatonin regulation may be a factor in the sleep onset difficulties seen in children with ASD. Although evidence supporting the use of synthetic melatonin for sleep onset and insomnia is growing, there is a need for randomized controlled trials for this agent. Low-dose melatonin (1 mg) given a couple of hours before bedtime can improve sleep. Many children require higher doses up to 3 mg, though safety and efficacy of this nutritional supplement at any dose have not been established. Side effects include daytime sleepiness, dizziness, nausea, and headaches. An increase in seizure frequency in vulnerable children is reported.

2. **Gastrointestinal problems.** Gastrointestinal complaints including constipation, vomiting, diarrhea, and abdominal pain occur frequently in children with ASD. Children with these symptoms should receive thorough evaluations and treatment, as would children without ASD. There is no evidence that supports specific gastrointestinal pathology (such as an "autistic enterocolitis" or a "leaky gut syndrome") to be associated with ASD. Common gastrointestinal problems may not always have obvious symptoms in children with ASD (e.g., abdominal pain, gastroesophageal reflux) and may manifest as sleep disturbances, irritability, self-injury, aggression, or stereotypy, for example. Children with limited or no language and unexplained behavioral changes should be evaluated for occult gastrointestinal pathology or other source of pain.

3. **Nutritional concerns.** Children with ASD frequently have very restricted diets, often preferring to eat certain colors, textures, or types of food, to the exclusion of all others. Such highly selective diets can lead to nutritional deficiencies. Prescription of a multivitamin is a practical first-line treatment in primary care. In addition, parents frequently choose to put their children with ASD on restrictive diets (see discussion of gluten-free/casein-free diet in Chapter 27, Complementary and Alternative Medicine in Autism Spectrum Disorders in this volume), further limiting dietary intake. As a result, the primary care provider must investigate potential nutritional deficiencies (especially of calcium, vitamin D, iron, and protein) and consult with a pediatric nutritionist if concerns arise.

4. **Epilepsy.** Reports indicate that children with ASD with intellectual disability and motor delays have a 42% prevalence of seizures, compared to 6%–8% prevalence among children with ASD without intellectual disability or associated medical problems. There is a bimodal distribution in age of onset of seizures, one in the first years of life and one in adolescence. A high degree of suspicion is indicated when behaviors such as staring spells (in which the child does not respond to touch) might be explained by a seizure, and referral to a neurologist and an electroencephalography should be considered.

5. **Comorbid symptoms.** Higher rates of bipolar disorder, depression, anxiety, hyperactivity, and irritability have been reported among children with ASD. Up to 45% of children and 75% of adults on the autism spectrum are prescribed a psychotropic medicine. To date, no medications have been shown to directly treat the core symptoms of autism. It is important for the primary care provider to rule out occult medical and dental causes of behavioral changes prior to initiating psychopharmacological treatment. In addition, the pediatric provider should ensure that all behavioral and educational treatments have been optimized prior to considering medications to treat behavioral problems in ASD, as the nonpharmacologic treatments should be the first-line approach to behavioral problems in ASD. However, psychopharmacologic agents can be used successfully as an adjunct to the educational and behavioral interventions, requiring collaboration between medical, psychiatric, and educational providers.

Children with autism often have idiosyncratic reactions or unacceptable side effects to psychopharmacologic agents, which limit their usefulness. Few placebo-controlled trials have been done in the pediatric population with ASD to support the use of these medications, although they are widely prescribed. Listed below are some of the most commonly targeted symptoms and commonly used medications. Primary care providers are strongly advised to seek consultation (at a minimum by telephone, but ideally with direct evaluation of the patient) with a developmental/behavioral pediatrician, child neurologist, or child psychiatrist prior to starting psychotropic medications for a child with ASD. In all cases, initial doses should be as low as possible and increases should be gradual and in response to data collected by parents and teachers regarding target symptoms and side effects. In many cases, parents choose to discontinue medications because the side effects or idiosyncratic reactions are actually worse than the symptoms they were prescribed to treat. Parents must be informed when psychopharmacologic agents prescribed are "off label" and of potential side effects. Details of dosing for brand name formulations of psychotropic medications are found in Chapter 25 on ADHD and Chapter 20 on Psychopharmacology in this volume.

a. **Inattention/hyperactivity.** Recent studies have demonstrated the efficacy of methylphenidate in inattention, hyperactivity, and impulsivity among children with ASD. However, the response rate for children with ASD treated with stimulants is lower than that in typical children, and there are reports of idiosyncratic reactions, such as irritability. Side effects include abdominal pain, increased heart rate, increase in blood pressure, delayed sleep onset, and appetite reduction. Trials of short-acting stimulants, at the lowest dose possible, can be done with frequent feedback from parents (and school, when appropriate) about observed response and side effects. Increase in height and weight must be followed carefully in children on stimulants, and stimulant-induced anorexia can be particularly challenging to manage in a child with ASD who has a limited diet, even before initiation of medication.

b. **Aggression and disruptive behavior.** Haloperidol has been shown to effectively reduce aggressive behavior, but the side effects of typical neuroleptics (e.g., tardive dyskinesia) limit its appeal today. An atypical antipsychotic, **risperidone** has been approved by the Food and Drug Administration for the treatment of children and adolescents with ASD. Target behaviors include irritability, aggression self-injury, and temper tantrums. Several randomized controlled trials support the short-term use, and several open-label trials have demonstrated long-term efficacy. Secondary effects that bear watching include excessive weight gain due to increased appetite, hyperprolactinemia, and QTc prolongation. Atypical antipsychotics have much lower rates of tardive dyskinesia and neuroleptic malignant syndrome when compared with typical antipsychotics. Often even low doses of risperidone (0.25 mg/day) can be effective, and, when given at night, can also improve sleep patterns. As doses increase, the medication "acts" like a typical antipsychotic with higher levels of potential toxicity, so consultation with a psychopharmacologist, developmental/behavioral pediatrician, or neurologist is advised whenever this medication is prescribed in the primary care setting.

An alpha adrenergic antihypertensive agent, **clonidine** has been found to be useful in treatment of hyperarousal symptoms including irritability, impulsivity, and repetitive behaviors in children with ASD. Alpha agonists have the potential to be dangerous in overdose, and side effects include sleepiness, hypotension, dry mouth, dizziness, and constipation. The longer-acting alpha adrenergic medication guanfacine, in regular and long-acting forms, may be a safer alternative, with less blood pressure lability. Only one alpha adrenergic agent, a long-acting guanfacine, has been approved for use in children with ADHD, but it is a new agent and has not been well studied in children with ASD. These agents should be used with caution in the primary care setting.

c. **Symptoms of anxiety/obsessive compulsive disorder.** Selective serotonin reuptake inhibitors (SSRIs) such as fluoxetine and fluvoxamine have been demonstrated to be helpful in the treatment of repetitive and maladaptive behaviors, depression, anxiety, aggression, and certain aspects of social interaction and language in individuals with ASD. Adverse effects of SSRIs include headache, dry mouth, fatigue, agitation, behavioral activation, sexual dysfunction, and nausea. These medications do not have specific indications for ASD. Care must be taken when choosing an SSRI for children with ASD, as SSRIs with the longer half-lives (e.g., fluoxetine) may not be advisable, because if idiosyncratic side effects occur, they will be more prolonged. SSRIs with more moderate half lives (e.g., sertraline, citalopram) may be a better choice, in case they need to be discontinued because of adverse effects.

IV. **Clinical pearls and pitfalls.**
- Parents of children with ASD need guidance in evaluating the quality of information available on the Internet and in the lay press. They require support from providers and community organizations in dealing with the stress caused both by the diagnosis of ASD and by the difficulties of navigating the process of obtaining services for their child.
- The primary care provider should ask about the educational services of the patient with ASD and should raise concern if the program is not intensive and using well-established educational methods as outlined in this chapter. The best way to assess whether an educational program is appropriate is by asking, *"Is your child making progress in school?"* If the answer is no, it is likely that either the program is not adequate, or there are other factors interfering with progress that need to be identified.
- Routine review of symptoms in a child with ASD should include questions about sleep, nutrition, and changes in behavior that could signify an underlying medical illness or pain.
- In older children with ASD and in those with milder symptoms, review of symptoms should include questions about social functioning with peers, mood, and bullying.
- Working with a developmental/behavioral pediatrician, child psychiatrist, or psychopharmacologist to manage behaviors or comorbid mental health concerns will optimize care of

the child with ASD over time. Careful psychopharmacological management with frequent communication with parents while medications are initiated and adjusted is critical for safety and success.

BIBLIOGRAPHY

For parents

Greenspan S, Wieder S. *Engaging Autism: Using the Floortime Approach to Help Children Relate, Communicate, and Think*. Cambridge, MA: Da Capo Books, 2006.

Harris S, Weiss MJ. *Right from the Start: Behavioral Interventions for Young Children with Autism*. Bethesda, MD: Woodbine House, 2007.

For professionals

American Academy of Pediatrics. *Caring for Children with Autism Spectrum Disorders: A Resource Toolkit for Clinicians*. Elk Grove Village, IL: American Academy of Pediatrics, 2007. Available from the American Academy of Pediatrics at AAP.org.

Buie T, Campbell D, Fuchs GJ III, et al. Evaluation, diagnosis, and treatment of gastrointestinal disorders in individuals with ASDs: a consensus report. *Pediatrics* 125:S1–S18, 2010.

Liptak GS, Stuart T, Auinger P. Health care utilization and expenditures for children with autism: data from US national samples. *J Autism Dev Disord* 36:871–879, 2006.

Myers SM, Johnson CP. The Council on Children with Disabilities. Management of children with autism spectrum disorders. *Pediatrics* 120:1162–1182, 2007.

Web sites

American Academy of Pediatrics. http://www.aap.org/healthtopics/autism.cfm

Autism, Asperger's syndrome, and related developmental disorders. http://www.autism-help.org/index.htm

29

Bad News in the Media

Marilyn Augustyn
Betsy McAlister Groves

I. **Description of the problem.** Over the last 30 years, media coverage of world events has changed, as has children's exposure to the media.
   - In 1965, American children spent 30 hours/week with their parents; in 2002 they spent 17 hours/week with their parents and 40 hours/week on average watching TV, using the computer, listening to the radio or CDs, and playing video games. In 2010, with technology, children have nearly 24-hour access to media with 8–18-year-olds devoting an average of 7 hours and 38 minutes for using entertainment media across a typical day (more than 53 hours a week). If "media multitasking" (using more than one medium at a time) is included, they average 10 hours and 45 minutes worth of media content into those $7\frac{1}{2}$ hours of media access.
   - Televisions are also commonly present in bedrooms, with 19% of infants, 29% of 2–3-year-olds, 43% of 4–6-year-olds, and 68% of children 8 years and older having a television in their bedrooms.
   - TV news coverage may be primarily *episodic* (focused on events) or *thematic* (including attention to trends, data on other conditions, providing context for an event). Ninety percent of network crime stories are framed episodically, and it has been hypothesized that this episodic presentation makes the viewer more likely to blame the victim and less likely to think of the larger context in which these events take place.
   - Studies of stories about violence on local news programs suggest that they overemphasize violent crime, distort issues of race, and cultivate fear of urban areas in heavy viewers. Both children and adults who watch a lot of TV come to believe that the world is a far more dangerous place than it really is.
   - Children are influenced by media—they learn by observing, imitating, and adopting behaviors. Extensive research evidence indicates that media violence can contribute to aggressive behavior, desensitization to violence, nightmares, and fear of being harmed. Because children younger than 8 years cannot discriminate between fantasy and reality, they may be especially vulnerable to some of these learning processes and may, thereby, be more influenced by media violence.

II. **Making the diagnosis.**
   Take a media history. The American Academy of Pediatrics recommends at least two media-related questions at each routine healthcare maintenance visit.
   1. **From parents.** This is particularly important if parents are concerned about how a child may be responding to an event. Key trigger questions include the following:
      - *"Does your child have a TV/Internet connection in his room?"*
      - *"Do you watch TV with your child or know what your child is watching?"*
      - *"Do you monitor Internet or online computer use?"*
      - *"How much screen time (including television, videos, computer, and video games) does your child have each day?"*
   2. **From the child.** After 4 years of age, children are often good historians about their favorite TV show, what they like to do on the computer, what they understand about current world events, etc.

III. **Advice for families.**
   A. Limit the child's (particularly young children's) access to TV, newspapers, and magazines with graphic images of violence and trauma.
   B. Talk to your child about what he/she sees on television. Maintaining open communication with children about the news or world events is very important. Your explanations and reassurance indicate that you are open to discussion and willing to engage. Take children's questions seriously and be prepared to answer the same questions repeatedly.
   C. Before talking to your child about a potentially distressing event in the media, take stock of your thoughts, beliefs, fears, and reactions. Children are great readers of emotional messages and will respond to verbal and nonverbal messages parents send about their

Table 29-1. Developmental perspectives

Age	Child's understanding	Interventions
Toddlers (2 yr and younger)	They will have no understanding apart from the reactions of their caregivers. Their only concern may be how it will impact their world.	Details may frighten them. Shield the child when possible from exposure to the news. Reassure them that their caregivers will keep them safe.
Preschoolers	Their capacity to distinguish real from fantasy is limited. Their main worry will be about their own safety and the safety of their parents.	Keep the TV off and stay close to home during the days surrounding an event. Show your child some things that may help keep him safe like smoke alarms or door locks.
School-aged children	It's best to start with a question to find out how much your child may know and begin from there. As they have a sense of right and wrong, they are often focused on why an event occurred.	It may be helpful to show the child that people are not powerless in this situation; for example, helping the child in an act to aid the situation, donating food to tragedy victims, etc. It is also a prime time to help the child understand how they too deal with anger.

own feelings. For some children, parental distress may be more upsetting than the event itself.

D. Children communicate their thoughts and worries in both verbal and nonverbal ways. Young children may draw pictures, use dramatic play or themes to share their feelings. Use these to elicit supportive discussions between parent and child.

E. Spend extra time with your children during times of stress. Maintain the daily routine. Predictability and structure are often comforting for children in times of stress.

F. **Developmental perspectives.** Table 29-1 presents suggestions of how to talk to children of different ages about world events.

BIBLIOGRAPHY

For parents

Web sites

American Academy of Pediatricians. http://www.aap.org/patiented/talkingAboutDisasters.htm

For professionals

AAP. Policy statement on media violence. *Pediatrics* 124(5):1495–1503, 2009. doi:10.1542/peds. 2009–2146.
AAP. Policy statement on disaster planning for schools. *Pediatrics* 122(4):895–901, 2008. doi: 10.1542/peds.2008–2170.
Generation M^2. Media in the lives of 8–18 year olds. http://www.kff.org/entmedia/mh012010pkg.cfm

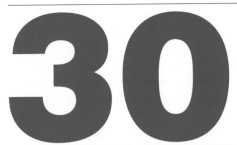

Bipolar Disorder in Children

Janet Wozniak
Joseph Biederman

I. **Description of the problem.** Childhood or pediatric-onset bipolar disorder is now the focus of an increasing number of research studies due to the high degree of disability associated with the symptoms and the suggestion of a higher prevalence than once thought. Up until the mid-1990s, the condition was thought to be so uncommon that it was generally not included in the training of child and adolescent psychiatrists or pediatric clinicians and was not considered in the differential diagnosis of a moody child. Because of an increase in diagnoses and medication prescriptions, there are concerns that the diagnosis may be over used, inappropriately subjecting some children to mood-stabilizing medications. The increase in diagnoses may be an accurate reflection of the prevalence of bipolar disorder in children. In fact, it may be an underestimate of real psychiatric illness in youth, and many children who could benefit from psychiatric intervention may never come to clinical attention. Factors such as symptom overlap with attention-deficit/hyperactivity disorder (ADHD) and developmentally different presentation from the classic form of bipolar disorder have led to its underdiagnosis in the past.

A. **Epidemiology.** The true epidemiology of childhood bipolar disorder is not known as no definitive epidemiologic studies have addressed the question.
- One study of adolescents suggests **that 1% are affected, with up to 15% suffering from a subthreshold (but highly disabling) form of bipolar disorder.**
- Other studies that indirectly address the prevalence of bipolar disorder in youth by examining rates in clinic, depressed and ADHD populations, generally confirm that **1% of children and adolescents are affected.**
- As research on the pediatric subtype of bipolar disorder increases, new evidence addressing the various subtypes of bipolar disorder present in adults, especially those with dysphoria, mixed states, and complex cycling, suggests that the **prevalence of bipolar disorder in the adult population may be 4%–5%,** also higher than previously thought.

B. **Etiology/contributing factors.** As in all psychiatric conditions, a complex interplay of environmental influences and genetic factors is responsible for the development of bipolar disorder in adults as well as in children. **There is no evidence that "bad parenting" or traumatic experience is responsible for the dramatic mood swings present in bipolar children** and adolescents. However, **parenting techniques, which focus on flexibility and decreased rigidity are gaining acceptance as essential in reducing the frequency and intensity of the rage aspect of bipolar disorder.**
1. Family studies increasingly implicate the role of genetics as important in the development of bipolar disorder, but a **complex, polygenetic etiology** is more likely than a single gene. Neuroimaging studies implicate the **limbic structures of the brain** as the site of the neurobiologic abnormality.

II. **Making the diagnosis. There is no definitive test for bipolar disorder.** Despite advances in neuroimaging and in identifying candidate genes, there are currently no biological markers for this disorder. Like other psychiatric disorders, the diagnosis is made clinically, by asking about the specific symptoms in a developmentally appropriate manner. Research studies often use the Young Mania Rating Scale, but this scale was designed for use in adult inpatients and is not as useful in children and adolescents.

A. **Signs and symptoms.** Bipolar disorder is a mood disorder, and therefore the diagnosis is anchored by the presence of abnormal mood states that fluctuate between depression and mania. Please see the chapter on depression for information regarding the symptoms of depression.
1. Mania is characterized by two types of abnormal mood: **euphoric and irritable.** To be diagnosed as having bipolar disorder, it is necessary to have had an **episode of mania that lasts 1 week or longer** (hypomania refers to episodes of mania lasting less than a week, but at least 4 days). Most individuals who have episodes of mania also have depression.

2. **Depression can cycle in an alternating fashion** with mania (a week or more of mania followed by an episode of depression). Some such individuals will then experience an **intermorbid period of good functioning,** free from abnormal mood states, although this type of alternating mood states and return to good functioning is rare in pediatric cases.

3. Others experience **"mixed" states in which mania and depression occur together.** In such states, an individual may be euphoric for part of a day, rageful/irritable for another part of the day, and depressed/suicidal for another part of the day. **Children and adolescents tend to present with mixed states and complicated cycling patterns** rather than classic episodes of mania alternating with depression. A return to a high-functioning, euthymic (even/normal) mood appears to be rare in bipolar youth. Many adults also present with mixed states, and most adults with bipolar disorder spend more time depressed than manic.

4. **Euphoric states** are characterized by a feeling of being high or hyper, being "on top of the world" or being powerful and able to "accomplish anything."

5. The irritable mood of mania is distinctly different from the irritability associated with depression, ADHD, age-appropriate tantrums, or "bad days." The **irritability of mania is extreme, persistent, threatening, attacking, and out of control. Rage episodes** can occur with long episodes (20–60 minutes or more) of destructive, out of control and dangerous anger.

6. In addition to abnormal moods, the diagnosis of mania requires at least three (or four in the absence of euphoria) additional symptoms, often remembered with the mnemonic DIGFAST (**D**istractibility, **I**ncreased activity/energy, **G**randiosity, **F**light of ideas, **A**ctivities with bad outcome, **S**leep decreased, **T**alkativeness).

B. **Differential diagnosis.**
1. With **unipolar depression**. Irritability can characterize both mania and depression. However, the irritability of depression is milder, more complaining/whining/grouchy and is associated with low self-esteem, self-denigrating and self-destructive feelings, joylessness, and hopelessness. The **irritability of mania is more severe and dramatic with aggression and explosiveness.**
2. With **ADHD.** Mania and ADHD share the symptoms of distractibility, increased energy or hyperactivity, and talkativeness. In addition, ADHD can be associated with irritability and decreased frustration tolerance, although the irritability of ADHD is of lower intensity. Both disorders can be characterized by impulsivity. In general, **the symptoms of mania are much more disabling and of a greater severity than ADHD.** It is important to note that ADHD frequently co-occurs with mania, and both disorders can be present.

C. **History: key clinical questions.**
1. To **assess overall moodiness.** *"How often (How much of each day? How many days out of the week?) and how severe are the child's abnormal mood states? How often do you see age-appropriate moods?"*
2. To **assess mania.** *"How common and how severe are angry mood states? How often does grouchy, cranky, whining behavior occur? How common is hitting, kicking, biting, spitting? How common (many times per day, once per day, a few times per week) are rage episodes or explosions? Do rages last a long time (20–60 minutes or more)? Are the rages threatening, aggressive, attacking, or dangerous? How common and how severe are euphoric or goofy/giddy/silly mood states? While all children can be silly, does your child take jokes too far? Does the child alienate others with immature behavior or excessive laughing fits?"*
3. To assess **depression and cycling.** *"How common are depressed, sad, blue or hopeless/joyless mood states? Do these moods occur on the same days as the manic mood states noted above? Do depressed moods occur during weeks or months separate from the manic mood states? Is the child self-destructive, self-abusive, or suicidal?"*
4. To assess **DIGFAST symptoms.**
   a. *"Is the child easily distracted from tasks by noise, sights, or internal thoughts?"*
   b. *"Does the child have high-energy states with increased motor activity? Is it difficult to calm or slow down the child?"*
   c. *"Is the child grandiose? Does he have inflated sense of self-esteem or does he overestimate his ability to do things? Does the child act or feel stronger/smarter/more powerful than others? Take on big projects? Does the child demonstrate a flagrant disregard for adult authority, acting like the boss? Is the child a braggart or show-off?"*
   d. *"Does the child jump from idea to idea quickly or go off on tangents that are hard to follow when they talk? Does the child complain of 'racing thoughts' or thoughts that occur so rapidly they are hard to keep track of?"*

e. *"Does the child show poor judgment in activities? Is the child reckless? Does the child want to buy or spend money excessively? Is the child sexually inappropriate (e.g., excessive bathroom humor, preoccupation with genitals or sexual matters, excessive or public masturbation, touching others' breasts or private parts, exposing self to others)?"*

f. *"Does the child function with less sleep than most other children of the same age? How many hours less? Has the child ever functioned on little or no sleep or just a few hours?"*

g. *"Is the child talkative? Does the child have pressured speech? Is the child difficult to stop or interrupt?"*

III. **Management.** Although some children may "grow out" of bipolar disorder symptoms (longitudinal studies are underway), bipolar disorder is generally considered to be a chronic, lifelong condition. Longitudinal studies of children suggest a pattern of partial recovery, with frequent relapse.

A. **Pharmacotherapy** is the mainstay of treatment of bipolar disorder and a combined pharmacotherapy approach (using medications in combination) is typically required. **Mood-stabilizing medications** spanning various categories are the first-line treatment. Mood stabilizers include **atypical antipsychotics** (risperidone, olanzapine, quetiapine, ziprasidone, and aripiprazole), **lithium,** and **certain anticonvulsants** (valproate, carbamazepine, oxcarbazepine, and lamotrigine).

- Clinical trials and clinical experience have suggested that atypical antipsychotics work the fastest and most effectively in youth to control the disabling symptoms of mania as compared to the more traditional agents (lithium and anticonvulsants).
- Pediatric bipolar disorder is difficult to treat and often requires combination therapy using more than one mood stabilizer at a time. Mood stabilizers may control mania, but leave depression untreated, requiring the cautious addition of an antidepressant (cautiously using low doses, as antidepressants can cause worsening of mania). Lamotrigine can also be useful for bipolar depression.
- Because bipolar disorder is highly comorbid with ADHD and anxiety disorders, medications addressing these conditions are often required. Stimulant medications must be used cautiously as they can exacerbate mania, but frequently improve the functioning of the child who has both mania and ADHD.

B. **Other therapies including cognitive behavioral therapy, dialectical behavioral therapy, family therapy, group therapy, and individual psychodynamic therapy** can all be helpful for various individuals. An approach combining medication treatment with these other therapies tailored to the needs of the individual is generally recommended for the treatment of bipolar disorder.

- Helping the bipolar individual develop insight into his condition and to recognize the early signs of relapse aids in treatment.
- Therapy is helpful to ensure medication compliance, which is important in preventing relapse.

C. **Psychiatric hospitalization** is frequently required in the management of bipolar disorder due to the **dangerous behaviors associated with mania, the suicidal behavior of depression** or **psychosis** associated with either. Many children improve with the containment and structure of hospitalization or residential treatment programs.

D. **The presence of comorbid conditions** can complicate the management and course of bipolar disorder in youth.

- In bipolar children younger than 12 years, **comorbid ADHD** is almost always present (90% or more).
- In adolescents with bipolar disorder, **comorbid ADHD** occurs in 50%–60%.
- **Conduct disorder or antisocial personality disorder** (criminal behaviors) may occur in as many as 40% of youth with bipolar disorder and may or may not improve when the bipolar disorder is treated.
- **Anxiety disorders** are present in 50%–60% of youth with bipolar disorder and may be easy to miss, as it may seem counterintuitive to be disinhibited from mania and ADHD but fearful and inhibited from anxiety simultaneously.
- **Alcohol and drug abuse and addiction** commonly occur in youth with bipolar disorder, with adolescent-onset bipolar disorder carrying the greatest risk. Random drug screening is recommended even in youth professing abstinence.

IV. **Clinical pearls and pitfalls.**

- Pediatric bipolar disorder may be a difficult diagnosis to make because it presents atypically rather than in classic manner with a developmental picture characterized by (1) more irritability (than euphoria); (2) mixed states and complex cycling; (3) chronicity rather than interepisode high functioning; and (4) high levels of comorbidity especially with ADHD. Adults also report this type of bipolar disorder.

- Parents often feel unfairly blamed by mental health professionals, pediatric clinicians, teachers, and family members for "causing" the disorder by not being strict enough or disciplining "bad behavior" effectively. In fact, a genetic etiology is most likely.
- Pediatric bipolar disorder is a neurobiologic disorder affecting thinking, feeling, and behavior in children in a dramatic way. It is characterized by out of control mood swings and frequent episodes of rage, irritability, and poor judgment.
- Some children present with different symptoms in different arenas. At certain stages of the disorder and at certain ages, rage and depression may only be evident to those family members closest to the child and not apparent to teachers, friends, or pediatric clinicians. The reasons for this are unclear but may relate to the progression of the disorder (most evident to parents initially, later spilling over into other arenas). This feature does not mean that parents are "doing something wrong" and should not discourage parents from seeking professional treatment.
- Although medications used to treat bipolar disorder in children carry many potentially serious side effects, not treating bipolar disorder in children can lead to worsening of the condition and/or the complications of suicidal behavior, substance abuse, or criminal arrest due to disinhibited behaviors in public.

BIBLIOGRAPHY

For parents

CABF (Child and Adolescent Bipolar Foundation). www.bpkids.org

Greene R. *The Explosive Child: A New Approach for Understanding and Parenting easily Frustrated, "Chronically Inflexible" Children.* New York, NY: Harper Collins, 1998.

McDonnell MA, Wozniak J, Brenneman JF. *Positive Parenting for Bipolar Kids.* New York: Random House, 2008.

Papolos D, Papolos J. *The Bipolar Child and Reassuring Guide to Childhood's Most Misunderstood Disorder.* New York, NY: Broadway Books, 2002.

For professionals

Birmaher B, Axelson D, Goldstein B, et al. Four-year longitudinal course of children and adolescents with bipolar spectrum disorders: the Course and Outcome of Bipolar Youth (COBY) study. *Am J Psychiatry* 166(7):795–804, 2009.

Findling RL, Calabrese JR. Rapid-cycling bipolar disorder in children. *Am J Psychiatry* 157(9): 1526–1527, 2000.

Geller B, Craney JL, Bolhofner K, et al. Two-year prospective follow-up of children with a prepubertal and early adolescent bipolar disorder phenotype. *Am J Psychiatry* 159(6):927–933, 2002.

Geller B, Tillman R, Bolhofner K, et al. Child bipolar I disorder: prospective continuity with adult bipolar I disorder; characteristics of second and third episodes; predictors of 8-year outcome. *Arch Gen Psychiatry* 65(10):1125–1133, 2008.

Moreno C, Laje G, Blanco C, et al. National trends in the outpatient diagnosis and treatment of bipolar disorder in youth. *Arch Gen Psychiatry* 64(9):1032–1039, 2007.

Wozniak J, Faraone SV, Mick E, et al. A controlled family study of children with DSM-IV bipolar-I disorder and psychiatric co-morbidity. *Psychol Med* 6:1–10, 2009.

Web sites

www.bpkids.org
arielslegacy.net
www.ryanlichtsangbipolarfoundation.org
www.stepup4kids.com

31

Biting Others

Barbara Howard

I. Description of the problem.

A. Epidemiology.

1. Almost all children bite at some time during the first 3 years. For example, 50% of toddlers in childcare are bitten three times every year. Bites constitute 6% of injuries to males and 3% to females in childcare.

2. As with most other aggressive behaviors, boys are more likely than girls to bite.

3. Biting is more severe or persistent in children with family dysfunction, where physical punishment is used, or when there is chronic stress.

4. Acceptability or modeling of violence predisposes to aggressive behaviors, such as biting.

B. Contributing factors.

1. **Environmental.** Children are more likely to bite others when they are in social situations beyond their coping abilities. Biting in these situations is usually intended to obtain objects, to gain attention, or to express frustration. It is also a powerful way of acquiring attention from adults. For example, some parents remove the child from the childcare setting for the day after a biting incident. Such *secondary gain* from the environment may prolong the biting phase.

2. **Developmental.** Biting emerges at predictable developmental stages.

   a. The first peak, at the **time of tooth eruption,** is rarely reported as a problem since caregivers interpret it as normal experimentation. Interestingly, breastfed infants generally learn very quickly not to bite the breast, probably because of their mother's shriek, her affective distress, and the prompt removal of the infant from the breast.

   b. The next peak in biting occurs around **8–12** months when infants bite as an expression of excitement. A strong negative emotional response by caregivers accompanied by putting down the infant generally leads to rapid extinction.

   c. The **second year of life** is normally a time when skills develop unevenly, and there is a strong desire to act autonomously. Fledgling or delayed abilities in expressive language and fine motor skills serve to cause frustration and set the child up for aggressive outbursts. Biting in toddlers may be used to dominate, to acquire an object, or to express anger or frustration. In addition, children undergoing stressful separation experiences (such as to go to childcare) may get emotional relief from causing distress in others by biting. This phase of biting typically disappears quickly.

   d. Biting in children **older than 3 years** should occur only in extreme circumstances (e.g., if they are losing a fight, perceive their survival to be threatened, or are very stressed).

II. Recognizing the issue.

A. History: key clinical questions.

1. *"When did the biting start? What else was different around that time"?* Look for recent stress (such as new childcare or a new sibling).

2. *"In what situations does it occur?"* Look for situations in which frustration is common and the child has poor coping skills. This may be a clue to developmental weaknesses such as fine motor delay (e.g., if biting occurs when coloring with crayons is expected). Biting that occurs when there has been a long period between meals may suggest hunger as a cause.

3. *"How have you handled it so far?"* Determine the previous measures used to address the problem and whether there is any secondary gain for the child to continue to bite (such as increased attention). Parental ambivalence about steps they have taken may need to be acknowledged to implement a better plan.

4. *"What other concerns do you have about your child's behavior or development?"* Other signs of aggressive behavior or specific developmental delays may point to an important contributing cause.

     5. *"How is anger expressed in your home?"* Children may model other family members' behaviors around expression of anger and violence.

     6. *"Have you had any concerns about how your child is cared for?"* Abuse, neglect, violence, or poor-quality care may contribute to the problem.

III. Management.

   A. Information for the family. Adults view biting as a very primitive behavior that elicits strong emotional reactions, especially in childcare settings. Families need to understand that biting by toddlers is usually a normal developmental phase and does not predict later aggression.

   B. Treatment (see Table 31-1).

     1. Determination of cause. Before formulating a treatment plan, the clinician must determine the reason for the child's biting. Developmental assessment will dictate the need for management of specific delays. Children who are frustrated by their relative weaknesses in skills compared with peers, for example, often do better when placed with younger children or in a less demanding setting. Other children push themselves to perform beyond their abilities. Such children may need support by arranging same-age peer play, placement in smaller groups, and avoidance of difficult tasks.

     2. Aversive reinforcement and redirection. The chronic biter will need to be observed closely so that appropriate social interactions can be praised and biting encounters interrupted quickly with a shout that declares the seriousness of the offense. The child should then be put in time-out, with a short explanation such as, "I know you are angry, but people are not for biting." Sympathizing with the victim is helpful and may also serve to avoid secondary gain for the biter. Later, the incident can be reviewed with the child and alternatives discussed for negotiating conflict and for expressing feelings. A teething ring to bite can be offered or attached to the clothing, allowing the child expression of the feelings through an acceptable alternative outlet.

Table 31-1. Techniques to diminish biting in toddlers

Directed to the child
- Provide close supervision.
- Ensure attention to positive behaviors.
- Redirect when anger or frustration appears.
- Verbalize feelings for the child.
- Assess all skill areas and habilitate deficiencies.
- If a bite occurs, shout a loud "NO!" and place child in time-out.
- Be sure that the child receives no interaction in time-out.
- Offer lots of positive attention to the child who was bitten.
- Offer teething ring or cloth to bite.
- If most bites are toward a certain peer, separate the children.
- If biting persists, remove to home or smaller childcare.

Directed to the caregivers
- Set consistent limits, especially on aggressive acts.
- Avoid physical punishment or exposure to violence.
- Express negative emotions verbally and stay in control.
- Avoid interfering in the partner's discipline: Whoever starts handling an event should finish.
- Do not bite back. This models the undesirable behavior, elicits fear and anger in the child, and makes the adult feel so guilty that his or her effectiveness in limit setting is diminished.
- Ensure that the child is not the least competent in his or her group.
- Ensure that all caregivers are properly responsive and not using physical punishment.

Directed to the parents if the child is about to be removed from daycare
- Meet with childcare staff.
- Determine exactly how incidents are being handled.
- Establish a consistent plan for managing incidents (which does not include taking the child home, if possible).
- Consider a shorter day in the childcare if the child tires.
- Negotiate a time-limited trial of intervention, documenting incidents to determine improvement.
- If necessary, move the child to home or a smaller, closely supervised, structured setting or one with younger or less aggressive children, or staff who are more open to dealing with biting.

3. **Parental attitudes toward aggression.** Parental attitudes toward aggression need to be discussed. Since corporal punishment is a contributor to persistent biting, it should be eliminated. Parents often need coaching to develop appropriate expression of negative affect. Counseling regarding reasonable limits for the child's behavior and nonphysical ways to attain them are the centerpiece of treatment. When parents interfere or criticize the other's discipline, the child experiences the tension and mixed feelings and may become unusually aggressive, including biting.

4. **Childcare setting.** When biting occurs in a childcare setting, a crisis often ensues. Having the parents of the victim meet the equally distraught parents of the biter (or even a meeting of the entire center) can help defuse these situations. The nature of the supervision and activities should be evaluated. Young children need an active curriculum focused on small-group play with responsive adults who are positive in their interactions and able to redirect untoward behaviors. There also should be enough toys to discourage disputes. Larger toys for shared play are associated with fewer struggles. A child in group care who persists in biting often will do better at home or in a family childcare setting. Corporal punishment, mistreatment, or neglect in the childcare should also be considered.

BIBLIOGRAPHY

Block RW, Rash FC. *Handbook of Behavioral Pediatrics.* Chicago, IL: Year Book, 1981.

Solomons HC, Elardo R. Biting in day care centers: incidence, prevention and intervention. *J Pediatr Health Care* 5:191–196, 1991.

32

Breath Holding

Barry Zuckerman

I. **Description of the problem.** Breath-holding spells (BHS) involve the involuntary cessation of breathing in response to a painful, noxious, or frustrating stimulus. If prolonged, they can lead to loss of consciousness and/or seizures. There are no reported long-term adverse outcomes associated with breath holding.

A. **Epidemiology.**
- Simple breath holding without loss of consciousness may be seen in up to 25% of children.
- True BHS with loss of consciousness has been reported in approximately 4%.
- The peak frequency is between 1–3 years of age, although they may begin in the newborn period.
- BHS after 6 years of age are unusual and warrant further investigation.
- They occur equally in males and females.
- There is a positive family history in approximately 25% of cases.
- 50% resolve by the age of 4 years; 90% by the age of 6 years.

B. **Etiology.** The etiology of BHS is speculative.
- Pallid spells may be facilitated by an overactive vagus nerve; cyanotic spells may be related to a more central nervous system inhibition of breathing in response to stress.
- Hematologic differences (iron deficiency, transient erythroblastopenia) have been reported.

C. **Types.**
1. **Cyanotic spells.** The most common type of BHS is a cyanotic spell, which is precipitated by anger or frustration. A short burst of crying, usually less than 30 seconds, leads to an involuntary holding of the breath in expiration, resulting in cyanosis that can lead to a loss of consciousness and occasionally a seizure (Table 32-1).
2. **Pallid spells.** The second type is precipitated by fright or minor trauma (e.g., occipital trauma due to a fall). Following the precipitating event, there is an **absence of crying** or a single cry, followed by pallor and limpness. This sequence of events is thought to be due to a hyperresponsive vagal response that results in bradycardia (and even asystole), causing pallor and loss of consciousness. Some of these children (about 15%) go on to faint when they are injured or frightened as adults.

Table 32-1. Progression of breath-holding spells

Cyanotic spell
Precipitating event (anger or frustration associated with temper tantrums)
Period of crying (frequently less than 20 sec)
Holding of breath in expiration
Cyanosis
Progressive loss of consciousness
Occasional twitching, opisthotonos, or clonic movements

Pallid form
Precipitating event (minor trauma, especially occipital trauma or fright)
Absence of crying or single cry
Bradycardia and often asystole
Simultaneous loss of consciousness and breath holding
Pallor
Occasionally generalized seizure or twitching

Table 32-2. Distinguishing breath-holding spells from seizures

	Severe breath-holding spells	Epilepsy
Precipitating factor	Always present	Usually not present
Crying	Present before convulsion	Not usually present
Cyanosis	Occurs before loss of consciousness	When it occurs, it is usually during prolonged seizure
Electroencephalogram	Almost always normal	Usually abnormal but may be normal
Incontinence	Uncommon	Common

II. **Making the diagnosis.**
- History is the mainstay of diagnosis; videotape documentation may be possible. The key to diagnosis is to differentiate BHS from seizures (Table 32-2). The presence of a precipitating factor followed by crying and cyanosis before the loss of consciousness and/or seizure is specific to BHS.
- An electroencephalogram is rarely necessary unless a clear precipitating event is not apparent.
- A blood count to rule out iron deficiency may be warranted in severe cases.

III. **Management.**
- A. **Information for parents.** BHS need to be explained and demystified for parents. The clinician should explain, in simple, concrete terms, the sequence of events leading to the loss of consciousness and seizure. The benign nature of these events should be emphasized because parental concerns about epilepsy, brain damage, or death are common.
- B. **Management strategies.**
  1. **Medications** are generally neither indicated nor helpful. Atropine has been tried in some cases of pallid spells. Iron supplementation may be tried in cases with hematological abnormalities.
  2. For cyanotic spells, an **intense stimulus** (e.g., a cold cloth on the face) may terminate the breath holding if applied before or within the first 15 seconds of apnea. Although the window of opportunity for this intervention is brief, many parents find it comforting to have *something* to try, rather than just feeling helpless.
  3. If the event progresses for either type of BHS, the **child should be placed on the floor to prevent falling.**
  4. When the child awakes (usually immediately after the seizure or loss of consciousness) **parents should not fuss over the child** so that inadvertent secondary gain does not occur.

BIBLIOGRAPHY

For parents

http://www.webmd.com/parenting/tc/breath-holding-spells-topic-overview.

For professionals

Breningstall GN. Breath holding spells. *Pediatr Neurol* 14(2):91–97, 1996.
Evans OB. Breath holding spells. *Pediatr Ann* 26(7):410–414, 1997.

33

Bullying

Douglas Vanderbilt

I. **Description of the problem.** Bullying is the assertion of power through aggression that involves one or more children repeatedly and intentionally targeting a weaker child through social, emotional, or physical means. The key features to this behavior are a power imbalance between the stronger bully and the weaker victim, intent to harm, and repetition of the behavior toward a single victim. It is on a continuum with teasing on one end and violent assault on the other. Teasing involves mild aggression and humor that creates social embarrassment but does not have the intent to harm seen in bullying. Clearly behaviors such as physical assault and "hate speech" are criminal and subject to the law.

Bullying can come in two forms:

- **Direct bullying** is overt. It can involve physical aggression such as hitting, stealing, and threatening with a weapon or verbal aggression such as name-calling, public humiliation, and intimidation.
- **Indirect bullying** is the covert type that is relational in nature. It involves spreading rumors, social rejection, exclusion from peer groups, and ignoring. A subtype of this, "emotional bullying," is an especially salient concern of youth today.

A. **Epidemiology.**
1. **Prevalence.**
   a. National Survey of Children's Exposure to Violence (2008) found a rate of 20% for being bullied in the last year and 30% lifetime risk.
   b. 55% of 8–11-year-olds and 68% of 12–15-year-olds rated teasing and bullying as big problems for kids of their age.
   c. 30% of middle and upper school students are involved in bullying as perpetrators and/or victims.
   d. Among sixth graders of low socioeconomic status students in LA, 7% were bullies, 9% victims, 6% bully-victims, 22% borderline, and 56% uninvolved.
   e. Types of bullying experienced or committed over the last 2 months include: 21% physically, 54% verbally, 51% socially, or 14% electronically.
2. **Age.**
   a. Bullying peaks in middle childhood (second grade) and decreases with age as more intense forms of victimization rise.
   b. Older children are less likely to talk about their victimization with only 50% of all children confiding in anyone.
3. **Gender.**
   a. Boys are twice as likely as girls to be bullies, more than three times as likely to be bully victims, and twice as likely to be victims.
   b. Boys are more likely to use and receive direct bullying.
   c. Girls are more likely to use and receive indirect bullying.
4. **Culture.** Intercultural comparisons are subject to social and community biases. The United States prevalence ranks near the middle of 40 countries studied.

B. **Etiology/contributing factors.**
1. **Settings.** Bullying occurs most frequently at school at any time or in any place where there is minimal supervision. Common times are during breaks, recess, and lunch. Common places are playgrounds, hallways, and en route to and from school. In addition to the real-world settings of the school and neighborhood, "cyberbullying" is becoming another manifestation of this behavior through Internet social networking sites, e-mail, text messaging, and blogs.
2. **Risk factors.**
   a. **Social.** Families may encourage bullying by showing a lack of consistent consequences, using discipline that is negative or physical, and modeling bullying behaviors to their children. Peer bystanders can also support bullying through acceptance or encouragement of the behavior. Schools have more episodes of bullying if they ignore or tolerate such behavior through weak supervision. Communities

with more social chaos and community violence have worse problems. Media images and societal values can promote aggression and violence as normative and appropriate methods of social behavior and conflict resolution.

b. **Individual.**

(1) **Characteristics of victims.** There are two types of victims. The passive type is physically weak and emotionally vulnerable, such as those with a learning disability or autism. Although less prevalent, the provocative type is reactive and fights back when attacked. They are more likely to have attention-deficit/hyperactivity disorder or oppositional defiant disorder. Overall, both victim groups are anxious, insecure, lonely, and lack social skills, but their external characteristics do not set them apart from others. Being bullied results in lower social status and higher social marginalization, poor self-esteem, and isolation. They have more emotional disorders, psychosis, and suicides. Long-term consequences in adulthood of being bullied as a child include increases in depression, abusive relationships, and poor physical health outcomes.

(2) **Characteristics of bullies.** Bullies have higher rates of conduct disorders and social standing. They have the lowest rates of adjustment problems because of their higher social status/prestige but are avoided by peers. Bullies, who self-identify, have higher rates of depression and psychological distress as compared with those who deny their behavior. They have more drug use and negative attitudes toward school. Childhood bullies have a four-fold increase in criminal behavior by their mid 20s. They are at higher risk of dropping out of school, carrying weapons, and fighting.

(3) **Characteristics of bully-victims.** These are individuals who have been bullied and then become perpetrators of similar behavior often for revenge. This group has the most problems with peer relationships and highest rates of depression, loneliness, substance use, and psychosis. Equally troubling is the fact that among intended or conducted perpetrators of school shootings, two-thirds were bullied and had violent ideation prior to their violent acts.

(4) **Characteristics of bystanders/uninvolved.** Fear of bullying distracts bystanders from learning and takes up teachers' time and resources. This group can encourage or discourage bullying by their reaction to the bully and victim. They can serve as an intervention point for programs to change peer social dynamics by increasing empathy for victim and censoring the bully.

II. **Making the diagnosis.** The clinician has four roles to address bullying:
- Proactive identification of the problem
- Screen for psychological comorbidities
- Counsel the families and children
- Advocate for bullying prevention

A. **Signs and symptoms.**

1. **Identifying the victim.** Bullying is often not a presenting complaint and requires proactive screening. Signs of a child being bullied include physical complaints such as insomnia, stomachaches, headaches, and new onset enuresis. Psychological symptoms may occur such as depression, loneliness, anxiety, and suicidal ideation and gestures. Behavioral changes are common such as irritability, poor concentration, school refusal, and substance abuse. School problems can also occur like academic failure, social problems, and lack of friends. Additional vigilance must be made for those children with chronic medical illnesses, physical deformities, and students in special education who may be potential targets.

2. **Identifying the bully.** Signs of a child being a bully are more difficult to discern due to the bully's desire to obscure the behavior. Children who are aggressive, overly confident, lack empathy, and are having oppositional or conduct problems may need careful screening. These children are at high risk if they come from families who use physical punishment or model violent behavior in conflict resolution.

3. **Differential diagnosis.** Care must be made not to miss psychological disorders that pose safety issues such as suicidal ideation and plans, substance abuse, and risk-taking behaviors. The physical, behavioral, emotional, and school symptoms of bullying may overlap with other conditions such as medical illness, learning problems, and psychological disorders. Serious disorders may need mental health screening and management.

B. **History: key clinical questions (See Table 33-1).**

III. **Management.**

A. Management for bullying involves interventions with parents, victims, bullies, bystanders, and school personnel. Interventions should include giving information

Table 33-1. Sample screening questions to investigate whether a child is being bullied

Questions for children
1. Have you ever been teased or bullied at school?
2. Do you know of other children who have been teased?
3. How long has this been going on?
4. Have you ever told the teacher about the teasing?
5. What kinds of things do children tease you about?
6. Have you ever been teased because of your illness/handicap/disability?... for not being able to keep up with other children?... about looking different from them?
7. At recess do you usually play with other children or by yourself?
8. Have you ever changed schools because you had problems with the other students?

Questions for parents
1. Do you have any concern that your child is having problems with other children at school?
2. Does your child go to the school nurse frequently for physical complaints?
3. Has your child's teacher ever mentioned that your child is often by himself or herself at school?
4. Do you suspect that your child is being harassed or bullied at school for any reason? If so, why?
5. Has your child ever said that other children were bothering him or her?

regarding the current research in bullying, supporting families, victims, and bullies, referring those children in need of further mental health services, and expecting behavioral change from the bully and social change from the school environment.

B. Individual.

    1. Victims. The clinician should empathetically listen to the parent and child to help empower them. The child and family need reassurance; do not blame the victim or trivialize the child's/parent's concern. For example:

    "No one deserves to be treated this way."

    "You are not alone."

    "Your parents and I will work together to help things get better for you."

    "The bullying will stop very soon."

    Suggestions should include having the child seek social support from teachers and friends and avoid situations where the bullying may occur. The phrase: **"Walk, Talk, and Squawk"** can help a child to deal with the bully. The child should "Walk" by ignoring the hurtful remarks, "Talk" by making confident yet nonprovocative statements to the bully, and "Squawk" by disclosing the episodes to adults. Role-playing can be helpful in problem solving these techniques with the child. Strategies can be used to help to bolster the child's insecurities and increase self-esteem such as extracurricular activities like drama clubs and sports.

    2. Bully. Once a bully is identified and appropriate screening for risk factors is completed, the clinician should educate the parents and child about the seriousness of the behavior and its potential consequences. Care must be made to label the behavior and not the child as the problem. The first step in changing the bully's behavior is helping the family and the child to acknowledge the behavior as hurtful. For example:

    "Do you feel bad when other children hurt your feelings?"

    "Bullying hurts other children's feelings."

    Interventions should include clear accountability of the child's behavior through observations at home by parents and at school by teachers and administrators.

C. Systemic. Bullying occurs in a permissive and encouraging environment. Successful interventions activate the bystander to protect the victim and censor the bully. Clinicians should encourage broad-based programs that simultaneously include school-wide rules and sanctions, teacher training, classroom curriculum, conflict resolution training, and individual counseling. The clinician must collaborate and engage with stakeholders in the school and community to inform practices and encourage interventions to change social norms regarding violence and access to firearms.

BIBLIOGRAPHY

For parents

Web sites

http://stopbullyingnow.hrsa.gov/adults/

http://www.education.com/topic/school-bullying-teasing/
http://www.bullying.org/

Books

Olweus, D. *Bullying at School: What We Know and What We Can Do.* Williston, VT: Blackwell Publishers, 1994.

For professionals
Web sites

http://www.aap.org/ConnectedKids/
http://www.safeyouth.org/scripts/topics/bullying.asp
http://pediatrics.aappublications.org/cgi/reprint/peds.2009-0943v1

For children
Web sites

http://stopbullyingnow.hrsa.gov/kids/
http://kidshealth.org/teen/school_jobs/bullying/bullies.html

Books

Berenstain S, Berenstain J. *The Berenstein Bears and the Bully.* New York, NY: Random House, 1993.
Romain T. *Bullies are a Pain in the Brain.* Minneapolis, MN: Free Spirit Pub, 1997.

34

Cerebral Palsy

Frederick B. Palmer
Alexander H. Hoon

I. **Description of the problem.** Cerebral palsy (CP) is a disorder of movement and posture, causing activity limitation, due to a static defect or lesion of the developing brain. Rather than a specific diagnosis, it encompasses a spectrum of neurodevelopmental syndromes characterized by persistent motor delay, abnormal neuromotor examination, and often an extensive range of nonmotor-associated disabilities in cognitive, neurobehavioral, neurosensory, orthopedic, and other areas. These associated disabilities reflect the fact that motor centers of the brain are rarely affected in isolation. CP, a clinical diagnosis, may be due to a wide range of genetic and environmental insults to the developing brain. When the clinical diagnosis of CP is established, it is important to investigate the etiology, which may be important to treatment, prognosis, risk of recurrence, and parental understanding. Although the brain lesion is, by definition, nonprogressive, its motor and nonmotor manifestations can be expected to change with the child's development. Therefore, careful ongoing medical and rehabilitation surveillance is necessary.

A. **Epidemiology.**
- About 2–3 per 1000 live births (half-born at term, half-born preterm)
- Evidence over the 1980s of an increase in CP birth prevalence in very low-birth-weight babies (with a decrease in mortality in this group), and a probable decrease during the late 1990s.

B. **Classification.** Clinical classification is based on the nature of the movement disorder, muscle tone, and topography. Classification by type is essential to management and anticipation of associated disabilities (Table 34-1) and future needs.
1. **Spastic CP** (65% of children with CP). Most children with CP have spasticity, an upper motor neuron syndrome consisting of persistent velocity-dependent hypertonus (increased muscle tone of clasp-knife character), increased deep tendon reflexes, pathologic reflexes, spastic weakness, and loss of motor control and dexterity. Spastic CP is further classified on the basis of topography:
   a. **Hemiplegia** (30% of children with CP). Primary unilateral involvement, often with the arm more involved than the leg.
   b. **Quadriplegia** (5% of children with CP). Four-limb involvement with legs often more involved than arms but with functionally limiting arm involvement.
   c. **Diplegia** (30% of children with CP). Four-limb involvement with legs much more involved than the arms (which may show only minimal impairment and no functional limitation). Diplegia should be distinguished from "paraplegia," which implies entirely normal arm function and suggests a spinal cord lesion, not CP.
2. **Dyskinetic CP** (19% of children with CP). The other major physiologic category is designated "dyskinetic" due to the prominent involuntary movements, fluctuating muscle tone, or both. Choreoathetotic and dystonic are the two most common subtypes. Most children with dyskinetic CP have relatively symmetric four-limb involvement and require no further topographic designation.
3. **Ataxic CP** (up to 10% of children with CP). This type of CP often has genetic underpinnings and is associated with significant comorbidities in vision, hearing, cognition, feeding, and epilepsy.
4. **Worster-Drought syndrome (bulbar CP)** should be considered in the child whose motor disability is primarily of a cranial nerve distribution. It may be associated with underlying perisylvian microgyria on neuroimaging and may be familial.

C. **Etiology/contributing factors.** Despite more than a century of research, specific etiologic factors responsible for the motor impairment remain uncertain in many children with CP, especially in children born at term. Large studies have shown that brain injury occurring at birth is the cause in only 8%–12% of cases. Developmental brain anomalies or prenatal insults are the most common etiologies. In premature children, both prenatal and perinatal factors are felt to play a role in what is most commonly a spastic diplegia or quadriplegia. Postneonatal etiologies (e.g., traumatic brain injury, meningitis) account

Table 34-1. Selected nonorthopedic-associated disabilities in cerebral palsy

Cognition

Intellectual disability (present in 30%–77%)

The most important factor influencing habilitation

Hemiplegia and diplegia associated with higher cognition

Easy-to-underestimate cognition in choreoathetosis

Epilepsy associated with lower cognition

Language disorder, learning disability (present in about 40%)

Heterogeneous group with deficits due to oromotor dysfunction, dysphasia, hearing loss

Often "superimposed" on intellectual disability

Very high risk for learning disability in child with CP and "normal" IQ

Neurobehavior (present in up to 50%)

Entire spectrum of neurobehavioral disorders (attention-deficit/hyperactivity disorder to autism) seen

No symptom is "typical"

Behavior dysfunction may be primarily a neurologic symptom or reflect discomfort from underlying medical problems (e.g., GERD, hip subluxation, skin breakdown)

Sensation

Visual disorders (present in 50%–90%)

Most common ones amenable to treatment

May have a bearing on education (acuity, field deficits)

Hemianopsia in 25% of hemiplegia (easily missed as gaze may compensate to side of field cut)

Refractive errors seen in 50% overall, 67% in diplegia; amblyopia develops in 14%

Hearing disorders (present in 10%) easily missed

Higher prevalence (45%–60%) in postkernicteric

Choreoathetosis and TORCH etiologies

Somatosensation (present in up to 50% of hemiplegia)

Deficits in stereognosis most common

May be the limiting factor in arm/hand functioning in hemiplegia

Repeated clinical examination essential to recognition

Associated with linear undergrowth but not muscular atrophy

Seizures (present in 30%–40%)

Often associated with spasticity and lower cognition

Growth failure

Undernutrition a frequent problem

Empiric nutritional goal of 10% weight for height

Multifactorial in origin: increased caloric needs, oromotor dysfunction, gastroesophageal reflux, chronic infection, "neurogenic," syndromic

Limb length asymmetry associated with hemisensory abnormalities

Other health problems

Genitourinary complaints common; pathogenesis unclear

Drooling a major cosmetic problem: may be exacerbated by antispasticity drugs; treatment with anticholinergics, surgery, and biofeedback disappointing

TORCH, toxoplasmosis, other, rubella, cytomegalovirus, herpes simplex; GERD, gastroesophageal reflux disease.

for about 10% of CP. Maternal and/or fetal infection/inflammation has been noted as an important antecedent of CP in term and preterm infants. Thrombophilia, including the Factor V Leiden mutation, the most common cause of familial thrombosis in neonates, infants and children, may be an important contributor to intrauterine stroke and hemiplegic CP. Advances in neuroimaging and molecular genetics are greatly improving our understanding of etiology and options for prevention.

  II. **Making the diagnosis.** Attention should be given to both developmental diagnosis (type and severity of CP) and etiological diagnosis.

    A. **Symptoms.** CP usually presents with significant motor delay, although the delay may not be recognized in the first months of life. Common presenting concerns include poor head control, hypertonia (especially during activities such as bathing or diapering), generalized hypotonia, early preferential hand use, absent weight bearing, and feeding problems. Experienced observers may note abnormalities in spontaneous general movements during the first weeks of life.

The nonprogressive nature of "the lesion" is essential to the diagnosis of CP. If etiology is not clear or if an atypical clinical picture includes loss of skills, hepatosplenomegaly, sensory disturbances, or other unusual findings, then evaluation for a progressive process (metabolic, structural, neurodegenerative, etc.) should be undertaken. This generally requires assistance from a subspecialist.

B. Neurologic signs.

1. Sole reliance on the neuromotor examination in diagnosing CP can lead to both under- and overdiagnosis. Instead, the clinician should initially focus on the presence or absence of motor delay.

   If there is no delay, CP is unlikely even if the neuromotor examination is abnormal (although children with such "minor neuromotor dysfunction" may have other neurodevelopmental disabilities, such as intellectual or learning disability). An exception to this "no motor delay, no CP" rule is seen in hemiplegia, in which the prominent upper extremity disability may cause substantial neuromotor asymmetry rather than gross motor delay. Focusing on upper extremity function will clearly identify these children.

2. On neuromotor examination, muscle tone may vary from excessive hypotonia to hypertonia (spastic, dystonic, or mixed in character). Hypotonia in an infant may be manifest as head lag on pull to sit, slip through at the shoulders, or an exaggerated curve in ventral suspension. Hypotonia with significant weakness and diminished tendon reflexes is uncommon in CP and suggests a neuromuscular disorder. Early hypotonia may persist, normalize, or evolve into hypertonia.

3. Recognition of abnormal spontaneous general movements during the first weeks of life may provide a sensitive tool for early detection of CP based on the continuing studies in the Europe.

4. Spastic hypertonia—persistent clasp-knife catch or "hitch" is a component of the upper motor neuron syndrome and is brought out by rapid movement of the limb by the examiner.

5. The hypertonus seen in dyskinetic forms is variable in nature and can usually be "shaken out" by the examiner with rapid movements of the limb. Involuntary movements, such as choreoathetosis, dystonic posturing, and tremor, may be associated. Facial and oromotor involvements are often prominent.

6. All children are born with a constellation of primitive (e.g., Moro) and "pathologic" (e.g., Babinski) reflexes, probably mediated at the brainstem level. In normal infants, brain maturation leads to the disappearance of these reflexes and the emergence of postural and equilibrium reactions that precede the attainment of motor skills. In infants with CP, primitive reflexes are often increased in intensity and delayed in disappearance. Recognition of these phenomena may aid in diagnosis, especially in the first 6–12 months of life when motor delay is less apparent.

7. The examination should include a careful assessment of oromotor and ocular function and a search for orthopedic abnormalities, including scoliosis and joint contractures. The general physical examination should focus on dysmorphic features, neurocutaneous signs, retinal abnormalities, organomegaly, and other findings that could suggest a specific etiology. Ophthalmologic and genetic consultations may be helpful.

C. Tests. Table 34-2 lists the indications for various tests in CP. Neuroimaging in the neonates and young infants known to be at risk for CP is an important step in the early detection of CP. An initial neuroimaging study in the older children may not directly affect management but may provide a structural correlate of the motor impairment and insight into the timing of the brain insult. Often parents find this information quite useful as they try to come to terms with their child's impairment.

In children with *atypical* clinical findings, especially choreoathetosis, metabolic disorders should be suspected. Plasma lactate, plasma amino acids, urinary organic acids, and selective use of other tests can be important. A karyotype, chromosomal microarray, or targeted fluorescence in-situ hybridization may be revealing in children with apparent prenatal onset of CP and additional, even minor, malformations.

III. Management.

A. Primary goals.

1. To work with the child and family to **help the child with CP to function as effectively and normally as possible in the home, school, and community.**

Table 34-2. Suggested indications for diagnostic or screening tests in children with motor disorders

Magnetic resonance imaging of the brain
  Cerebral palsy or motor asymmetry
  Abnormal head size or shape
  Craniofacial malformation
  Loss or plateau of developmental skills
  Multiple somatic anomalies
  Neurocutaneous findings
  Seizures
  IQ <50
  Low-birth-weight infant at term age equivalent

Cytogenetic studies—karyotype, chromosomal microarray, and/or targeted FISH
  Microcephaly
  Multiple (even minor) somatic anomalies
  Family history of intellectual disability
  Family history of repeated fetal loss
  IQ <50
  Skin pigmentary anomalies (mosaicism)
  Suspected contiguous gene syndromes (e.g., Prader–Willi, Smith–Magenis)

Metabolic studies
  Dyskinetic CP (choreoathetosis, dystonia, ataxia)
  Episodic vomiting or lethargy
  Poor growth
  Seizures
  Unusual body odors
  Somatic evidence of storage
  Loss or plateau of developmental skills
  Sensory loss (e.g., retinal abnormality, hearing loss)
  Acquired cutaneous disorders

FISH, fluorescence in-situ hybridization; CP, cerebral palsy.
Adapted from Palmer FB, Capute AJ. Mental retardation. *Pediatr Rev* 15:473–479, 1994.

    2. To provide a foundation for the child to **function independently as an adult,** minimizing the activity limitations imposed by the neurodevelopmental and associated disabilities.
    3. To **assist the parents in accepting and assuming their roles as primary advocates** for their child's needs.
    4. To **coordinate the recommendations of the many medical and other providers** into an integrated healthcare plan. Table 34-3 outlines common clinical indications and goals for referral to *nonmedical* professionals. These guidelines and comments reflect personal experience rather than rigid rules and should be interpreted in the context of available resources.
    5. When needed, to assist adolescents, young adults, and their families to **transition care to adult providers** in as efficient, effective, and coordinated manner as possible.
  B. General principles of treatment.
    1. The severity of disorder should help determine the aggressiveness of the treatment. For example, an infant with a motor quotient below 0.5 generally requires complete evaluation by a physical or occupational therapist, or both, and ongoing intervention. Children with milder delays (motor quotient 0.5–0.7) may only need a one-time consultation and suggestions for home management. The Gross Motor Function Measure (GMFM) and five-level Gross Motor Functional Classification System (GMFCS) provide a standardized approach to determining motor prognosis.
    2. Although some traditional interventions and motor therapies are not of clearly proved efficacy, they can be useful if used with clear indications and objective goals in mind.
    3. **Parents should be included in any therapy** and should incorporate techniques into their everyday activities with the child.
    4. **Therapists and intervention programs should be kept informed** about the child's health and, in turn, should keep the clinician informed of their activities.

Table 34-3. Suggestions for use of nonmedical specialties

Service	Common useful indications	Comments
Special nutrition services	Weight for height less than 5% or declining Suspected insufficient caloric intake due to poor swallow, gastroesophageal reflux	Nutritional problems require extensive medical workups Significant gastroesophageal reflux common in severe CP Reactive airway disease in CP is chronic aspiration until disproved; pursue dysphagia and gastroesophageal reflux Gavage or gastrostomy feeding may be needed to meet caloric requirements Reasonable weight is tenth percentile for height
Occupational therapy	Fine motor delay (DQ <0.50)[a] Presence or- risk of contractures in the upper extremities Overdependence on others for activities of daily living for child's cognitive and motor level Oromotor dysfunction, excess drooling, poor oral intake, excessive feeding time Equipment needs	Constraint-induced therapy should be considered in hemiplegia
Physical therapy	Gross motor delay (MOQ <0.50)[b] Difficult or inefficient ambulation in the absence of prominent delay Abnormalities of tone or reflexes interfering with function or management Presence or risk of contractures in the lower extremities Equipment needs	Videotaping motor function, or formal gait analysis, may be helpful in assessment Helpful to have physical therapist present for orthopedic and other subspecialty evaluations Short-term therapy for children with MOQ 0.50–0.70 may be useful
Audiology	All patients with CP due to high prevalence of hearing loss Recommend and apply amplification, if indicated	Office-based hearing screening is unreliable and insensitive Brainstem auditory evoked responses (BAERs) provide nonspecific measures of hearing loss in high-risk premature infants in the newborn period; more specific results using BAERs, behavioral audiometry, and acoustic impedance audiometry are obtained after 6 months of age Early treatment of hearing loss can significantly improve outcome
Speech and language	Global language delay Isolated expressive language delay Dysarthria Assist in diagnosis and management of feeding concerns	Receptive language may be surprisingly better than expressive language Language may be underestimated in patient with oromotor involvement Repeat evaluations necessary Isolated articulation lessons usually not rewarding

(continued)

Table 34-3. (*Continued*)

Service	Common useful indications	Comments
Psychometric testing	All children with CP due to high prevalence of cognitive disorder Reevaluate in patients with suspected plateau, degeneration, or difficulty in school	Academic achievement testing may be handled by school Parent and teacher input needed in assessing discrepancies between IQ and achievement Special testing methods for children with severe motor or sensory impairment
Special education (private or school-based)	Upon entering first grade or when change in placement is suggested To develop an individualized educational plan (IEP)	Classroom teacher input is invaluable Evaluation in conjunction with psychometric testing advised
Behavioral psychology	Parent or teacher difficulty in managing behavioral problems Concerns about parental discipline practices	Behavior techniques may be enhanced by medication (e.g., stimulants) Teachers and other caretakers should be involved in the program Planned management should be adaptable to home, school, and community
Social work	Often useful at initial diagnosis When difficulties in parent adaptation are noted Suspected child abuse When services are not easily accessed	To aid the clinician in attending to the many details involved in supervising care by the intricate network of agencies Respite care services may enhance the long-term outlook for family-provided care Evaluation in suspected child abuse is essential

[a]Developmental quotient (DQ) = Fine motor age (milestone-based) divided by chronologic age.
[b]Motor quotient (MOQ) = gross motor age (milestone-based) divided by chronologic age.
CP, cerebral palsy.
Adapted from Rosenblatt M, Palmer EB. Cerebral palsy. In Johnson RT (ed), *Current Therapy in Neurological Diseases* (3rd ed), Philadelphia: Decker, 1991.

5. Clinicians must **be familiar with available local intervention programs,** their services, and ever-changing details of eligibility, access, and payment.
6. Assistance in identifying needs and appropriate intervention options is often available through neurodevelopmental disability programs in tertiary centers.
7. Where tertiary services are not available or accessible, the physician should create and lead a virtual interdisciplinary team of available professionals to serve the child. Accountable healthcare roles require effective, family-centered coordination by the primary care provider when tertiary services are not provided.

C. Criteria for referral.
1. An **orthopedic evaluation** is needed for any child with limitation in range of motion of any joint(s). Orthopedic surgery may be indicated when function is impaired; care is limited; or pain is caused by deformity, contracture, or muscle imbalance. Goals of surgery should be clearly understood by families. The common parental expectation for unreasonable functional gains should be anticipated. Orthopedic and neurodevelopmental pediatric consultants should work closely with physical and occupational therapists in nonsurgical interventions. Therapists can assist in prescribing appropriate adaptive equipment and bracing. Such equipment includes seating and positioning devices and transportation implements.
2. **Neurosurgical interventions in CP have a long history.** Intrathecal baclofen (ITB) and selective dorsal rhizotomy (SDR) are employed in many centers for children with spastic diplegia. Both are costly procedures and require surgeons with expertise. When patients are carefully selected and followed in a specialized program, there may be benefits both in ease of care, as well as functional benefits. An important difference is that an ITB pump may be removed, whereas SDR is permanent. However, ITB requires

close, ongoing management, whereas SDR is a single procedure. ITB is an important therapeutic approach for children with refractory spasticity or dystonia. The pump delivers baclofen into the intrathecal space via an implanted, programmable system. ITB allows titratable reductions in spasticity using doses of baclofen in microgram amounts, rather than milligram amounts with oral use. It avoids the adverse effects often associated with higher doses of oral baclofen. Specific goals for functional improvement should be clear before deciding on surgical interventions. Stereotactic ablation surgery and implanted stimulators have been unrewarding and are seldom indicated.

3. If **pharmacological adjuncts** are to be used, specific treatment goals are essential and should include functional improvement, not just reduction in tone. It is generally best to have the child's physical or occupational therapist assist in objective measurement of agreed-upon outcomes to avoid basing dosage decisions solely on "he's better [or worse] today" reports from family or treatment programs.

Medication is sometimes effective in reducing hypertonus in spastic and mixed forms of CP. However, striking functional improvement is rarely seen. Benzodiazepines, especially diazepam, are most commonly used. Baclofen, a γ-aminobutyric acid agonist, is also used (usually in older children). Botulinum toxin, a long acting blocker of transmission at the myoneural junction, can be injected directly into the muscle and has resulted in reduction of tone. Again, functional goals should be identified and monitored in pharmacologic interventions. Medications to control involuntary movements are sometimes useful as an effective adjunct in severe dyskinetic CP. Dopamine agonists and anticholinergics have been employed in treating dystonia and rigidity.

Although the range of side effects to oral medications is beyond the scope of this chapter, several generalizations can be made. Some medications have recognizable side effects, such as sedation from diazepam and seizures from acute baclofen withdrawal. Others may be more subtle, such as cognitive or personality changes with trihexyphenidyl and benztropine. Periodic drug weans should be considered to determine whether benefits are persistent. As always, clinicians should listen carefully to parental/caregiver concerns about any changes in their children after medication initiation or dosage change. It is often helpful to keep community therapists masked to onset and dosing of medications, utilizing their unbiased opinions about changes in function (or side effects) with medication changes.

BIBLIOGRAPHY

For parents

Organizations and Web sites

American Academy for Cerebral Palsy and Developmental Medicine, 555 East Wells, Suite 1100 Milwaukee, WI 53202. (414) 918-3014. www.aacpdm.org

Association of University Centers on Disabilities, 1010 Wayne Avenue, Suite 920, Silver Spring, MD 20910; (301) 588-8252. www.aucd.org/

The Council for Disability Rights, 205 West Randolph, Suite 1650 I Chicago, IL 60606; (312) 444-9484. www.disabilityrights.org

Disabled Sports USA, 451 Hungerford Drive, Suite 100, Rockville, MD 20850; (301) 217-0960. www.dsusa.org

Exceptional Parent Magazine, 555 Kinderkamack Road, Oradell, NJ 07649-1517. Also see www.eparent.com for an extensive online resource for parents of children with disabilities compiled by *Exceptional Parent Magazine*.

United Cerebral Palsy Associations, 1660L Street, NW, Suite 700, Washington, DC 20036; (800) 872-5827. www.ucp.org

Publications

For parents

Batshaw ML, Pelligrino L, Roizen NJ. *Children with Disabilities* (6th ed), Baltimore: Paul H Brookes, 2007.

Miller F, Bachrach SJ. *Cerebral Palsy: A Complete Guide for Caregiving* (2nd ed), Baltimore: The Johns Hopkins University Press, 2006.

For professionals

Accardo PJ (ed). *Capute and Accardo's Neurodevelopmental Disabilities in Infancy and Childhood* (3rd ed), Baltimore: Paul H Brookes, 2008.

Keogh JM, Badawi N. The origins of cerebral palsy. *Curr Opin Neurol.* 19:129–134, 2006.

Liptak GS. Complementary and alternative therapies for cerebral palsy. *Ment Retard Dev Disabil Res Rev* 11:156–163, 2005.

Ment LR, Bada HS, Barnes P, et al. Practice parameter: neuroimaging of the neonate: report of the Quality Standards Subcommittee of the American Academy of Neurology and the Practice Committee of the Child Neurology Society. *Neurology* 58:1726–1738, 2002.

Nelson KB. The epidemiology of cerebral palsy in term infants. *Ment Retard Dev Disabil Res Rev* 8:146–150, 2002.

Rosenbaum PL, Walter SD, Hanna SE, et al. Prognosis for gross motor function in cerebral palsy: creation of motor development curves. *JAMA* 288:1357–1363, 2002.

Rubin IL, Crocker AC (eds). *Medical Care for Children and Adults with Developmental Disabilities* (2nd ed), Baltimore: Brookes, 2006.

Schaeffer GB. Genetic considerations in cerebral palsy. *Semin Pediatr Neurol* 15:21–26, 2008.

Shimony JS, Lawrence R, Neil JJ, et al. Imaging for diagnosis and treatment of cerebral palsy. *Clin Obstet Gynecol* 51:787–799, 2008.

Tosi LL, Aisen ML (eds). Adults with cerebral palsy: a workshop to define the challenges of treating and preventing the secondary musculoskeletal and neuromuscular complications in this rapidly growing population. *Dev Med Child Neurol* 51(s4)1–184, 2009.

35

The Child with Dysmorphic Features

John C. Carey

I. **Description of the problem.**
   A. **Epidemiology.**
   - Approximately 3%–4% of all infants have a medically significant congenital malformation (see Table 35-1 for definition of terms).
   - About 30% of all children have a single minor anomaly or mild malformation.
   - An additional 10% show two or more of these physical findings.
II. **Making the diagnosis.**
   A. **The diagnosis of a multiple congenital anomaly syndrome** is significant for the child, the family, and the healthcare professionals, for a number of reasons.
      1. **Recurrence chances in genetic counseling.** The recognition of an established disorder of known etiology provides information on the cause and heritable aspects of the condition, as well as potential prenatal options for future pregnancies.
      2. **Relative prediction of prognosis.** Each disorder has its own particular natural history, risks for problems, and outcomes.
      3. **Appropriate laboratory testing and screening.** Precise diagnosis informs medical management and eliminates the need for unnecessary tests; appropriate screening can be planned according to the particular natural history of the syndrome.
      4. **Treatment and management issues.** Knowledge of the natural history of a condition allows for the establishment of guidelines for routine care, including suggestions for educational interventions.
      5. **Coping with the disorder.** In many families, the knowledge of a condition helps in dealing with the uncertainty of the situation.
   B. **Data collection.** The importance of a thorough history in the evaluation of a child with a potential syndrome cannot be overemphasized. Information on the gestational and birth history should include history of fetal movement, drugs and medications taken during pregnancy including alcohol consumption, intrauterine positioning, status of amniotic fluid, and maternal medical history. Documentation of a complete family history with a three-generation pedigree (including inquiry regarding consanguinity) is essential. Key clinical questions include the following:
      1. Does the child in question have an **organized pattern of malformation** (i.e., a syndrome or sequence), or does the child exhibit a constellation of features that are consistent with the family and/or ethnic background (variant familial developmental pattern)?
         a. If the child has a pattern, do the findings consist of multiple **primary** malformations or dysplasias (a syndrome), or do the findings represent **secondary** manifestations (deformations or disruptions) comprising a sequence?
         b. If the child has a pattern, does the pattern represent a **known syndrome** (or sequence), or is it a **previously unidentified, provisionally unique pattern?**
      2. What is the **date of the onset** of the physical abnormalities? Are they prenatal or postnatal? Some physical signs that are clues for syndromes are of postnatal onset and often provide signs for a metabolic disorder (e.g., the facial changes and joint contractures of the mucopolysaccharidosis and other storage disorders).
   C. **Physical examination of the craniofacies.** The ability to **recognize and interpret minor anomalies and mild malformations** is the most important skill required in approaching the child with a potential syndrome. The practitioner needs to be observant and skilled in describing physical variations and deciding what, in fact, is a useful clue and what is not (Fig. 35-1). The **evaluation of the face and hands** is particularly important since most malformation syndromes have phenotypic variations in these regions. The common frustration of clinicians in approaching the potentially dysmorphic child probably helped lead to that pejorative, stigmatizing term, the "FLK" (funny-looking kid), which should be eliminated from the clinical vocabulary.

Table 35-1. Definitions of commonly used terms

Term	Definition
Malformation	A primary morphologic defect of an organ or body part resulting from an intrinsically abnormal developmental process (e.g., cleft lip)
Deformation	An alteration of the form, shape, or position of a previously normally formed body part caused by mechanized forces (e.g., club foot due to oligohydramnios)
Sequence	Pattern of multiple anomalies derived from a single known anomaly; a primary defect with its secondary changes (e.g., Pierre Robin sequence)
Syndrome	A recurring pattern of multiple defects due to a single etiology (e.g., Williams syndrome)
Dysmorphic	abnormally formed; more conventionally, used to refer to the presence of multiple minor anomalies or mild malformations, as in *dysmorphic* facial features

Source: Adapted from the recommendations of the International Working Group. Spranger J, Benirschke K, Hall JG, et al. Errors of morphogenesis: concepts and terms. *J Pediatr* 100:160–165, 1982.

1. **The examination.** The clinician should examine the face as he or she would examine the heart or abdomen, looking at it in general and then examining each feature systematically (hair, forehead, eye slant, eyebrows, ears, etc.) to determine what about this face makes it look different. Does one feature make the face look distinctive or unique, several features, or one area of the face? The gestalt should be noted (the

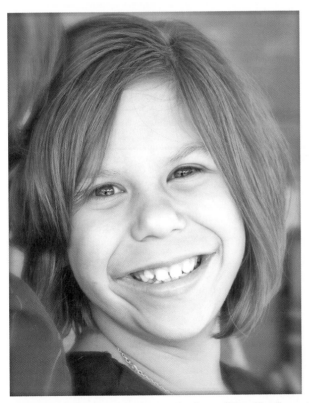

Figure 35-1. Child with Williams Syndrome. Note the General Facial Gestalt, Which is Characteristic. Also, Note that all of the Features Fall into the Category of Continuous Features; None is a True Malformation, Minor or Major. The Mouth Size Measures Above the 90th Percentile, but Otherwise the Features are not Abnormal in the Statistical or Embryologic Sense of the Word. (Courtesy of Kevin and Monaca Seamans.)

Table 35-2. Types of variations and malformations of the craniofacies

	Definition
Major malformations	Medically significant defects (e.g., cleft lip, microtia)
Mild malformations	Structural alterations that have no intrinsic medical significance (occur in <4% of population, e.g., helical ear pit, preauricular tag)
Minor anomalies	
Continuous features with measurable alterations	Features that lend themselves to measurement and can be defined on standard curves (e.g., small ears) using the graphs in *Smith's Recognizable Patterns of Human Malformation*
Continuous features, not defined by measurements	Features that shade into normal variation and do not have a defined threshold (e.g., micrognathia, depressed nasal bridge, prominent nasal tip[a])

[a]For updated descriptions of minor anomalies see Elements of Morphology: Standard Terminology, entire January 2009 issue of the *American Journal of Medical Genetics* 149A:1–127.

whole is more than the sum of the parts). If the ears appear low set, the clinician should consider why they look that way. Are they small, posteriorly rotated, or over-folded, or does the low placement, in fact, represent an illusion? If the ears appear large, measurements should be taken and plotted on available curves.

2. **Classification.** Table 35-2 presents a classification of types of variations of the face. It is of note that most of the features of a child with Down syndrome fall into the minor anomaly category. This is the class of features that usually requires comparison to family members, especially parents and siblings, and consideration of ethnic background. Photographing the patient is important for documentation. The pictures can be placed in the chart for future review or assuming parent permission evaluation by a clinical geneticist.

3. **The approach.** Table 35-3 summarizes the practical steps that can be used in approaching the dysmorphic child.

   The most useful and easily available reference source for looking up features and attempting to make a diagnosis is *Smith's Recognizable Patterns of Human Malformation* by Jones. In addition, a number of computer programs (London Dysmorphology and POSSUM) have been designed to assist in the diagnostic process.

D. **Laboratory evaluation.**

1. After initial evaluation of the child, if no secure diagnosis has been reached and the child has multiple congenital anomalies, a **chromosome analysis** should be considered. Currently, this investigation is best accomplished by performing **comparative genomic hybridization microarray.** There is a 5%–15% yield of positive microarray analysis among children with dysmorphic features and developmental delay.

2. If there is suspicion that the child's features are suggestive of the fragile X syndrome (Chapter 45), then a **DNA analysis of fragile X** is warranted.

3. If one of the microdeletion syndromes is clinically likely (e.g., Prader–Willi syndrome, Williams syndrome), then targeted **FISH** (fluorescence in-situ hybridization) is indicated.

4. **TORCH (toxoplasmosis, other, rubella, cytomegalovirus, herpes simplex) titers** are usually not indicated in an infant who has multiple primary defects that are alterations in embryogenesis (e.g., cleft lip, polydactyly, or even minor anomalies).

Table 35-3. Practical steps in the approach to the dysmorphic child

1. *Examine the child's family members.* Compare features to parents' or siblings'. When possible compare to photographs of family members at the same age as the index case.
2. *Consider ethnic background.* Certain features have different frequencies in different ethnic groups (e.g., eye measurements are different in African Americans vs. persons of Hispanic descent vs. European Caucasians).
3. *Measure areas where standards exist* (e.g., ear size, palpebral fissure length). Do not trust the gestalt in deciding whether a feature is large or small; have plastic rulers available in the clinic setting.
4. *Look up the most distinctive and/or rarest defect for quick identification* (e.g., the white forelock suggesting Waardenburg syndrome).
5. *Become acquainted with the terminology and ways to describe the face and hands.*

5. **Amino acid studies and other investigations of intermediary metabolism** are not indicated in an infant with multiple primary malformations since none of the known aminoacidopathies or disorders of fatty acid oxidation is consistently associated with structural anomalies of prenatal onset. However, there are some inborn errors of metabolism that will have associated congenital or early onset physical abnormalities that can raise the question of the child having a dysmorphic syndrome. Examples include the abnormal "kinky" hair of an infant with Menkes syndrome and the specific dysmorphic features of Smith–Lemli–Opitz syndrome. Imaging studies and referrals to subspecialists are indicated according to the presence of accompanying problems.

III. **Management.**
   A. **Specialty referral.** Consultation with a dysmorphologist or clinical geneticist skilled in syndrome recognition is indicated for any child who has dysmorphic features. Referral for consultation is also appropriate for any family with questions about the diagnosis, the natural history of the disorder, the recurrence chance, the genetic aspects, prenatal options, issues of reproductive decision making, and psychological support.
   B. **Health maintenance and anticipatory guidance.** Once the diagnosis of a particular syndrome is made, the clinician can review the natural history of the disorder and establish a plan for follow-up and screening.
   C. **Psychological support.** The process of evaluating a child for a syndrome can, in and of itself, be overwhelming and even stigmatizing for the family. Families often perceive the meticulous detail of the examination as a "picking-apart" process. Discussion of the benefits for making a diagnosis is helpful, and acknowledging these potential reactions are important in the initiation of the referral process.

IV. **Clinical pearls and pitfalls.**
   - **The null hypothesis strategy.** The diagnosis of a syndrome should be approached in a hypothesis-generating manner. The clinician should state the null hypothesis—"This child does not have a dysmorphic syndrome"—and then review the evidence. This approach attempts to avoid overdiagnosis and puts the burden of proof on the person who makes the diagnosis. It also demands a certain amount of critical thinking about the use of the minor anomalies in the diagnostic thought process.
   - **The eye does not see what the mind does not know.** This often-cited axiom underscores the importance of the knowledge of the disorder, as well as the need for astute observation. Recognition of the subtleties of physical variation, as well as clinical variability of a disorder, is crucial in the evaluation.
   - Children who have syndromes are not necessarily unusual or different in appearance. What is usually present is a **difference from their unaffected family members,** rather than a clear-cut abnormality. In many syndromes, the features are consistent and show difference from the family background but are not very distinctive or striking.
   - "You know my method. It is founded upon the observance of trifles." Sherlock Holmes, *The Boscombe Valley Mystery.*

BIBLIOGRAPHY

For parents

Genetic Alliance. Offers links to several hundred support groups for various disorders. 1–800-336-GENE http://www.geneticalliance.org

For professionals

Aase JM. Dysmorphologic diagnosis for the pediatric practitioner. *Pediatr Clin North Am* 39(1):135, 1992.
Cassidy SB, Allanson JE. *Management of Genetic Syndromes* (3rd ed), Hoboken, NJ: Wiley-Blackwell, 2010.
Jones KL. *Smith's Recognizable Patterns of Human Malformations* (6th ed), Philadelphia, PA: Saunders/Elsevier, 2006.
London Dysmorphology Database. An electronic reference requiring purchase. The program is found in many medical libraries and is often located in the office of a dysmorphologist or clinical geneticist. Available from http://www.lmdatabases.com
POSSUM (Pictures of Standard Syndromes and Undiagnosed Malformations). An electronic reference requiring purchase. The program is found in many medical libraries and is often located in the office of a dysmorphologist or clinical geneticist. Available from:http://www.possum.net.au

Chronic Conditions

Ellen C. Perrin

I. **Description of the problem.** The federal Maternal and Child Health Bureau (MCHB) defines children with special healthcare needs (CSHCN) as: *"those who have a chronic physical, developmental, behavioral, and/or emotional condition and who require health and related services of a type or amount beyond that required by children generally."*

A. **Epidemiology.** Children with chronic health conditions are of increasing interest and importance to primary care clinicians because of (1) their increasing prevalence; (2) the growing recognition that these children and their families are at higher than usual risk for family stress, social isolation, and difficulties with social and psychological adjustment; and (3) the additional challenges they present for comprehensive pediatric care and coordination.

B. **Prevalence.** The true prevalence of chronic health conditions in childhood is unknown because of varying definitions used for the presence of a "chronic health condition":
   - Very different numbers of children are identified if parents are asked using the definition above; versus if the child is limited in participating in the usual activities for a child of similar age; or if they are asked to identify the presence of specific diagnoses.
   - The National Survey of CSHCN identified 12.8% of children in 2001 and 13.9% of children in 2005 as having an SHCN. Among children aged 5 years and less the prevalence was 9%, whereas among children aged 6 years and older it was 16%.
   - The National Survey of Children's Health identified 22% of parents who reported their children to have an SHCN in 2005. These differences are based on slightly different definitions of what constitutes an SHCN and the level of severity of the condition.
     - 13.6% of the children surveyed were reported to have one of the 16 specific conditions listed, whereas 8.7% had two or more conditions.
     - 10.6% of children had conditions rated as "moderate" or "severe," whereas 11.6% were rated as "mild."
   - Among children aged 6–17 years, health conditions were reported to "interfere with the child's ability to attend school regularly, participate in sports and other activities, and/or make friends" in 17.2%
   - Overall, the prevalence of chronic health conditions in children has increased considerably over the past 25 years. A few specific conditions have decreased in prevalence because of greater availability of prevention (e.g., spina bifida); others have increased because of improvements in survival (e.g., leukemia); a few new conditions have emerged (e.g., HIV/AIDS); but the largest proportion of recent growth has been driven by a few high-prevalence conditions. Asthma now affects almost 10% of children and adolescents; obesity well over 15%; and behavioral/mental health conditions are now estimated at more than 15%.
   - Children with chronic physical illnesses have more than their share of emotional, behavioral, educational, and social difficulties. For example, 12.7% of parents who report that their child has a special healthcare need also report "a behavioral or conduct problem," compared with only 0.8% of parents who do not report an SHCN. Similarly, 11.4% of parents who report that their child has an SHCN also report "anxiety" and 8.3% report "depression," in comparison to 0.6% and 0.3%, respectively among parents who do not report an SHCN.

II. **Salient issues.** There are considerable commonalities among the experiences of children who have various types of chronic health conditions, and in the experiences of their families (Table 36-1). In addition to those issues they share, important differences in characteristics of children themselves, of parents and families, and of their specific health conditions have considerable effects on the experience of having a chronic condition (Table 36-2).

A. **Characteristics of children.**
   1. The age at which a child develops a chronic health condition and the child's age at any particular time, independently contribute to the child's experience of the condition

Table 36-1. Issues common in the presence of chronic health conditions

For children

Limitations in usual childhood activities because of the condition itself and medical care requirements

Need for medications, other treatments

Experience with doctors, nurses, and other providers

Pain and discomfort

Experience with hospitalization

Feeling different from peers

Loneliness

Worry about the future

Dependency, loss of control

Stigma

For families

Extra burden of care

Financial drain

Interactions with complex medical system

Multiple doctors, nurses, and other professionals

Restricted social networks

Difficulties with childcare, short and long term

Special requirements of school

Necessity to inflict pain and discomfort

Interference with needs of other family members and of family system

Worries about long-term care, insurance

Uncertainty in daily life planning

Loneliness

Guilt

Anger

Stigma

Table 36-2. Factors affecting children's experience of a chronic health condition

Characteristics of the child	Characteristics of the family
Age of onset	Marital status
Personality/temperament	Number and ages of children
Intelligence	Parents' education
Self-concept	Parents' occupations
Gender	Financial situation
Ethnic background	Strength of parents' relationship
Developmental level	Parents' self-esteem
Understanding of illness	Extended family support
Locus-of-control beliefs	Social support network
	Ethnic background
Characteristics of the illness	
Age of onset	
Stable or unpredictable	
Prognosis	
Interference with mobility	
Interference with normal activities	
Visibility	
Academic effects	
Medications and other treatments	
Intensity of care requirements	
Discomfort	
Nervous system involvement	

Table 36-3. Challenging tasks for children with chronic health problems

	Primary task	Challenges
Infants and toddlers	Development of trust and security	Parental grief Altered eating/feeding experiences Restriction of movement Hospitalizations Painful procedures Chronic discomfort
Preschoolers	Development of autonomy	Medication requirements Dietary restrictions Mobility restrictions Need for adult supervision Repeated separations Impaired limit setting Limitations on peer interactions Differences from peers
School-aged children	Development of sense of mastery Restrictions on independence	Dependence on medical care Requirements for adult monitoring Medication and dietary requirements Activity restrictions School absence Altered body image Decreased growth

Adolescents	Development of personal identity
	   separate from family
		Visible deformity
		
		Requirements of medical
		   supervision
		Medication and dietary
		   requirements
		Vocational limitations
		Challenges to sexuality
		Enforced dependency

and the particular issues associated with its management (Table 36-3). For example, congenital conditions generally are associated with greater resiliency than conditions whose onset is during early adolescence.

2. Children's ability to manage their condition is related not only to their age but also to their understanding of the illness. Children with chronic health conditions are no more sophisticated than their healthy peers in their conceptual sophistication about the processes of illness causation and treatment. Healthy children and their peers with a chronic condition gain conceptual understanding of the processes of bodily functioning and of the prevention, causation, and treatment of illness along a predictable sequence of developmental stages parallel to those described in other domains by Piaget and others (Table 36-4).

3. It is important to assess the level of the child's cognitive sophistication about illness prior to instituting specific health education efforts, providing information about the condition, or determining appropriate expectations for the child's participation in the care and management of the condition. The child's intelligence, temperamental style, locus-of-control beliefs, self-concept, gender, and ethnic background all contribute to his/her resiliency in adapting to the extra stresses of a chronic health condition.

B. Characteristics of conditions.

1. Certain kinds of health conditions present children with greater risks for difficult adjustment than do others. Neurological conditions, especially those that involve cognitive dysfunction, and conditions that are associated with unpredictable exacerbations (e.g., asthma) appear to present special challenges to children and families.

Table 36-4. Typical progression in children's understanding of illness concepts

Cognitive level	Approximate age (years)	Understanding of illness	Typical responses to How do children get sick?	Typical responses to How do children keep from getting sick?	Typical responses to How can children get better?
1		No response; does not know; inappropriate or off-task response			
2	4–6	Phenomenism: circular or phenomenistic response	"By catching something"; "sometimes you just do"; "from throwing up"	"Stay healthy"; "go to doctor for checkups"	"Go to the doctor"; "take medicines"
3	7–9	External agents: concrete, external causes cited; no explanation of how the agents interact with the body to result in, prevent, or cure illness	"If you go out in the rain without your boots"; "eating bad foods"; "from other people"	"Get shots"; "stay away from sick people"; "eat good foods"; "rest enough"	"Eat foods that are good for you"; "rest a lot"; "do what the doctor says"
4	10–13	Internalization: internalization and/or relativity in understanding of illness; once agent is internalized, illness follows invariably	"Germs get in and spread all over your body"; "when you breathe in sick people's germs"	"Take special vitamins that will keep your body strong"; "rest/food/ exercise … give your body what it needs"	"Do different things for different illnesses"; "get more sleep than usual"; "take the right kind of medicine to give your body what it needs"
5	10–13	Interaction: interaction of host and agent described; some effect of agent on body	"Germs get in your system and start to eat/kill your cells"; "interference with normal body parts"	"If your body is strong from eating what you should, it will be able to resist the germs"; "exercising keeps the bones in place so they can work right"	"Resting allows your body not to waste its energy so it can fight the germs better"; "vitamins help the body to repair what is not working right"
6	>14	Mechanisms: processes of illness causation, prevention, or treatment described; includes notion of bodily response	"Germs take away food from the body and then the body has nothing to use for power"; "eat something that messes up your muscles so your heart does not work right"	"The right foods nourish the fighting cells so they are powerful enough to kill germs that get inside you"	"Good food/vitamins help your body to make more blood so the cells can fight off the germs"; "make your heart stronger so your body has better defenses"

179

2. The adjustment of children, of their siblings, and of their parents cannot be predicted simply from the severity of the condition. Some children with only moderate disease experience a greater impact on their lives and challenges to their psychological and social adjustment than do children who are more severely affected. The confusing experience of marginality, in which a child is neither clearly sick (and in need of special services and attention), nor clearly well, may result when a health condition is not obvious to peers and important adults and does not interfere noticeably with normal activity but still requires a special diet, medication, or medical care.

C. **Characteristics of families.** Parents, siblings, and extended family interactions play a very major part in children's successful adjustment.

   1. Parental reactions to a diagnosis of a chronic health condition and their adaptation to its long-term implications affect the coping resources of the child and his siblings. The risk of parental discord and divorce is somewhat greater for families that include a child with a chronic health condition, reflecting the additional stresses presented by the parenting and care of these children.

   2. Siblings are at risk to feel neglected in comparison with the child toward whom so much worry and attention is directed. Some may feel resentful or develop evidence of anxiety and/or depression.

   3. The development of children's positive views of themselves is supported by their family's perception of their health condition as an incidental difficulty requiring shared problem solving, rather than as an intrusion on the family's functioning. The family's ability to attend to each member's needs for nurturance and attention, to express and deal with conflict, to support the independence of all members, and to provide both structure and flexibility are critical to children's successful adaptation.

III. **Management.** Maintaining optimal growth and development in the presence of a chronic health condition is a challenge to families, to primary care clinicians, and to the children themselves. Although there is a somewhat greater risk of psychological, social, and educational difficulties for children with chronic health conditions, most of them and most of their families adapt successfully to the extra challenges they confront.

A. Primary care clinicians have the opportunity—and therefore also the responsibility—to be available to families over a long period of time. They are often the first professional person consulted about issues of concern to children and their parents. Thus, they are in a unique position to **support families and to help them to coordinate their child's care.** In addition to ensuring that these children receive all usual preventive and acute illness care and health supervision, the primary care clinician should serve as an effective interface among subspecialty and surgical teams, early intervention and family support programs, schools, third-party payers, nursing services, and a large variety of other care providers.

B. Primary care clinicians also should provide regular **monitoring** of the child's development; the emotional and social adaptation of children, parents, and siblings; and **referral** for appropriate mental health services when indicated. Such comprehensive attention to overall healthcare supervision for children with ongoing health conditions has been made easier in some states with new coding guidelines that allow supplemental third-party reimbursement for extended office visits, case conferences, and sometimes lengthy telephone-assisted care.

C. Primary care clinicians need to know the **resources available** in their own community. They should have, or be able to develop, effective contacts with local school systems, the resources of the Department of Public Health, home nursing and respite care services, and sources of specialty medical and surgical care. In addition, they should provide community-specific information regarding supportive networks of children with health conditions and of their parents and their siblings.

D. Clinicians also have a responsibility to **assure appropriate education** of children and their families about the health condition and its management. This may require repeated discussions with children and parents as children grow in their ability to understand their illness and its care. Clinicians should guide gradual transfer of responsibility for monitoring and care of the illness from parents to children as they reach adolescence. In addition, they should help parents to plan for an appropriate school program, with attention to the integration of the child's medical and educational needs. Excessive school absences that result from the course of a condition itself and from requirements for its care can be made less disruptive by home tutoring services for long-term and for predictable short-term absences. Effective communication among the school system, the pediatric clinician, and the family can make overall healthcare management and transitions between school and home care efficient and effective.

BIBLIOGRAPHY

General resources

National Information Center for Children and Youth with Disabilities (NICHCY). National information and referral center on disabilities and disability-related issues; offers state resource information. www.nichcy.org

DisabilityInfo.gov. Information and resources for children and adults with special needs, and their families. Information on education, health, housing, technology, and much more. www.disabilityinfo.gov

Exceptional Parent. Monthly publication for families, addressing a wide range of topics related to children and youth with disabilities. www.eparent.com

Family Village. Wide variety of specific resources for families who care for children and adults with disabilities. Spanish resources available www.familyvillage.wisc.edu

Family Voices. National grassroots organization of families and friends of children with special health needs. State chapters and coordinators. Many publications on healthcare issues and resources. Spanish resources available www.familyvoices.org

Federation for Children with Special Needs. Provides advocacy and support for families in the areas of health, education, early childhood, and transition for children and young adults with special needs. www.fcsn.org

Professional resources

National Survey of Children's Health. http://www.nschdata.org/Content/Default.aspx/. Accessed October 1, 2010.

National Survey of Children with Special Health Care Needs. http://cshcndata.org/Content/Default.aspx. Accessed October 1, 2010.

Bethell CD, Read D, Blumberg SJ, et al. What is the prevalence of children with special health care needs? Towards an understanding of variations in findings and methods across three national surveys. *Matern Child Health J* 12:1–14, 2008.

Inkelas M, Raghavan R, Larson K, et al. Unmet mental health needs and access to services for children with special health care needs and their families. *Ambul Pediatr* 7:431–438, 2007.

Lavigne JV, Faier-Routman J. Psychological adjustment to pediatric physical disorders: a metaanalytic review. *J Pediatr Psychol* 17:133–157, 1992.

McMenamy JM, Perrin EC. Filling the GAPS: care of children with chronic health conditions in pediatric practice. *Ambul Pediatr* 4(3):249–256, 2004.

Perrin EC, Gerrity PS. Development of children with chronic illness. *Pediatr Clin North Am* 31:19, 1984.

Perrin EC, Schott J. Somehow we'll make it work: interviews with children with a chronic condition and their families. DVD available from the author (eperrin@tuftsmedicalcenter.org).

Witt WP, Riley AW, Coiro MJ. Childhood functional status, family stressors, and psychosocial adjustment among school-aged children with disabilities in the United States. *Arch Pediatr Adolsec Med* 157:687–695, 2003.

37

Colic

Steven Parker
Tracy Magee

I. **Description of the problem.** There is no reliably objective definition of colic. It is often characterized as persistent, excessive, paroxysmal crying in an otherwise well, thriving infant; colic begins at about 3 weeks of age, peaks at 6–8 weeks of age, and dissipates by 4 months of age. However, the length of time spent crying to qualify as excessive crying continues to be debated and alters true estimates of the prevalence. Using the most restrictive definition, Wessel's rule of threes (*more than 3 hours per day, for 3 or more days per week for more than 3 weeks of excessive crying*), colic is thought to affect 10% of all full-term infants, whereas using the least restrictive definition, *problematic crying*, colic is thought to affect up to 40% of all full-term infants. In addition, parental tolerance for infant crying is quite variable: some are stoic in the face of constant crying, whereas others come to the primary care clinician for the occasional whimper. The best definition of colic may be a purely clinical one: colic is *any recurrent inconsolable* crying in a *healthy and well-fed infant* that is experienced by the parents or caregivers as a problem.

A. **Epidemiology.**
- Estimates range from 7%–40%, depending on the criteria for diagnosis
- No differences by gender, breast- versus bottle-fed, full-term versus preterm, or birth order
- Two times increased risk if maternal smoking during pregnancy
- Whites > nonwhites
- Parents older and more educated
- Industrialized countries > nonindustrialized
- More frequent the farther away from the equator
- Increased incidence of physical abuse in colicky infants especially shaken baby syndrome

B. **Clinical features.**
1. Colic typically begins at **41–42 weeks of gestational age** (including preterm infants).
2. **Two patterns** of colic have been noted.
   a. **Paroxysmal fussing** typically occurs between 5–8 PM. The infant is contented and easily soothed at other times of the day. These infants do not cry more frequently over 24 hours; rather, they sporadically cry for a longer period of time.
   b. **The hyperirritable infant** is one whose crying occurs at all hours of the day, often in response to ambiguous external or internal stimuli. They may also exhibit increased tone and other signs of hyperarousal.
3. Colic **stops as mysteriously as it starts,** by 3 months in 60% and by 4 months in 80%–90% of infants. Infants crying past the 4-month period are at higher risk for developmental delays.
4. There are **no predictable long-term infant outcomes** (behavioral, temperamental, or psychological) that emerge from a colicky infancy, although later sleep problems are often seen, and parents and caregivers with a colicky infant may have more depression, anxiety, and marital difficulties.

C. **Etiology.** Theories of causation abound (Table 37-1), but evidence for any one is scant. It appears likely that there is no single cause of colic and that it represents the final common pathway for a number of etiologic factors.

II. **Making the diagnosis.**

A. **History: key clinical questions.**
1. "*When does the crying occur?*" The timing of the cry provides useful information. For example, if it occurs directly after a feeding, aerophagia, or gastroesophageal reflux may be considered. If it occurs reliably 1 hour after feedings, a formula intolerance is possible. If the crying occurs only from 5–7 PM everyday, it is difficult to posit an organic problem that would cause pain at only one time of the day.
2. "*What do you do when your baby cries?*" It is important to determine how the parents have tried (successfully and unsuccessfully) to console the infant. In some cases, their

Table 37-1. Theories of the etiology of colic

Gastrointestinal

Cow's milk protein intolerance (an equal number of studies have found an association of cow's milk with colic as have not)

Gastroesophageal reflux

Lactose intolerance (higher breath H_2 level in some colicky infants)

Immature gastrointestinal system (ineffective peristalsis; incomplete digestion; gas)

Faulty feeding techniques (e.g., under- or overfeeding, infrequent burping)

Hormones causing enterospasm

Increased motilin levels (one study showed higher levels of motilin, but not vasoactive intestinal peptide or gastrin, in colicky infants)

Decreased cholecystokinin levels ($\rightarrow$ gallbladder contractions)

Hormonal

Increased circulating serotonin (hypothetical only but an attractive hypothesis because serotonin has a circadian rhythm in infancy, which could explain the curious timing of paroxysmal fussing)

Progesterone deficiency (one study in 1963, never repeated)

Neurological

Imbalance of autonomic nervous system (parasympathetic $\gg$ sympathetic)

Immature neurotransmitters

Nonestablished circadian rhythm

Temperamental

Difficult temperament (but there is poor correlation of colic and later temperament)

Hypersensitivity (crying at end of day represents discharge after a long day of shutting out intrusive environmental stimuli, parents may be overstimulating)

Parental behaviors/handling

Most studies do not show a relationship between parental anxiety, psychopathology, and/or emotional difficulties and colic; at most, nonoptimal handling may exacerbate but not cause the symptoms

techniques may have inadvertently worsened the situation (e.g., anxiously overstimulating a hypersensitive infant); in other cases, the technique may be inappropriate (e.g., giving half-strength formula or dangerous/suspect home/folk remedies).

3. *"What does the cry sound like?"* Most parents can distinguish a cry of pain from that of hunger. In addition, the description of the cry provides insight into parental distress, empathy, or anger with the cry. Research suggests that colicky cries have a higher pitch and are described as "urgent" or "piercing."

4. *"Tell me how and what you feed your baby."* Underfeeding, overfeeding, air swallowing, and inadequate burping have all been implicated in colic.

5. *"How does it make you feel when your baby cries?"* *"What worries you most about the crying?"* History taking is an opportune time to begin the process of parental support. Opening up the subjects of parental guilt, helplessness, and anxiety sends the message that these topics merit discussion. Some parents are especially worried about their anger toward the screaming child, believing that such anger is the mark of a bad parent. Others seek pediatric attention because they are afraid of actually harming the infant during a crying spell or that the infant has a mysterious illness.

6. *"How has the colic affected your family?"* Colic is a *family* issue. In some cases, it may disturb the parents' relationship with each other, cause distress in a sibling, or serve as a forum for blaming the parents (e.g., by grandparents).

7. *"What is your theory of why the baby cries?"* To support the family, their hypotheses for the crying must be understood. Some may view it as a curse, others as a rebuke to their parenting skills, and others as a sign that something is terribly wrong with the baby.

B. **Physical examination.** A thorough physical examination serves to rule out medical problems that cause pain or discomfort, as well as to reassure the parents that the infant is physically well. However, in only about 5% will a definable medical cause be found. Any problem that causes pain can lead to hyperirritability (but rarely to paroxysmal fussing).

- Infections (otitis media, urinary tract infection, oral herpes)
- Gastrointestinal (diarrhea, constipation, gastroesophageal reflux)

- Genitourinary (posterior urethral valves)
- CNS (intra- or extracranial hemorrhage, hydrocephalus)
- Ophthalmologic (corneal abrasion, glaucoma)
- Cardiac (supraventricular tachycardia)
- Narcotic withdrawal syndrome (especially methadone)
- Fracture, hernia, anal fissures
- Tourniquet (on toe or finger)

  The diagnosis of colic is predicated on the infant being healthy and well fed. Only after a thorough history and physical examination do not reveal an obvious source of pain should the diagnosis of colic be considered.

III. Management.

A. Shotgun approach.
Because the cause of colic is rarely clear, a shotgun approach is often helpful. Table 37-2 lists suggestions for parents to help them deal with colic. The history and physical examination may point to one line of treatment as potentially more useful than another. As a general rule, **most treatments for colic work in 30% of infants, but none works for all infants.** It is best to try only one or two interventions at a time. This allows for the effective measure to be more easily identified. In addition, since *nothing* may work very well, it is helpful to keep a few suggestions in reserve, at least until the process runs its course at 3–4 months.

B. Parental support.
Colic is a benign, self-limited problem with no untoward sequelae for the infant. Its impact on the early parent–child relationship should be of primary concern. Long after the crying abates, the consequences of an impaired parent–infant relationship can do damage. Therefore, the primary role for the clinician in the management of colic is to support the family through a difficult period and ensure that no untoward interactions are set up.

1. **Inform the family.** The mysterious but benign nature of colic should be reiterated. The family will need constant reassurance that nothing is physically wrong with the infant. This is best accomplished by frequent physical examinations to assure the family that nothing has been missed and an emphasis on the otherwise normal growth and development of the infant. The usual time course should be explained but not to downplay the family's current distress (e.g., *"I know how distressing it is to care for an inconsolable infant. I've seen a lot of colicky babies, and fortunately it almost always disappears by 3–4 months. In the meantime, let's see what we can do to help things here and now"*).

2. **Lessen parental feelings of guilt.** Most parents (especially inexperienced ones) feel that the crying occurs because of something that they are doing wrong. They require reassurance that this is not the case and that colic occurs with even the most attentive, loving, and experienced caregivers. *"You aren't doing anything wrong. This is coming from your baby."*

3. **Empathize and depathologize parental feelings of resentment and anger.** Many parents are mortified by the ambivalent and frankly negative feelings engendered by their crying infant. They should be reassured that *all* parents feel some resentment and anger toward their colicky infant, that it does not make them bad parents, and that these feelings are short-lived. In some cases, parental fear of harming the baby during an episode should be taken seriously and a brief hospitalization may be indicated to provide respite. *"All parents have these feelings. Just let me know if you are ever so worried you could be at the breaking point and could get so mad you could hurt the baby."*

4. **Provide close and consistent follow-up.** Parents should call the clinician within 48 hours of the first visit to report on progress. If no progress is evident, a second visit can be scheduled within a week for further discussion and to reassure them that there is no organic problem. The parents need to be able to count on the clinician's availability during this difficult time. *"Let me see you back in a week to see how things are going. And call any time. Let me know how it is going. I have many tricks for colic up my sleeve. If one doesn't work, we'll try another. Don't worry, we'll get through this."*

5. **Remind the beleaguered parents that it is permissible to take breaks from the baby.** If the baby cries inconsolably despite all reasonable interventions, it is permissible to put the baby down and let him or her cry for increasingly longer periods of time before attempting another consoling maneuver. *"You've tried everything and she's still crying. Why not put her down for a while and let her cry without you holding her and see if she can calm down on her own."*

   - Parents can be reassured that crying is healthy for the lungs, that (especially since the infant is crying anyway) it is not emotionally damaging for the infant to cry alone for a while at this age, and that such isolation teaches some infants how to

Table 37-2. Suggestions for parents to help colic

	Strategy	Comments
Feeding/ nutritional	Change formula from cow's milk to soy based	Emphasize to parent that it is a clinical trial, that it might not work, and that changing formulas does not mean that there is anything physically wrong with the baby.
	Change formula from soy based to predigested	Expensive but sometimes effective
	If breast-feeding, have mother stop cow's milk, caffeine, etc.	One study showed increased bovine IgG in the breast milk of mothers of colicky babies. Ask the breast feeding mother which foods seem to be associated with increased irritability.
	Change nipple or bottle; feed in upright position with frequent burping	Try to decrease air swallowing (e.g., by using bottle with a plastic liner)
	Probiotics	Newest line of research may help (*One study showed Lactobacillus reuteri decreased crying in 95% of infants*)
Alternate sensory stimula- tion	Supplemental daytime carrying	One study found little benefit of supplemental carrying for truly colicky infants (Front carrier, e.g., Snugli, allows hand to be free while carrying)
	Car seat on dishwasher or drier	Must be observed, because the seat can shift
	Ride in the car	Not advisable in the middle of the night if driver is sleepy
	Change of scenery or no scenery	New sights can distract from the distress or baby may be overstimulated and no scenery may be needed
	Pacifier	In Herman Meyer's words, "If for no other reason than to obstruct the opening from which the cacophonous sound emanates."
	Swing	Rarely allows more than 30 min of relief
	Belly massage	Use a lubricating lotion
	Swaddling	Especially good for babies who are hypersensitive to body movements or touch
	Heartbeat tape or white/ pink noise generator	Especially good for babies who are hypersensitive to noise
	Hot-water bottle on belly	Should not be too hot
	Sleep tight (device that generates white noise and vibrates the bed)	Some pediatric practices have the device available to loan to patients. (Two controlled studies, however, have shown disappointing benefits)
	Warm bath	
Medications	Herbal tea (e.g., chamomile, spearmint, fennel)	A study of chamomile/verbena/licorice/ fennel/mint tea found improvement in 57% of colicky infants, though amount needed to get effect could affect nutrition.
	Simethicone	Probably harmless, dubiously helpful
	Antispasmodics	**Should not be used.** Despite some evidence of efficacy, there have been case reports of respiratory arrests associated with their use in infants

self-console. Some parents find letting their infant cry unattended to be intolerable. They should be supported in handling the problem in the way that is most comfortable to them.

- Parents should also be encouraged to take breaks from the baby by letting a friend, family member, or babysitter attend to him or her for a few hours while the parents go out of the house for some unrestricted free time. They should be reminded that the crying is not as emotionally wrenching for a nonparent to hear and that they can best serve their baby when they themselves are refreshed. *"You know it's okay to leave her with someone else for a while. You both could use a break from each other every now and then."*

BIBLIOGRAPHY

For parents

Web sites

http://children.webmd.com/guide/could-be-colic

For professionals

Brazelton TB. Crying in infancy. *Pediatrics* 29:579–588, 1962.

Clifford TJ, Campbell MK, Speechley KN, et al. Sequelae of infant colic: evidence of transient infant distress and absence of lasting effects on maternal mental health. *Arch Pediatr Adolesc Med* 156:1183–1188, 2002.

Barr RG, Paterson JA, MacMartin LM, et al. Prolonged and unsoothable crying bouts in infants with and without colic. *J Dev Behav Pediatr* 26:14–23, 2005.

Wessel MA, Cobb JC, Jackson EB, et al. Paroxysmal fussing in infancy, sometimes called "colic." *Pediatrics* 14:421–434, 1954.

38 Depression

Brian Kurtz
Michael Jellinek

I. **Description of the problem.** Childhood major depressive disorder (MDD) is characterized by a significant, often recurrent emotional and behavioral change from baseline to a dysphoric or irritable mood; loss of pleasure or fun; and with decreased functioning in the home, in school, and with peers. MDD in adolescence is sometimes less obvious or hidden compared with that in the childhood.

   A. **Epidemiology/incidence.** Point prevalence figures vary, since criteria for diagnosis are hard to measure precisely.

   1. **MDD in the pediatric population.**

      a. **Infants and preschoolers.** 1%. Seen as failure to thrive, as well as attachment, separation, and behavioral problems.

      b. **School-aged children.** 2%–3%. Closer fit to adolescent/adult criteria. Typically heralds a more protracted, recurrent, or severe course. Suicide attempts and completions uncommon to rare and often in the context of multiple family and environmental stressors.

      c. **Adolescents.** 5%–6% +. Presents more like the adult syndrome and typically requires evaluation of suicidal behavior and substance use. Depressive symptoms, transient, and not meeting criteria for MDD are quite common.

   2. **MDD in specialized populations.**

      a. As many as 7% of general pediatric inpatients (especially with chronic disease) and 28% of child psychiatry clinic patients.

   3. **Comorbid diagnoses in children with MDD.** 60%–80% of children meeting criteria for MDD have additional or comorbid disorders, such as anxiety, attention deficit disorder, substance abuse, and conduct problems, including lying, stealing, vandalism, and truancy. Comprehensive treatment planning must include and integrate comorbid disorders.

   B. **Etiology/contributing factors.**

   1. **Genetic.** The biologic offspring of depressed adults are up to three times more likely to have MDD, which may present earlier and recur more frequently. Research in the past decade implicated a polymorphism in the serotonin transporter promoter region (5-HTTLPR) as contributing to vulnerability to depression, although a recent meta-analysis has called this into question. Genome-wide linkage scan studies have identified areas of interest on chromosomes 15q, 17p, and 8p. There is also emerging evidence that adverse early life events can exert epigenetic effects, such as methylation status of gene regulatory regions. If confirmed, this study suggests a pathway for interaction between environmental and genetic factors influencing behavior and mood. In general, research suggests polygenetic inheritance, and interaction between genetic factors and life stress, in the development of depression.

   2. **Environmental.** Distinguishing etiologic environmental factors that cause MDD from those that are coincidental to or a consequence of MDD is difficult. Children identify with, learn from, and share the mood of their parents and siblings. They are greatly affected by losses, especially parental death and divorce, and other stresses including trauma and abuse. The boundary between extended bereavement and MDD requires careful monitoring. From a neurobiological perspective, environmental factors affect stress hormone reactivity along the hypothalamic–pituitary–adrenal axis and may thereby exert an influence on the development of depression.

   3. **Organic.** It is hypothesized that a biochemical imbalance in norepinephrine may contribute to the fatigue of MDD; an imbalance in serotonin may cause the problems of irritability and anxiety. Many acute medical conditions (including toxic ingestions, metabolic disturbances, and central nervous system infections) and several chronic medical illnesses can lead to changes in appetite, weight loss, decreased energy, or irritable mood.

4. **Developmental.** Adolescence is a time of change, of puberty, of separation, of transition from the familiar childhood family unit in the context of evolving autonomy. Intrapsychic depressive experiences become more differentiated and specific as emotional, language, cognitive, and social development proceed. Depressive symptoms are more common and the adolescent's increasing self-centered perspective and sense of autonomy sometimes interferes with a clinical relationship. Young children with MDD may simply experience a vague and overwhelming discomfort, whereas older children may come to use *stomachache, headache,* or feeling fearful as words for internal mood states. Such abstract terms as depression and age-appropriate symptoms like *blue, bored, empty, down and bothered, angry, or irritable* are more likely to be used in early adolescence.

5. **Transactional.** The interaction of environmental contributions from school, home, and peers differs at different developmental stages and is influenced by genetic and organic factors. Some factors such as a special skill, relationship, or intellectual strength may foster resiliency; other factors such as family tension may act as a stressor. Some school-aged children with MDD lose their ability to concentrate in school, causing performance and peer relationships to suffer. Other children are able to control their mood swings while at school, only to collapse into a depressed or irritable mood on safe arrival home.

II. **Making the diagnosis (see Table 38-1).**
   A. **Signs, symptoms, and behavioral observations.** The *Diagnostic Statistical Manual for Primary Care (DSM-PC)* gives a range of presentations typical in primary care settings and is organized by symptoms rather than only by diagnosis.
      1. **Infant/toddler.** Both the persistently passive, unresponsive infant and the irritable, unsoothable, crying infant may suffer from the mood dysregulation associated with depression. Their clinical presentations may evolve into a quiet, inhibited toddler with arrested social development or an overactive, impulsive, and irritable preschooler. Key features may include anhedonia, fatigue, excessive guilt, and diminished cognitive abilities.
      2. **School age.** In school-aged children with MDD, the expected pride associated with industry and enthusiasm may be overwhelmed by humiliation, defeat, irritability, and self-doubt. The child may become sad, isolated, rejected, and accident prone. Temper tantrums or morbid preoccupations with bodily injury, illness, abandonment, or death might emerge. There may be pediatric office visits for multiple somatic complaints. Bereavement may not gradually ease to normal functioning, but instead persist to a full depressive state.
      3. **Adolescents.** May have difficulty containing intense negative feelings. Experiencing a crushing defeat or rejection, they both have the passion and the means to act on self-destructive urges. They may have direct negative actions inward against themselves by disregarding food, sleep, and hygiene. Some turn to alcohol and drugs for numbing symptomatic relief or engage in destructive behaviors. Instead of appearing sad and eliciting sympathy (as adults with MDD might), adolescents with MDD often seem irritable, angry and resentful. Given the danger of depression and substance use, especially the high mortality of teenage accidents, this age group merits special attention, especially direct questions, in private, concerning their mood and behavior.
   B. **History: key clinical questions.**
      1. *"How is your child's mood? How does the child feel about himself or herself? For how many days, weeks, months, has this been the case?"* Diagnosis of MDD requires at least a 2-week period of prominent mood-related symptoms, but pediatric clinicians may see shorter periods of sadness or milder persistent symptoms. Parental depression can have an environmental as well as genetic impact on children; most parental depression goes unrecognized and untreated.
      2. *"Has there been a recent change in your child's behavior, school performance, or peer relationships?"* A decrease in functioning or significant change in behaviors can be a key indicator of mood-related stress and disability (and should be evident in all areas of daily functioning).
      3. *"Does your child have a past history of feeling down, or has he ever seen a mental health professional in the past?"* Studies indicate a high risk for recurrence for MDD.
      4. *"Does anyone in the extended family have a history of depression, mania, anxiety, attention deficits, or alcohol or substance use?"* Family psychiatric history is an important predictor of childhood risk. The incidence of depression in mothers, in general, is approximately 5%; mothers of young children or those facing marital discord are at higher risk.

Table 38-1. Criteria for child and adolescent major depressive episode

Depressed mood or loss of interests or pleasure in activities at home, at school, or with peers for at least 2 weeks or more than 50% of the time. Coincident with depressed mood, changes in *at least four* of the following	Including sad, blue, bored, empty, oppositional, irritable, angry, and rageful feelings
Appetite or weight	In relation to expected weight gain; may present in infants and preschoolers as a feeding difficulty and in adolescents as anorexia or obesity
Sleep patterns	Including insomnia, hypersomnia, and frequent wakenings
Agitation	Including restlessness and aggressiveness; infants may be fussy and school-aged children hyperactive
Social withdrawal	In infants and preschoolers, problems of attachment and separation or loss of spontaneous play; in school-aged children, school reluctance, school phobia, or a sudden drop in school performance or after-school activities
Energy loss	Including listlessness, fatigue, and lethargy
Self-esteem	In school-aged children, feelings of stupidity, clowning around, or engaging in self-reproachful boasting; in adolescents, expressions of guilt, self-deprecation, helplessness, or hopelessness
Concentration	In infants and preschoolers, speech and motor delays or regression; with children or adolescents in school, sustained change in ability to attend in class, complete assignments out of class, concentrate, or make decisions
Dangerousness	In infants, possibly head banging; in school-aged children, accident proneness; in adolescents, stealing, lying, and truancy
Somatic symptoms	In infants and preschoolers, failure to thrive and rumination; in school-aged children, enuresis, encopresis, and vague complaints; in adolescents, complaints of abdominal or head pain
Suicidal ideation	Recurrent thoughts or death or morbid preoccupation with illness, accidents, and/or death
Substance use	

5. *"Is your child often intensely worried? Profoundly anxious? Impulsive or inattentive? Prone to lie or steal?"* Identifying and clarifying comorbid diagnoses makes for more effective treatment.

6. *"If depressed, has your child ever brought harm to himself, even accidentally? Has the child ever talked or threatened to hurt himself or others?"* (And to the child: *"Have you ever felt so bad that you wanted to hurt yourself?"*). Self-destructive acts or threats must be taken seriously and should automatically lead to a careful suicide assessment and referral for psychiatric evaluation and follow-up. (See chapter on suicide.)

III. Management.

A. Primary goals. Most children with MDD can be safely cared for as outpatients. Initial management of depression includes education and counseling to patients and families about depression and options for treatment, development of a treatment plan with specific goals in key areas of functioning, establishing links with mental health resources available in the community, and development of a safety plan. For mild to moderate depression, pediatric clinicians wishing to include this work in their practice can consider assessing family history of MDD, noting short-term stressors, and encouraging more support for the child. For moderate to severe MDD or where watchful waiting has seen the child's mood state persist or worsen, the comprehensive treatment of childhood MDD is beyond the expertise of most primary care clinicians and should be referred to a mental health professional. The primary care clinician should monitor the treatment through the ongoing relationship with the family. Urgent psychiatric consultation is indicated whenever the child or adolescent might be psychotic, acutely suicidal, abusing substances, or otherwise difficult to manage safely.

B. Aids to clinical management. Public health initiatives have been developed to aid primary care clinicians in assessing depression and working with depressed children and adolescents. These include Bright Futures in Practice: Mental Health and the Guidelines for Adolescent Depression—Primary Care. The materials for both programs are available free of charge on the Internet, and include tool kits with information for providers, patient and parent information sheets, and rating instruments. The Bright Futures tool kit includes the Pediatric Symptom Checklist (PSC) and the Center for Epidemiological Studies Depression Scale for Children (CES-DC). The Guidelines for Adolescent Depression in Primary Care (GLAD-PC) tool kit includes the Columbia Depression Scale (CDS), the Patient Health Questionnaire-9 (PHQ-9), the Kutcher Adolescent Depression Scale (KADS), and the Beck Depression Inventory (BDI).

C. Treatment strategies. The strategies listed below are often integrated by experienced clinicians as clinically indicated. The pediatric clinician faces the difficult challenge of defining the symptoms, issues, and convincing parents to accept and complete a mental health referral.

1. **Psychodynamic therapy** attempts to provide a safe and supportive environment for the child to explore, understand, and learn to express inner feelings and conflicts. It is often most effective for children and adolescents with low self-esteem. Play therapy is used in younger children who do not yet effectively use words to convey inner feelings.

2. **Cognitive-behavior therapy** reviews and challenges negative thoughts, actions, and feelings in a systematic and logical way.

3. **Family therapy** views the family as a system unto itself and attempts to identify behavioral patterns and alliances that keep the family from developing or changing. It is often best for multiply stressed families and can be an important avenue for early detection of depression in other family members.

4. **Group therapy** views the child in a social and interactive context. It is often useful for developing social skills and social support.

5. **Parent guidance** helps parents to learn to deal with depression in their children or in themselves. Parents who feel personally overwhelmed or confused by the parental role may find this approach helpful. Depressed parents should be referred for psychiatric evaluation.

6. **Environmental interventions** aim to support academic performance and raise a child's self-esteem through the use of role models and positive experiences that foster industry, responsibility, and pride. A carefully chosen summer or after-school activity, hobby, or encouragement of a friendship can be invaluable.

7. **Medications** focus on correcting biochemical imbalances. Selective serotonin reuptake inhibitors (SSRIs) such as fluoxetine, sertraline, and citalopram or escitalopram are first-line for pharmacotherapy; fluoxetine is Food and Drug Administration (FDA)-approved for depression in children and adolescents and escitalopram is FDA-approved in adolescents. Among other factors, parental responsiveness to a particular medication may guide medication choice. In most patients, these medicines are well-tolerated. However, many children experience mild side effects, such as gastrointestinal effects, headaches, and changes in sleep, and some experience more distressing effects such as restlessness and behavioral activation. The issue of whether antidepressants increase the risk of suicidal behaviors in certain individuals has received a great deal of attention, especially since the FDA issued a "black box warning" about this issue in 2003. Following this, prescription of SSRI medications to children and adolescents, particularly by primary care providers, declined, and this in turn was correlated at least temporally with an increase in the suicide rate in youth. It appears that the link between antidepressants and suicidal behavior is complex; one clear issue is that an assessment of safety prior to starting an antidepressant and close follow-up are needed. The FDA recommends weekly contact for a month, followed by contact every 2 weeks for another month when an antidepressant is started.

D. Primary care follow-up. The clinician should follow specific psychological symptoms over time, monitor safety, watch for side effects of medications, monitor patient compliance, and encourage appropriate child psychiatric follow-up. A suggestion for the primary care clinician for the initial management of depression is to see a patient weekly, even if very briefly, to monitor safety, side effects, and improvement. If there is no change or a worsening in the first 6 weeks, a referral to a mental health specialist becomes more necessary.

BIBLIOGRAPHY

For parents

AACAP (American Academy of Child and Adolescent Psychiatry) Depression Resource Center. www.aacap.org/cs/Depression.ResourceCenter

National Alliance on Mental Illness. www.nami.org/Content/NavigationMenu/Mental_Illnesses/Depression/Depression_in_Children_and_Adolescents.htm

National Institute of Mental Health. www.nimh.nih.gov/health/topics/child-and-adolescent-mental-health/index.shtml

ParentsMedGuide for Depression from the American Psychiatric Association and AACAP. www.ParentsMedGuide.org

For professionals

Bright Futures at Georgetown University. Bright Futures in Practice: Mental Health. Available at: www.brightfutures.org/mentalhealth/

Cheung AH, Zuckerbrot RA, Jensen PS, et al. Guidelines for Adolescent Depression in Primary Care (GLAD-PC): II. Treatment and ongoing management. *Pediatrics* 120(5):e1313–e1326, 2007.

Luby JL. Early childhood depression. *Am J Psychiatry* 166(9):974–979, 2009.

The Reach Institute. Guidelines for Adolescent Depression—Primary Care. Available at: www.glad-pc.org

Wolraich ML, Felice ME, Drotar D (eds). *The Classification of Child and Adolescent Mental Diagnoses in Primary Care; Diagnostic and Statistical Manual for Primary Care (DSM-PC) Child and Adolescent Version.* Elk Grove Village, IL: American Academy of Pediatrics, 1996.

Zuckerbrot RA, Cheung AH, Jensen PS, et al. Guidelines for Adolescent Depression in Primary Care (GLAD-PC): I. Identification, assessment, and initial management. *Pediatrics* 120(5):e1299–e1312, 2007.

39

Down Syndrome

Siegfried M. Pueschel

I. **Description of the problem.** The child with Down syndrome has recognizable physical characteristics and limited intellectual functioning due to the presence of an extra chromosome 21 or part of the long arm of chromosome 21.

A. **Epidemiology.**
- Estimated incidence of Down syndrome is between 1 in 800–1200 live births.
- 3000–5000 children with Down syndrome are born each year in the United States.
- There has been a slight decrease in the birth prevalence due to the increased utilization of prenatal screening (alpha fetoprotein, unconjugated estriol, free beta human chorionic gonadotropin, pregnancy-associated plasma protein-A (PAPP-A), inhibin-A, and ultrasonography) and diagnostic techniques (chorionic villus sampling, amniocentesis, and other procedures), leading to subsequent termination of the pregnancy.
- There is a higher prevalence in the population because of an increased life expectancy.

B. **Genetics.** There are four main types of chromosome abnormalities in Down syndrome.
1. **Trisomy 21** is observed in the vast majority (93%–95%) of children with Down syndrome.
2. **Translocation** occurs in 4%–6% of children with Down syndrome. Most translocations involve the attachment of the long arms of the supernumerary chromosome 21 to chromosome 14, 21, or 22. If a translocation is identified in a child with Down syndrome, the parents' chromosomes need to be examined, since in about one-third of the cases a parent may be a balanced carrier of the translocation. Genetic counseling is recommended.
3. **Mosaicism** occurs in approximately 1%–2% of children with Down syndrome.
4. A rare chromosome aberration, **partial trisomy 21,** is noted in some persons with Down syndrome.
5. Much progress has been made in molecular genetics. Recent genome studies revealed that there are more than 420 genes encoded on chromosome 21 of which 145 have been studied well.

C. **Etiology.** Many etiologies of Down syndrome have been posited including radiation, viral infections, genetic predisposition, autoimmune processes, and others. It is well known that advanced maternal age is a definite risk factor that may be associated with problems in production line, persistent nucleoli, hormonal imbalance, delayed fertilization, and relaxed selection. Most of these theories are tentative. Recent investigations suggest that the absence or reduced proximal recombination appears to predispose to nondisjunction in meiosis I and the presence or increase of proximal exchanges predisposes to nondisjunction in meiosis II. In addition, some studies indicate an increased incidence of Down syndrome in diabetic mothers and in females with only one ovary.

II. **Making the diagnosis.**

A. **Signs and symptoms.** There is a wide variability in the characteristics of children with Down syndrome. Some individuals have only a few signs, whereas others show most of the features as listed in Table 39-1.

B. **Differential diagnosis.** The main features of Down syndrome are often recognized by the clinician in the neonatal period. However, on rare occasions children with other chromosomal aberrations may display a similar phenotype (e.g., newborns with 49, XXXXX syndrome may have similar facial features). Conformation by chromosome analysis is mandatory.

C. **Medical concerns.** Some of the medical concerns of newborn children with Down syndrome may be life-threatening and require immediate correction, whereas others may only become apparent during subsequent days and weeks or in later life.
1. **Neonatal medical problems.**
   a. **Congenital heart disease** is diagnosed in 40%–50% of children with Down syndrome (most often atrioventricular canal, followed by ventricular septal defect, Tetralogy of Fallot, patent ductus arteriosus, and atrial septal defect). All newborns

Table 39-1. Percentage of phenotypic findings in a group of 114 infants with Down syndrome (abbreviated list)

Sagittal suture separated	98
Oblique palpebral fissures	98
Wide space between first and second toes	96
False fontanel (widening of sagittal suture at the parietal area)	95
Plantar crease between first and second toes	94
Increased neck tissue	87
Abnormally shaped palate	85
Hypoplastic nose	83
Brushfield spots	75
Mouth kept open	65
Protruding tongue	58
Epicanthal folds	57
Single palmar crease	53
Brachyclinodactyly	51
Short stubby hands	38
Flattened occiput	35
Abnormal structure of ears	28

with Down syndrome should be examined by a pediatric cardiologist and undergo echocardiography. A child with congenital heart disease who is in heart failure will require appropriate medical treatment. Many of these children will undergo heart surgery during the first year of life.

b. **Anomalies of the gastrointestinal tract** including tracheoesophageal fistula, esophageal atresia, pyloric stenosis, duodenal atresia, duodenal stenosis or webs, annular pancreas, aganglionic megacolon (Hirschsprung's disease), imperforate anus, and others occur in about 5%–12% of infants with Down syndrome. Many of these congenital anomalies require immediate surgical attention.

c. **Congenital cataracts** are identified in approximately 3% of newborns with Down syndrome. These cataracts are usually very dense and need to be extracted soon after birth followed by correction with glasses, contact lenses, or lens implants.

2. **Medical problems during childhood.**

a. **Nutritional aspects.** During infancy, feeding problems and poor weight gain may be observed, especially in infants with significant congenital heart disease. On the other hand, excessive weight gain often becomes a problem in later childhood and during adolescence. Parents need to be informed with regard to appropriate dietary practices, proper eating habits, avoidance of high caloric foods, and regular physical exercise starting in early childhood.

b. **Infections.** Children with Down syndrome have a high prevalence of respiratory infections, especially those with congenital heart disease. Otitis media also has been noted to occur more frequently. Skin infections are often seen in adolescents with Down syndrome, mainly at the thighs, buttocks, and perigenital area.

c. **Dental concerns.** Problems with tooth eruption, tooth shape, and sometimes absence or fusion of teeth are observed. The most devastating dental problems relate to gingivitis and periodontal disease. It is important that persons with Down syndrome practice appropriate dental hygiene, follow good dietary habits, and are examined regularly by a dentist.

d. **Visual impairment.** Many children with Down syndrome have ocular disorders including blepharitis, strabismus, nystagmus, hypoplasia of the iris, and refractive errors. It has been reported that up to 40% of children are myopic and another 20% are hyperopic and 2%–5% have keratoconus and about 12% have amblyopia. Children with Down syndrome should be examined by a pediatric ophthalmologist annually.

e. **Audiologic dysfunction.** Numerous reports from the literature indicate that about 60% of children with Down syndrome have some form of middle ear pathology, often resulting in a hearing deficit. Most of these deficits are due to a conductive hearing loss, and some children have neurosensory hearing impairment or a mixed hearing loss.

f. **Seizure disorders.** There is an increased frequency (6%–10%) of seizure disorders in individuals with Down syndrome. Infantile spasms may be observed at a higher frequency in young children with Down syndrome during their first year of life, grand mal seizures as well as complex partial seizures are more often noted during adolescence and late adulthood.

g. Sleep apnea. Approximately 60% of children with Down syndrome have sleep apnea, most often due to upper airway obstruction. These children usually present with noisy breathing, snoring, frequent apnea during sleep, sleepiness during daytime, and behavior disorders.

h. Thyroid dysfunction. Up to 20% of children with Down syndrome have some form of thyroid dysfunction, usually compensated or uncompensated hypothyroidism. Also, hyperthyroidism has been observed in some children with Down syndrome. Because of the high prevalence of thyroid dysfunction, thyroid function tests should be carried out annually.

i. Atlantoaxial instability. Atlantoaxial instability is due to increased ligamentous laxity at the upper cervical spine. Approximately 15% of children with Down syndrome have this disorder, although only 1%–2% have symptomatic atlantoaxial instability, and they usually require surgical intervention. Children with Down syndrome should have radiologic assessment of the cervical spine starting at the age of 3 years; before entering Special Olympics sport activities; and if indicated during adolescence. If asymptomatic atlantoaxial instability is present, it is recommended that the individual refrain from participating in sport activities that potentially could lead to injury of the neck and spinal cord compression. It is of utmost importance to prevent symptomatic atlantoaxial instability because of its devastating neurologic consequences.

j. Orthopedic problems. There is an increased prevalence of hip dislocation, patellar subluxation, and metatarsus valgus in children with Down syndrome.

k. Dermatological concerns. There are dermatological concerns such as alopecia, folliculitis, xerosis, cheilitis, onychomycosis, and others.

l. Hematological diseases. Immunologic and hematologic issues (e.g., increased prevalence of leukemia) have been observed in children with Down syndrome.

m. Gastrointestinal disorders. Gastroesophageal reflux and celiac disease occur at a higher frequency in children with Down syndrome.

III. Management.

A. Primary goals. The main objective of appropriate management is to provide optimal medical and surgical care to all persons with Down syndrome. No form of treatment should be withheld from any child with Down syndrome that would be given unhesitatingly to a child without this chromosome disorder.

B. Information for families.

1. Initial counseling. Although there is no completely satisfactory way of giving "bad news" to parents, the clinician's positive approach, tact, compassion, and truthfulness will have a vital influence on the parent's subsequent adjustment. The clinician's style and manner of counseling parents during the initial traumatic period is of utmost importance and sets the tone for the atmosphere that will prevail in future years.

a. Use proper terminology and inform both parents together in a sensitive and honest way as soon as the clinical diagnosis has been made.

b. Time your remarks to coincide with increasing parental adaptation.

c. Schedule follow-up sessions for review of basic considerations and communication of more details (chromosome analysis, developmental expectations, etc.).

d. Spend extra time in talking about various health concerns and developmental issues that will make the parents aware of your sincere interest in helping them and their child.

e. Stress that most observable characteristics do not cause significant disability in the child. For example, the slanting of the palpebral fissures and the presence of Brushfield spots do not interfere with the child's vision. However, other abnormalities such as congenital heart disease or duodenal atresia are serious and require prompt medical attention.

2. Treatment. It is important to let parents know that there is no cure and no effective medical treatment available for children with Down syndrome at the present time. Numerous "medications" have been recommended to improve the mental capacity of children with Down syndrome, but none have been found to be of benefit.

3. Education. Parents should be informed about early intervention programs and inclusive educational strategies in integrated school programs that are available to children with Down syndrome. With appropriate education and positive learning experiences, many children with Down syndrome will be able to function well in society. Most individuals will be able to hold a job and many will be gainfully employed later.

BIBLIOGRAPHY

For parents

Organizations

National Down Syndrome Congress. www.ndsccenter.org
National Down Syndrome Society. www.ndss.org

Books

Pueschel SM. *A Parent's Guide to Down Syndrome: Toward a Brighter Future.* Baltimore, MD: Brookes Publishing, 2001.
Pueschel SM, Sustrova M. *Adolescents with Down Syndrome.* Baltimore, MD: Brookes Publishing, 1997.

For professionals

Mégarbané A, Ravel A, Mircher C, et al. The 50th anniversary of the discovery of Trisomy 21: the past, present and future. *Genet Med* 11(9):611–616, 2009.
Skotko BG, Capone GT, Kishnani PS, Down Syndrome Diagnosis Study Group. Postnatal diagnosis of Down syndrome: synthesis of the evidence on how to best deliver the news. *Pediatrics* 124(4):e751–e778, 2009.

Encopresis

40

Laura Weissman
Leonard Rappaport

I. **Description of the problem.** Encopresis is defined as repeated passage of stool into inappropriate places in a child older than 4 years, chronologically and developmentally. The behavior is not due exclusively to the direct physiological effects of a substance (e.g., laxatives) or a general medical condition, except through a mechanism involving constipation.

A. **Epidemiology.**
- Encopresis reportedly affects 2.8% of 4-year-olds, 1.9% of 6-year-olds, and 1.6% of 10–11-year-olds.
- Encopresis usually presents in children younger than 7 years although it can present at any age.

B. **Etiology/contributing factors.**
- More than 90% of encopresis is due to functional constipation where retained stool distends the rectum, resulting in stool leaking around a stool mass. Distention of the rectum results in abnormal feedback to the stretch receptors in the bowel concerning the need to stool resulting in leakage. As a result the child often does not receive a signal to defecate until soiling is nearly complete.
- Encopresis is not generally caused by underlying psychopathology but can be associated with emotional distress. In addition, encopresis itself can result in considerable embarrassment, humiliation, punishment, and bullying.
- Rare cases of encopresis are due to damaged corticospinal pathways or anorectal dysfunction such as that seen after pull through surgery. This can also be seen in the case of undiagnosed Hirschsprung disease or after surgical correction of this disorder.
- A small subset of children with encopresis may impulsively pass stool due to anxiety or other emotional stressors, without underlying constipation.
- There are a small number of children who soil on purpose, but they are rare and it is best to assume a physiological reason and treatment as an initial approach.

II. **Making the diagnosis.**
A. **History: key clinical questions.**
1. *"Was there a time when the child's bowel movements seemed typical?"* History starts at birth with specifics surrounding bowel function and any treatments used. Past medical and surgical history may identify systemic diseases or medical causes of constipation that indicate treatments other than laxatives and maintenance of stool regularity.
2. *"Did your child have a period of stooling into the toilet? How old was he or she? Did he or she feel the stool coming and get to the bathroom by her- or himself regularly?"* Distinguishing delayed toilet training, where the child never consolidated the ability to stool independently into the toilet and is essentially afraid to use the toilet to stool, from encopresis is essential. Treatment will vary, depending on whether or not constipation underlies the stooling accidents, rather than toilet refusal (although toilet refusal is often associated with constipation as well).
3. *"How often does your child stool and urinate into the toilet now? How often into underwear? Are the stools large? Hard? Liquid? Do they hurt?"* Review details of present urinary and bowel patterns, such as frequency of stool evacuation into the toilet, stool accidents, stool consistency, and the urge to defecate. More severe, prolonged constipation generally will require more aggressive treatment. Any history of abuse or other trauma should be sought as well. Children who have been abused may become incontinent in times of stress or as part of regressive behavior and are less suitable candidates for rectal suppositories or enemas. They may also soil their underwear to keep someone away from them.
4. *"Often stool problems coexist with wetting accidents. Has he or she had any urinary tract infections? Does she or he have urine accidents in the day or at night?"* Urinary patterns, daytime wetting and nocturnal enuresis, and symptoms of urinary tract infection must be elicited and may indicate neurological abnormalities or urine contamination. Constipation and especially encopresis may be associated with urinary

tract infections, especially in females, due to poor hygiene. Even without infection, enuresis can be caused by a dilated rectum pushing on and irritating the bladder, thus causing bladder spasms.

5. *"I see lots of kids who have poop accidents and don't like having them. If you and your parents help me figure out what is going on, I think I can help so the accidents get better."* History taking provides an essential opportunity to communicate with the child. The child must be an active participant for the treatment to be effective, and often children with encopresis are overwhelmed and embarrassed when encopresis is discussed. The child often appears to not even be listening to the discussion, but they certainly are. When treatment is successful, the clinician often observes a drastic change in positive affect in the patient. Developing a sense of the child's perspective can create a connection between caregiver and patient and should include questions about present school and family functioning.

B. Signs and symptoms. A child with functional constipation and consequent encopresis will report uncomfortable and infrequent stooling into the toilet with uncontrolled stool accidents into underwear or pull-ups. Physical examination of the child with encopresis includes the following:

- Growth parameters.
- Attention to signs of systemic disease.
- Neurological assessment including a close look for skin abnormalities overlying the spine.
- Examine the anal opening. Anal fissures will cause ongoing pain with defecation; tags may reflect inflammatory bowel disease, and an absent anal wink may indicate neurological abnormality.
- Rectal examination can be useful in assessing for Hirschsprung disease and may provide an indication of the degree of rectal impaction to guide treatment.

C. Differential diagnosis. Any disorder that can cause constipation can cause encopresis. A detailed history and physical examination is required to rule out systemic or organic causes of constipation or incontinence, such as spinal cord dysplasia or tethering, hypothyroidism, and a history of abnormal stools such as a meconium ileus seen in the case of cystic fibrosis.

D. Diagnostic assessment. For most children, no further diagnostic assessment is necessary beyond thorough history and physical examination. Laboratory investigation is indicated only as history or physical examination suggests: rarely laboratories may include thyroid function tests, electrolytes, calcium, and magnesium. An abdominal radiograph may be useful when the history is vague or the child is uncooperative with the abdominal or rectal examination and also can be used to educate families. Lumbosacral spine films or magnetic resonance imaging are indicated when lower extremity neurological examination is abnormal or sacral abnormalities are visualized.

III. Management.

A. Psychoeducation. Demystify the shame and blame around stool accidents. Use the child's abdominal radiograph or an illustrated explanation (or both) to review the process of retained stool that leads to a distended colon and especially rectum, allowing stool to "sneak out without warning." Discuss that retained stool has to be cleaned out with medication and that there will likely be a lot of stool to clean out. Empathize with the stress and frustration that everyone has experienced, and emphasize the need to break the cycle of failure that may have developed. Clarify that now the child truly cannot control the stool leaking out and should not be blamed. On the other hand, to cure encopresis, the child needs to commit to following your suggestions for treatment.

B. The initial clean out of retained stool. The first part of treatment includes a clean out of the retained stool that is dilating the rectum and impacting stool continence. There are many different choices for clean out regimens and this often depends on the child and the family. Children aged 7 years and older without a history of trauma may opt for a fast and direct choice: a 14-day cycle of sequential Day 1—Fleets® enema, Day 2—bisacodyl pills, Day 3—bisacodyl suppository, which is then repeated four times over 12 days. To get compliance, it is helpful to explain to children that the enemas and suppositories are necessary since the muscle has been stretched by the stool and is not strong enough to get the stool out easily from oral medicine. Starting with the enema makes sense since the pill is likely to give the child a stomach ache if the bowel is full. Younger children (younger than 7 years developmentally) or those who cannot tolerate suppositories or enemas, may require polyethylene glycol without electrolytes, starting at one capful (17 g) in 8 ounces of fluid per day along with a stimulant medication such as senna or bisacodyl. Impaction that is present for many months may require higher dosing. During the initial clean out, the child and the family should expect a large amount of stool output and are reminded of the radiograph full of stool. The frequency of accidents may increase initially during the clean out but then should subside. The child should return at the end of the clean out and at that time, there should really be no accidents. If there are still accidents either there is retained stool remaining in the rectum or the child is being given too much laxative resulting in accidents that are iatrogenic.

C. **Regular bowel patterns must be established.** This requires medication and a behavior plan. It makes sense to meet with the child and family after the clean out is complete to ensure complete clean out and to plan the next stage of treatment. Polyethylene glycol without electrolytes is used frequently. The maintenance dose of polyethylene glycol without electrolytes generally ranges from $\frac{1}{2}$ capful (8.5 g) every other day to 1 capful (17 g) twice a day. Dosing is adjusted to maintain soft regular stools. As the child may not develop the urge to defecate for 6–9 months after constipation is treated, a regular sitting time is necessary. It is helpful to schedule that sitting time about 20–30 minutes after a meal to take advantage of the gastrocolic reflex.

The goal is to stool before the sensation of needing to stool develops since we want to keep the rectum as empty as possible so that it can come back to its normal size. The family must work to eliminate any negative associations around toileting that may have developed. Limiting conversation about toileting can be helpful. A reward program as an incentive is also important to increasing motivation for engaging in toileting behavior. This can include stickers or other tokens as rewards for sitting on the toilet or taking care of his or her bodily needs. Older children may benefit from having games or activities that can only be used in the bathroom as well.

IV. **Clinical pearls and pitfalls.**
- Most families of a child with encopresis have never met anyone with the same problem. Reassuring them that encopresis is not so unusual and can be treated successfully is a vital first step.
- Parent and child education around the mechanism of encopresis to increase understanding and decrease blame is essential for treatment.
- Constipation and encopresis are often long-term issues, recurring intermittently after great initial improvement with treatment. Children may require medications such polyethylene glycol without electrolytes, and/or high-fiber supplements for extended periods (months to years).
- Reviewing signs of stool backup (e.g., hard stools, skipping days between bowel movements, stomach aches, and/or smears) and developing a rescue plan (e.g., increased polyethylene glycol without electrolytes, the addition of a stimulant such as senna, increased sitting, and/or increased fiber) empowers the child and family to anticipate, tolerate, and treat recurrences. If you do not warn them, they may be embarrassed to come back and tell you on account of the perceived shame around encopresis.

BIBLIOGRAPHY

For parents

Web sites

Children's Medical Center, University of Virginia. http://www.people.virginia.edu/~smb4v/tutorials/constipation/encotreat.htm

For professionals

Brazzelli M, Griffiths P. Behavioural and cognitive interventions with or without other treatments for defaecation disorders in children. *Cochrane Database Syst Rev* (4):CD002240, 2001.
Loening-Baucke V. Encopresis. *Curr Opin Pediatr* 14(5):570–575, 2002.

41 Enuresis (Incontinence)

Leonard Rappaport
Laura Weissman

I. **Description of the problem.** Incontinence is defined as a lack of urinary continence.
  * Beyond age 4 years for daytime continence.
  * Beyond age 5 years for nocturnal continence.
  * The loss of continence after at least 6 months of dryness.
  A. **Definitions.** The International Children's Continence Society classifies urinary incontinence into two categories **continuous incontinence** defined as continuous wetting (more likely with congenital malformations) and **intermittent incontinence** defined as intermittent wetting. Intermittent incontinence can be further subdivided into daytime incontinence and nocturnal incontinence. Intermittent nocturnal incontinence is now synonymous with the term **enuresis.**
    1. Another classification distinguishes between enuresis (intermittent nocturnal incontinence) with and without bladder symptoms as individuals in these categories differ clinically. **Monosymptomatic enuresis** is wetting without lower urinary tract symptoms or daytime symptoms, whereas **nonmonosymptomatic enuresis** is wetting with lower urinary symptoms such as severe frequency, urgency, or daytime symptoms.
    2. Enuresis can also be divided into **primary enuresis** (incontinence in a child who has never obtained continence) and secondary enuresis (when a child has been continent for at least 6 months and becomes incontinent).
    3. Nonmonosymptomatic wetting is associated with a greater degree of organic pathology.
  B. **Epidemiology.** Although the development of urinary continence varies by culture, gender, race, and country, the prevalence of daytime wetting in 7-year-old children is approximately 2%–3% for boys and 3%–4% for girls. For nighttime wetting or enuresis the prevalence is 10%–15% in 7-year-olds.
  C. **Familial transmission/genetics.** There is a genetic predisposition to enuresis. If one parent had enuresis, 44% of his or her children will have enuresis. If both parents had enuresis, 77% of their children will have enuresis. Identical twins have the highest concordance rate (68%). Several genetic loci have been located by intensive family studies.
  D. **Etiology.** In the vast majority of cases, the etiology of incontinence is unknown. There are, however, causes that should be considered.
    1. **Nocturnal incontinence or enuresis.**
      a. **Contributing factors to primary monosymptomatic enuresis.**
        (1) **Maturational delay is a** commonly accepted but unproven cause of nocturnal incontinence. This refers to the enuretic child's inability to send, perceive, or respond to information about a filled bladder during the night. Support for this theory comes from the spontaneous cure rate and relationship between enuresis and maturation of motor systems.
        (2) **Sleep and arousal factors.** Originally, it was thought that enuresis was a non-rapid eye movement dyssomnia (like sleepwalking and night terrors). Data suggest that enuresis occurs in *all* stages of sleep and that there is no difference in sleep patterns between children with enuresis and their nonenuretic peers. Obstructive sleep apnea (OSA) can be associated with nocturnal enuresis. In some cases, interventions for OSA including a tonsillectomy and adenoidectomy can result in resolution of enuresis symptoms.
        (3) **Central nervous system factors.** Continuing research has focused on the possible role of antidiuretic hormone secretion in children with nocturnal enuresis, leading to an increase in urinary output and suggests that this may be a contributing feature in enuresis. Although desmopressin acetate (DDAVP) is a recognized and approved treatment for enuresis, considerable data have accumulated that make this etiology less likely.

(4) Psychopathology/stress. There are no data to support enuresis as a neurotic disorder. Similarly, although stress may exacerbate or contribute to enuresis, it is not a primary etiologic factor. However, certain conditions, such as attention-deficit/hyperactivity disorder (ADHD) are related to an increase in enuresis. However, the ADHD itself may not be causal but representative of a neurochemical marker.

b. Causes of secondary enuresis with and without daytime symptoms.

(1) Increased bladder irritability. A common cause of secondary enuresis is increased bladder irritability, usually due to a urinary tract infection. In addition, any mass impinging on the bladder (e.g., severe constipation) can increase bladder irritability.

(2) Increased urinary output. Any process that increases urinary output can cause enuresis (e.g., diabetes mellitus, diabetes insipidus, and sickle cell disease).

(3) Bladder capacity. Bladder capacity tends to be decreased in children with enuresis compared with their nonenuretic siblings. This reflects differences in functional, rather than absolute, bladder capacity, with contractions occurring earlier in filling.

2. Daytime incontinence.

a. Known causes.

(1) Increased bladder irritability (see above).

(2) Micturition deferral. A common cause of daytime wetting in preschool children is due to holding of the urine and ignoring the urge to void, usually during play. Incontinence results when detrusor contraction cannot be suppressed. Children with short attention spans often fail to respond to body signals until it is too late. This type of wetting can be more common in children with behavioral issues.

(3) Abnormal sphincter control. Although abnormal urinary sphincter control is rare, insidious pathology (e.g., spinal cord abnormalities) can cause abnormal sphincter control. Some hypothesize that there is a group of children with decreased sphincter strength without obvious cause who may have a higher incidence of diurnal enuresis.

(4) Structural abnormalities. Girls with ectopic ureters, which empty into the vagina, have constant wetting with no recognized episodes of incontinence. Partial labial fusion may develop after inflammation, allowing urine to collect in a pocket behind the fused labia minora and subsequently leak.

(5) Vaginal reflux. Overweight girls or girls who sit with their legs together when urinating, can reflux urine into the vagina. The urine will then leak out over the next several hours without the urge to void. This causes almost constant daytime wetting without nighttime episodes.

b. Contributing factors.

(1) Urge syndrome. Children with daytime and nighttime wetting, as well as urgency and frequency, often have unstable detrusor contractions early in bladder filling. They often squat, sitting asymmetrically on one heel in an effort to prevent a detrusor contraction. Symptoms resolve with time, usually by 10–12 years.

(2) Giggle incontinence. Emptying the bladder entirely while laughing may be familial. It is common in school-aged girls and generally resolves with maturity.

(3) Stress incontinence. With increased abdominal pressure, such as during coughing, some children's bladders empty.

(4) Postvoid dribble syndrome. Children may sense wetness after a void but without actual incontinence.

II. Making the diagnosis.

A. History: key clinical questions. A complete history should be obtained with a particular focus on a family history of enuresis, the child's pattern of wetting, and the previous interventions.

1. *"Has the child ever been dry at night?"* It is important to differentiate primary from secondary enuresis.

2. *"Does the child have accidents during the day, as well as at night?"* Treat the daytime wetting first if it coexists with nocturnal incontinence.

3. *"Has the child been constipated? How many days does he typically go between bowel movements? Are bowel movements hard, particularly large, or painful to produce?"* Treat constipation prior to more invasive investigation, unless history or physical examination suggests otherwise.

4. *"Was anyone else in the family late in achieving dryness at night or day?"* A positive family history may make the family more sympathetic to the child's feelings. It may be helpful to elicit the parents' own experience with enuresis and how it affects their response to their child.

5. *"What methods have you tried to fix the problem?"* Evaluate the positive and negative interventions. Determine if they were appropriately implemented and their secondary effects (e.g., on the child's self-esteem).

6. [To the child] *"How much of a problem is this to you?"* The child must be motivated to be cured if treatment is to be successful.

7. *"Are there other symptoms your child is describing such as pain or needing to use the bathroom frequently?"* Symptoms such as urgency, frequency, urine leaking, or daytime and nighttime symptoms should result in further investigation of organic pathology.

B. **Physical examination.** A complete physical examination should be performed, with emphasis placed on the spinal, neurologic, and genital examinations as well as examination for constipation.

C. **Social history.** A social history should focus on history of stress and abuse.

D. **Tests.** The laboratory evaluation should be very limited. A urinalysis is recommended in all children, and a urine culture should be obtained in all girls or in boys if there are symptoms or suspicion for a urinary tract infection. Further workup should be directed by findings in the history and physical examination. There is no indication for the use of imaging techniques or urodynamic studies unless suggested by the history or physical examination.

III. **Management.**

A. **Primary goals.** The primary goals in the treatment of incontinence are to alleviate the problem and to limit its impact on the child's self-esteem and interpersonal relationships. Although a cure is possible for most children, a small percentage may have to learn to live with this problem. Initial interventions should be directed both at helping the child cope with the problem and working on a solution.

B. **Information for the family.** The family should be told how common enuresis is and made to understand that it is usually a developmental problem over which the child has little to no control. Punishments only lower the child's self-esteem without improving the symptoms. Finally, parents should understand that effective treatments are available and that most treatments require cooperation between them, the child, and the primary care clinician.

C. **Treatment strategies.**

1. **Nocturnal enuresis.** The spontaneous remission rate for nocturnal enuresis is 15% per year.

   a. **Alarms** have become the preferred treatment for nocturnal wetting or enuresis because of their high efficacy, low cost, ease of use, and low regression rate. However, their use requires a considerable commitment from the parents (at least for the first week or two) when the child may not awaken to the alarm. Children must be motivated, and are generally older than 7 years with the exception of younger, mature, highly motivated patients. The parents and child should be instructed in its use.
   - Use the alarm every night for at least 2 to 3 months and sometimes as long as 6 months.
   - Both parents and child need to be involved.
   - The child should be instructed to visualize the steps necessary before going to sleep at night, such as waking when the alarm sounds, going to the bathroom, changing into dry clothes, replacing the alarm, and pulling off wet sheets. The child should then act out these steps before going to sleep.
   - Parents should wake the child when the alarm rings and take the child to the bathroom (even if an accident has already occurred). After a week or two, the child usually will awaken independently when the alarm sounds.
   - Restart the alarm after the underwear is changed.
   - Use a reward incentive chart for dry nights (sticker or stars).
   - Most children who respond to alarms do so within 4 months. Fifty percent of those who achieved dryness with alarm therapy remained accident free after the therapy was discontinued.

   b. **Medications.**

      (1) **DDAVP** is a synthetic analog of 8-arginine vasopressin and has shown to be effective in the treatment of nighttime enuresis by decreasing urine production at night.

- Studies have shown that children who use DDAVP have an average of around 1.3 dryer nights per week but there is a very high relapse rate when discontinued.
- There are concerns about hyponatremia from water intoxication while taking DDAVP, so excessive nighttime fluid intake should be avoided.
- There is currently a black box warning for the intranasal form on account of water intoxication given the long half-life so it is not recommended and the oral formulation is preferred.

(2) **Imipramine,** a tricyclic antidepressant, has been shown to be successful in the treatment of nocturnal enuresis with reported decrease in one wet night per week, although the mechanism for this improvement remains uncertain. There are two problems with imipramine in the treatment of enuresis: the high relapse rate when stopped and the very high toxic index if taken in overdosage. As a result, this is not recommended as a first-line therapy.

(3) Anticholinergic medications such as oxybutynin work by increasing bladder capacity and decreasing overactivity. There is some research using uncontrolled trials, which suggest that this may result in improvement by increasing bladder capacity.

Side effects include constipation, flushing, dizziness, increased temperature, and urine retention after voiding.

- Some clinical experience suggests that children with reduced bladder capacity might benefit from a combination of DDAVP and an anticholinergic agent; however, given the side effects of this combination (constipation and residual urine volume), it should only be used with close monitoring.

c. **Behavioral therapy.** The research is currently inconclusive regarding the use of other behavioral interventions for incontinence, but some suggests a potential benefit as does clinical experience.

(1) **Bladder stretching exercises** are not found to be a successful form of treatment.

(2) **Bladder relaxation exercises** are found to be a successful form of treatment. This includes behavioral techniques, which teach the child to be more aware and relax muscles related to urination.

(3) **Motivational incentives** (e.g., star charts and other reward systems) generally provide a positive focus on a child's remaining dry at night. Their relatively low efficacy makes them a useful adjunct but not a primary treatment of nocturnal wetting.

2. **Daytime incontinence.** When a child has both nocturnal enuresis and daytime incontinence, the daytime component should be addressed first. It is recommended to treat the underlying pathology. If no organic cause is identified, the following is recommended. In most children, the daytime incontinence will resolve over several months.

a. **Treatment of constipation.**
- Implementation of a regimen to ensure the treatment of underlying constipation is essential. This includes dietary interventions, laxatives if needed, and behavioral interventions to encourage stool evacuation.
- Encourage physical activity.

b. **Behavioral interventions** can be extremely useful. These include the following:
- **Timed voiding.** Encourage voiding every 2 hours and allow for easy access to restrooms. Utilize a reward incentive for remaining dry during intervals and complying with the voiding schedule.

c. **Use of appropriate voiding methods.**
- Encourage liberal fluids during the day but discourage fluids prior to bedtime.
- Discourage the child from holding urine.
- Encourage good voiding technique, which allow for relaxation of the pelvic floor.

d. **Medications** for diurnal enuresis are rarely indicated. Potential agents include anticholinergics (oxybutynin and tolterodine tartrate), which work to decrease bladder spasms, and alpha blockers (doxazosin and tamsulosin), which work by relaxation bladder sphincter and decreasing the resistance. However, these medications have many side effects commonly including constipation from the anticholinergics, which can exacerbate enuresis.

D. **Improving self-esteem/family function.** Self-esteem is best preserved by a nonpunitive response to the incontinence. The child and family should be made aware that wetting is common and that it is usually not a sign of emotional, psychological, or medical dysfunction. The child can be empowered to take responsibility for dryness at night following an accident via the "double bubble" technique.

- Place a plastic sheet over the mattress, followed by the usual sheets and blankets.
- Place another plastic sheet over those sheets, again followed by another set of sheets and blankets.
- Keep a dry set of pajamas by the bedside.
- During the day, rehearse with the child how to take the wet set of sheets off the bed, uncovering the dry second set, and how to change pajamas.
- This technique can defuse family tensions by allowing the child to handle his own needs at night and not awaken the parents. It is not for punishment but to help the child take responsibility for his own bodily functions.

   E. **Criteria for referral.** The child should be referred to a urologist when genitourinary pathology is suspected. Psychological counseling should be sought when the child's social function appears to have been impaired by the enuresis or when the family's response appears to be unduly punitive.

IV. **Clinical pearls and pitfalls.**
- *Always* obtain a complete history and physical examination when beginning the treatment of a child with enuresis, even if they are your primary care patient and you think you know them well.
- Parents may have not shared with the clinician all the information pertaining to incontinence unless they are asked directly. Parents need to be asked about previous interventions and, in particular, how these interventions were instituted. Frequently parents will have tried an intervention inappropriately.
- Involvement of the child is essential. No intervention will be successful without the motivation and commitment of the child.
- Always pay attention to the evolution of the child's self-esteem. Punitive techniques should be avoided at all costs.
- Do not forget to ask. Many families are ashamed to tell their pediatricians that their child has enuresis. Sadly, sometimes the more a family likes a pediatric clinician, the less likely they are to share a shameful subject.

BIBLIOGRAPHY

For parents

Mack A. *Dry All Night.* Boston, MA: Little, Brown, 1989.

For children

Boelts M. *Dry Days, Wet Nights.* Morton Grove, IL: Albert Whitman & Company, 1994.

For professionals

Cayan S, Doruk E, Bozlu M, et al. Is routine urinary tract investigation necessary for children with monosymptomatic primary nocturnal enuresis? *Urology* 58(4):598–602, 2001.

Graham KM, Levey JB. Enuresis. *Pediatr Rev* 30:165–173, 2009.

Neveus T, Von Gontard A, Hoebeke P, et al. The standardization of terminology of lower urinary tract function in children and adolescents: report from the Standardization Committee of the International Children's Continence Society. *J Urol* 176:314–324, 2006.

Rappaport L. The treatment of enuresis: where are we now? *Pediatrics* 92:464, 1993.

Robson WL, Leung AK. Daytime wetting. *J Pediatr* 139(4):609–610, 2001.

Robson WLM. Evaluation and management of enuresis. *N Engl J Med* 360(14):1429–1435, 2009.

von Gontard A, Schaumburg H, Hollmann E, et al. The genetics of enuresis: a review. *J Urol* 166(6):2438–2443, 2001.

Wille S. Comparison of desmopressin and enuresis alarms for nocturnal enuresis. *Arch Dis Child* 61:30, 1986.

Web sites

American Academy of Family Physicians. http://familydoctor.org/366.xml
American Academy of Family Physicians. http://www.aafp.org/afp/20030401/1499.html

Selected enuresis alarms

Nite Train'r Alarm Koregon Enterprises, 9735 Southwest Sunshine Court, Beaverton, OR 97005, 1-800-544-4240.

Nytone Medical Products, 2424 South 900 West, Salt Lake City, UT 84119, 801-973-4090.

Wet Stop Alarm, Palco Laboratories, 8030 Soquel Avenue, Santa Cruz, CA 95062, 1-800-346-4488.

42

Failure to Thrive

Deborah A. Frank

I. **Description of the problem.** Failure to thrive (FTT) refers to children, usually younger than 5 years, whose growth persistently and significantly deviates from the norms for their age and sex on the National Center for Health Statistics (NCHS) growth charts.

A. **Epidemiology.** Nutritional growth failure is seen in 8%–12% of children of low-income families. However, the prevalence of FTT in the general population is unknown.

B. **Family transmission/genetics.** Familial short stature may be considered when the child's weight is appropriate to height and when linear growth velocity parallels the normal curve on the growth chart. It is, however, perilous to assume that poor growth, particularly low weight for height, in children is secondary to familial predisposition for several reasons:

- Parental height may be a poor guide of the child's growth potential if parents themselves were nutritionally deprived as children and therefore did not attain their optimal growth (as is often the case with immigrant and impoverished families).
- The parents may have an eating disorder and be excessively concerned with obesity.
- The child may share an organic problem with the parents (e.g., celiac disease).

C. **Etiology.**

1. **"Organic" versus "nonorganic."** Traditionally, the etiology of FTT was considered either organic or nonorganic. However, this dichotomy is of limited use since children with so-called nonorganic FTT are suffering from malnutrition, a serious organic insult, whereas children with major organic diagnoses may, in part, have growth failure attributable to social and nutritional factors. Diagnostically and therapeutically, it is useful to assess each child and family along four parameters: (1) medical, (2) nutritional, (3) developmental, and (4) social. Problems in any or all of these areas may interact to produce growth failure. For example, a temperamentally passive child with iron deficiency may fail to receive frequent enough feedings from an exhausted mother who has other more demanding children.

2. **Psychosocial causes.**

   a. Child may fail to thrive in families of any social class **when parents' emotional and material resources are diverted or not available from for the care of the child**. This can occur because of poverty, parental depression, maladaptive parenting practices, family discord, substance abuse, domestic violence, or acute reaction to a recent loss or trauma (such as death of grandparent or unemployment), or depletion of a caregiver's energy by another chronically ill family member of any age, but including other children with special healthcare needs.

   b. **FTT does not necessarily imply parental neglect or pathology.** Feeding disorders can reflect numerous medical stressors (see below) or can develop in physically well children when not eating serves other purposes (e.g., to express anger, to exert autonomy from overly intrusive caretakers, to gain the attention of otherwise abstracted caretakers, or to divert adults from conflict with each other).

   c. Children with **preexisting minor developmental deficits** (e.g., subtle oral motor difficulties, hypersensitivity to stimulation) may develop feeding problems that lead to nutritional FTT. Apathy and irritability associated with malnutrition may exacerbate parent–child interactional dysfunction and lead to further feeding difficulties.

   d. Children **living in poverty** are often at nutritional risk because of inadequate food supplies in the home ("food insecurity"), homelessness, overcrowding, and the inability of federal feeding programs (e.g., SNAP (Supplemental Nutrition Assistance Program-formerly food stamps) supplemental food program for women, infants, and children (WIC), child care, or school meals) to reach many of the eligible families. In other cases, the benefit levels of such programs are insufficient to meet the nutritional needs of at-risk children.

Table 42-1. Often inapparent medical causes of FTT

Infectious
Giardiasis (other parasites, e.g., nematodes)
Chronic urinary tract infection
Chronic sinusitis
HIV

Mechanical
Adenoid and/or tonsillar hypertrophy
Dental lesions
Vascular slings
Gastroesophageal reflux

Neurologic
Oral motor dysfunction (gagging, tactile hypersensitivity, decreased or increased oral tone)

Toxic/metabolic
Lead toxicity
Iron deficiency
Zinc deficiency
Rickets
Inborn errors of metabolism

Gastrointestinal
Celiac disease
Malabsorption (various causes including cystic fibrosis)
Chronic constipation

Allergic
Food allergies (often presents as FTT with atopic dermatitis)

3. **Medical causes.**
   a. The **organic causes** of FTT encompass a whole textbook of pediatrics. Usually most are suggested by a careful history and physical examination, but some are occult (Table 42-1). Inborn errors of metabolism are rare but catastrophic cause of FTT, often with an associated history of seizures, recurrent dehydration, or developmental regression.
   b. **Perinatal risk factors** include prematurity and intrauterine growth retardation (IUGR). IUGR with dysmorphic features suggests a growth-retarding syndrome (genetic, congenital, or related to teratogen exposure).
D. **Long-term outcomes.** FTT is a major risk factor for later developmental and behavioral difficulties, usually reflecting both the nutritional deprivation of the developing nervous system and the environmental experiences of the child.
II. **Making the diagnosis.**
   A. **Signs and symptoms.** Although there are no universally accepted anthropometric criteria, the following are frequently used:
      1. **Weight less than 5th or 3rd percentile.**
      2. **Failure to maintain previously established growth trajectory, particularly after 18 months of age,** with parameters crossing two major percentiles (e.g., 75th to below 25th).
      3. **Decreased rate of daily weight gain for age** (Table 42-2).

Table 42-2. Average daily weight gain for age

Age	Median daily weight gain (g)
0–3 mo	26–31
3–6 mo	17–18
6–9 mo	12–13
9–12 mo	9
1–3 yr	7–9
4–6 yr	6

   4. **Depressed weight for height,** which always reflects inadequate nutritional intake for the child's metabolic requirements. (Short stature with a weight that is proportionate to height may reflect chronic malnutrition or may be genetic/syndromal or endocrinologic in origin.)
B. **History: key clinical questions.** It is important first to scrutinize the growth chart to ascertain the timing of onset of growth failure.
   1. *"What were the changes in your family's or child's life around the time the child's growth slowed?"* Perhaps a parent returned to work and the child was placed in daycare at the time; perhaps there was a family loss.
   2. *"What, when (how often), where, why, and by whom is your child fed?"* It is useful to ascertain a 24-hour dietary recall. In addition, the child's behaviors and affect at mealtime should be elicited.
   3. *"How much low-calorie liquid (e.g., juice, soda, iced tea, coffee, soup, Kool-Aid, water) does your child drink each day?"*
   4. *"Does your child choke on food, have trouble chewing or swallowing, vomit, or spit up or take a few bites and then stop eating."* Oral motor problems, gastroesophageal reflux, sometimes with associated food allergies, and painful teeth usually present with one or more of these symptoms.
   5. *"What are your child's bowel movements like?"* Frequency and nature of stools may be a clue for occult gastrointestinal disease. Both constipation and diarrhea should prompt further evaluation and intervention.
   6. *"Do you ever run out of food?"* If the clinician does not ask, the parents may never tell.
   7. *"Does your child snore, even when there is no cold?"* Tonsillar and/or adenoidal hypertrophy is a frequently missed cause of poor oral intake.
   8. *"Are there any foods to which your child is allergic or which he is not allowed to eat for religious or other reasons (e.g., vegetarian)?"*
   9. *"Do you and the child's other caretakers see eye to eye about the growing and eating problem?"*
   10. *"Are there any significant stresses in the house?"*
C. **Behavioral observations.**
   1. The clinician can **observe the child while eating or being fed** in his or her office (or ideally during a home visit by trained observer):
      • Is the child adaptively positioned to eat?
      • Are the child's cues clear, and does the caretaker respond appropriately?
      • Are there oral motor difficulties?
      • Does the caretaker permit age-appropriate autonomy and messiness?
      • What is the affective tone at the feeding interaction for both the feeder and the child?
      • Is the child easily distracted during the feeding?
      • Is the child fed in front of television?
   2. The clinician should also observe the **quality of the *nonfeeding* interactions:**
      • Is the caretaker irritable, punitive, depressed, disengaged, or intrusive?
      • Is the child apathetic, irritable, noncompliant, or provocative?
D. **Physical examination.** A careful history and physical examination should be performed to identify medical contributants to the FTT. In addition, all children with FTT should have formal developmental testing, with particular attention to cognition, language, and subtle fine motor difficulties.
E. **Tests.**
   1. Testing should be performed on the basis of the history and physical examination. **Basic screening laboratory tests** should include complete blood cell count with differential, lead, free erythrocyte protoporphyrin, urinalysis, urine culture, electrolytes, blood urea nitrogen, and creatine. Clinicians should have a low threshold for obtaining urine cultures, liver function tests, HIV screening, sweat tests, and measurements of immunoglobulin A, and antitransglutaminase antibody to rule out occult celiac disease.
   2. If the child is a new immigrant or recent traveler, lives in a homeless shelter, has been camping, or is in daycare and has a history of diarrhea or abdominal pain, **evaluation for enteric pathogens** (e.g., *Giardia lamblia, Heliobacter pylori*) should be considered and screening for hepatitis should be considered. A purified protein derivative should be considered for children with immigration or travel history, homelessness, or an experience of visiting incarcerated adults.
   3. If the child is short but is an appropriate weight for height, a **bone age** may be useful to distinguish the constitutionally short child (with a bone age equivalent to chronological age) from a child with endocrine or nutritional derangement (with a

---

Try to keep mealtimes and snack times about the same each day. Children work well with schedules.

Children need to eat often, not constantly. Offer something every 2–3 hours, to allow three meals and two to three snacks per day.

Make sure your child can reach the food. Use a high chair, telephone book, or a small table.

Allow your child to feed himself or herself. Try very small amounts at first. Offer seconds later. *Expect messiness.*

No force feeding, bribing, or cajoling! This will backfire.

Variety is not important. Total *calories* and *protein* are.

Offer solids before liquids.

Limit juice, water, and carbonated drinks. Offer milk or formula instead.

Offer foods that are easy for your child to handle: "finger foods" such as Cheerios®, french fries, slices of banana, cut-up burger, hot dogs, or peas.

Add margarine, mayonnaise, gravies, and grated cheese. For snacks, use peanut butter, cheese, pudding, bananas, or dried fruit.

Junk foods (soda, doughnuts, candy, etc.) have little protein and fewer calories than some other food choices. Junk foods will not help growth; they only take up valuable space in the stomach.

Eat with your child when possible, or allow your child to eat with others, so meals and snacks can be fun.

Figure 42-1. Effective Feeding Checklist for Parents.

delayed bone age). Evidence of rickets on wrist films or physical examination mandates evaluation of calcium, phosphorous, alkaline phosphatase, and vitamin D parameters.

III. **Management.**
   A. **Primary goals.** The primary goal is for the child to attain catch up growth at a rate faster than average for age to repair the growth deficit. This typically requires a calorically dense diet that provides 1.5–2 times the recommended daily allowance of calories and protein. In addition, other identified medical and socioemotional difficulties must be specifically addressed.
   B. **Treatment strategies.**
      1. **Instruct the parents in high-calorie/high-protein diet** (Figs. 42-1 and 42-2). This diet may violate current norms since increased fat may be necessary to provide adequate calories in small volume.
      2. **Feed the child three meals and three snacks** on a consistent schedule.
      3. Give a **multivitamin** with iron and zinc (and therapeutic dosages of iron if indicated).
      4. **Meet with** *all* **caretakers** involved in feeding the child to reduce conflict, to prevent the child from playing one caretaker against another, and to ensure consistency in the feeding regimen.
      5. **Discuss adaptive feeding interactions** (e.g., allowing the child to self-feed even if messy, decreasing power struggles at meals, and fewer distractions in the environment). Encourage turning off the television at mealtimes, eating with other family members, and pleasant conversation not related to food. Discourage grazing and constant sipping on low-calorie liquids which decrease appetite.
      6. **Ensure access to resources** (e.g., WIC, food stamps, food pantries).
      7. **Give all immunizations** (including influenza vaccine); aggressively **treat intercurrent infections and chronic conditions such as asthma, atopic dermatitis, or gastroesophageal reflux.**
      8. **Follow growth weekly to monthly,** depending on age and severity of malnutrition. Success is manifested as faster than normal rate of weight gain for age.
      9. Depending on the needs of the family, **mobilize community services,** including mental health, substance abuse treatment, housing advocacy, and job training.
      10. **Ensure that the child receives developmental intervention** through Head Start, early intervention, or public school programs.

24-calorie per ounce formula
    1 can (13 oz) formula concentrate
    8 oz water
Note: Don't make the formula more concentrated than this: overconcentrating can be harmful to a child's kidneys.

Super fruit
    1 jar (4 oz) strained fruit
    1 scoop formula powder

Super milk (use instead of whole milk; 28 calories per ounce)
    1 cup dry milk powder
    4 cups whole milk

Super pudding
    2 cups whole milk
    ½ cup dry milk powder
    1 pkg. instant pudding mix
Mix whole and dry milk together. Then follow package directions for making pudding. Yield: 4 servings (116 calories per serving)

Super shake
    1 cup whole milk
    1 pkg. Carnation® Instant Breakfast
    1 cup ice cream
Mix together in blender. (430 calories)

Note: If making any of these changes causes your child to have diarrhea, stop and call your pediatrician.

Figure 42-2. Recipes for Children.

  C. Criteria for referral.
    1. Children whose **growth rate fails to respond in 2–3 months** should be referred to a multidisciplinary team in an appropriate center.
    2. Children with **severe malnutrition, risk of abuse, serious intercurrent illness, or extreme parental impairment or anxiety** should be hospitalized.
  IV. Clinical pearls and pitfalls.
    • Failure to correct for prematurity in plotting growth may lead to a factitious diagnosis of FTT. The chronologic age should be corrected for prematurity until 18 months for head circumference, until 24 months for weight, and until 40 months for height. Even after correcting for prematurity, very low-birth-weight children may remain short for corrected age, but weight for height should be proportionate.
    • Children with symmetrical IUGR whether from unknown causes or prenatal exposure to alcohol may remain short but should not be underweight for height. Following most intrauterine exposures, except alcohol, children in adequate caregiving environments usually show postnatal catch up in both height and weight.
    • Depressed height for age may be genetic/syndromic, endocrine, or nutritional, but depressed weight for height always reflects primary or secondary malnutrition.

BIBLIOGRAPHY

For parents

Texas Children's Hospital, article on high calorie diet. http://216.239.53.104/search?q=cache:fOjriwdNl_cJ:www2.texaschildrenshospital.org/internetarticles/uploadedfiles/145.pdf+CHILDREN+HIGH+CALORIE+FOODS&hl=en&ie=UTF-8

For professionals

Blenner S, Wilbur MA, Frank DA. Food insecurity and failure to thrive. In Wolraich ML, Drotar DD, Dworkin PH, et al. (eds), *Developmental-Behavioral Pediatrics: Evidence and Practice.* Philadelphia, PA: Mosby-Elsevier, 2008, 768–779.

Ficicioglu C, An Haack K. Failure to thrive: when to suspect inborn errors of metabolism. *Pediatrics* 124:972–979, 2009.

Frank DA, Blenner S, Wilbur MA, et al. Failure to thrive. In Reece RM, Christian CW (eds), *Child Abuse: Medical Diagnosis and Management* (3rd ed), Elk Grove Village, IL: American Academy of Pediatrics, 2009, 465–511.

Gahagan S. Infant feeding processes and disorders. In Wolraich ML, Drotar DD, Dworkin PH, et al. (eds), *Developmental-Behavioral Pediatrics: Evidence and Practice.* Philadelphia, PA: Mosby-Elsevier, 2008, 757–767.

43

Fears

Marilyn Augustyn

I. **Description of the problem. Fear** is an unpleasant emotion with cognitive, behavioral, and physiological components. It occurs in response to a consciously recognized source of danger, either real or imaginary. From an evolutionary perspective, fear is a key to survival.

A **phobia** is a persistent and compulsive dread of and preoccupation with the feared object or event. Phobias may interfere with the child's functioning in a way that fears do not.

A. **Epidemiology.**
- Fears are present at various times in the lives of *all* children.
- Between 2–6 years, most children experience more than four fears.
- Between 6–12 years, they experience an average of seven different fears.
- Fears often peak at the age of 11 years and then decrease with age.
- Studies of identical twins suggest a genetic predisposition to fearfulness in some children.
- Females report fears more often than do males.
- Mothers often underreport (by up to 40%) the fears of their children.
- Unconfronted fears are more likely to persist.
- Phobias are seen in 7% of adults (disabling phobias in 2%); the prevalence in children is unknown.

B. **Familial trends.**
1. **Fearful, anxious parents tend to have fearful, anxious children,** probably through a combination of genetic predisposition and social learning.
2. **Simple phobias appear to run in families,** although individuals rarely share the same specific phobic stimulus.

C. **Etiology/contributing factors.**
1. **Environmental.**
   a. Although fears in childhood reflect a universal developmental tendency, the **onset often relates to a triggering event.** For example, a child may become fearful of dogs following a startling experience with an unleashed large dog. The (perhaps) innate human fear of large animals is intensified by a developmental level that does not allow a nonthreatening explanation of the event.
   b. New **stimuli from the media** join the roster of later childhood fears (e.g., school violence, sexual abuse, environmental toxins, terrorist attacks) even as old ones have dissipated (e.g., the communists). Sensationalistic news flashes during commercial breaks from programming can often heighten children's fear of exposure.
   c. Significant fears may reflect an **accurate assessment of a truly harmful situation** or represent a **displacement of feeling** from another environmental stressor (e.g., physical or sexual abuse).
2. **Developmental.** Fears change and evolve as cognitive development becomes more sophisticated. Fear of falling and loud noises are the only fears children have at birth. The emergence of other common fears reflects a child's increasing awareness of the world around him. Early childhood fears center on the environment. Exposure to real world dangers intensifies and expands fear. Table 43-1 provides the timing of selected fears throughout early development.

II. **Making the diagnosis.** The most useful way to differentiate a fear from a phobia is **the degree to which the fear interferes with the child's daily activities** (Table 43-2). If the child is developing normally in all other aspects, most often the behavior is a simple fear. If the fear impinges on important activities, it may have progressed to a phobia and requires specialized attention.

A. **History: key clinical questions.** The primary care clinician must determine if the symptoms represent a simple fear, a response to significant environmental pathology, or a displacement of other stresses in the child's life.
1. *"Does your child's fear interrupt his or her daily schedule more than three times per day?"*

Table 43-1. Common fears in childhood and adolescence

Fear	Age (Years)							
	1	2	3	5	7	9	12	14
Separation	X	X			X			
Noises		X			X			
Falling	X				X		X	
Animals/insects	X		X	X				
Toilet training	X	X						
Bath	X	X						
Bedtime		X	X		X			
Monsters/ghosts			X	X				
Divorce				X				
Getting lost			X	X				
Loss of parent				X				
Social rejection						X	X	X
War						X		
New situations						X		
Adoption						X		X
Burglars							X	X
Injections	X	X	X	X	X	X	X	X
Sexual relations								X

2. *"Can anyone recall a specific trigger to the fear?"*
3. *"How do you* [the parents] *usually respond to the child's fear?"*

III. **Management.** Management will depend on whether the problem is a simple fear, a mild phobia, a debilitating phobia, or a response to environmental pathology. In most cases, simple parental support and empathy will suffice. Fears are ubiquitous throughout childhood. The goal is not to *banish* all of them but to help the child learn positive ways of coping with and transcending them. In the words of Selma Fraiberg, "The future mental health of the child does not depend upon the presence or absence of ogres in his fantasy life.... It depends upon the child's solution to the ogre problem."

A. **Information for parents.** Parents should understand that simple fears are normal and do not necessarily represent a problem in the child or in the environment. The complexity and overwhelming nature of the world, coupled with a child's limited cognitive resources, conspire to create fears in *all* children, even those in the most secure and loving of homes.

B. **Supportive strategies.** Parents can exacerbate children's fears by using them as a threat (e.g., *The doctor is going to give you a shot if you are not good*), by humiliating the child (e.g., *Only babies are afraid of bugs*), by indifference to the child's distress, by unrealistic expectations to master the fear, and by overprotectiveness (thereby confirming the child's hypothesis that the stimulus is to be feared). They should follow these guidelines:

1. Parents should **respect the child's inclination to withdraw from that which is feared**.
2. **The parents and the clinician should not exaggerate the fear or belittle it. They should also not overreact.**
3. **Support should be provided to the child as he develops an increased mastery of the fearful object. Do not cater to a fear.** This may involve initial avoidance of the fearful stimulus, planned discussions about the fear with attempts to correct cognitive misconceptions, and a gradual introduction to the feared stimulus with much family support, "bibliotherapy," that is, reading a book together about the feared stimulus

Table 43-2. Differentiation of fears and phobias

	Fears	Phobias
Response to reassurance	Yes	No
Plausible event as cause	Yes	No
Distractible	Yes	No
Impinges on play/development	No	Yes

can be useful. Watching reassuring videos together (such as *Monsters, Inc.*) can also lessen anxiety.

4. In young children, some fears cannot be reasoned away. **Parents may have to resort to comprehensible and concrete actions,** such as "monster proofing" the bedroom.

5. **Unconfronted fears can last.** Although many fears will disappear as quickly as they came, some persist and may become ingrained.

6. **Coping with a fear often involves breaking fear into its parts:** physical aspects, cognitive aspects, and behavioral aspects. Different techniques may help in fear mastery for each but useful techniques for overcoming fear include imagination, information, observation, and exposure.

C. **Criteria for referral.** The child/family should be referred to a mental health professional for a phobic condition when fears begin to generalize from the situation of origin or the fears significantly hamper the child's activities of daily living or if the fears are felt to represent a realistic response to a truly threatening environment. Mental health professionals may use such techniques as behavioral modification with systematic desensitization or psychopharmacology to treat severe phobias.

BIBLIOGRAPHY

For parents

Books

Garber SW, Freedman Spizman R, Daniels Garber M. *Monsters Under the Bed and Other Childhood Fears: Helping Your Child Overcome Anxieties, Fears and Phobias*. New York: Villard Books, 1993.
Schachter R, McCauley CS. *When Your Child Is Afraid*. New York, NY: Simon & Schuster, 1988.

Web sites

American Academy of Pediatrics/Keep Kids Healthy. http://www.keepkidshealthy.com/cgi-bin/extlink.pl?l=http://www.aap.org/pubserv/fears.htm
http://www.keepkidshealthy.com/parenting_tips/fears.html

For children

Viorst J. *Alexander and the Terrible, Horrible, No Good, Very Bad Day*. New York, NY: Simon & Schuster Children's Books, 1972.
Spinelli E. *When Mama Comes Home Tonight*. New York, NY: Simon & Schuster, 1998.
Waddel M. *Owl Babies*. Cambridge, MA: Candlewick Press, 1996.

For professionals

Egger H, Costello E, Angold A. School refusal and psychiatric disorders: a community study. *J Am Acad Child Adolesc Psychiatry* 42(7):797–807, 2003.
Johansson K, Hasselberg M, Laflamme L. Exploring the neighborhood: a web-based survey on the prevalence and determinants of fear among young adolescent girls and boys. *Int J Adolesc Med Health* 21(3):347–359, 2009.
Ollendick T, Neville J, Muris P. Fears and phobias in children: phenomenology, epidemiology, and aetiology. *Child Adolesc Ment Health* 7(3):98–106, 2002.

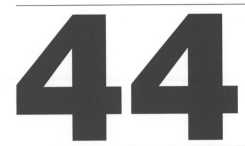

Fetal Alcohol Spectrum Disorders

Yasmin Senturias
Carol C. Weitzman

I. **Description of the problem.** Fetal alcohol spectrum disorder (FASD) is an umbrella term that describes the range of effects that can occur in an individual whose mother drank alcohol during pregnancy. Fetal alcohol syndrome (FAS) is a distinct cluster of facial dysmorphia, growth problems, and central nervous system (CNS) abnormalities associated with maternal alcohol use during pregnancy. Other categories within the spectrum include partial FAS, alcohol-related neurodevelopmental disorder, and alcohol-related birth defects (ARBD). The absence of facial dysmorphia does not guarantee that the CNS abnormalities are of less severity, and there is a significant continuum of impairment along the FASD spectrum. These effects can include physical, mental, behavioral, and/or learning disabilities that may have lifelong implications for individuals with FASD. FASD is considered the leading preventable cause of intellectual disability and developmental disabilities in the western world.

A. **Epidemiology.**
   • The Centers for Disease Control (CDC) reports FAS prevalence to be from 0.2 to 1.5 cases per 1000 live births but the broader profile of FASDs are reported to occur in up to 9 to 10 per 1000 live births, which translates to about 40,000 alcohol affected births per year in the United States.
   • FAS occurs in all racial and socioeconomic groups. Certain groups such as American Indians and Alaskan Natives have been documented to have prevalence rates of up to 3–5 cases per 1000 children. The foster care population has reported prevalence rates as high as 15 cases per 1000 children. FAS is also highly prevalent in the juvenile justice system with 200 per 1000 or a full 20% found to have either FAS or a related disorder. Alcohol consumption is a global public health issue and countries with high rates of alcohol consumption also have high rates of FAS. For example, in Russia, FAS among children in orphanages is estimated to be 15 cases per 1000 children. In South Africa, the birth prevalence for FAS has been reported to be as great as 41–46 cases per 1000 live births and as high as 4–7 cases per 1000 children in Italy.

B. **Etiology/contributing factors.**
   1. **Dose.** The more a pregnant woman drinks, the greater the risk of FAS. However, as reflected in the U.S. Surgeon General's advisory, there is no known safe amount of alcohol during pregnancy Prenatal alcohol exposure to one or more drinks per day is associated with reduced birth weight and intrauterine growth retardation, spontaneous abortion, preterm delivery, and stillbirth.
   2. **Pattern.** Drinking patterns that create high peak blood alcohol level pose the greatest risk. Binge drinking is felt to be particularly risky. A binge is defined as the consumption of four alcoholic drinks per drinking occasion. One drink is defined as 12 oz of beer or wine cooler, 5 oz of wine, or 1.5 oz of liquor.
   3. **Timing.** First trimester exposure poses risks to major structures; second trimester exposure poses risk of spontaneous abortion; and third trimester exposure has the greatest impact on height, weight, and brain growth. However, no period of pregnancy appears to be safe for drinking since damage can occur at any point after conception. The brain can be affected by alcohol in all the three trimesters.
   4. **Genetic sensitivity or effects of metabolism.** There may be genetic differences in a woman's ability to metabolize alcohol and in how a fetus is affected. The fetus is limited in its ability to metabolize alcohol and alcohol levels in the fetus are thought to be higher and present for a more prolonged period when compared with maternal levels.
   5. **Maternal nutrition.** Alcohol intake can have direct or indirect effects on the nutritional status of the fetus either because alcohol abusers often have a poor diet or because alcohol can interfere with the absorption or processing of nutrients such as thiamine, magnesium, zinc, and folate.
   6. **Maternal age.** Children of mothers who are older than 30 years have a higher risk of negative outcomes following prenatal alcohol exposure.

7. **Parity.** Studies suggest that the risk of having a child with FAS increases with each successive pregnancy. The rate increases from 0.2–1.5/1000 to 771/1000 live births for the younger sibling of a child with FAS.

II. **Making the diagnosis.**
A. **Signs and symptoms.** The FAS diagnosis requires all three of the following:
   1. **Documentation of three facial abnormalities; smooth philtrum, thin vermillion border, and small palpebral fissures.** These features should be assessed using a standardized method such as the University of Washington Lip-Philtrum Guide (www.fasdpn.org) and a palpebral fissure normogram standardized for age and racial norms.
   2. **Documentation of growth deficits (weight and/or length, at or below the 10th percentile).** The CDC guidelines state that the weight or height growth deficit can occur at anytime beginning in the prenatal period (adjusted for age, sex, gestational age, and race/ethnicity).
   3. **Documentation of CNS abnormality** (structural, neurological, or functional) CNS abnormalities may be structural, neurological, or functional. Structural abnormalities have been described in a number of ways and include the following: (1) The CDC 2004 Guidelines includes a head size at or below 10th percentile adjusted for age and sex, (2) the University of Washington Diagnostic Guide includes microcephaly or an occipital-frontal circumference less than two standard deviations, and/or (3) abnormalities on neuroimaging that are believed to have occurred prenatally (e.g., reduction in size of corpus callosum, cerebellum, or basal ganglia). Neurological findings include seizures not attributable to postnatal insults or fever, poor coordination, or visual motor difficulties. CNS dysfunction includes deficits in cognition, executive function, motor function, attentional control, social skills, adaptive skills, memory, and language, among others. There can be a wide range of severity of these challenges. About 25% of children with FAS have IQs below 70. Those who have higher IQs may have persistent neurobehavioral problems that result in learning difficulties (e.g., mathematics disorder), poor comprehension, slow processing speed, sleep disorders, cognitive rigidity, and impaired problem-solving abilities. The relatively higher IQs of these individuals, coupled with absence of gross facial dysmorphology, makes them more prone to be labeled as aggressive, oppositional, willful, or lazy rather than neurobehaviorally challenged.
   4. **Documentation of alcohol exposure.** Although it is important to document alcohol exposure, this is often difficult to obtain. Birth mothers may be hesitant to provide the information, and when the child is adopted, exposure to prenatal alcohol may be unknown. When the FAS diagnostic criteria is met on the basis of the characteristic facial growth and CNS abnormalities, confirmation of maternal alcohol exposure is helpful but not essential for the diagnosis. There are clinical criteria to identify the other FASDs, but for the individuals who do not meet full facial growth and CNS criteria for FAS, there should always be confirmed prenatal alcohol exposure.
B. **Differential diagnosis.** A careful history that includes maternal alcohol use is needed to differentiate the effects of alcohol from those of other teratogens. There could also be growth retardation, facial dysmorphology, and/or CNS disturbance in other disorders such as fetal valproate syndrome, fetal hydantoin syndrome, maternal phenylketonuria (PKU), and velocardiofacial syndrome. It may be helpful to consult with a geneticist if questions about alternative or comorbid diagnoses arise. It is also important to rule out other problems that can contribute to the CNS dysfunction, such as early negative child experiences, comorbid mental illness, etc.
C. **History: key clinical questions.**
   1. **Pregnancy history.** *"During this pregnancy, how many times a week did you drink beer, wine, or liquor? How many cans, glasses, or drinks each time?"* (Or in the case of a foster or adopted child, *"Do you know how much alcohol was consumed during this pregnancy?"*). Remember to ask about alcohol consumption prior to knowledge of the pregnancy, as some women may not have had knowledge until several weeks to months into the pregnancy (e.g., certain women with irregular periods, or who become pregnant while on a contraceptive). Binge drinking (consuming four or more standard drinks on a single occasion) is considered particularly harmful, and so is chronic drinking throughout the pregnancy.
   2. **Past medical history.** Ask about the child's general health and then about specific medical problems seen in FAS/FASD. Inquire about the child's vision (e.g., refractive problems due to small globes) and hearing (i.e., sensorineural/conductive hearing loss). Also ask about a history of heart murmurs (e.g., atrial/ventricular septal defects),

kidney problems (e.g., horseshoe kidneys), or spinal abnormalities (e.g., scoliosis), which can occur in children with an FASD.

3. **Developmental history/educational function.** *"Does your child show unusual sensitivity to touch (overreaction to injury, tags in the back of clothes, hugs), light, or sound (says things are too bright or too loud)? Does the child have difficulty behaving at large, noisy gatherings or at recess or lunch?"* Sensory hypersensitivity is a frequent but poorly recognized feature of FAS causing children to become easily overstimulated.

"Does your child understand cause and effect, abstract thinking? Can he generalize information learned in one context to another? Does your child seem to "learn" and "forget" the same piece of information over and over?" Children with FASD may have trouble with academics (specifically mathematics or subjects requiring abstract reasoning), problem solving, memory, and even language comprehension.

4. **Social skills.** *"How does your child relate to peers?"* Individuals with FASD may be indiscriminately friendly or unheedingly fearless and exhibit poor judgment and impulse control. They may be more susceptible to being used or manipulated (even into wrongdoing) by other individuals.

5. **Adaptive Skills.** Inquire about self-care skills. Many children with FAS/FASD have executive dysfunction. Some children with FASD may have a normal IQ and yet have significantly deficient adaptive skills.

6. **Maladaptive behavior.** Inquire about problem behaviors. Children may have behavioral problems due to poor comprehension and cause-and-effect reasoning, with subsequent frustration, and externalizing behaviors. Some children are very hyperactive and impulsive, which can readily contribute to these problem behaviors. They may also act out more in noisy places (e.g., cafeteria or gymnasium).

D. **Physical examination.** A complete physical and neurologic examination is necessary and should evaluate growth, facial dysmorphology, and neurological function not only as it pertains to FAS but also to rule out comorbid or alternative diagnoses. Children exposed to valproate may have some similar features to children with FAS including wide-spaced eyes, short palpebral fissures, long philtrum, and thin vermillion border. Children with velocardiofacial syndrome may have short palpebral fissures and a thin vermillion border. Maternal PKU effects and toluene embryopathy have all three facial characteristics that characterize children with FAS but could be ruled out by obtaining a good history (maternal diagnosis of PKU, maternal toluene abuse). Additional information on the differential diagnoses can be found in the *Fetal Alcohol Syndrome: Guidelines for Referral and Diagnosis* (Bertrand et al., 2004).

Physical examination and/or subsequent diagnostic tests may be able to identify potential ARBD such as cardiac (e.g., septal defects or aortic anomalies), renal (e.g., horseshoe kidneys), ocular (e.g., optic nerve hypoplasia), otologic (e.g., sensorineural hearing loss), skeletal/spinal (e.g., clinodactyly, spina bifida), or oral (e.g., cleft palate).

E. **Tests.** The diagnosis of FAS relies on fulfillment of the diagnostic criteria. Developmental, neurological, and psychological, and speech-language evaluation can assist in establishing the presence of CNS dysfunction, identifying alternative/comorbid conditions, and planning appropriate services. Genetic evaluation may help establish the diagnosis, rule out comorbid syndromes, or recommend alternative diagnoses.

III. **Management.**

A. **Information for the family.**

1. Symptoms are not the result of "poor parenting" or a "bad personality." The child is "unable" not "unwilling."

2. Individuals with FASD have a CNS abnormality that is permanent but not degenerative. The CNS abnormality often presents as neurocognitive dysfunction with associated difficulty in learning, self-care, behavior, and self-regulation. Persons with FASD and their families, as well as educators and care providers can help by providing accommodations that take into consideration the individual's strengths and weaknesses.

3. There is a spectrum of effects related to prenatal alcohol exposure—from subclinical effects to mainly neurobehavioral effects to full FAS. FAS/FASD is often characterized as a hidden disability because the physical abnormalities may not be as obvious and yet brain-based challenges can be profound.

4. Early diagnosis and developmental intervention as well as a nurturing environment can improve outcomes and can be protective against secondary disabilities.

B. **Treatment.**

1. **Early intervention.** Some children with FASDs may have obvious developmental disabilities as early as infancy or toddlerhood. Early intervention services can be provided

to children 0–36 months with significant developmental delay in one or more areas (e.g., language, motor skills, and social skills).

2. **Educational intervention.** Some individuals with FASD may have more subtle neurodevelopmental weaknesses that can be easily overlooked until school-age years, when they are expected to learn by integrating from a wide knowledge base and to generalize from one learning situation to another. School-based services are important for many individuals with FASD because they may have specific learning disabilities or brain-based difficulties (attention-deficit/hyperactivity disorder or executive functioning deficits, etc.). Currently, FASD is not one of the categories in the Individuals with Disabilities Education Act (IDEA) for which one can obtain special education services (http://www.nichcy.org). Since FAS is a medical diagnosis that can cause trouble with educational functioning, some school districts may also categorize it under "Other Health Impairment." School systems may benefit from educational sessions geared toward understanding students with FASD.

3. **Social skills training.** As many children with FASD have difficulty reading and accurately interpreting social cues, it is important that social skills are taught, practiced, and reinforced. Learning to curtail indiscriminate social approach can be challenging for many of these children and may place them in vulnerable positions if not addressed.

4. **Parenting strategies.** Parenting a child with an FASD can be challenging due to the outlined neurobehavioral deficits. Children with FASD benefit from a structured environment where there are reasonable rules, routines, and supervision. They benefit from instructions that are concrete, consistent, simple, and specific and visual aids may help. They may need several repetitions in order for them to master concepts. Children with FASD need help with transitions and may require multiple cues.

5. **Medication management.** Stimulants (methylphenidate, dextroamphetamine) and alpha adrenergics (clonidine or guanfacine) can be helpful for hyperactivity, impulsivity, and inattention. Selective serotonin reuptake inhibitors (e.g., fluoxetine, fluvoxamine, sertraline); anticonvulsants (e.g., carbamazepine, valproic acid); and antipsychotics (e.g., risperidone, quetiapine (Seroquel)) may help address depression, anxiety, or other mood disorders. It may be helpful to address medication questions with a developmental pediatrician, or child psychiatrist with expertise in these issues.

6. **Advocacy issues.** Individuals with FASD will benefit from support, apprenticeship, and advocacy in the home, school, and workplace in order that they receive adequate preparation for adult life. Individuals will need help in the transition between the school and the workplace. There may also be need for an advocate to navigate the legal system as the brain-based cognitive challenges experienced by individuals with FASD may make them more prone to victimization, poor judgment, and poor cause-and-effect reasoning.

7. **Identification of risk and protective factors.** There are several protective factors that have been shown to improve functioning for individuals with prenatal alcohol exposure. These include a stable and nurturing environment; early diagnosis; absence of violence; stable home placements; and eligibility for social, developmental, and educational services (i.e., developmental intervention or special education). Conversely, risk factors for poor outcomes also have been identified, including multiple caregiving placements, early or continued exposure to violence, and failure to qualify for disability services.

IV. **Clinical pearls and pitfalls.**
- Diagnosis at any point, but especially before the age of 6 years, is a predictor for better outcomes Diagnosis is not the end point, but helps start the process of identifying the individual's inherent strengths and neurobehavioral challenges, and the provision of appropriate intervention.
- Not all children with FASD will have facial or growth abnormalities. Even in children with FAS, facial features can be subtle.
- Only 20%–25% of children with FAS have intellectual disability and a normal or average IQ does not mean that a child does not have an FASD. IQs range from 20–120 in FAS and 49–142 for the other FASDs.
- Learning difficulties that are not remediated or for which there are no accommodations/interventions can lead to longstanding frustration and either internalizing or externalizing symptoms. It is important to address the primary disabilities (learning/language problems, etc.) as this is the best way to prevent secondary disabilities (substance abuse, school failure, mental illness, criminal involvement).
- Many children with FAS have troubles with low self-esteem due to the neurobehavioral challenges they encounter on a day-to-day basis. It may be helpful to refer to a therapist

with knowledge on FASD who can support the child and who can guide parents and teachers on appropriate strategies.
- Adolescence is a challenging time for many individuals but for individuals with FASD, especially for those who are identified late, there may be more significant behavioral problems such as inappropriate sexual behavior, aggression, lying, and criminal activity.
- The clinician can help the biologic mother to understand that the diagnosis of FASD does not mean that she drank during pregnancy out of the intent to hurt her child and that both she and the child are victims of the disease of alcoholism. If the parent is suffering from continued addiction, the clinician should refer a parent for substance abuse evaluation and treatment.

BIBLIOGRAPHY

For families

Books

Kleinfield J, Wescott S (eds). *Fantastic Antone Succeeds: Experiences in Educating Children with Fetal Alcohol Syndrome*. Fairbanks: University of Alaska Press, 1993.

Kleinfeld JS, Morse BA, Wescott S (eds). *Fantastic Antone Grows Up: Assisting Alcohol Affected Adolescents and Adults*. Fairbanks: University of Alaska Press, 1998.

Malbin D. *Fetal Alcohol Spectrum Disorders: Trying Differently Rather Than Harder* (2nd ed), Portland, OR: FASCETS, 2002.

Streissguth AP. *Fetal Alcohol Syndrome: A Guide for Families and Communities*. Baltimore, MD: Paul H. Brookes Publishing, 1997.

Web sites

Centers for Disease Control and Prevention (CDC). www.cdc.gov/ncbddd/fas

FASD Center for Excellence. http://fasdcenter.samhsa.gov

Fetal Alcohol Syndrome Consultation, Education and Training Services. www.fascets.org

Fetal Alcohol Syndrome: Support, Training, Advocacy, and Resources. www.fasstar.com

National Organization on Fetal Alcohol Syndrome. www.nofas.org

FAS Community Resource Center. www.come-over.to/FASCRC/

The Arc of the United States. http://www.thearc.org

For professionals

Astley SJ, Stachowiak J, Clarren SK, et al. Application of the fetal alcohol syndrome facial photographic screening tool in a foster care population. *J Pediatr* 141(5):712–717, 2002.

Bertrand J, Floyd RL, Weber MK, et al. *Fetal Alcohol Syndrome: Guidelines for Referral and Diagnosis*. Atlanta, GA: Centers for Disease Control and Prevention, 2004.

Green JH. Fetal alcohol spectrum disorders: understanding the effects of prenatal alcohol exposure and supporting students. *J Sch Health* 77(3):103–108, 2007.

Lupton C, Burd L, Hardwood R. Cost of fetal alcohol spectrum disorders. *Am J Med Genet C Semin Med Genet* 127C:42–50, 2004.

National Institute on Alcohol Abuse and Alcoholism. *Helping Patients Who Drink too much: A Clinician's Guide* (updated 2005 ed.). Bethesda, MD: U.S. Department of Health and Human Services, 2005. NIH Publication No. 07-3769.

Senturias Y, Asamoah A, Allard A, et al. Fetal alcohol spectrum disorders (FASD): what medical professionals need to know. *J Ky Med Assoc* 2009.

Streissguth AP. *Fetal Alcohol Syndrome: A Guide for Families and Communities*. Baltimore, MD: Paul H. Brookes Publishing, 1997.

45

Fragile X Syndrome

Randi Hagerman

I. **Description of the problem.** Fragile X syndrome (FXS) is the most common inherited form of mental retardation. It causes a spectrum of developmental problems, ranging from learning disabilities and emotional problems (in those with a normal IQ) through all levels of mental retardation. The fragile X premutation can also be associated with developmental problems including attention-deficit/hyperactivity disorder (ADHD) and social deficits in addition to problems with tremor and balance difficulties in aging.

A. **Epidemiology.**
- Causes intellectual disability in approximately 1 in 2500–4000 in the general population.
- Responsible for approximately 20%–30% of all cases of X-linked mental retardation.
- Approximately 1 in 130–259 females and 1 in 250–810 males in the general population carry the premutation (55–200 CGG repeats).
- No known racial or ethnic differences; identified in all racial groups tested.
- Both males and females can be unaffected carriers although ADHD, anxiety, and social deficits including autism spectrum disorders (ASDs) can occur in premutation carriers. Approximately 40% of older male carriers and 16% of older female carriers can develop the fragile X-associated tremor ataxia syndrome (FXTAS). Primary ovarian insufficiency (POI) occurs before 40 years of age in about 20% of female carriers.

B. **Genetics.** FXS is caused by a mutation in the fragile X mental retardation-1 gene (*FMR-1*), which is located on the bottom end of the X chromosome. The mutation causes a fragile site or break in the chromosome at that location. The *FMR-1* gene was identified and sequenced in 1991. An unusual expansion of a cytosine, guanine, guanine (CGG) nucleotide repetitive sequence was found to be the mutation. Within the *FMR-1* gene, normal individuals have a nucleotide CGG sequence that repeats up to 45 times, **carriers with a premutation have an expansion of the CGG sequence between 55–200 repeats**, and **individuals affected with FXS have a CGG repeat number greater than 200 (termed a full mutation).** When this occurs, the gene usually becomes methylated or turned off so that little or no *FMR-1* protein (FMRP) is made, and the full FXS occurs.

A carrier male will pass only X chromosome to all of his daughters, who will be obligate carriers and pass the mutation to 50% of their offspring. A significant expansion of the mutation will often occur in their children so that males and females with intellectual disability are common. A detailed family tree must be drawn to sort out possible carriers and other extended family members who may be affected by FXS or by premutation involvement including FXTAS and POI.

II. **Making the diagnosis.** Both behavioral and physical features are included in the fragile X checklist (Fig. 45-1), which serves as a reminder for clinicians of the signs and symptoms of FXS.

A. **Signs and symptoms in males.**
1. **Early signs and symptoms.**
   - Infants with FXS may appear to be normal, although behavior and feeding difficulties have been described including recurrent vomiting.
   - **Recurrent otitis media** begins in the first year of life for the majority of males affected by this syndrome.
   - **Hypotonia** is also notable in young boys, with subsequent mild delays in motor milestones.
   - Most boys with FXS and significantly affected girls with fragile X **are delayed in the onset of language.** Phrases or short sentences are usually delayed until the age of 3 years or older. The language delays in addition to hyperactivity or tantrums are the typical initial concerns leading to medical consultation.
   - **Prominent ears** with occasional ear cupping, **hyperextensible finger joints, double-jointed thumbs, flat feet,** and soft skin are seen in the majority of boys

SCORE:	0	1	2
		Borderline or present	
	Not present	In the past	Definitely present
Mental retardation			
Hyperactivity			
Short attention span			
Tactilely defensive			
Hand flapping			
Hand biting			
Poor eye contact			
Perseverative speech			
Hyperextensible finger joints			
Large or prominent ears			
Large testicles			
Simian crease or Sydney line			
Family history of mental retardation or autism			

TOTAL SCORE _____

A score > 15 has a 45% chance of FXS

Figure 45-1. Fragile X Checklist. (Modified from Hagerman RJ, Amiri K, Cronister A. Fragile X checklist. *Am J Med Genet* 38:283–287, 1991.)

with fragile X in early childhood. These physical findings are considered to be part of a connective tissue dysplasia that is related to the absence of FMRP.
- Young boys with FXS may also have a broad or prominent forehead and a large head circumference.

2. **Later signs and symptoms.**
- **Macroorchidism** becomes prominent in males with FXS during the early stages of puberty. Usually the testicular volume is at least twice the normal size, with an adult range in FXS of 40–100 cc. Although the spermatic tubules are tortuous by histological studies, fertility has been reported in several males with FXS.
- In addition, a long **face and prominent jaw** are often noted after puberty.
- Other diagnoses such as Soto syndrome, Tourette syndrome, Pierre-Robin sequence and other congenital defects such as cleft palate or hip dislocation may be associated with FXS because of the connective tissue problems and behavioral difficulties that occur in this disorder.

B. **Behavioral problems in males.** Behavioral problems are a common presenting complaint in young boys with FXS. These include hyperactivity; impulsivity; an extremely short attention span; perseveration in speech and actions; hand flapping with excitement; hand biting with anger or frustration; oversensitivity to touch, noises, and textures of food or clothing; shyness; poor eye contact; self-talk; and tantrums. These behaviors are often described as "autistic-like," and 30% of boys with FXS have autism and an additional 30% have pervasive developmental disorder-not otherwise specified.

Table 45-1. Associated medical problems in fragile X syndrome in males

Medical problem	Frequency in males
Flat feet	80%
Scoliosis	<20%
Mitral valve prolapse	50%–80% in adulthood
Recurrent otitis	60%
Strabismus	8%–30%
Nystagmus	Occasional
Refractive errors	20%
Seizures	20%
Macroorchidism	80% at puberty

C. **Signs and symptoms in girls. Approximately 70% of females who carry the full mutation will have a borderline or intellectually impaired IQ (IQ < 70).** The other 30% will have a normal IQ but may have significant learning disabilities, including attentional problems (with or without hyperactivity), math deficits, and language delays. **Significant shyness** is very common, often accompanied by poor eye contact. Females with FXS may be given a psychiatric diagnosis of avoidant disorder or ASD because of their social deficits. Schizotypal features (i.e., oddness in social interactional skills and appearance), depression, mood lability, anxiety, impulsive behavior, ADHD, or emotional problems have also been reported in women affected by FXS.

D. **Tests.** All children with intellectual impairment or autism of unknown etiology should have **fragile X DNA testing.** If a learning disabled or carrier individual is suspected, fragile X (*FMR-1*) DNA testing should be carried out. Once a proband is diagnosed with FXS, other family members should be assessed with *FMR-1* DNA testing, including all siblings of the proband and of the carrier parent and grandparent. Premutation carriers older than 50 years, especially males, are at risk for FXTAS and should be referred to a neurologist if symptoms of tremor, neuropathy, cognitive decline, or gait instability occur.

III. **Management.**

A. **Goals and initial treatment strategies.** The goals of the primary care clinician are to provide appropriate medical therapy and to coordinate a team of professionals who will provide optimal treatment for the child with FXS. Speech and language therapy and occupational therapy are essential for all young children affected by FXS. A developmental preschool setting can usually provide these therapies, in addition to special education. Whenever possible, mainstreaming or full inclusion with typical peers is preferable since children with FXS usually model their behavior after their peers.

B. **Follow-up.** Medical follow-up includes recognition and treatment of connective tissue problems and associated complications of FXS (Table 45-1). **Since ophthalmological problems** are common, referral to an ophthalmologist prior to the age of 5 years will facilitate early treatment. Orthopedic referral is appropriate if scoliosis or joint dislocations occur. Mitral valve prolapse is usually noted in the older child or adult, so referral to a cardiologist for evaluation and echocardiogram is necessary if a murmur or click is heard in auscultation. Vigorous treatment of recurrent otitis media in early childhood is indicated and usually includes the use of pressure equalizing tubes, so that a fluctuating hearing loss does not interfere with optimal language development.

C. **Psychopharmacology.** The most common behavioral problem is hyperactivity, which is seen in approximately 80% of affected boys and 30% of affected girls. Therefore treatment of ADHD symptoms in these children is a main focus of intervention (see Chapter 25). A common concern of families of adolescent children with FXS is treatment of outbursts or aggression, a significant problem in approximately 30% of male adults and adolescents with FXS. Episodic dyscontrol usually occurs during or after significant environmental overstimulation (such as shopping in a busy store), or it may be precipitated by anger or frustration. A variety of medications have been used with some success (including clonidine, selective serotonin reuptake inhibitors (SSRIs), risperidone, aripiprazole, and anticonvulsants), but controlled studies have not yet been performed. SSRIs such as fluoxetine, sertraline, and citalopram can improve anxiety obsessive compulsive behavior and irritability, although 20% may have significant behavioral activation. SSRIs are also helpful for premutation carriers who experience anxiety or depression. Aripiprazole in low dose is usually helpful for anxiety, attention, mood lability, and aggression. New targeted treatments are being studied to reverse the neurobiological abnormalities in

FXS including metabotropic glutamate receptor 5 antagonists and γ-aminobutyric acid agonists.

D. Other therapies. Sensory integration therapy by an occupational therapist with a specific focus on calming techniques may be helpful. Significant behavioral problems may also respond to a behavioral modification program organized by a psychologist who can also provide support and guidance for the parents. If autism is diagnosed, behavior intervention treatment for autism should be carried out.

E. Criteria for referral. All families with FXS should be referred to a geneticist or genetics counselor for a detailed discussion regarding the inheritance of this mutation throughout the family tree. A clinical and genetic assessment of other family members who may be affected by the fragile X-associated disorders including FXTAS, FXS, and POI is indicated.

BIBLIOGRAPHY

For parents

National Fragile X Foundation. Has produced many educational pamphlets, books, and videotapes regarding FXS; has resource centers associated with parent support groups in the United States and internationally; supports research and organizes conferences for parents and professionals. 1615 Bonanza Street, Suite 320 Walnut Creek, CA 94596 1-800-688-8765. www.FragileX.org

FRAXA Research Foundation. Has a network of support groups and funds research. P.O. Box 935, West Newbury, MA 01985-0935 978-462-1866. www.fraxa.org

Braden ML. *Fragile, Handle with Care: More About Fragile X Syndrome, Adolescents and Adults.* Dillon, CO: Spectra Publishing Co., 2000.

For professionals

National Fragile X Foundation. Identifies laboratories that carry out DNA testing. 1-800-688-8765 or 925-938-9300.

Hagerman R, Berry-Kravis E, Kaufmann WE, et al. Advances in the treatment of fragile X syndrome. *Pediatrics* 123:378–390, 2009.

Chonchaiya W, Schneider A, Hagerman RJ. Fragile X: a family of disorders. *Adv Pediatr* 56(1):165–186, 2009.

Web sites

National Fragile X Foundation. http://www.fragileX.org
FRAXA Research Foundation. http://www.fraxa.org
Conquer Fragile X. http://www.CFXF.org
http://dante.med.utoronto.ca/Fragile-X/linksto.htm

46 Gay, Lesbian, Bisexual, and Transgender Youth

Ellen C. Perrin
Nicola J. Smith

I. **Recognition of sexual orientation and gender identification.** Before adolescents are able to self-identify with any form of sexual orientation, they often question what their feelings, fantasies, and behaviors mean, and if they are transient or an intrinsic part of themselves. Rather than relying upon a stringent categorization of individuals as heterosexual, homosexual, or bisexual, sexual orientation should be viewed as a continuum ranging from absolute heterosexuality to absolute homosexuality. Adolescents have come to recognize and acknowledge their sexual orientation at younger ages recently, presumably due to the increased visibility and social acceptance of the diversity of sexual orientation and sexual expression. Given appropriate information and support, individuals generally will resolve uncertainty about sexual orientation by late adolescence through self-exploration of feelings, fantasies, and experiences. Children may also be coming to recognize discomfort with their anatomic sex and explore the implications of a transgender identity at younger ages than was previously believed.

II. **Definitions of terms.**
   - **Sexual orientation.** A persistent pattern of physical and emotional attraction to members of the same and/or opposite sex. Components include sexual fantasies, emotional and romantic attractions, sexual behavior, and self-identification.
   - **Homosexuality.** A persistent pattern of same-sex arousal accompanied by weak or absent arousal to members of the opposite sex.
     Lesbian: Popular term for homosexual female.
     Gay: Popular term for homosexual male.
   - **Bisexuality.** A pattern of arousal toward people of either sex.
   - **Transgenderism (transsexuality).** A strong and persistent cross-gender identification, not merely a desire for sociocultural advantages of being the other sex. Individuals describe feeling "trapped" in the body of the opposite sex and may seek to alter their physical appearance accordingly. May be heterosexual or homosexual.
   - **Transvestism.** Dressing in the clothing usually characteristic of the opposite sex; this is not an indication of sexual orientation.
   - **Homonegativity** is a discomfort, dislike, or critical judgment about people who are not heterosexual.
   - **Homophobia** is an irrational fear or hatred of homosexual individuals.
   - **Heterosexism** is the belief that only a heterosexual orientation is "natural" and normal.

III. **Epidemiology.** Evidence suggests that homosexuality has existed in all societies and cultures, but the stigma associated with it is so powerful that it has remained largely unmentionable and secret. Most of the published information is based on reports from middle-class, well-educated, Caucasian populations, as the stigma of homosexuality is even greater among people of color, certain religions, and developing nations.
   - The percentage of teenagers reporting predominantly homosexual attractions steadily increases with age, with a peak of 6%–10% among 18-year-old students. Up to 35% of students report sexual experiences with a partner of the same sex.

IV. **Factors contributing to sexual orientation.**
   A. **Environmental/social process theory.** There is no scientific evidence that certain parenting practices and/or other environmental factors lead to homosexual orientation. The early theory of "dominant mother–passive uninvolved father" is no longer accepted. Sexual orientation is considered innate.
   B. **Organic/hormonal theory.** The biological theory of sexual orientation suggests that sexual orientation is a consequence of the early biological environment and/or events. Neuroanatomically, investigations of brain activity by magnetic resonance imaging (MRI), functional MRI, and positron emission tomography scans demonstrate differences in functioning in sexually dimorphic areas depending on sexual orientation, most showing that brain functioning of homosexual males is more similar to that of heterosexual females than of heterosexual males, or are intermediate. Fewer studies have been

performed on homosexual females. Some studies suggest that prenatal hormone levels that are sex atypical may be responsible for various structural and behavioral differences, although studies of hormonal differences in heterosexual and homosexual adults have not yielded consistent differences.

C. **Genetic etiologies.** There have been few studies on the heritability of homosexuality and bisexuality. Most genetic studies are awaiting replication or have failed to be replicated. Twin studies and pedigree investigations have shown that there is a higher concordance in sexual orientation between monozygotic twins than dizygotic, higher concordance in dizygotic twins than nontwin siblings, and that there may be a higher incidence of homosexuality among family members of homosexual individuals than among family members of heterosexual individuals. Although genetic studies focusing on identifying causal genes are slowly increasing in number, no single gene or set of genes has been reliably indicated, and evidence suggests that the development of sexual orientation is a complicated and most likely multifactorial process.

D. **Can sexuality be changed?** Despite numerous assertions that psychosocial interventions could "cure" homosexuality, there is little empirical evidence. While sexual practices, behavior, and identity may have been changed in some investigations, there is no evidence of change in sexual orientation. In addition, there is evidence that the interventions sometimes result in psychological harm. Since 1993, medical associations such as the American Academy of Pediatrics (AAP), American Medical Association (AMA), and American Psychological Association (APA), have been increasingly vocal against such attempts to change sexual orientation, stating that therapeutic attempts to change sexual orientation are contraindicated and ethically inappropriate.

V. **Stages in the formation of a homosexual identity.** A typical progression in stages of understanding and acceptance of sexual orientation was developed by Richard Troiden in relation to homosexual males, and may differ for females.

Stage I: sensitization. The prepubertal stage is not within the realm of sexuality, but rather refers to generalized feelings of being different from same-sex peers. This is recognized largely by gender-neutral or gender-atypical interests and behaviors.

Stage II: identity confusion. The realization in early adolescence that his/her feelings and/or behaviors may be identified as homosexual/bisexual often surprises the youth and clashes with previously held self-images. This results in confusion and uncertainty about sexual identity. Youths may respond to identity confusion in one of several ways:

Denial: ignoring the feelings/behaviors.

Repair: attempting to eradicate the feelings/behaviors.

Avoidance: actively avoiding learning about homosexuality out of fear that the information will confirm their suspicions.

Redefining: viewing the feelings/behaviors as temporary or evidence of bisexuality.

Acceptance: resolution of confusion as the youth acknowledges that the feelings, behaviors, and fantasies may be homosexual, and the seeking out of information.

Stage III: identity assumption. Begins with self-definition as homosexual and may include regular association with other homosexual teens, sexual experimentation, and embarking on the lengthy and complex process of sharing his or her identity with others ("coming out"). Adolescents usually confide in a sibling, friend, or teacher before informing their parents or professionals.

Stage IV: commitment. Usually marked by self-acceptance, emotional intimacy, and a clear recognition of sexual orientation. Commitment occurs when the youth's homosexual identity is internalized and integrated. This stage is generally reached during adulthood.

VI. **Psychosocial and medical risks.** Although homosexual youth have many of the same medical concerns and needs as heterosexual teenagers, some are also at increased risk for a variety of psychosocial and medical problems, based on sexual activity and the experience of growing up in a society without widespread acceptance of sexual minorities. The increased risk is not inherent to sexual orientation, as some gay, lesbian, bisexual, and transgender (GLBT) youth navigate this transition without apparent difficulty. However, social ostracism, stigma, stress, and lack of social support and acceptance may result in mental illness, risky behaviors, and increased healthcare needs. The challenge for pediatric clinicians is to direct youth and their parents to appropriate information and social supports and to be alert to special needs expressed by those GLBT youth who are at increased risk for negative outcomes.

Heightened risks exist for sexually active GLBT youth for both medical and psychosocial problems (see Table 46-1).

A. **Traumatic injury.** Homosexual sexual activity may result in injuries to anogenital and oropharyngeal systems.

Table 46-1. Special risks faced by GLBT youths

Medical	Psychosocial
• Gastrointestinal conditions, hepatitis • Anogenital conditions, urethritis • STIs, including HIV/AIDS • Unanticipated pregnancy • Traumatic injury	• Depression, anxiety, and suicidality • Substance abuse • Eating disorders • Pregnancy • Homelessness and prostitution • Violence (as perpetrator and as victim)

B. **HIV and sexually transmitted infections (STIs).** In the CDC's 2008 estimates of HIV prevalence in the United States, 5.1% of 13–24-year-old youth were living with HIV, and 48.1% of overall HIV-positive cases were men who have sex with men. In both men and women, racial and ethnic minorities are at substantially higher risk of HIV. Syphilis also is disproportionally prevalent in GLBT adults and adolescents. Although lesbian adolescents with only same-sex partners may be at lower risk for HIV and other STIs, the large amount of experimentation in sexual activities/partners by GLBT youth precludes making any assumptions based on stated orientation alone.

C. **Pregnancy.** Sexual experimentation and heterosexual activity are common among both heterosexual and nonheterosexual youth. Studies report that between 50%–80% of GLBT youth have had heterosexual intercourse, sometimes initiated in association with denial and/or avoidance of homosexual feelings. Healthcare providers should not assume that pregnant teenagers are heterosexual, or that lesbian adolescents do not need counseling about contraception.

D. **Family conflicts** and possible rejection based on a teen's sexual orientation and/or gender identification exacerbate risks for GLBT youths, leading to shame, guilt, and challenged self-esteem. Up to one quarter of GLBT teens who disclose their sexual orientation to their parents are told to leave the home.

E. **Depression, anxiety, and suicidality.** GLBT youth often experience depression and anxiety along with their confusion and uncertainty about their emerging sexual identity and its implications. They often feel isolated, which may be intensified by an openly hostile environment. Deciding when to "come out" to friends and family can heighten anxiety and may be the time of greatest risk for suicidal ideation. Increased rates of suicide, particularly among male homosexual adolescents, have been reported repeatedly, with 25%–40% of gay and bisexual male adolescents admitting having *attempted* suicide. Lesbian and bisexual girls do not differ significantly from the generally high rates of suicidality in young women, irrespective of sexual orientation. The risk factors that predict suicide attempts in heterosexual youth are also the best predictors for suicidality among GLBT youth (e.g., depression, hopelessness, loss of support, abuse, prior suicide attempt, and substance use).

F. **Substance abuse** may represent an attempt to escape from the stigmatization, shame, and discrimination that GLBT youth face. GLBT adolescents have almost two times the likelihood of early marijuana, cocaine, and alcohol use, and are more likely to initiate tobacco use at a younger age and to report ongoing tobacco use than their heterosexual peers.

G. **Truancy and underachievement.** As a result of heterosexism, homophobia, and pervasive stigma, GLBT youths may underperform in school and eventually may resort to truancy and dropping out. School-based support from teachers, counselors, and other students (e.g., Gay-Straight Alliances) has been helpful in reducing these secondary consequences.

H. **Eating disorders.** There is an increased risk of eating disorders in homosexual men and male adolescents, presumed to be due to the desire to appear physically attractive to men. Gay and bisexual males are more likely to engage in both binging and purging, as compared to heterosexual peers.

I. **Homelessness and prostitution.** GLBT youth are at risk of being ejected from their homes due to their homosexuality, especially if the disclosure occurs without support and advice. About 25% of homeless youth identify themselves as GLBT. They are exposed to multiple medical and psychosocial risks, including drugs, sexual abuse, and prostitution or "survival sex," which in turn place them at high risk for HIV, STIs, suicide, and trauma.

J. **Violence.** GLBT youth are at increased risk for suffering and/or perpetrating verbal, physical, and sexual violence compared with heterosexual peers, starting in early

Table 46-2. Predictors of resilience

Parental acceptance and support
Sibling support
Extended family support
Community youth groups
School-based "Gay-Straight Alliances"
Religious communities

adolescence. This threat may further isolate youth and increase their feelings of vulnerability, anxiety, isolation, and/or depression.

VII. Resilience among GLBT youth. Over the past decade, the increasing social recognition and acceptance of diversity in sexual orientation and gender identity, and a number of specific societal and school-based efforts have increased the available resources for GLBT teens. The Internet also has created safe and anonymous opportunities for youth to explore their emerging sexuality. Table 46-2 summarizes some of the factors that assist in creating resilience among these youths.

VIII. Clinician's role.

A. Office environment. Many GLBT youth fear discrimination from healthcare clinicians, which delays disclosure and seeking of medical care. This fear is not unfounded, as at least 20% of physicians acknowledge homophobic attitudes. Pediatric clinicians must be proactive in counteracting these fears and attitudes, to best serve and be available to GBLT youth.

   1. Physical environment. Pediatric clinicians should foster a safe environment by letting patients and their families know directly that the office supports GLBT youth. Confidentiality policies should be prominently posted in office waiting areas and examination rooms.

   2. Intake form. Intake questionnaires in paper or electronic format may be useful as a way for youth to indicate a subject they would like to discuss, in a way that may be less intimidating. Once an indication is made that the teen has questions or concerns about sexuality, it is the responsibility of the pediatric clinician to initiate further conversation. Also, all forms and questionnaires should be reviewed for assumed heterosexuality and rewritten using gender-neutral language.

   3. Documentation. Clinicians should consider using an internal code to document information about sexual orientation, so that the information does not become public without explicit consent.

B. Information-gathering.

   1. Behavioral observations. Healthcare providers should avoid making assumptions of sexual orientation on the basis of observation of gender-neutral or gender-atypical behaviors, as this is not a reliable indicator of sexual orientation.

   2. History: key clinical questions. With all adolescent visits, establishing confidentiality at the outset is key. Patients should be told that questions about sexuality are asked of all adolescents. They should also be informed that when they do not need to answer all questions, the clinician is always available for questions or discussions, and that providing honest answers allows the clinician to deliver the best care. Clinicians should ask all questions nonjudgmentally. Using the same approach for all patients increases clinician comfort and performance, which in turn increases youth comfort.

   Care should be taken that questions about sexuality do not assume heterosexuality. Asking only about opposite-sex relationships may suggest that the clinician is not open to a discussion about non-heterosexual orientation. Some examples of gender-neutral questions about sexual behavior are provided in Table 46-3.

   In addition, it is important to understand the extent of the teenager's sexual activity, since medical management should be guided by the adolescent's sexual *behaviors*, not *orientation*. For example, *"How do you protect yourself and your partner against sexually transmitted diseases and pregnancy?"* It is especially important to assure that *all* teenagers have a thorough understanding of HIV/AIDS and its prevention. Counseling should emphasize on education in transmission and prevention of HIV and stress the wisdom of limiting the number of sexual partners, avoiding the exchange of bodily fluids, and the regular use of condoms during all forms of sexual intercourse. Reviewing the correct way to use a condom is also helpful, as is reminding the adolescent that abstinence is another option. It is important to remember that even those youth who identify as gay/lesbian may engage in heterosexual activity.

Table 46-3. Gender-neutral questions about sexuality

Do you have a boyfriend or a girlfriend?

Some of my patients your age date—some boys, some girls, some both. Are you interested in dating?

Have you ever been attracted to boys or girls or both?

There are many ways of being sexual with another person: petting, kissing, hugging, as well as having sexual intercourse. Have you had any kinds of sexual experiences with boys or girls or both?

Do you have any concerns about your sexual feelings or the sexual things you have been doing?

Do you consider yourself gay, lesbian, bisexual, or heterosexual (straight)?

The practitioner should attempt to understand the level of support that the youth has both inside and outside of the home. For example, *"Have you discussed these concerns with your parents or any other adult? Any of your friends or siblings?"* Practitioners can also offer assistance and guidance to youth and their family around the disclosure process.

It is important to keep in mind that sexual behavior does not necessarily reflect sexual orientation. Also, some youth are resistant to traditional labels and have developed new terminology that they may see as less restrictive. Examples include heteroflexible, omnisexual, transboi, half-dyke, bi-dyke or boidyke, queer, unlabeled, questioning.

C. Medical management.
  1. Testing for STIs. Young males participating in sex with other males should be tested for all STIs, including syphilis and oral, anal, or urethral gonorrhea at intervals as suggested by their sexual history. All sexually active youth should be immunized against hepatitis B and all youth should be counseled extensively about HIV and AIDS. Since many adolescents are sexually active with both males and females, discussion of both pregnancy and STIs may be indicated.
  2. Assessing risk. Practitioners should attempt to understand the level of support that the youth has both inside and outside of the family, as less support is associated with more risks to health and emotional well-being. Risk for suicidal ideation, depression, substance use, and abuse should be assessed if circumstances warrant.
  3. Counseling. Healthcare providers are a unique source of information and support for GLBT youth. Besides providing medical information and dispelling myths, clinicians can offer advice to youth who have not yet disclosed their sexual orientation to parents or other family members. Because youths are disclosing their sexual orientation to their parents at increasingly younger ages, when they are still financially and emotionally dependent on their parents, they may be at increased risk for conflict and even rejection. For some youths, it may be prudent to wait until they are less financially dependent upon their parents. Healthcare providers may be able to offer assistance and supportive information for both the youth and parents.
  4. Referral. Healthcare providers should refer GLBT youth to mental health colleagues, as they would all youth, with
    a. Suicidal ideation, depression, chemical dependency, or other severe psychiatric symptoms.
    b. Serious social situations, including abuse, homelessness, school dropout, and prostitution.
    c. Difficulties with interpersonal adjustment that does not respond to education and social support.
D. Supporting the family.
  1. Parents' experience. For many parents, the disclosure of homosexuality or of transgender identification only confirms their own recognition; for others finding out that their son or daughter is GLBT is shocking, discomforting, and difficult. Most parents' initial reactions include fear for their son or daughter's health and well-being, grief at the loss of the adult child they had anticipated, and guilt about their own imagined role in the genesis of their child's sexual orientation. They may initially be reluctant to share information even with their other children, grandparents, and siblings or close friends. It is also not uncommon for two parents to have different reactions (e.g., one being accepting and the other ambivalent or rejecting), leading to parental conflict.

2. **Support and advice.** Healthcare providers should be available to answer questions and dispel myths for parents, just as they are available for the youth. Many parents equate sexual experience with sexual orientation, thinking that their child does not have enough information or experience to truly decide orientation. Clinicians should help educate parents about this difference and the innate basis of sexual orientation. To address parental fears about their child's future, it is helpful to provide examples of successful GLBT role models, either local or on large-scale.

3. **Referral/resources.** Encouraging parents to learn as much as they can about GLBT issues is an important first step to helping them cope and eventually advocate for their child. Clinicians should build a list of referral sources, including local resources and parenting groups for GLBT youth, as well as reliable Web sites, organizations, and books.

E. **Community advocacy.** Clinicians of GLBT youth have an important role in raising awareness and acceptance of diversity in sexuality within their communities. Encouraging families and communities to form Gay-Straight Alliances in schools is an important evidence of social support. Pediatricians may serve as advisers to schools, making sure that tolerance policies and curricular materials at every age convey an appreciation of diversity and foster a safe environment. School and community libraries should contain books that describe the range of sexual orientation and the spectrum of family constellation for children of all ages. Physicians provide an effective presence in local and national politics, as well as a valuable voice within professional associations and medical education programs. The clinicians' commitment to learning more about GLBT youth via continuing medical education (CME) is an important element of providing high-quality care.

BIBLIOGRAPHY

Organizations

Gay and Lesbian National Hotline 1-888-THE-GLNH (1–888-843–4564). Non-profit organization providing nationwide toll-free peer-counseling, information, and referrals.

Gay, Lesbian, Straight Educational Network (GLSEN), 90 Broad St., 2nd Floor, New York, NY 10004, 212-727-0135. http://www.glsen.org/templates/index.html

National AIDS Hotline 1-800-CDC-INFO (1-800-232-4636) 24 hours/day and 7 days/week; in English and en Español; email: cdcinfo@cdc.gov; http://www.cdc.gov/hiv/default.htm

Parents and Friends of Lesbians & Gays (P-FLAG), 1726M Street NW, Suite 400 Washington, DC 20036, 202-467-8180. www.pflag.org

National Gay and Lesbian Task Force, 1325 Massachusetts Ave NW, Suite 600, Washington, DC 20005, 202-393-5177. http://thetaskforce.org/

National Youth Advocacy Coalition (NYAC), 1638 R Street NW, Suite 300, Washington, DC 20009, 1-800-541-6922. http://nyacyouth.org

For teenagers and young adults

Bass E, Kaufmann K. *Free Your Mind: The Book for Gay, Lesbian, and Bisexual Youth and Their Allies*. New York: Harper Collins, 1996.

Bauer MD (ed). *Am I Blue? Coming Out From the Silence*. Minneapolis, MN: Harper Collins Children's Books, 1994.

Gray M. *In Your Face: Stories from the Lives of Queer Youth*. Binghamton, NY: Haworth Press, Inc., 1999.

Heron A (ed). *Two Teenagers in Twenty—Writings by Gay and Lesbian Youth*. Boston, MA: Alyson Publications, 1994.

Huegel K. *GLBT: The Survival Guide for Queer and Questioning Teens*. Minneapolis, MN: Free Spirit Publishing, 2003.

For parents

Bernstein R. *Straight Parents, Gay Children: Keeping Families Together*. New York, NY: Thunder's Month Press, 1995.

Jennings K, Shapiro P. *Always My Child: A Parent's Guide to Understanding Your Gay, Lesbian, Bisexual, Transgendered or Questioning Son or Daughter*. New York, NY: Fireside, 2003.

Richardson J, Schuster MA. *Everything You Never Wanted Your Kids to Know About Sex (But Were Afraid to Ask)*. New York, NY: Crown Publishing, Random House, Inc., 2003.

Savin-Williams RC. *Mom, Dad. I'm Gay. How Families Negotiate Coming Out*. Washington, DC: American Psychological Association, 2001.

For professionals

Brill S, Pepper R. *The Transgender Child: A handbook for Families and Professionals*. San Francisco, CA: Cleis Press, 2008.

Frankowski BL, Committee on Adolescence. American Academy of Pediatrics, clinical report. Sexual orientation and adolescents. *Pediatrics*. 113(6):1827–1832, 2004.

Makadon HJ, Mayer KH, Potter J, et al. (eds). *The Fenway Guide to Lesbian, Gay, Bisexual, and Transgender Health*. Philadelphia, PA: American College of Physicians, 2008.

Meininger E, Remafedi G. Gay, lesbian, bisexual, and transgender adolescents. In Neinstein LS (ed), *Adolescent Health Care: A Practical Guide* (5th ed), Philadelphia, PA: Lippincott Williams & Wilkins, 2007.

Perrin EC, Cohen KM, Gold M, et al. Gay and lesbian issues in pediatric health care. *Curr Probl Pediatr Health Care* 34:355–398, 2004.

Perrin EC. *Sexual Orientation in Children and Adolescents: Implications for Health Care*. New York, NY: Kluwer Academic/Plenum, 2002.

47

Gender Identity Disorder

Laura Edwards-Leeper
Norman P. Spack

I. Description of the issue.

- *Gender* refers to the psychological and societal aspects of being male or female and *sex* refers to the physical aspects.
- *Gender identity* refers to one's inherent sense of being male or female, regardless of anatomic make-up, and should not be confused with *sexual orientation*, which refers to the individuals to whom one is sexually or romantically attracted (i.e., to one's heterosexuality, homosexuality, or bisexuality).
- *Gender dysphoria* refers to the discomfort individuals experience with their biological sex and/or with the gender role assigned to it.
- *Gender variance* is a behavioral pattern of intense, pervasive, and persistent interests and behaviors characterized as typical of the other gender. Gender-variant behaviors in children include play activities, toys and hobbies, clothing and external appearance, identification with role models of other gender, preference for other-gender playmates, and statements that indicate a wish to be of the other sex. This pattern is described in the *Diagnostic and Statistical Manual of Mental Disorders, Fourth Edition (DSM-IV)* as "gender identity disorder" (GID), although some question whether this diagnostic label is appropriate based on current knowledge.
- *Transgender* is not a formal diagnosis but is an umbrella term that describes individuals whose gender identity is different from their biological sex.
  Prepubescent boys with gender variance may, for example, be consumed by an interest in Snow White, or want nothing for their birthday except a new Barbie doll. Their interests tend to be restricted to those that are typically feminine. They may show observable discomfort with typically masculine pursuits and avoid rough-and-tumble play. Similarly, prepubescent girls with marked gender variance typically show distinct discomfort with activities that are typically associated with girls, they may refuse to wear skirts and dresses, and insist that they "want to be a boy."
  Transgender adolescents often appear androgynous, but those who have already transitioned socially may present convincingly as the other gender, wearing opposite gender clothes, including underwear. Biological females may bind their breasts tightly, wear multiple layers to hide breasts, and choose a short haircut. Biological males may wear their hair long and fold their genitalia in an effort to hide or avoid contact with their phallus or testicles. The more physically developed the adolescent is, the more difficult it is for him or her to "pass" as the desired gender without medical intervention.
  - **A. Etiology.** GID does not result from a dysfunctional family system, childhood abuse, trauma, or an emotional disorder. However, the debate continues whether GID should remain a psychiatric disorder and be included in the next edition of the *DSM*. No known anatomical or biochemical disorders exist in transgender individuals, and although some evidence does suggest a biological explanation for transgenderism, a specific biological explanation is elusive.
  - **B. Natural history of gender variance.** Gender variance often becomes evident during the preschool period, and most adolescents seeking treatment for the first time have experienced gender dysphoria from an early age. Some report not having had the courage to express their gender dysphoria openly until later because of shame, embarrassment, or fear of others' reactions. A subset of transgender adolescents does not report gender dysphoria in early childhood. This late onset of transgenderism is somewhat atypical and should be evaluated carefully, but it does not preclude consideration of medical treatment. Research has found that most (80%) preadolescent children with GID are likely to "desist" from a transgender identity when they enter adolescence; many go on to identify as gay or lesbian.
    In the past, healthcare professionals saw fewer girls than boys experiencing gender dysphoria; however, this trend has been changing with a ratio closer to 1:1 appearing in recent years. The higher prevalence of genotypic males presenting for treatment previously

could be due to the fact that the range of acceptable gendered behaviors in most modern societies is broader for girls than for boys.

II. **Significance of the issue.** Transgender children and adolescents are at high risk of anxiety and depression before receiving a medical intervention. Many engage in self-harming behavior and report suicidal ideation and attempts. They often exhibit low self-esteem and a lack of self-worth and report being socially isolated or bullied by peers and adults. Psychological problems typically intensify when transgender children reach puberty, when they cannot escape the reality of their biological sex, which is at odds with their gender identity. Although there are cases of co-occurring psychiatric disorders (e.g., depression, anxiety), these psychological symptoms are often a result of the discomfort transgender individuals feel in their own bodies and the social rejection they experience. It is common for these symptoms to decrease and even disappear after the adolescent begins a social or physical transition to the other gender. Diagnoses of major disorders, especially mood disorders (e.g., major depressive disorder, bipolar disorder) should therefore be reevaluated in this context.

III. **Management.**
  A. **Children.** Although the gender identity and sexual orientation of individual children with gender variance cannot be predicted with certainty, many of these children will identify themselves as gay, lesbian, bisexual, or transgender (GLBT) as adults. The serious risks that GLBT adolescents often face, such as being misunderstood, harassed, and rejected by others, which often leads to increased psychological problems, may be partly averted if children have the clear knowledge early in childhood that they are loved and accepted for who they are. Therefore, an important role of the pediatric clinician is to provide parents with information and support for diversity in gender roles and behavior, as well as sexual orientation, from early childhood onward. Heterosexual parents may initially know little about or harbor negative views about transgenderism, homosexuality, or bisexuality. However, many, if not most, parents will be able to modify their attitudes over time to support their child. This support will bolster the child's self-esteem and his or her ability to cope with social stigma. Parents who maintain persistently negative, harsh, and judgmental beliefs should be counseled about the potential effects of their attitudes on their children's long-term well-being.

  When parents initially express concerns about their child's gender-variant behaviors, pediatric clinicians traditionally have offered reassurance (*"Don't worry, he'll outgrow it"*). But this approach may not be in the best interest of the child and the family. Denial of the child's differentness deprives families of an opportunity to fully understand and support the child's needs.

  1. **Recommended assessment for children.** It is often helpful to refer gender variant children to a mental health therapist who has experience working with these issues. However, parents should confirm that the therapist perceives his or her role as one of supporting the child's development into the gender identity that the child deems as appropriate. A therapist who aims to alter the child's self-affirmed gender identity will likely cause more psychological and emotional harm than good.

  B. **Adolescents.** Adolescents first presenting with gender dysphoria who report a longstanding cross-gender identification often persist in their transgender identification. In addition, these patients have likely worked to keep their gender identity hidden from parents and peers, for fear of their responses. Therefore, maintaining confidentiality is of utmost importance until the adolescent is ready to disclose his or her gender identity concerns to parents.

  Adolescents who began experiencing gender dysphoric feelings **after** puberty warrant a complete evaluation, but their ultimate gender identification is less certain. All adolescents presenting with cross-gender feelings are at increased risk for psychological problems, as a result of their gender identity concerns. Self-harming behaviors (e.g., cutting), suicidal ideation, and suicide attempts are not uncommon. In addition, symptoms of anxiety, depression, poor body image, and low self-esteem often coexist.

  1. **Recommended assessment for adolescents.**
    a. **Psychological evaluation.** Initial assessment requires the involvement of an adolescent mental health professional trained in child and adolescent development, gender identity development, and the recommended best practices for treating transgender youth, as outlined in the *Endocrine Society Manual of Clinical Practice for Treatment of Transsexual Persons*. This relationship serves to help patients and their families clarify whether the patient is transgender, a process that may require many sessions over the course of months, or even years. Throughout the process, the mental health professional can encourage patients and families to understand and accept behaviors that fall outside the cultural norms for biologic sex, emphasizing that gender nonconformance is possible without necessarily having

to alter one's gender identity or body. The therapist can also help families advocate for their children in school and in the community, writing letters of support and advising school counselors.

If it is determined that the patient fulfills the *DSM-IV* criteria for GID, the mental health clinician's role shifts to supporting the patient and family in deciding whether a formal social and/or medical transition to the other gender is in the patient's best interest. Ideally, the mental health professional connects the family with a comprehensive, interdisciplinary clinic to provide further evaluation. The importance of a long-term relationship with a qualified and supportive mental health professional cannot be overstated.

b. **Interdisciplinary evaluation.** The initial evaluation in an interdisciplinary medical clinic is usually completed by a psychologist and includes the following:
   - A comprehensive clinical interview with the adolescent and parent(s) together and individually to obtain information about the following: (a) adolescent's gender identity development, (b) psychosexual functioning, (c) current wishes regarding medical interventions, (d) body image concerns, (e) mental health history and current status, (f) information about the family system, psychiatric history, and support, (g) school/educational information, and (h) social history and peer relationships.
   - A battery of measures to formally assess the adolescent's gender identity.
   - A battery of measures to formally assess the adolescent's psychological functioning.

   This evaluation aims to determine whether the following key criteria are met:
   - Fulfillment of the *DSM-IV* criteria for a GID diagnosis.
   - The absence of any underlying untreated psychiatric disorders.
   - Agreement to continue participating in ongoing supportive psychotherapy.
   - The presence of a supportive family system.

c. If the above criteria are met, the patient should be referred to a **pediatric endocrinologist or adolescent medicine specialist** for the next part of the evaluation, to determine if the patient is a candidate for a medical intervention.

   Medical treatment of the transgendered adolescent following careful psychometric assessment. A goal of **initial medical therapy** is to allow the patient to complete the assessment without developing permanent physical characteristics of the natal sex, and to delay initiation of development of permanent characteristics of the affirmed gender. This is accomplished by suppressing puberty and deferring the use of cross-sex steroids and surgeries until later adolescence when the patient is old enough to fully understand the implications, including infertility.

   Ideal treatment involves the use of pubertal suppression via GnRH (gonadotropin-reheasing hormone) analog at Tanner 2 genital development in genotypic males (doubling or tripling of gonadal size to 4–8 cm without phallic or other evidence of testosterone effects), and at Tanner 2 breast budding in genotypic females. The benefits of this approach include the following:
   - prevention of a need for mammoplasties in genotypic females,
   - prevention of menarche and menses, which can be psychologically traumatic,
   - allowing a longer period of growth in genotypic females via delayed epiphyseal closure,
   - prevention of skeletal changes in genotypic males, especially facial bones that accentuate the brow, zygoma, and mandible, and to prevent an Adam's apple,
   - prevention of unwanted phallic growth and disturbing spontaneous erections,
   - prevention of permanent male voice and virilized hair pattern, including temporal balding,
   - GnRH-induced pubertal suppression is totally reversible, with retained ovulatory and sperm production, should the patient "desist" from gender transition.

d. **Definitive therapy.** Around the age of 16 years, following repeat intensive psychometric evaluation, appropriate candidates can begin to take cross-sex steroids to develop the secondary sexual characteristics of the affirmed gender. Ideally, the steroids (parenteral testosterone, oral or patch estrogen) would be gradually introduced while the GnRH analog is continued to restrain the endogenous gonad. Unfortunately, the lack of insurance coverage for medical and surgical therapy for GID in the United States compromises the ability to provide ideal GnRH analog therapy. Often less effective agents with more side effects (such as high-dose progesterone, either oral or in depot intramuscular form) must be substituted.

Patients aged 16 years or older may be considered for mammoplasty, with letters of support from the treating mental health professional and prescribing clinician. Female-to-male transgender individuals rarely seek genitoplasty because of lack of functionality and limited cosmetic result. Bilateral oophorectomy and hysterectomy are increasingly being sought. Any castrating procedure, including feminizing genitoplasty, is deferred in the United States and in most other countries until the age of 18 years, and then only with strong letters of support.

C. Parents and families. It is important to not to minimize the considerable challenge of parenting a gender-variant child in most families and communities and the role of the pediatric clinician in supporting families along this road. Siblings, grandparents, aunts, and uncles may need information, support, and guidance to come to a new understanding and acceptance of the gender-variant child.

Parents of a child with GID face considerable uncertainty about how best to help their child. Some general principles are clear.

1. It is beneficial to:
   a. Help children feel more secure about their affirmed gender identity regardless of whether it matches their genotypic sex.
   b. Work to diminish, as much as possible, peer ostracism and social isolation.
   c. Identify and treat evidence of associated behavioral or emotional distress.
2. Attempts to alter the early developmental pathway toward a particular gender identity and sexual orientation are unlikely to be effective and very likely to send of message of disapproval and nonacceptance to a child who has little or no real control over his or her gender-variant behaviors.

D. Roles of the primary care clinician are the following:
- Encourage parents to reexamine their own beliefs about gender roles and to embrace a less rigid notion of what is appropriate for males and females.
- Parents should be encouraged to focus on loving their child for who he or she is and the qualities the child possesses.
- Parents and clinicians should advocate for the child or adolescent in the school system, community, etc. Letters of support by medical and mental health providers often hold significant weight in these advocacy efforts.
- Help the family determine if or when a social and/or a physical transition should occur and help them prepare for all aspects of this (e.g., school issues, reactions of extended family members, friends, neighbors, religious community).
- Educate parents about the current knowledge regarding prevalence of gender dysphoric children becoming transgender adults. Relay the various treatment options available and emphasize the importance of the parents taking their child's lead, allowing for the possibility of their child changing his or her mind at any point.
- As the clinician, be aware of the impact of the adolescent's gender identity crisis on the other family members—provide support and offer mental health referrals when appropriate. Parent-to-parent support through support groups may be invaluable, either locally or using electronic technology. Clinicians can be influential as a source of support, information, and guidance for all members of the family.

BIBLIOGRAPHY

Brill S, Pepper R. *The Transgender Child: A Handbook for Families and Professionals.* San Francisco, CA: Cleis Press, Inc., 2008.

Brown ML, Rounsley CA. *True Selves: Understanding Transsexualism.* San Francisco, CA: Jossey-Bass Publishers, 1996.

Ettner R, Monstrey S, Eyler AE (eds). *Principles of Transgender Medicine and Surgery.* New York, NY: The Haworth Press, 2007.

Hembree WC, Cohen-Kettenis P, Delemarre-van de Waal HA, et al. Endocrine Treatment of Transsexual Persons: An Endocrine Society Clinical Practice Guideline. *J Clin Endocrinol Metab* 94(9):3132–3154, 2009.

Gooren L. The biology of human psychosexual differentiation. *Horm Behav* 50:589–601, 2006.

Suggested Web sites

Gender Identity Resource and Education Society of UK (GIRES). http://www.gires.org.uk
Gender Spectrum Education and Training. http://www.genderspectrum.org
International Foundation for Gender Education. www.ifge.org
Parents, Families, and Friends of Lesbians and Gays (PFLAG). http://community.pflag.org
Trans Youth Family Allies (TYFA). http://imatyfa.org
World Professional Association for Transgender Health (WPATH). http://www.wpath.org

Movies/Videos

Ma Vie en Rose (My Life in Pink). A film by Alain Berliner; Sony Picture Classics. (For older children and adults.), 1997.

The Dress Code. A film by Shirley MacLaine; MGM/UA Studios. (PG-13), 2000.

Oliver Button Is a Star. Directed by John Scagliotti and Dan Hunt, with Tomie de Paola and others. www.oliverbuttonisastar.com, 2001.

For children

de Paola T. *Oliver Button Is a Sissy*. New York: Voyager Books, Harcourt Brace, 1979. (Reading levels 4–8).

Fierstein H, Cole H (illustrator). *The Sissy Duckling*. New York, NY: Simon & Schuster, 2002 (Reading levels 4–8).

Harris R. *It's Perfectly Normal*. Cambridge, MA: Candlewick Press, 1994. (Ages 10 and up).

Bell R, Alexander RB. *Changing Bodies, Changing Lives*. New York, NY: Random House, 1998. (Teenage level).

48

The Gifted Child

Michele Rock

I. **Description of the issue.** How "giftedness" is defined continues to be debated. Some suggest that it is primarily determined by an individual's intelligence quotient based on standardized testing. Given this more restrictive definition, the "cut off point" for giftedness may still vary. However, usually a child with an IQ 2.0 standard deviations or more above the mean (i.e., IQ 130) would be considered gifted. At some point, parents of gifted children will likely need to understand how the U.S. Department of Education defines giftedness: "... students, children, or youth who give evidence of high achievement capability in areas such as intellectual, creative, artistic, or leadership capacity, or in specific academic fields, and who need services and activities not ordinarily provided by the school in order to fully develop those capabilities." In 1993, the U.S. Department of Energy (DOE) revised this definition and stated that "outstanding talents are present in children and youth from all cultural groups, across all economic strata, and in all areas of human endeavor."

Giftedness determined solely on standardized IQ tests may exclude children from disadvantaged socioeconomic backgrounds. Children with diverse cultural backgrounds or those with learning or physical disabilities are also less likely to be identified as gifted. Given the diversity of children, schools, and communities, a "local" definition of giftedness is often proposed.

II. **Epidemiology.** The number of children in the United States identified as gifted depends on the definition applied and methods employed to screen and assess gifted children. The most recent data from the National Center for Education Statistics in 2006, estimates approximately 3 million U.S. children are considered gifted. This is likely an underestimate as many children go unrecognized and there are no systematic assessments for children for creative/artistic gifts.

III. **Making the diagnosis.** Parents may first raise the question of their child being gifted at routine healthcare maintenance while discussing developmental milestones. When children master developmental milestones early, parents may begin to wonder if their child will continue to exhibit early acquisition of skills or "giftedness." For the school-aged child, parents may present to primary care clinicians after the school raises the idea of giftedness or if their child is having difficulties at school that the parent feels is attributable to a curriculum that is not challenging enough for their child.

A. **Signs/characteristics (see Table 48-1).** In addition to early acquisition of developmental milestones, parents of gifted children may describe their child as having an excellent memory, imagination, and curiosity. Parents may also report that their child has a large vocabulary, strong phonemic awareness, and reading skills and exhibits other preacademic skills ahead of expectations. Precocious infants do not necessarily become precocious children. No single characteristic or group of characteristics is considered pathognomonic for "giftedness."

B. **Assessment.** Prior to school age, assessments will often require advocacy on the part of the parent and clinician to find a psychologist in their community; it may be especially difficult to find one with training and/or experience in evaluating gifted children. For the school-aged child, parents may find it helpful to access general information on their state and local policies on gifted and talented educational programming, available funding, and resources prior to requesting the school evaluation. It is important before any formal assessment to explore with parents what "giftedness" means to them. Early high performance on psychological and/or academic achievement testing is not necessarily predictive of future performance.

IV. **Management.**

A. **Home.** Although some literature has endorsed an increased occurrence of emotional and behavioral difficulties in gifted children, other research reports no increased risk. Regardless, parents may seek support and benefit from guidance in the following areas:

1. **Parental expectations.** Exceptionality in one or more areas does not mean a child may not have difficulties in other areas. Asynchronous development is common for gifted

Table 48-1. Characteristics of gifted children

Asynchrony across developmental domains
Advanced language and reasoning skills
Conversation and interests like older children
Insatiable curiosity; perceptive questions
Rapid and intuitive understanding of concepts
Impressive long-term memory
Ability to hold problems in mind that are not yet figured out
Ability to make connections between one concept and another
Interest in patterns and relationships
Advanced sense of humor (for age)
Courage in trying new pathways of thinking
Pleasure in solving and posing new problems
Capacity for independent, self-directed activities
Talent in a specific area: drawing, music, games, math, reading
Sensitivity and perfectionism
Intensity of feeling and emotion

Adapted with permission from Robinson NM, Olszewski-Kubilius PM. Gifted and talented children: issues for pediatricians. *Pediatr Rev* 17:427, 1996.

children, and parents may find it challenging if their child seems to struggle in other areas of their development. Parents may set too high expectations and pressure their child to demonstrate "exceptionality" in all areas. There may also be a tendency to "over schedule" a child rather than nurture specific interests that the child would like to explore. Remind parents to praise and help their gifted child focus on "process" over performance and outcomes.

2. **Siblings.** Comparison between siblings by parents and the siblings themselves can be unavoidable. Consider counseling parents to discuss a sibling's feelings openly and recommend parenting children as unique individuals with strengths and weaknesses rather than gifted or not gifted. Parenting a gifted child can require a significant amount of time. Designated special time with each child can help alleviate sibling discord.

3. **Peer relationships.** Gifted children may feel they are perceived as "different" or "nerdy" by classmates especially if they are not matched in interests and abilities. If the gifted child had accelerated advancement, they may not have social skills at the level needed to develop appropriate peer relationships in their current classroom. Parents may need to encourage and facilitate their child finding same age and older friends who share their interests. Gifted children can benefit from having friendships with children who are at a similar social-emotional level and those who match their abilities.

B. **School.** For parents of a school-aged child, it is important for them to be aware of their state and local school boards' definition of a gifted child. Each state is different whether gifted and talented programming is mandated and if funding is available. Information on educational options can be accessed through each state's Department of Education Web sites and by contacting local school boards and special education departments. For any educational option to address a gifted child's special needs, careful consideration should be given to the "fit" of the option to the child's unique needs. Options may include early kindergarten placement, use of pullout programs and resource rooms, multiage classrooms, curriculum modifications, access to accelerated courses, and grade advancement. For schools with limited resources, curriculum modification may need to be requested by the parent. If so, parents should first request educators provide this but if unsuccessful may consider providing the necessary information and materials themselves or through private resources.

C. **Other considerations.** Be cognizant that gifted children may also present with a specific learning disability and "average" performance may cause educators to overlook the child's academic needs. In addition, gifted children may exhibit behaviors consistent with attention-deficit/hyperactivity disorder. When considering this diagnosis in a gifted child, careful evaluation of the fit between the child and academic expectations and supports should take place.

V. **Clinical pearls.**

A. As clinicians, be aware that gifted children are present in every racial/ethnic and socioeconomic group and many remained unidentified.

B. Unrecognized gifted children may not realize their potential because of lack of opportunities and support, which can put them at risk for underachievement and low self esteem.
C. Recognize and inform parents when children exhibit signs of precociousness. Offer information and guidance early to parents. Be ready to provide links to community and national resources.
D. Gifted children have unique needs and are still as "at risk" as nongifted peers for social and emotional difficulties.

BIBLIOGRAPHY

For parents and professionals

Organizations

Council for Exceptional Children, 1110 North Glebe Rd., Suite 300, Arlington, VA 22201, 703-620-3600. http://www.cec.sped.org
National Association for Gifted Children, 1707 L Street, N.W. Suite 550, Washington, DC 20036. Telephone: (202) 785-4268. Fax: (202) 785-4248. www.nagc.org

Additional Web sites

The ERIC Clearinghouse on Disabilities and Gifted Education. http://www.ericec.org/
The National Research Center on Gifted and Talented. http://www.gifted.uconn.edu/nrcgt/
The United States Department of Education. http://www.ed.gov
Supporting Emotional Needs of the Gifted. http://sengifted.org/
John Hopkins University Center for Talented Youth. http://cty.jhu.edu
Support and advice for parents of gifted children. http://www.hoagiesgifted.org
GT World is an on-line support community for individuals with intellectual giftedness. http://gtworld.org/
Duke University Talent Identification Program. http://www.tip.duke.edu/resources/parents_students/parenting_tips.html

Books

Webb J, Gore J, Amend E, et al. *A Parent's Guide to Gifted Children*. Scottsdale, AZ: Great Potential Press, Inc., 2007.
Smutny J. *Stand Up for Your Gifted Child*. Minneapolis, MN: Free Spirit Publishing, 2000.
Walker SY. *The Survival Guide for Parents of Gifted Kids: How to Understand, Live With, and Stick Up for Your Gifted Child*. Minneapolis, MN: Free Spirit Publishing, 2002.

49

Headaches

Martin T. Stein

I. Description of the problem.
A. Epidemiology.
- Headaches represent the most common recurrent pain pattern in childhood and adolescence.
- 40% of children and 70% of adolescents have experienced a headache at some time.
- Chronic recurrent headaches occur in 15% of children and adolescents. Chronic daily headache occurs in 2% of middle school–aged girls and 0.8% of middle school–aged boys; in high school, it occurs in 4% and 2%, respectively.

B. Etiology.
Children experience headaches from many causes, but only a few pathologic mechanisms induce head pain:
- Inflammation, traction, and direct pressure on intracranial structures.
- Vasodilation of cerebral vessels.
- Sustained contractions, trauma, or inflammation of scalp and neck muscles.
- Sinus, dental, and orbital pathologic processes.
- The brain parenchyma, most of the dura and meningeal surfaces, and the ependymal lining of the ventricles are insensitive to pain. Central nervous system causes of headache result from stretching or inflammation of a limited number of pain-sensitive intracranial structures.

II. Making the diagnosis.
Most headaches are brief and do not significantly alter a child's life. Recurrent headaches may be accompanied by fears and anxieties about brain tumors and other life-threatening diseases. The diagnostic challenge for the primary care clinician is multifaceted:
- To differentiate benign, self-limited headaches from those that suggest a serious organic disease.
- To explore the potential relationship between headaches and a child's home, school, and social environment.
- To recognize patients with headaches secondary to internal stressors (depression, anxiety, phobias) and those with environmental causes.
- To develop a therapeutic plan consistent with the cause, severity, and significance of the headaches for the child and family.

A. Differential diagnosis.
A useful clinical model to differentiate the large variety of headaches in children and adolescents focuses on four categories: (1) tension headaches, (2) migraine headaches, (3) extracranial headaches, and (4) intracranial headaches (Table 49-1). Tension-related and migraine headaches occur most frequently. An alternative model of headaches in children deemphasizes the migraine–tension dichotomy and places greater emphasis on a headache continuum. Migraine with associated anatomic nervous system symptoms is at one end of the continuum and muscular tension headache at the other end. Symptoms and signs of both tension and migraine headaches in children are often nonspecific compared with the less common causes. Headaches in younger children, especially infants and toddlers, are more likely to have a specific organic cause. A focused clinical interview, coupled with age-appropriate behavioral observations and a comprehensive physical examination, will result in the probable diagnosis at the initial office visit for most patients.

B. History: key clinical questions.
Whenever possible, questions should be directed to the patient, inquiring of the parent only after the child or adolescent has had an opportunity to describe the headache to the clinician. Most recurrent forms of pediatric headaches are associated with a behavioral diagnosis (in the presence or absence of migraine). The clinical interview should develop in a manner that raises questions simultaneously about both organic and behavioral causes. An open-ended question (*"Tell me about your headaches."*) will allow the child and parent to explore what seems important to them and may lead to further exploration in the direction of either organic or behavioral etiologies. Focused

questions that may suggest common (sinusitis, migraine) or uncommon (increased intracranial pressure, chronic infection) organic etiologies should be directed to the patient or parent.

The history should begin with a description of the headache pattern. In infants and toddlers, nonspecific symptoms may reflect a headache (e.g., irritability, inconsolability, sleep disturbances, poor appetite, head banging, or repetitive placing of a hand to the head or face). In older children and adolescents, an open-ended question may yield important information about the location, quality, onset, duration, and frequency of the headache.

An aura, unilateral location and throbbing pain will be present in some children with migraine. Those with a "common migraine" may have a generalized aching headache with nausea or vomiting but without an aura. A morning headache; awakening with

Table 49-1. Classification of headaches

	Mechanism	Features/etiology
Tension headaches (muscle contraction headaches)	Contraction of scalp and neck muscles	Sensation of tightness or pressure over frontal, temporal, occipital regions, or generalized Life-event change/stress: home, school, social relations, activity overload, depression Normal physical examination (occasional tightness or tenderness of posterior cervical muscles)

Migraine headaches	Vasoconstriction and/or vasodilation of cerebral vessels	Family history (70%–80%)
		Paroxysmal attacks
		Gender: in childhood, boys and girls equally; in adolescence, girls more than boys
		Common migraine
		  Unilateral or generalized
		  Throbbing or aching
		  Nausea/vomiting
		  No aura
		Classic migraine
		  Aura (visual)
		  Nausea/vomiting
		  Unilateral
		  Throbbing
		Complex migraine
		  Ophthalmoplegia
		  Hemiparesis
		  Acute confusional state
		  Cyclic vomiting
		  Paroxysmal vertigo

Extracranial sources	Inflammation or trauma of structures or sustained contracture of scalp and neck muscles	Typically regional pain in area of pathology but often generalized in young children Otitis media and mastoiditis Sinusitis (chronic purulent rhinorrhea and/or nocturnal cough) Dental infection Tonsillopharyngitis (streptococcal) Refractive errors and strabismus Cervical spine osteomyelitis or discitis Systemic infection with fever Temporomandibular joint syndrome Severe malocclusion

(continued)

Table 49-1. (*Continued*)

	Mechanism	Features/etiology
Intracranial sources	Inflammation	Meningitis, encephalitis, cerebral vasculitis, subarachnoid hemorrhage
	Traction	Central nervous system tumor
		Cerebral edema
		Abscess
		Hematoma
		Postlumbar puncture
		Pseudotumor cerebri
	Toxic substances	Lead-Alcohol
		Carbon monoxide
		Hypoxia
		Foods and food additives (nitrates, nitrites, monosodium glutamate, phenylethylamine)
		Paint, glue (including model glue)
		Oral contraceptives
		Renal disease
	Direct pressure	Hydrocephalus
		Trauma
	Vascular (nonmigraine)	Hypertension
		Arteriovenous malformation
		Fever
	Miscellaneous	Noise
		Sensory overload

vomiting; worsening of pain with coughing, sneezing, and straining; and progression of pain in severity and frequency should suggest an intracranial source.

The clinical interview begins the therapeutic process. Detailed, focused, and empathic questions give the child and family a sense of security that the symptoms are being evaluated by a concerned, knowledgeable clinician. It also gives the child and parents the opportunity to explore the interpersonal, educational, and family aspects of their lives that may provide insight into the headache formation.

1. *"Tell me about your headaches. What do they feel like?"* The child who has difficulty describing the headache can be asked to *"draw a picture of what the headache feels like."* The drawing may be concrete (a person or family) or abstract with designs or color. The child's description of the drawing, as well as the parents' and clinician's emotional responses, may provide useful information about the nature of the pain.

2. *"What seems to bring on a headache?"* (or) *What are you doing when the headache starts?* The emotional or physical environment in which the headache occurs may provide a clue to etiology.

3. *"What do you do to stop the headache?"* Common migraine typically resolves with sleep. Tension headaches resolve gradually during the awake state.

4. *"Do others in your family experience headaches?"* A history of episodic throbbing headaches in adults will suggest familial migraine headaches. Positive or negative reinforcement of headaches within the family may give an important clue to the etiology of recurrent headaches.

5. *"What is a headache?"* (To the preschool child) *Where do headaches come from?* (School-aged child) *What causes your headache?* (Adolescent) *Why do you think you get headaches?* These developmentally appropriate questions give a clue to the child's explanatory model of headache formation. Responses provide clinical insight into a patient's development, a clue to cognitive adaptation to the headache, and a source for improved communication between clinician and child through empathic connections.

6. *"Why do you think that your headaches are more frequent or more severe?"* For most children who experience headaches, it is helpful to explore the child's developmental understanding of headaches. A perceived cause of a headache will be linked to the child's cognitive and developmental stage (Table 49-2). The child is given an

Table 49-2. Developmental conceptions of headache

Cognitive stage	Answer to "How do people get headaches?"
Prelogical (3–6 yr)	
Phenomenism	"From God" or "From the weather"
Contagion	"From foods, like chocolate"
Concrete-logical (7–12 yr)	
Contamination	"From running and getting hot"
Internalization	"Eating or doing certain things that make inside your head hurt" or "From thinking too hard in math class"
Formal-logical (>13 yr)	
Physiological	"From things happening to you that cause too much blood flowing to your head; that's why it feels like a hammer pounding in your head"
Psychophysiological	"When people get nervous or do too much, this causes their body to react with a headache"

Modified with permission from Marcon RA, Labb EE. Assessment and treatment of children's headaches from a developmental perspective. *Headache* 9:586–592, 1990.

opportunity to reflect on the symptoms. The response may provide a clue to self-esteem, ego integration, superego formation, and interpersonal relationships.

7. *"How are things going at school . . . at home . . . with your friends?"* The structure of the family (and a family medical history), friendships, and the school environment are critical to understanding the etiology of and response to the headache and potential therapeutic interventions.

   a. **Family stress.** Is the child living with someone who experiences headaches? The family constellation should be explored for recent changes in parental relationships, a new sibling, emotional illness in family members, economic stress (lost job, homelessness, and child support), and family violence.

   b. **Social stress.** When factors such as inherent shyness, bullies, class and racial differences, and physical or mental dysfunction affect social relationships, psychophysiological reactions are common. Recurrent frontal, generalized, or temporal headaches (both with and without associated symptoms of pallor, malaise, nausea, and vomiting) are seen in these situations. Importantly, common migraine headaches as well as tension headaches may be associated with social or familial stress.

   c. **School stress.** Stress that originates in the classroom may be associated with headache formation. The school may act as an environmental stressor by placing demands on both cognitive achievement and social behavior. Children's adaptive potential to a variety of school pressures varies significantly.

      The clinical interview should explore the nature of the classroom (number of students, where the child sits), the relationship between the child and the teacher, the quality and quantity of academic work, the child's response to homework, and the parents' attitudes about learning. Parents can be asked when they last spoke to the child's teacher, the content of the conference, whether the child is learning, and if the child is happy at school.

8. *"What do you think we can do together to help the headaches go away?"* This question engages the child in a therapeutic alliance and opens the possibility of managing the problem together.

C. **Physical examination and further testing.** Narrating normal physical findings to the child during a comprehensive physical examination is reassuring and helps to demystify the medical evaluation. Organic causes for a child's headaches are usually apparent after a complete history and physical examination. Routine diagnostic studies are not indicated when the clinical history has no associated risk factors (recent onset of severe headache, absence of family history of migraine) and the physical/neurological examination is normal (absence of abnormal neurological finding, gait abnormality, seizures). When the signs and symptoms of organic causes of headache are vague or subtle and a specific diagnosis remains elusive, a specialty consultation may be useful.

III. **Management.**

A. **Primary goals.** The clinician's goals for management should be to provide a developmentally appropriate understanding of the cause of headaches for both parent and child. The working assumption is that through a greater understanding of the physical and behavioral causes and triggers for headaches, both the child and the parent will be able to cope with and adapt to the pain as well as collaborate in recommended therapies.

B. Treatment strategies.

1. **Information.** When migraine or tension headaches are present, the anatomic mechanisms of pain should be illustrated by means of a descriptive narrative and schematic drawings. Visual images of the abnormal anatomic structures may help some children to gain control over the symptoms. Simple drawings of a blood vessel contracting and dilating with an explanation of pain-sensitive nerve endings within the blood vessel illustrates the physical nature of migraine headache and the associated symptoms.

2. **Relaxation exercises.** For tension headaches, children may respond to a progressive relaxation exercise that teaches them to relax specified areas of the body. The exercise may be followed by teaching the child to focus on a pleasant image of his or her choosing. Other children respond to an explanation directed at "tight muscles around the head" that cause pain at times of stress and tension ("worry," "nerves," and "daily hassles"). The clinician can demonstrate this phenomenon by tensing her or his biceps and asking the child to mimic that maneuver. This should be followed by an explanation that the biceps muscle is similar to the thin muscles around the head, which tighten at the point where the headache occurs. The child can learn to image—through visual imagination—the tense, painful cranial muscles' relaxing gradually and voluntarily as the pain diminishes.

   These forms of voluntary relaxation follow the principles of self-regulation that have been successful in the elimination of migraine and tension headaches in school-aged children and adolescents (see Chapter 19). Controlled studies of children with headaches have shown that relaxation therapy and imaging (with or without biofeedback) significantly decreases headache frequency with lasting effects. It is a safe and simple intervention that can be practiced by the primary care clinician.

3. **Headache diary.** A headache diary may be a useful adjunct intervention. The older child or parent is asked to chart the headaches (time of day, intensity on a 1–10 scale, associated symptoms, intervention, and duration) and record any stressful events that occur in the life of the child or family around the time of the headache. This exercise may encourage parents and children to talk about environmental triggers for headaches specifically and improve parent–child communication in general. Following an initial treatment period, it may be useful to shift the emphasis of the diary to headache-free days, which can shift family focus to successes rather than failures.

4. **Medication.** A pharmacologic approach to acute, chronic, and recurrent headaches may be beneficial for pain relief and prevention. Most children and adolescents with occasional migraine and tension-related headaches respond to acetaminophen and ibuprofen when the pain is of mild to moderate severity. Parenteral medication is available for the very severe migraine. More severe recurrent headaches respond to prophylactic suppression therapy, although there are few controlled drug studies in children. The primary care clinician will rarely need to resort to suppression therapy because episodic, severe headaches are uncommon in children and adolescents.

C. Follow-up. In general, a child with recurrent headaches should always be followed up within 2–4 weeks after the initial office evaluation. Support for behavioral interventions, monitoring of headache frequency and functional severity, and reviewing the parent–child understanding of the symptoms are the goals for the follow-up visit. New information or clinical observations may either alter the initial diagnosis or provide a new direction for management.

BIBLIOGRAPHY

McGrath PJ, Reid GJ. Behavioral treatment of pediatric headache. *Pediatr Ann* 24:486–491, 1995.

Lewis D, Ashwal S, Hershey A, et al. Practice parameter: pharmacological treatment of migraine headache in children and adolescents. *Neurology* 63:2215–2224, 2004.

Quality Standards Subcommittee of the American Academy of Neurology and the Practice Committee of the Child Neurology Society. Practice parameter: evaluation of children and adolescents with recurrent headaches. *Neurology* 58:1589–1596, 2002.

Stafstrom CE, Rostasy K, Minster A. The usefulness of children's drawings in the diagnosis of headache. *Pediatrics* 109:460–472, 2002.

Galli F, Patron L, Russo PM, et al. Chronic daily headache in childhood and adolescence: clinical aspects and a 4-year follow-up. *Cephalalgia* 24(10):850–858, 2004.

http://www.mjn.com/newsletterimages/v8s8pp2.html. Accessed June 14, 2010.

50

Hearing Loss and Deafness

Laurel M. Wills
Karen E. Wills

I. **Description of the condition.** A broad understanding of childhood deafness or hearing loss goes beyond traditional medical or audiological definitions to include developmental, linguistic, and sociocultural implications as well. Advances in communication therapies, progressive special education policy, and "high-tech" devices, such as cochlear implants or frequency modulation (FM) listening systems, have dramatically changed the developmental outlook for children with hearing loss. Individualized care management decisions must account for the following characteristics:

A. **Degree or severity of hearing loss.**
  - "Normal" hearing is defined as the ability to detect a full range of environmental and speech sounds at a whispering volume of 10 to 20 decibels (dB), whereas conversational speech typically registers at 50 to 60 dB.
  - Mild (25 to 40 dB range), moderate (41 to 55 dB), moderately severe (56 to 70 dB), severe (71 to 90 dB), and profound (90 dB or higher) degrees of deafness are associated with diminishing capability to detect and discriminate speech and environmental sounds.
  - The configuration or profile of hearing loss, depicted as an *audiogram* (Fig. 50-1), varies for each child, with better hearing in certain frequencies than in others, and with separate profiles displayed for the right and left ears.
  - The audiogram may or may not accurately reflect the *functional* listening level. For example, one child with moderate hearing loss might be able to comprehend what she hears better than a second child with only mild hearing loss. Deafness is not simply "turning down the volume" on normal hearing; it may also involve distortion of speech sounds that are heard. "Listening skills" are influenced by multiple factors including the child's biomedical status, cognitive and social-communicative skills, and past experiences (schooling, speech–language therapy, hearing aid use, family support, etc., as described further below).

B. **Type and anatomic location of lesion causing hearing loss.**
  - Conductive hearing loss commonly results from conditions that interfere with the functioning of the eardrum or ossicles, but leave the hearing *nerve* intact, such as middle ear infections, effusions, or cholesteatoma. Conductive hearing loss is generally in the mild to moderate range.
  - Sensorineural hearing loss is defined as a dysfunction of the cochlear hair cells in the inner ear or of auditory nerve itself (8th cranial nerve), preventing transmission of sound signals to the brain.
  - Auditory neuropathy refers to dysfunction at one or more points along the auditory pathway of the nervous system (8th nerve, auditory brainstem nuclei, central auditory cortex), with or without an otherwise normally functioning cochlea.
  - Mixed hearing losses involve both *peripheral* (outer and middle ear) and *central* (inner ear and neural) components of the auditory pathway.
  - Children with mild or unilateral hearing loss may have age-typical speech skills, and thus may go undiagnosed until well into their elementary school years. They may present with symptoms of inattention, distractibility, language or learning deficits, or irritable mood; thus, a basic hearing screen should be a standard part of developmental–behavioral pediatric assessments.
  - Children with fluctuating hearing loss (associated with chronic severe otitis media, or severe bilateral cerumen impaction) in early childhood may show distorted or delayed speech and language development, which sometimes can persist into later childhood.

C. **Age of onset of hearing loss.**
  - Children who are born deaf or who lose their hearing prior to acquiring spoken language (*"prelingual deafness"*), relative to those who lose their hearing later on (*"postlingual deafness"*), are usually at a communicative disadvantage with regard to developing and/or preserving spoken language skills.

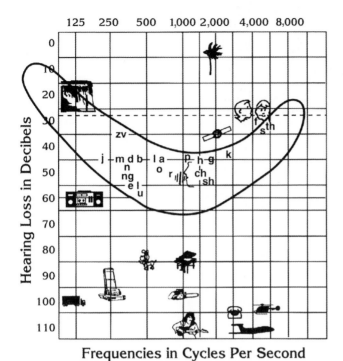

Frequencies in Cycles Per Second

Figure 50-1. Audiogram showing a comparison of the frequency and intensity of various environmental and speech sounds.

- Older children or adolescents who are *late-deafened* (e.g., from meningitis or progressive hearing loss), but still fluent in their native spoken language, are usually optimal candidates for restoration (rehabilitation) of oral–aural communication skills.
- Hearing loss that is *progressive* may be detected and treated later than *stable* hearing losses. Often, older children or adolescents attempt to minimize or deny the increasing severity of a progressive hearing loss, just as older adults often do, to avoid the psychosocial stigma of wearing hearing aids or acknowledging a "disability."

D. Age at (and interval between) identification and intervention.

- Prelingual or congenital deafness confers risk for loss of stimulation to the auditory pathways during sensitive early developmental periods, hence the recommendation to intervene *early* with hearing aids or cochlear implants, when appropriate. Similarly, in cases of acquired or postlingual deafness, early detection and expeditious intervention improves prognosis.
- Informal office methods of "testing" hearing in babies and young children (such as clapping or ringing a bell, and then watching for response) are considered unreliable, and can result in delayed diagnosis. When parents report concern about a child's hearing due to symptoms such as "not responding to sounds at home", "not listening", or "not talking" at the expected age, formal referral to a pediatric audiologist is indicated.
- Universal newborn hearing screening, now considered a standard of care, has dramatically improved the rate of early detection of childhood hearing loss, allowing for earlier intervention with strategies that improve access to oral–aural (spoken) and/or manual–visual (signed) language.
- Only ~10% of deaf babies are born to deaf parents, whereas ~90% of deaf babies are born to hearing parents. These "deaf-of-deaf" children are more likely to grow up as "native" signers, due to the rare natural circumstance of having exposure, since birth, to one or more fluent Sign Language models. In contrast to the reaction of most hearing parents, those who identify as culturally deaf may be pleased when their child is also born deaf; some may express concerns about raising a child with "normal" hearing.

E. Coexisting disabilities related to cause of hearing loss.

- Approximately one-third of children with hearing loss have additional medical or neurological diagnoses, as described below. The other two-thirds of children tend to be healthy, "typically developing" youngsters with "isolated" hearing loss, usually genetic in origin.
- Dual sensory loss (hearing and vision) occurs in a number of conditions, such as prenatal cytomegalovirus (CMV) infection or Usher Syndrome. In general, it is critically important to protect and optimize vision for purposes of speech (lip)-reading and/or signing. Thus, formal periodic evaluation with a pediatric ophthalmologist is strongly recommended for all hard of hearing and deaf children.
- Children born in developing countries (e.g., international adoptees and immigrant children) and low-income children with less access to healthcare are more likely to have late-identified hearing loss or multiple disabilities.

F. Psychosocial experience and home environment.

- Positive adjustment and social–emotional well-being among deaf children is closely linked to the quality of parent–child communication, (irrespective of modality), as well as to warm, responsive nurturing, and developmentally appropriate expectations within the parent–child relationship (see parenting resources in bibliography). Chronic frustration, conflict, and chaos in the home are linked to behavior and emotional problems in deaf children. Since 90% of deaf children are born to hearing parents who are likely to know little about deafness, the diagnosis of deafness can be a crisis that tries the family's coping resources, demanding support systems within their extended family and community, as well as support from healthcare and education professionals.

II. Epidemiology.

- Twenty million Americans of all ages have a hearing loss.
- Roughly 1 million children and adolescents have a "communicatively significant" hearing loss.
- 1 to 2/1,000 live births will have severe or profound deafness.
- 6 to 10/1,000 will have milder degrees of hearing loss.
- Males and females are equally affected.
- Preventative measures, such as vaccines against rubella, *Hemophilus influenza* B, and pneumoccal disease, as well as appropriate treatment of otitis media and neonatal hyperbilirubinemia, have all markedly reduced the incidence of childhood hearing loss in developed countries.
- Academic underachievement, functional illiteracy, and underemployment remain significant concerns for this population.

III. Etiology.

A. Genetic causes account for roughly 50% to 60% of all children with hearing loss, and of these genetic causes, about one-third are "deafness-related syndromes" and two-thirds are "nonsyndromic". Laboratory testing and DNA molecular analysis is now available for some of the more common gene mutations, such as Connexin 26 (*GJB2*). Malformations of the cochlea or other inner ear structures can result in hearing loss and, in some children, problems with balance or equilibrium. Other examples include Usher syndrome (sensorineural deafness associated with progressive vision loss from retinitis pigmentosa), Treacher–Collins syndrome (conductive or mixed hearing loss, associated with dysmorphic facies and eye findings), and Waardenburg syndrome (sensorineural deafness and pigmentary changes of the hair and irises). All of these are examples of syndromes usually associated with normal intelligence.

B. Nongenetic or "acquired" hearing loss can be separated into etiologies occurring in the prenatal, perinatal, and postnatal periods:

- **Prenatal:** Maternal infections, most commonly including CMV, toxoplasmosis, and rubella should be considered in the setting of a newborn with microcephaly, intrauterine growth retardation, seizures, or unusual eye findings. Newborns with CMV or toxoplasmosis may also be asymptomatic. Deafness from congenital CMV infection may be present at birth or can emerge and progress during early childhood. New laboratory techniques enable retrospective analysis for CMV on bloodspot specimens collected at birth in the nursery and kept in storage.
- **Perinatal:** Severe hyperbilirubinemia, also relatively rare in developed countries, can result in damage (kernicterus) to the auditory nuclei and other central, "retrocochlear" neurologic regions. Neonatal sepsis or severe neonatal cardiorespiratory compromise often requires treatment with ototoxic antibiotic or diuretic medications, thus newborn intensive care unit (NICU) graduates and premature babies have a much higher incidence of hearing loss than full-term healthy neonates.

- **Postnatal:** Chronic suppurative otitis media or other types of middle ear pathology can result in a transient or permanent conductive or mixed hearing loss. Bacterial meningitis, though much less common in this vaccine era, remains a common cause of acquired hearing loss. Ototoxic medications also include certain chemotherapeutic agents used in pediatric cancer therapy. Noise trauma or physical trauma can result in conductive or mixed hearing loss. Rare in childhood, acoustic nerve tumors can also cause deafness, usually unilateral.
- **Unknown etiology:** ~Twenty percent or more of children have a hearing loss of un-determined etiology, despite thorough evaluation.

IV. Making the diagnosis.

A. Newborn Hearing Screening is the ideal way to diagnose congenital hearing loss. **Developmental screening tools** that are standardized and validated, and used during routine healthcare maintenance to primary care practices, query parents about speech and language milestones. Parental observations and concerns should be taken seriously in order to make the diagnosis of hearing loss early.

B. History and physical examination. A thorough prenatal and birth history, past medical, developmental, and family (genetic) history may identify the cause of deafness and co-existing conditions. On the physical examination, particular attention should be given to facial features and other potentially syndromic markers (e.g., skin and hair pigment changes), appearance of the external and middle ear, eye exam and vision screen, and a complete neurologic exam, including muscle tone, coordination, gait, and balance. Additional subspecialty evaluation and input regarding treatment options is usually indicated, including: otolaryngology, clinical genetics, child neurology and/or psychology, infectious disease, among others.

C. Hearing and speech evaluations. It is important to realize that hearing acuity can be formally tested in the newborn period—no infant is too young! The testing methods discussed are performed or supervised by qualified audiologists, who have specific pediatric training:

- Physiologic measures (requiring no cooperation): Universal newborn hearing screening relies on noninvasive physiologic methods such as otoacoustic emissions (OAE) and/or brainstem auditory evoked response (BAER or ABR). OAE testing is performed by presenting a click stimulus via a soft-tipped probe in the external ear canal. The computer receiver then detects the "acoustic emissions" or echolike sounds produced by the hair cells of the cochlea. False-positive OAE tests can result from middle ear fluid or vernix in the external ear canal at birth. If these emissions are not detected, the baby or child is referred on for BAER testing, the current "gold standard" physiologic measure of hearing acuity. BAER testing involves placement of scalp electrodes to measure electrical waveforms produced along the auditory pathway in response to a sound stimulus presented by an earphone. Older children who are unable to cooperate with behavioral tests, such as some with developmental or autism spectrum disabilities, can also be evaluated with these types of "passive" hearing tests.
- Behavioral testing (requires cooperation or active participation): These include visual reinforcement audiometry (useful with older infants and toddlers), conditioned play audiometry (useful with older toddlers and preschoolers), and routine behavioral audiometry (useful with school-aged children and adolescents). As noted earlier, informal office methods, such as watching for a baby's response to a hand clap or bell ringing, can be deceptive and inaccurate because the baby may react to a visual cue, vibration, or movement, and the decibel level of the noise presented is uncontrolled.
- *Visual reinforcement audiometry* is performed by having the toddler sit facing outward on a parent's lap in a sound-treated room. The audiologist presents a series of tones at specific frequencies and volumes from a speaker at one or the other side of the room, watching for the child's reaction. Visual reinforcement is offered (e.g., with a dancing toy in one or the other corner of the room) when the baby clearly localizes and looks toward the sound source.
- *Conditioned play audiometry* is performed in a sound-treated room in which the preschooler is taught or "conditioned" to respond with a play activity (e.g., put a block in a box) in response to hearing a specific tone. When the child is too young or unable to tolerate headphones, hearing acuity can only be determined for "the better ear in a sound field", as opposed to more precise measures of hearing, in each ear, made possible by using headphones in older children and adolescents.
- *Routine behavioral audiometry* involves the older child simply raising a hand when a tone is heard through the right or left side of the headphones. School-and clinic-based hearing screens are useful tools, but can miss milder degrees of hearing loss. Referral

to an audiology clinic is recommended whenever hearing status is questioned, even for a child who has passed routine screening.

- Tympanometry and pneumatic otoscopy are measures of eardrum mobility and middle ear disease, which may be abnormal in the setting of conductive hearing impairment. These are performed by many primary care offices, as well as audiologists. It is not uncommon for parents to mistake an office-based tympanogram for a "hearing test". For example, a child with profound sensorineural deafness may have normal tympanograms.
- The audiologist will also perform measures of speech detection and discrimination, in addition to "pure tone" audiometry, at the initial hearing assessment and later, when testing hearing aid function. It is important to make a distinction among speech detection (knowing when one is being spoken to), speech discrimination (being able to recognize certain speech sounds or words), and comprehension of "connected" speech (being able to listen and understand the meaning of spoken phrases and sentences in conversation).
- In addition to audiology testing, children with hearing loss require assessment of communicative competence, that is, thorough evaluation of spoken, signed, and gestural communication abilities, by an experienced speech–language clinician and/or special educator.

V. Management.
- **Role of the primary care practitioner:** Pediatric management starts by creating a compassionate and conscientious "medical (or healthcare) home" for the child with hearing loss and for his or her parents. Fostering a realistic, but hopeful sense of the future and awareness of the many available resources is critical in energizing parents for the challenges ahead. For youngsters with cochlear implant(s), due to the increased risk of meningitis, it is critically important to maintain an up-to-date immunization status (specifically pneumococcal vaccine) and to treat all middle ear disease fairly aggressively, given the proximity of the implant to the nervous system.
- **Role of audiologist:** The majority of children will need regular follow-up with a "primary" audiologist in order to detect and document any change or progression in the hearing loss and to assess for fit and proper functioning of hearing aids, cochlear implants, or other assistive listening devices, for example, used at school.
- **Other medical subspecialists:** All deaf and hard of hearing children should have regular, thorough eye and vision examinations by a pediatric ophthalmologist, since visual acuity is so crucial to communication via speech-reading and visual–manual methods (e.g., American Sign Language, Cued Speech). In addition, the ophthalmologist may need to evaluate specifically for colobomata, chorioretinitis, or retinitis pigmentosa, depending on the individual patient's history.
- **Cochlear implants:** A cochlear implant is a surgically implanted, electronic device that has two main parts: an internal portion composed of an array of microelectrodes inserted into the turns of the cochlea, and an external portion that receives, processes, and transmits speech sounds to the internal portion via an ear level attachment. The FDA (Food and Drug Administration) has approved the surgery in babies as young as 12 months of age (since the cochlea is essentially full-sized at birth), and increasingly, bilateral implants are recommended (over unilateral) to improve binaural processing and sound localization. Team evaluation of potential implant candidates assesses the child's medical and developmental status, and the family's expectations and ability to follow through with the intensive process of auditory (re)habilitation. Many children show remarkably positive outcomes, becoming competent oral–aural communicators, and functioning well in mainstreamed school settings. Children with additional disabilities can be quite successful cochlear implant candidates or users, but the ultimate prognosis may be more guarded. School speech therapists, as well as those in private agencies, should be supported by collaboration with hospital-to-school liaison staff on the cochlear implant team. Many children and adults who make good use of cochlear implants also continue to use and benefit from either Cued Speech and/or American Sign Language (ASL) communication, following a bilingual–bicultural approach (e.g., see http://www.cochlearcommunity.com/aslciers). Of importance to the primary care clinician, case reports of postimplant site infections and meningitis warrant vigilance about maintaining immunization schedules and prompt treatment of any wound or ear infections in these children.
- **Communication options**
  - Oral–aural (spoken) communication entails intensive instruction and practice with speech, listening, and speech-reading skills and maximizes the child's use of his or her residual or restored hearing. Children who have milder hearing losses or a more successful experience with hearing aids or cochlear implant use will tend to communicate

orally. Some oral communication methods emphasize strong listening without use of visual cues or signs, whereas others represent an eclectic mix of approaches.

- Cued Speech is a system of hand shapes and hand positions ("cues") that assist in speech-reading. The hand "cues" visually represent specific sounds or "phonemes" that, when used during conversation, can remove the ambiguity between sounds that look alike to the lip-reader, for example, / p / and / b /, as in "pen" versus "Ben", or "red" versus "green". Even deaf individuals who are proficient "speech-readers" comprehend only about 40% to 50% of what is spoken, and "piece together" meaning from the context of the conversation. Cued speech is becoming more popular in schools because it seems to help children with hearing loss grasp important phonemic distinctions, an important foundation for literacy.

- ASL is considered the "native or natural language" of the Deaf Community in the United States. ASL uses hands, arms, facial expression, body position, and movement to convey meaning, with unique grammatical rules that are visually based and therefore quite different from English. Various Signed English "systems" employ ASL signs, paired with spoken English; many hearing teachers, hearing parents who learn to sign with their children, and others learning ASL as a second language, learn these "Pidgin Signed English" or "Conceptually Accurate Signed English" approaches. ASL is not a global language, but rather, is unique to most of North America.

- **Education and psycho-educational evaluation.** With such wide individual differences among children who are deaf, there is no one-size-fits-all educational program. School programs differ in the communication options that they offer (see above). They also differ in the extent to which children are mainstreamed or congregated.

  - Deaf and Hard-of-hearing (D/HH, in educational parlance) children may be included within a regular classroom, perhaps using an Oral, Cued Speech, Signed English, or ASL interpreter to better understand the teacher and classmates. Instruction that alternates or integrates use of ASL and spoken English is referred to as a "bilingual–bicultural approach". For example, a school using this approach might teach science or social studies using ASL for optimal comprehension, whereas English reading and writing might be taught by speaking, listening, and perhaps using Cued Speech or "Visual Phonics" hand gestures to assist lip-readers, by making speech sounds visually more distinct.

  - Many students use assistive listening devices, such as an FM system, in which the teacher wears a microphone that transmits speech sounds directly to the child's hearing aid. CART (computer-assisted real time) captioning, in which a typist transcribes a lecture using a computer, is becoming a popular option for D/HH high school and college students who can also study the printed English transcript of a lecture.

  - Psychological or psycho-educational evaluation of deaf children should be done by a clinician who is knowledgeable about cultural, educational, linguistic, and developmental issues associated with deafness and experienced in working with interpreters, or ideally, conversant in the child's primary communication mode. Tests of reasoning and problem solving using visual patterns and pictures are usually the most appropriate way to measure intelligence in children who are deaf. Verbal question-and-answer tests may be useful to assess proficiency with conceptualizing problems and articulating solutions in English, keeping in mind that the child's exposure to English language–based concepts and culture may be limited. A child's struggles with English speech or literacy cannot be ascribed to low intelligence when hearing is impaired. On the other hand, children with deafness, especially those who have other neurologic compromise, can also have developmental and learning disabilities, including language-processing disorders. Teachers and caregivers may mistakenly assume that a child's problems with learning, language, memory, attention, or emotional self-regulation occur "just because of his deafness." These children should be evaluated by a psychologist who is familiar with "typically developing" deaf children, who can assess whether the presenting concerns are consistent with deafness, *per se*, or represent an additional, potentially treatable, condition.

- **Community building and social support.** Parents need to understand that there are a variety of choices, but no "one right way" to raise a deaf child. However, parents should be forewarned that some professionals, other parents, books, and media will strongly advocate for one or another "right way." Parents are likely to need professional help and support to learn about, and select, communication options and educational programs for their child who is deaf. The bibliography lists contact information for agencies that help parents make these decisions, including ones with parent-to-parent support groups.

- **Mental Health.** In general, the parenting attitudes and skills that promote mental health, strong self-esteem, and prosocial behavior in all children are also associated with positive adjustment among children who are deaf. Specifically, a supportive, warm, family environment is associated with better social skills and happier mood in the child. The presence of harsh, critical, aggressive, or lax and inconsistent parenting is associated with children's aggressive and rule-breaking behavior. Establishing strong social support networks for deaf and hard of hearing children and adolescents is crucial to healthy development. Modern communication devices, such as text messaging and videophones, have been helpful in avoiding social isolation.

VI. Clinical pearls and pitfalls.

- A baby is never too young to test hearing acuity. If a parent or grandparent raises concern about hearing in a child, refer the family to a pediatric audiologist as soon as possible.
- Early identification of hearing loss can radically improve developmental outcome. Engage the family as soon as possible with local early intervention or D/HH educational services.
- Comprehensive evaluation of a deaf or hard of hearing child is a multidisciplinary pursuit best performed by clinicians experienced in working with deaf children and proficient in or knowledgeable about various communication modalities.
- Terminology in this field can be tricky. Many individuals take offense at the clinical term, "hearing impaired" (often because of the view that the signing Deaf Community represents a healthy, linguistic minority, rather than a disability group), while others do not like "hearing loss" when the condition has been present from birth. Thus, it is best to simply ask parents or older patients what words they use to describe themselves or their children.
- Think "eyes", not just "ears", when thinking about deaf children. They will learn about their world through their eyes, as much or more than hearing children, whether they communicate using speech-reading or manual–gestural methods. All deaf and hard of hearing children need to see the eye doctor for a thorough exam. Special services exist in many geographic areas and specialized national centers for children with deaf–blindness.
- Parent-to-parent support is vitally important as the parents of a child with hearing loss are coming to terms with the diagnosis and exploring treatment options, which can be confusing and controversial. Reliable, unbiased national parent resources, as well as local parent networks, exist in many regions. Forewarn parents that some professionals, agencies, books, and other parents may be strongly biased towards the view that there is only "one right way" to raise, educate, and communicate with a child who is deaf. Try to provide parents with a more balanced view, such as is represented in the bibliography that follows.

BIBLIOGRAPHY

For parents and clinicians

Bodner-Johnson B, Sass-Lehrer M (eds). *The Young Deaf or Hard of Hearing Child: A Family-Centered Approach to Early Education*. Baltimore, MD: Paul H. Brookes Publishing, 2003.

Candlish PM. *Not Deaf Enough: Raising a Child Who Is Hard of Hearing With Hugs and Humor*. Washington, DC: Alexander Graham Bell Association, 1996.

Dorros C, et al. Medical home for children with hearing loss: physician perspectives and practices. *Pediatrics* 120:288–294, 2007.

Medwid DJ, Chapman WD. *Kid Friendly Parenting With Deaf and Hard of Hearing Children*. Washington, DC: Gallaudet University Press, 1995.

Schwartz S (ed). *Choices in Deafness: A Parents' Guide to Communication Options* (3rd ed), Bethesda, MD: Woodbine House, 2007.

Web sites

Alexander Graham Bell Association, http://www.agbell.org
American Academy of Audiology, www.audiology.org
American Sign Language Think Tank, http://www.aslthinktank.com/
American Society for Deaf Children, www.deafchildren.org
Boy's Town Institute, www.babyhearing.org (English and Spanish)
Cochlear implant information, http://www.listen-up.org/implant.htm
Deaf Education Enhancement—Michigan State University: www.deafed.net
Early Hearing Detection and Intervention (from Centers for Disease Control), http://www.cdc.gov/ncbddd/ehdi (English and Spanish)
Family Voices, www.familyvoices.org
Hands and Voices, www.handsandvoices.org
Helen Keller National Center for Deaf-Blind Youth and Adults, http://www.hknc.org/
Laurent Clerc National Deaf Education Center (Gallaudet University), http://clerccenter.gallaudet.edu/

National Association of the Deaf, www.nad.org

National Dissemination Center for Children with Disabilities (formerly the National Information Clearinghouse for Handicapped Children and Youth), www.nichcy.org *The "State Resources Sheets" are an invaluable list of agencies in every state that provide parent support and governmental oversight of services related to hearing loss.*

Self Help for Hard of Hearing People, Hearing Loss Association of America, www.shhh.org

The National Center for Hearing Assessment and Management (Utah), www.infanthearing.org

51

Intellectual Disabilities: Behavioral Problems

Theodore A. Kastner
Kevin K. Walsh

I. Description of the problem.

A. Terminology. The term used to describe children and adults with what we have known as "mental retardation" is in a state of flux. The phenomenon of changes in terminology in this field is well-known, as terms over time often acquire negative connotations. The term "mental retardation" is rapidly being replaced by the term "intellectual disability" in America; in other countries, other terms have been selected. For example, in Great Britain, the term used to describe this group is "learning disability."

B. Epidemiology. The incidence of behavioral disorders in children with intellectual and other developmental disabilities is greater than in children without them, because any brain damage or dysfunction appears to increase the likelihood of behavioral or psychiatric disorders.

- Forty percent of people with intellectual disabilities experience a period of disturbed behavior and function at some time in their lives.
- The epidemiology of behavioral problems among children with intellectual and related developmental disabilities is unknown because of their cognitive and communicative limitations, and because appropriate diagnostic tools are not yet available.
- It is estimated that diagnosable psychiatric disorders exist in 5% to 10% of children with intellectual and developmental disabilities.

C. Etiology. There are four major causes of severe, challenging behaviors in children with intellectual disabilities: adaptive dysfunction, psychiatric disorders, medication side effects, and organic causes. In many cases, the etiology is of multiple origins (e.g., a psychiatric disorder accompanied by family dysfunction).

1. **Adaptive dysfunction** is a mismatch between the needs, abilities, and goals of the child and that of the environment (usually the school and/or family unit). In this model, the potential *communicative* nature of the behavior is often considered. For example, does a behavioral outburst always accompany a request to accomplish difficult tasks? In this case, the behavioral problem may be due to unrealistic environmental expectations or poor adaptive skills of the child or both. Adaptive dysfunction can often be distinguished from mental illness or an organic cause by a lack of vegetative signs (weight loss or sleep problem) and a consistent relationship between the behavior and various setting events.

2. **Psychiatric disorders** are more common in children with intellectual disabilities than in the general population. The most common psychiatric disorders associated with intellectual disabilities in children may be the mood disorders, such as depression and bipolar disease (often in atypical forms, e.g., rapid cycling and chronic mania). Mood disorders in children with intellectual disabilities can often be recognized by the presence of a sleep disturbance, change in weight or eating habits, overactivity or motor restlessness, mood lability (crying or laughing), and a behavioral history of cycling. Less commonly, anxiety disorders, psychosis, Tourette syndrome, attention-deficit/hyperactivity disorder (ADHD), and obsessive–compulsive disorder are seen.

3. **Medication side effects** are a common cause of behavioral morbidity among children with intellectual disabilities. For example, in a study of 209 people with mental retardation who presented with behavioral complaints, undiagnosed medication side effects were noted in 7%. These included akasthisia, tardive dyskinesia, and other side effects typically associated with the use of major tranquilizers.

4. **Health-related causes.** Occult medical illnesses have been found in about 20% of behaviorally disordered children with intellectual and developmental disabilities. The high prevalence is due to their greater healthcare needs, communication barriers around symptomatology, and a lack of effective healthcare services. Perhaps the most common medical cause of disturbed behavior is unrecognized or poorly treated epilepsy, especially partial complex seizures. Interictal irritability, for example, can exacerbate aggressive or self-injurious behaviors. Other undiagnosed medical causes

Table 51-1. Formulating a diagnosis in individuals with intellectual disabilities and behavioral problems

1. Rule out the presence of a medical disorder.
2. Evaluate the presence of environmental supports and stressors.
3. Look for a complex of behavioral symptoms.
4. Establish a psychiatric diagnosis using standard or modified criteria.
5. Develop treatment goals.
6. Monitor treatment with a predetermined methodology.
7. Establish a treatment end point.

of behavioral problems include thyroid dysfunction, premenstrual syndrome, and cardiac disease.

II. **Making the diagnosis.**

A. **Signs and symptoms.** Behavioral problems in children with intellectual disabilities include aggression, self-injury, overactivity, disruptive behaviors, and sleep disturbances. In addition, rumination, elopement, property destruction, and other behaviors are occasionally seen.

B. **Behavioral questionnaires.** Inventories or behavioral scales can be used to facilitate the evaluation of behavioral problems in children with intellectual disabilities. These include the *Reiss Screen for Maladaptive Behavior*, the *Reiss Scales for Children's Dual Diagnosis*, the *Psychopathology Instrument for Mentally Retarded Adults (PIMRA)*, and the *Aberrant Behavior Checklist*. There are also many specialized tools for specific disorders such as the *Childhood Autism Rating Scale* or the *Vanderbilt ADHD Diagnostic Scales* (parent and teacher versions). It is frequently of benefit to use two or more inventories and to have more than one caregiver complete the instrument.

C. **Physical examination.** The physical examination should be comprehensive and thorough. If an organic cause of behavioral problems (e.g., hypothyroidism in a child with Down syndrome) is missed by the clinician, it is unlikely that the disorder will be recognized by another childcare clinician. Laboratory testing should be conducted when clinical suspicions are aroused by the history and physical examination. Even when these produce no clues, however, the clinician should remain ever vigilant to the possibility of an occult medical problem.

D. **Diagnostic hypotheses.** The clinician should formulate a psychiatric diagnosis or etiologic hypothesis before prescribing a treatment. Steps needed to develop a diagnosis and treatment plan for children with intellectual disabilities and behavioral problems are outlined in Table 51-1. A recent volume that may be of assistance in this endeavor is the *Diagnostic Manual—Intellectual Disabilities* (DM-ID) that presents a systematic adaptation of most of the DSM-IV-TR diagnostic categories for individuals with intellectual disabilities.

Strict diagnostic criteria for psychiatric disorders may not be met due to a number of features related to intellectual disabilities, especially cognitive and communicative deficits. Frequently, a clear diagnosis cannot be made, and the clinician may resort to empirical trial-and-error treatments. The general points in Table 51-2 should be noted when considering the use of psychotropic medication in children with intellectual disabilities.

III. **Treatment.** The treatment of behavioral problems in children with intellectual disabilities may require changes in the child's environment (including behavioral intervention), psychoactive medications, medical interventions, or any combination of the three.

Table 51-2. Clinical concerns when using psychopharmacology in children with intellectual disabilities and behavioral problems

The diagnosis should guide treatment.

The more severe the behavior or the degree of intellectual disabilities, the more likely it is that the problem is of biological and/or psychiatric origin and will respond to appropriate medical treatment.

Anticonvulsants (such as carbamazepine and valproic acid) and antihypertensives (such as beta-blockers) are powerful psychotropic agents.

Treat multiple diagnoses with a single medication if possible (e.g., treat epilepsy and depression with carbamazepine and/or lamotrigine; treat hypertension and anxiety with a beta-blocker).

The end point in a trial of medication is remission of symptoms or intolerable side effects.

Table 51-3. Behavioral symptoms suggesting psychiatric diagnoses and treatment

Behavioral symptoms	Possible diagnoses	Potential psychoactive therapy
Overactivity, decreased sleep, poor attention, self-injury, aggression	Bipolar disorder	Mood stabilizers or atypical neuroleptics
Overactivity, poor attention, autism, self-injury, aggression	Anxiety disorders	Propranolol, buspirone, atypical neuroleptics, or selective serotonin reuptake inhibitors
Poor attention, fragile X syndrome	Attention-deficit/ hyperactivity disorder	Methylphenidate, tricyclic antidepressants, clonidine
Stereotypic behavior, self-injury, aggression	Obsessive compulsive disorder, depression	Atypical neuroleptics, or selective serotonin reuptake inhibitors
Social withdrawal, abnormal sleep pattern, poor attention, self-injury, aggression, rumination	Depression	Mood stabilizers, antidepressants

A. **The environment and behavioral intervention.** If the social milieu is nonoptimal, the behavior of the child with intellectual disabilities may represent an attempt to control or alter that environment or to avoid demands. Behavioral problems may then be reduced or eliminated as the child is taught appropriate replacement behaviors that can serve the same function. This intervention begins with *functional analysis* and is best conducted as part of a comprehensive behavioral diagnostic process that includes traditional medical and psychiatric evaluations. It is also possible that behavioral problems can arise from poor communication skills. In such cases, the functional analysis of the behavior needs to focus on any possible communicative intent in order to develop interventions that provide communication supports or alternatives.

B. **Psychoactive medications.** Given the vast number of psychoactive medications on the market, it is wise to be familiar with one or two drugs in each of the major classes of medications. This is generally sufficient to allow the clinician the flexibility to make appropriate choices between treatments. Specifically, the interested clinician should be comfortable using anticonvulsants (carbamazepine and valproic acid), antimanic drugs (lithium carbonate), tricyclic antidepressants (desipramine and imipramine), stimulants (methylphenidate and dextroamphetamine), antianxiety drugs (propranolol and bus-pirone), serotonin reuptake inhibiting antidepressants (sertraline and fluoxetine), and atypical neuroleptics. Risperidone and aripiprazole have both been approved to treat the irritability associated with autism spectrum disorders. The general indications for use of many of these medications are included in Table 51-3.

Many of the medications have multiple effects. Carbamazepine is an effective anticonvulsant with antidepressant, antimanic, and neuralgic effects. It can be an excellent first choice in the treatment of aggression and/or self-injury, particularly in the presence of overactivity or a sleep disorder. In addition to depression, selective serotonin reuptake inhibitors are valuable in the treatment of anxiety disorders and obsessive–compulsive disorder. The atypical neuroleptics are often a good first choice of treatment during an acute problem, although every effort should be made to find alternative treatments because of long-term side effects.

C. **The family.** The level of family stress and the family's ability to use the resources of the extended family or obtain alternative community supports are important predictors of outcome. For example, a recent study of children with epilepsy noted that family function was one of the most important predictors of behavioral problems. The primary care clinician should always remember that a strong family is a critical and effective treatment partner.

D. **Follow-up.** Interventions for children with intellectual disabilities and behavioral problems should be accompanied by careful follow-up. The behavioral response to the treatment plan should receive careful scrutiny. Children taking psychoactive medication may require periodic screening for drug levels, side effects, and behavioral changes, depending on the medication used. In addition, the diagnosis may need to be reconsidered in the light of the response to treatment. For example, when a trial of stimulant medication causes a worsening of behavior or ever-increasing dosages are required to maintain therapeutic effect, the diagnosis of bipolar disorder should be considered.

BIBLIOGRAPHY

For parents

Batshaw ML, Pelligrino L, Roizen NJ (eds). *Children With Disabilities* (6th ed), Baltimore, MD: Paul H. Brookes, 2007.

Web sites

Developmental Disabilities Health Alliance, Inc., www.ddha.com
The Arc (formerly the Association for Retarded Citizens), http://www.thearc.org
VOR at http://www.vor.net/

For professionals

Accardo PJ. *Capute and Accardo's Neurodevelopmental Disabilities in Infancy and Childhood* (3rd ed), Baltimore, MD: Paul H. Brookes, 2008.
Betz CL, Nehring WM. *Promoting Health Care Transitions for Adolescents With Special Health Care Needs and Disabilities*. Baltimore, MD: Paul H. Brookes, 2007.
Emerson E, et al. (eds). *The International Handbook of Applied Research in Intellectual Disabilities*. West Sussex, England: John Wiley and Sons, 2004.
Fletcher R, et al. *Diagnostic Manual-Intellectual Disability: A Textbook of Diagnosis of Mental Disorders in Persons With Intellectual Disability*. Kingston, NY: NADD Press, 2007.
Rubin IL, Crocker AC (eds). *Medical Care for Children and Adults With Developmental Disabilities* (2nd ed), Baltimore, MD: Paul H. Brookes, 2006.

Behavioral questionnaires

Aberrant Behavior Checklist http://www.slosson.com/onlinecatalogstore_c51452.html
Reiss Screen for Maladaptive Behavior, Reiss Scales for Children's Dual Diagnosis, and Psychopathology Instrument for Mentally Retarded Adults (PIMRA), http://www.idspublishing.com/screen.htm

52

Intellectual Disability: Diagnostic Evaluation

David L. Coulter

I. **Description of the problem.** According to the American Association on Intellectual and Developmental Disabilities (AAIDD), intellectual disability is defined as follows:
   A. **Definition.** "Intellectual disability is characterized by significant limitations both in intellectual functioning and in adaptive behavior as expressed in conceptual, social, and practical adaptive skills. This disability originates before age 18" (Schalock et al., 2010).
      1. Note that the term "intellectual disability" replaces the previous term of "mental retardation," and that the term intellectual disability covers the same population of individuals who were diagnosed previously with mental retardation in number, kind, level, type, and duration of the disability, and the need of people with this disability for individual services, and every individual who is or was eligible for a diagnosis of mental retardation is eligible for a diagnosis of intellectual disability (Schalock et al., 2010).
      2. Significant limitation in intellectual functioning means an IQ (intelligence quotient) score that is more than approximately two standard deviations below the mean, considering the standard error of measurement for the specific IQ test used.
      3. Significant limitation in adaptive behavior means an adaptive behavior score that is more than approximately two standard deviations below the mean, considering the standard error of measurement for the specific adaptive behavior test used.
      4. Classification of individuals with intellectual disability should not be based solely on the IQ score. Previously used subcategories of mild, moderate, severe, and profound (which were based solely on the IQ score) should not be used, since the IQ score often does not reflect the totality of the individual's functioning. Instead, *classification is based on the types and intensities of supports and services needed by the individual.* Instruments such as the Supports Intensity Scale (Thompson et al., 2004) can be used to classify support needs.
   B. **Etiology.** Intellectual disability may be the end result of *one or more* of the following categories of risk.
      1. **Biomedical.** These are factors that have had a deleterious impact on the child's CNS (e.g., genetic and metabolic disorders, environmental toxins, infections).
      2. **Social.** Inadequacies in the social and/or family environment (e.g., inadequate stimulation, social unresponsiveness) can diminish cognitive and social growth and functioning.
      3. **Behavioral.** The damaging behavior of others (e.g., trauma, maternal substance abuse) can lead to intellectual disability.
      4. **Educational.** The availability and quality of educational and training programs can affect intellectual development and influence whether or not a child functions in the range of intellectual disability.
      5. **Interactions between risk factors.** In any given case, multiple risk factors may be present and may interact at different ages or stages of development. This concept reflects the transactional approach to human development, in which reciprocal interactions between individuals and their environment influence the developmental outcome. Some risk factors may be more significant (principal or primary cause of intellectual disability), and others may be less significant (contributing or secondary cause), but the interaction between them is almost always important. For example, a child with phenylketonuria (a biomedical risk factor) may function at a lower level because of both environmental deprivation (a social risk factor) and poor parental compliance with the prescribed diet (a behavioral risk factor).

II. **Making the diagnosis.**
   A. **Signs and symptoms.** Intellectual disability should be suspected in any child who is significantly below the normative developmental milestones for his age. Many (but not all) children diagnosed with global developmental delay will eventually meet the criteria for a diagnosis of intellectual disability. In addition, children with an *established* risk (e.g., Down syndrome) are very likely to have intellectual disability.

B. **Evaluation of the etiology.**
   1. An understanding of the etiology of intellectual disability begins with a **complete medical and psychosocial history** and a **complete physical and neurologic examination.** This preliminary assessment results in a list of possible causes or differential diagnosis, which should include consideration of any and all potential risk factors.
   2. The differential diagnosis should be thought of as a set of **hypotheses about the etiology,** so that the subsequent workup is designed to test the most reasonable hypotheses. Table 52-1 is designed to help the primary care clinician design an appropriate workup based on the most likely hypotheses in a particular case. This table lists a series of possible hypotheses based on whether the potential risk occurred prenatally, perinatally, or postnatally. A set of possible strategies for testing each of these hypotheses is then suggested.
   3. **There is no single diagnostic workup that is appropriate to all cases.** In some cases, the workup will be very simple (as in chromosomal analysis when Down syndrome is suspected). In most cases, however, the etiology will not be obvious, and a careful workup will be needed. Such an evaluation, however, will result in identification of the principal or primary cause of intellectual disability in only about one-third of cases. Because new diagnostic measures for intellectual disability are emerging rapidly, the etiologic evaluation in "idiopathic" cases should be considered an ongoing process that can take advantage of the newest techniques and research.
      Most neurologists recommend the following studies for evaluation of the child with global developmental delay:
     a. **High-resolution chromosomal analysis and fragile X studies** are recommended because not all chromosomal abnormalities lead to obvious physical signs (diagnostic yield approximately 5% to 6%).
     b. **Chromosomal microarray** (genomic hybridization) studies are recommended, preferably using the newest and most sensitive versions available (additional diagnostic yield 5% to 10%).
     c. *Methyl CpG binding protein 2 (MeCP2)* **testing** is recommended by many specialists because the spectrum of conditions associated with this gene is now recognized to be broader than just classic Rett syndrome (e.g., the *MeCP2* duplication syndrome that is associated with autism in boys).
     d. **Radiologic imaging of the brain** is recommended, and MRI (magnetic resonance imaging) is preferred (diagnostic yield 55%) to CT (computed tomography) (diagnostic yield 39%).
     e. **Metabolic screening** for amino acid and organic acid disorders has a low diagnostic yield but may identify potentially treatable disorders, and so is recommended particularly when genetic studies and neuroimaging are unrevealing.

III. **Management.**
  A. **Conveying the diagnosis and prognosis.**
   1. **Diagnosis.** Primary care clinicians are often present when the diagnosis is first made. Unfortunately, parents often have unpleasant memories about how the diagnosis was first conveyed to them. To avoid this and to help ensure that the diagnosis is conveyed sensitively, clinicians can follow these guidelines:
     a. **Listen to what the parents say about the child.** This will give the clinician a sense of their level of sophistication, understanding, and emotional acceptance of the child's problems.
     b. **Ask the parents about which particular aspects of their child's problems bother them the most.** This will help to address the issues *most important to them.*
     c. **Review the results of the evaluation in a way that is easily understandable and unambiguous.** Avoid technical jargon and overly complex explanations. Assess parental understanding by asking them to rehearse how they will explain their child's problem to a family member.
     d. Parents will be all too eager to assume the responsibility and guilt for their child's problem. **Consistent and persistent reassurance that the condition was not their fault is always indicated.**
     e. **The clinician should respect the parents' preference for using an alternative term to "intellectual disability"** (such as "special needs" child). However, it may be useful for them to understand that their child meets the diagnostic criteria for intellectual disability when such a designation provides eligibility for important supports and services.
   2. **Prognosis.** The primary care clinician should help the family to prepare for the future. This requires an understanding of the child's prognosis for functioning as an

Table 52-1. Hypotheses and strategies for determining etiology of intellectual disability

Hypothesis	Possible strategies
Prenatal onset	
Chromosomal disorder	Extended physical examination Referral to geneticist Karyotype, chromosomal microarray, and fragile X study; consider *MeCP2* testing
Syndrome disorder	Extended family history and examination of relatives Extended physical examination Referral to clinical geneticist or neurologist
Inborn error of metabolism	Screening for amino acids and organic acids Quantitation of amino acids in blood, urine, and/or CSF (cerebrospinal fluid) Analysis of organic acids by GC–MS (gas chromatography–mass spectrometry) or other methods Blood levels of lactate, pyruvate, carnitine, and long-chain fatty acids Arterial ammonia and gases Assays of specific enzymes; consider mitochondrial genome studies; consider CSF neurotransmitter analysis Biopsies of specific tissue for light and electron microscopic study and biochemical analysis
Developmental disorder of brain formation	CT (computed tomography) or MRI (magnetic resonance imaging) scan of brain Detailed morphologic study of brain tissue (e.g., biopsy)
Environmental influences	Growth charts Placental pathology Maternal history and physical examination of mother Toxicologic screening of mother at prenatal visits and of child at birth Referral to clinical geneticist Review maternal records (prenatal care, labor, and delivery)
Perinatal onset	Review birth and neonatal records
Postnatal onset	
Head injuries	Detailed medical history Skull x-rays, CT or MRI scan (for evidence of sequelae)
Infections	Detailed medical history
Demyelinating disorders	CT or MRI scan; CSF analysis
Degenerative disorders	CT or MRI scan Evoked potential studies Assays of specific enzymes Biopsy of specific tissue for light and electron microscopy and biochemical analysis
Seizure disorders	Electroencephalography
Toxic-metabolic disorders	See "Inborn error of metabolism" Toxicologic studies Heavy metal assays
Malnutrition	Body measurements Detailed nutritional history Family history of nutrition
Environmental	Detailed social history Psychological evaluation Observation in new environment

adult. In general, pediatric clinicians tend to *underestimate* the level at which adults with intellectual disability can function in the community. The clinician must achieve the delicate balance of not giving overly optimistic predictions of the child's potential capabilities (thereby engendering intense disappointment over time) and not underestimating his long-term potential (thereby creating a negative self-fulfilling prophecy). The clinician should ensure, over time, that the family accepts the prognosis, incorporates it into their family planning (e.g., for guardianship and financial trusts), and has realistic expectations for the child's future.

B. Clinical issues.

1. Primary care issues include **health supervision, immunizations, nutrition and growth, gynecologic care, and sex education**. Some children with intellectual disability also have other problems that may require referral to a specialist (e.g., neurologist, psychiatrist, orthopedist, or physiatrist). The primary care clinician should work collaboratively with the family and with any specialists involved in the child's care.

2. The primary care clinician should closely monitor the **academic progress of the child** with intellectual disability. A young child (age <3 years) should be referred for early intervention services as soon as a developmental problem is identified (often before the diagnosis of intellectual disability is actually made). An older child should be referred to the public school system to ensure that a comprehensive evaluation is done and an appropriate educational plan is developed.

3. As the child gets older, the clinician will need to anticipate concerns about the **transition to adult living**: guardianship, living arrangements, work, sexuality, and family planning, among others.

4. The primary care clinician understands better than most specialists that the child with intellectual disability belongs to a family that may be extended and/or nontraditional. Improving the child's quality of life requires improving the family's quality of life. Particular attention should be paid to helping siblings of the child with intellectual disability understand and accept their role, which may become prominent during adulthood (as their parents age).

BIBLIOGRAPHY

For parents

Every state has a government agency responsible for providing services to people with intellectual disability, but available services may be limited by state-specific policy and budgetary factors.

The Arc is the largest organization for parents of children with intellectual disability. Many local Arcs have parent support groups as well as case advocacy and specific supports and services. Their website (www.thearc.org) has much useful information for parents and families.

For professionals

Associations

The American Association on Intellectual and Developmental Disabilities conducts workshops and publishes journals and books on intellectual disability. Their website (www.aaidd.org) is a useful source for professionals seeking further information.

The Association of University Centers on Disability coordinates a network of regional training and service programs. Their website (www.aucd.org) also has information on current policy perspectives relating to intellectual and other developmental disabilities.

Publications

Dykens EM, Hodapp RM, Finucane BM. *Genetics and Mental Retardation Syndromes: A New Look at Behavior and Interventions*. Baltimore, MD: Paul H Brookes, 2000.

Schalock RL, Borthwick-Duffy SA, Bradley VJ, et al. *Intellectual Disability: Definition, Classification and Systems of Supports* (11th ed), Washington, DC: American Association on Intellectual and Developmental Disabilities, 2010. [See especially Chapter 6 on Etiology and Chapter 10 on Prevention.]

Shevell M (ed). *Neurodevelopmental Disabilities: Clinical and Scientific Foundations*. London: Mac Keith Press, 2009.

Thompson JR, Bryant B, Campbell EM, et al. *The Supports Intensity Scale*. Washington, DC: American Association on Intellectual and Developmental Disabilities, 2004.

53

Language Delays

James Coplan

I. **Description of the problem.**
- **Language** is a symbol system for the storage or exchange of information.
- **Expressive language** refers to the ability to generate symbolic output. This output may be either visual (picture exchange cards, signing, writing) or auditory (speech).
- **Receptive language** refers to the ability to decode (i.e., extract meaning from) the language output of others. Receptive language encompasses visual (visual schedules, sign language comprehension, reading) and auditory (listening comprehension) skills.
- **Speech** refers to the mechanical aspects of sound production (articulation, rate, rhythm, volume, pitch, and vocal quality).
- **Language disorders** encompass any defect in the ability to encode or decode information through symbolic means.
- **Speech disorders** encompass any deficit in the production of speech sounds. Children with disordered *language* (as in autistic spectrum disorder—*ASD*) may have normal *speech*. Conversely, children with disordered *speech* (as in hearing impairment, dysarthria, or stuttering) may have normal *language*.

A. **Epidemiology.** Delayed speech or language development are the most common developmental disorders of childhood, occurring in approximately 10% of preschool children (Table 53-1).

B. **Development of language.**
1. Language acquisition results from a complex interplay of innate biological capabilities and environmental stimulation. Infants acquire language through observation and through listening to speakers in their environment. Vocalizations during the first six months of life (cooing, laughing, monosyllabic and polysyllabic babbling) are biologically programmed; they are universal across all cultures, and occur even in infants who are deaf. By the latter half of the first year of life, a hearing infant's vocalizations begin to reflect the vocal repertoire of his or her caregivers, with selective refinement of some sounds (the guttural "ch" for Germanic and Semitic speakers, the rolling "r" in Spanish, etc.), and the pruning away of others. This is also the age when vocalizations begin to dwindle in an infant with congenital deafness.

2. By age 12 months, normal infants have grasped the notion that an arbitrary set of sounds symbolically *represent* a specific object or action; the arbitrary sound "bottle" not only produces a bottle (courtesy of the baby's caregiver), but the sound "bottle" also *means* bottle. Likewise, a 12-month-old knows that he or she can signify a desired object by pointing to it rather than reaching for it. This ability to represent objects or actions in symbolic form constitutes the central feature of language. Two-word phrases appear by age 24 months, and complete sentences by age 36 months. The ability to respond to common "wh" questions (who, what, when, where, and why) is fully developed by 48 months. That is also the age by which a child's speech should be completely understandable (even though the child may make minor articulation errors).

3. Some consider language development to be just one aspect of overall cognitive development, marked by a general ability to infer rules and causal relationships. Alternatively, language acquisition may represent a highly *modular* skill, emerging simultaneously with, but independently of, general cognitive ability. There are theoretical and clinical examples to support both views: In children with normal development or global delay (intellectual disability), language proficiency correlates closely with overall cognitive ability. On the other hand, there are many examples of children with normal overall cognitive ability but selective impairment of language (Developmental Language Disorder—*DLD*; see below), as well as children with superficially preserved language skills but broader evidence of general cognitive impairment (Williams Syndrome).

Table 53-1. Causes of delayed speech or language

Disorder	Prevalence (per 1,000 children)
Hearing loss (HL)	
• Permanent, profound	1–3
• Permanent, mild to moderate	3–10
• Intermittent, mild to moderate (otitis media with effusion*)	30–50?
Intellectual disability	30
Developmental language disorders (DLD)[†]	50
Autistic spectrum disorders (ASD)	10
Dysarthria[‡]	1–3

*Up to 25% of children have chronic/recurrent otitis media with effusion (OME) during the first 3 years of life. The "attack rate" for speech and language delay due to OME remains unknown.
[†]Focal impairment of brain systems serving language, with sparing of the rest of the central nervous system (CNS).
[‡]Usually encountered within the context of cerebral palsy.

C. Etiology of language delays.
   1. Environmental.
   - In a typical home environment, lack of stimulation is seldom, if ever, the cause of speech or language delay. Suggestions that such parents become "more stimulating" may do more harm than good, either by instilling parental guilt or by delaying a search for an underlying organic disorder as the basis for the child's delay.
   - Bilingual upbringing does not cause speech or language delay. The bilingual child may intermix the vocabularies of both languages, but total vocabulary size and length of utterance should be equivalent to those of a child reared in a monolingual environment.
   - Birth order or having an older sibling who "talks for the child" do not cause speech or language delay.
   - Social or environmental risk factors for delayed speech or language (e.g., poverty, lack of parental stimulation) are frequently intertwined with organic risk factors such as nutritional status, low-level lead exposure, low-grade iron deficiency, or parental genetic endowment (language disorders have a strongly genetic component). Thus, a child may receive a multifactorial "hit" to speech or language development. (Conversely, some children will be fortunate enough to get a multifactorial "boost" from these same genetic, nutritional, cultural, and environmental factors.)
   2. Organic. Speech or language delay may occur in isolation, as in the case of developmental language disorders (DLD), or may occur as one facet of some other disorder, such as hearing loss (HL), intellectual disability, autistic spectrum disorders (ASD), or dysarthria (physical impairment of oral motor movement, typically seen within the context of generalized upper motor neuron impairment, i.e., cerebral palsy). DLDs are clinically heterogeneous, and may involve some combination of phonologic development (speech sound production), semantics (meaning), syntax (sentence structure), and pragmatics (use of language as a tool for social interchange).
   3. Developmental.
   - Laziness, twinning, and tongue-tie do not cause language delay.
   - So-called twin speech is often indicative of the fact that *both twins* have an organically based language disorder, rather than a private language.
   - **"Constitutional delay"** implies a normal long-term developmental outcome. Although constitutional delay of speech acquisition exists, this is a diagnosis that can be established only in retrospect. If a preschool child's speech pattern is deficient based on comparison with age norms, then action is called for. Adopting a wait-and-see attitude in the hope that the child will "outgrow" the problem is inappropriate.
II. Making the diagnosis.
   A. Signs and symptoms. Parents may express concerns regarding "delayed speech." The practitioner must determine whether it is speech alone, or language that is delayed (Table 53-2). The pattern of speech and/or language delay, coupled with an appraisal of development in other domains (fine motor, adaptive, play, personal/social), will often suggest a specific developmental diagnosis. Note the value of visual language development (eye gaze, joint visual attention, gesture games, pointing) as a distinguishing feature: visual language development is delayed in children with intellectual disability and ASD but normal in children with HL, DLD, and dysarthria.

Table 53-2. Signs of speech or language delay by type of disability

	Language feature			
	Auditory expressive			
Disability	Content	Intelligibility	Auditory receptive	Visual
Hearing loss (HL)	↓	↓	Variable	Normal
Intellectual disability	↓	↓	Variable	↓
Developmental language disorders (DLD)	↓	↓	↓	Normal
Autistic spectrum disorders (ASD)	↓	Normal	↓	↓
Dysarthria	Variable	↓	Variable	Normal

Clarity of speech. Unfamiliar adult can understand 25% of a 1-year-old, 50% of a 2-year-old, 75% of a 3-year-old, and 100% of a 4-year-old.

B. **History.** A well-taken developmental history is the most important diagnostic measure. The language history should encompass auditory expressive, auditory receptive, and visual language milestones. The Early Language Milestone Scale (ELM Scale-2; see Appendix B) is one useful guide for normal language development in very young children. The developmental history should also cover general cognitive development (tool use, self-care skills), motor development, and personal–social development (social interaction with caregivers and peers, atypical behaviors such as insistence on routines or stereotypies).

C. **Physical examination.** Elements of the history and physical examination pertinent to the assessment of the child with language delay are listed in Table 53-3.

D. **Tests.**

1. **Office screening.** The ELM Scale-2 (Appendix B) screens language development from birth to age 36 months and intelligibility of speech from ages 24 to 48 months. It is designed for childcare professionals with varying degrees of expertise in early child development and demonstrates excellent test–retest and interobserver reliability. A good general developmental screening test is the Parents' Evaluation of Developmental Status (http://www.pedstest.com/). The M-CHAT (Modified Checklist for Autism in Toddlers) (http://www.firstsigns.org/) is a useful screening tool for atypicality (see Chapters 11 and 12).

2. **Hearing.** Office hearing screening procedures used by clinicians are prone to yield false-negative results or are inappropriate for the very young child. All children with

Table 53-3. Assessing the child with language delay

Medical history
- Teratogenic exposure (alcohol, prescription or recreational drugs)
- Fetal growth (weight, length, head circumference, and percentile values)
- Risk factors for HL (hearing loss) (neonatal intensive care unit; recurrent otitis media)

Developmental history
- Oromotor: Problems with sucking, swallowing, chewing, excess drooling
- Fine motor/adaptive: Age at acquisition of tool use (spoon, crayon)
- Language: Auditory expressive, auditory receptive, visual
- Play: Banging and mouthing (9 mo); casting (12 mo); stacking and dumping (14 mo); scribbles with crayons (16–18 mo); imitative play ("helps" with housework, 24 mo); make-believe (36 mo); rule-based play (board games; 48 mo)
- Personal/social: Eye contact; rigid behavior, stereotypical movements, fascination with certain objects, sensory issues

Family history
- Educational attainment of parents and siblings
- Language delay, hearing loss, or other developmental disability

Physical examination
- Length, weight, head circumference, and percentile values
- Dysmorphic features
- Submucous cleft palate/bifid uvula
- Neurocutaneous lesions
- Neurologic exam: Hyper- or hypotonia, hyperreflexia, cognitive level

speech or language delay should have their hearing tested by a certified audiologist, regardless of the clinician's subjective impression of how well the child seems to hear.

3. **Formal developmental testing.** Language, cognitive, and behavioral function should be assessed with an eye toward the following questions: (1) "What is the child's overall cognitive level, and is the child's language ability commensurate to his or her overall cognitive level?" (2) "Are there any atypical features (poor socialization, impaired pragmatics, repetitious behaviors or stereotyped movements, sensory aversions or attractions)?"

4. **Referral.** The primary care clinician should refer children with suspected language delays to their local early intervention clinician (typically administered via the county health department), or other resource (university clinic, speech/language pathologist, developmental pediatrician) for further evaluation and treatment. If the results are negative, everyone will be appropriately reassured; if the results are positive, developmental intervention can be implemented in a timely fashion.

5. **Medical assessment.** All children with speech or language delay need formal audiologic evaluation. Additional testing may include genetic and metabolic studies (in the case of intellectual disability or ASD). CNS (central nervous system) imaging and EEG (electroencephalogram) are seldom informative, the principal exception being children with autistic regression or Landau–Kleffner syndrome (epileptic aphasia).

E. **Prognosis.**

1. Children with speech or language delay due to DLD typically present with impaired intelligibility of speech and delayed emergence of single words, phrases, and sentences. Comprehension often appears normal, at least initially. Speech gradually improves, and most children become functional oral communicators by the time of school entry. As speech improves, underlying deficits in language production, comprehension, or central auditory processing (discrimination of speech in the presence of background noise) often become evident. Children with DLD are at increased risk for language-based learning disabilities. The prognosis for children with other causes speech or language delay (HL, intellectual disability, ASD, dysarthria) is a function of the severity of the primary disability.

III. **Management.**

A. **Primary goals.** The primary goal of management is to minimize frustration for the child and parents, while promoting optimal development of language. Table 53-4 lists suggestions for parents to provide a linguistically enriched environment.

B. **Reading aloud.** Information on reading-aloud programs is usually available through the local public library. Not infrequently, a recommendation that parents read aloud with their child will lead the clinician to discover that the parent is semiliterate or illiterate. A remedial reading program for the parent can sometimes be instituted in conjunction with the reading-aloud program for the child.

C. **Information for the family.** Do not rush to judgment, giving parents either false reassurance ("Don't worry, your child will grow out of it") or needless anxiety ("He or she will never be able to..."). On the other hand, do not procrastinate once the outcome seems clear. If there is a developmental disability, this should be explained to the parents in a straightforward yet compassionate manner. ("Why didn't our doctor tell us before now?" is a common complaint). Above all, listen to the family. ("We tried to tell our doctor there

---

Table 53-4. Do's and don'ts for parents to promote language development

Don't

Try to make your child speak; it's unhelpful and demoralizing.

Use complicated language. Instead, expand a little bit on whatever your child says (e.g., Child: "Cookie!" Parent: "Oh, you want a cookie.")

Criticize pronunciation or grammatical errors.

Do

Talk to your child. Narrate daily events as you do them (e.g., "Okay, now I'm cleaning the floor. Oh, it's dirty. Can you see the dirt?").

Respond whenever your child speaks. It's important to reward every utterance.

Ask your child a lot of questions (e.g., "What's that? Where should we put that?").

Accompany your words with gestures to make them more comprehensible.

Read books aloud to your child.

Keep communication fun!

was a problem, but the doctor wouldn't listen to us" is another equally common complaint.) Following identification of a developmental disorder, the primary care clinician serves a key role by ensuring that the consultants who are involved have appropriately explained the issues and by regularly monitoring the child and the family's progress. With the explosion of information available on the internet, there are specific resources and support groups for virtually all developmental disorders. Connecting the family to other parents of similarly affected children is a source of great strength and comfort to most families.

D. Treatment.

- Treatment of speech or language delay is primarily educational. Infants and toddlers up to age 36 months are typically served in home-based programs.
- Enrollment in a special education program administered by the child's school district is often the best option for children of age 36 months or older, since a classroom setting will provide not just language instruction but practical experience in the use of language in a social setting.
- For all children with speech or language disorders, the first priority is to enable the child to *communicate*—whether verbally or by some other means. Signing or picture card systems are commonly employed for children with severe speech delay due to DLD, as well as for children with ASD, who are typically visually oriented. Parents can be assured with confidence that signing does not delay speech. On the contrary, sign language exposure may actually promote oral language development.
- Language therapy for the child with intellectual disability will be integrated into an overall program stressing adaptive, play, and social development, in addition to language.
- Augmentative communication devices (picture boards, electronic communication devices) are also widely available for children with persistent, severe deficits of speech and language due to cognitive or motor impairment.
- Therapy for the child with HL will vary, depending on the degree of hearing loss, but may include some combination of orally based speech therapy plus signing, as well as amplification or cochlear implantation.
- Therapy for the child with ASD is multimodal, including intensive behavioral intervention, language therapy, and a program designed to enhance cognitive flexibility, social skills, and sensory processing (see Chapter 28).

IV. Clinical pearls and pitfalls.

- Parents may say, "My child's speech is delayed, but he understands everything," but they are frequently incorrect. The child with delayed speech often does not understand everything that is being said, but relies instead on contextual cues and set routines, or depends on the parents to break everything down into a series of one-step commands. These strategies may be highly adaptive for a child with limited comprehension, but the ability to follow even a very large number of one-step commands is no better than approximately 18–24 months, developmentally.
- Clinical detection of hearing loss, even severe to profound loss, is astonishingly difficult on physical examination, since children "cheat" by observing visual cues. If the child's speech or language is delayed, if the parents question hearing loss, or if there are elements in the medical history, family history, or physical examination that put the child at risk for HL, the clinician should get an audiogram, no matter how well the child seems to hear in the office.

BIBLIOGRAPHY

For parents

Beginning with Books. Information on reading aloud. Carnegie Library of Pittsburgh, Homewood Branch, 7101 Hamilton Avenue, Pittsburgh, PA 15208, 412-731-1717.

Hulit LM, Howard MR. *Born to Talk: An Introduction to Speech and Language Development*. Allyn & Bacon, Inc., Boston, MA, 2005.

Speech and Language; National Institute on Deafness and Other Communication Disorders: http://www.nidcd.nih.gov/health/voice/speechandlanguage.asp

For professionals

Batshaw ML, Pellegrino L, Roizen NJ (eds). *Children With Disabilities* (6th ed), Paul H. Brookes, Baltimore, MD, 2007.

Beukelman DR, Mirenda P. *Augmentative and Alternative Communication: Supporting Children and Adults With Complex Communication Needs*. Paul H. Brookes, Baltimore, MD, 2005.

Coplan J. *Making Sense of Autistic Spectrum Disorders*. New York: Bantam-Dell, 2010.

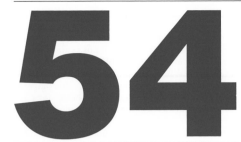

Lying, Cheating, and Stealing

Nerissa S. Bauer
Martin T. Stein

I. **Description of the problem.** The significance of three related behaviors in children—lying, stealing, and cheating—can be identified in the context of developmental tasks. Imagination and symbolic thinking in the preschool child followed by the formation of a conscience, understanding cause and effect, and self-esteem in a school-aged child determine and modulate the meaning of these behaviors. Every child lies and cheats at sometime, and many children steal something before adolescence. The challenge for the pediatric clinician is to unravel the significance of these events for an individual child—to clarify a normal developmental experience from disruptive, developmentally inappropriate misbehavior. These behaviors may be grouped under the general term: disruptive behavior disorders, but may have implications toward the development of *Diagnostic and Statistical Manual of Mental Disorders, Primary Care (DSM-PC)* disorders such as oppositional defiant disorder, conduct disorder, and attention-deficit/hyperactivity disorder (ADHD), especially if untreated or if it goes undiagnosed in its earliest stages.

A. **Epidemiology.**
1. These behaviors are seen occasionally in all children. A precise prevalence is unknown for the normal population.
2. Estimate of gender difference: three to four times more common in boys.
3. When occurring frequently in association with aggressive behaviors and impacting adversely on development and function:
   a. Oppositional defiant disorder: 2%–16%
   b. Conduct disorder: 6%–16% (males); 2%–9% (females)
   c. Significant stealing: 5%
4. Risk factors: inappropriate parental response to or unrealistic expectations for behavior, family disharmony, coercive discipline, difficult temperament, excessive exposure to violence (in home, community, television, movies), and cognitive deficiency.

B. **Familial transmission.** Both environmental and genetic components are found in the most severe forms when there is consideration of a disruptive behavior disorder.

C. **Etiology/contributing factors.**
1. **Environmental.** The child's immediate environment may be a contributing factor. When a preschool child expresses a developmentally appropriate "untruth," parental overreaction (e.g., expression of guilt or excessive discipline) may contribute to repetition of the behavior. Situational stress may come from school (recent change in grade, new school, bullying, or victimization), home (parental unemployment, poor housing conditions, parental illness, exposure to violence), or community (child abduction, natural disaster, violence in media).
2. **Developmental.** Temperament, the stable, individual differences in emotional reactivity, activity level, attention, and self-regulation may in some children be associated with excessive lying, stealing, and cheating. Both behavioral inhibition or low self-regulation and the "difficult child" may predispose to these behaviors especially in the context of a parent or teacher whose own temperament is not adaptable to the child.

   Characteristics of a developmental stage clarify many behaviors. In the 3- and 4-year-olds, an active imagination can generate "tall tales" or **"white lies."** They reflect developmentally appropriate processing of events. Young children often have a difficult time distinguishing between fantasy and reality during the toddler and preschool years. Young children cope with stressful situations by reflection—how a child wishes things were or how they should be. In the school-aged child, there is an awareness of societal expectations and the gradual emergence of a conscience (usually by the age of 8 years) with the cognitive and emotional maturity to differentiate a truth from an untruth. **Cheating** is seen occasionally in the school-aged child and more often in middle school. Winning games and academic success in school may overcome the child's sense of what is right and desire to be part of a team. Prior to the age of 7 years, children will often "bend" rules to win board games and not have a true understanding that rules are not to be broken. **Stealing** may begin with a toddler/preschool child whose actions are guided by egocentrism and who does not understand that taking something that does not belong to her is wrong. "What's mine is mine" and "What's yours is mine" is reflective of the typical mindset of these young children. In school-aged children, isolated stealing is usually an impulsive act. At this age and in middle school, stealing may develop out from the child's desire for possessions or a result of attention seeking or revenge. It may reflect poor parental role modeling or ill-defined rules/boundaries.

3. **Parenting and other role models.** Considering the frequency of lying, stealing, and cheating during early development, the parental response to an event is a critical factor. Each of these behaviors is a potential opportunity to teach a child about their role in society—a preschool child who steals a candy bar, a school-aged child who lies about a grade, or a middle school youth who cheats on an examination. The manner in which parents, teachers, and other adults respond to these events is important. In addition, the way parents live their own lives models significant behaviors for children each day.

4. **Organic:** Neurobehavioral disorders may be associated with poor self-regulation and lead to excessive lying, cheating, and stealing. It may be seen in children and youth with oppositional behaviors as a component of depression, anxiety, or conduct disorder. Genetic disorders and fetal drug exposure (e.g., fetal alcohol syndrome) may predispose to repetitive and chronic lying, cheating, or stealing.

II. **Making the diagnosis.** The assessment should take place in a supportive environment that allows for a thorough history and physical examination, review of pertinent supporting documents (i.e., teacher narratives, past psychoeducational testing), and time to address specific parental concerns. The pediatric clinician should (1) distinguish if the misbehavior is normal in terms of the child's overall cognitive development or abnormal; (2) evaluate potential risk or protective factors that may be contributing or can readily extinguish the misbehavior; and (3) provide guidance to parents that encompass both preventive, as well as, practical parenting strategies to be utilized "in the moment."

A. **Signs and symptoms.** Parents and clinicians usually (or eventually) know when a child has lied, cheated, or stolen something. The recognition of these behaviors begins the process of a behavioral diagnosis. An isolated symptom in the absence of other behavior problems or developmental delay suggests that the behavior may be consistent with normal developmental expectations. First and foremost, the pediatric clinician should obtain an understanding of the misbehavior in concrete terms, utilizing the ABC framework.

   a. Antecedent to misbehavior (any triggers or patterns)
   b. Behavior (concrete, discrete behavior)
   c. Consequence (parental response to misbehavior)

   Pediatric clinicians who rely upon this type of behavioral history taking framework will find it easier to understand the parent's perspective of the misbehavior, as well as, be better prepared to counsel the family on management. If parents have limited insight into the issue, asking the parent to describe the last time the misbehavior of concern occurred can help the clinician gather the necessary information.

   In addition to the specifics of the behavior, assessment should also include the following:
   • Developmental milestones with an emphasis on language, cognitive capacity, and social interactions. Developmental mastery at specific stages is protective against persistent disruptive behaviors.
   • Family role modeling and parental response to behaviors.
   • Experience with peers in context of social role models; peer pressure.
   • Educational achievement, including family and child's expectation for performance.
   • Low self-esteem.

B. **Differential diagnosis.** When the behaviors cannot be explained in the context of normal developmental stages, consider more pervasive type of disorders. Lying, cheating, and stealing may be associated with a specific behavioral disorder, including oppositional defiant disorder, conduct disorder, ADHD, anxiety, depression, posttraumatic stress disorder, an adjustment disorder, or pervasive developmental delay. Or it may be reflective of a child's lower cognitive functioning. These behaviors may reflect aggression manifested by words or actions that seem intended to harm another person or oneself. Lying, for example, is seen in bullying behavior and stealing may be a part of retaliatory or reactive behavior.

C. **History: key clinical questions.** Start with an inventory of possible risk and protective factors.

   1. **Individual risk factors.** Prenatal history (exposure to drugs, alcohol, cigarettes, lead), birth history (resuscitative events or prolonged neonatal intensive care unit

experience), quality of early attachment experiences, temperament (poor adaptability, distractible, intense reaction to change), immature social skills, vulnerable peer groups, developmental regression.

2. **Familial and relational risk factors.** Poor temperament match between parent and child, ineffective parenting practices, marital conflicts, parental separation, divorce, domestic violence, family history of psychopathology (e.g., alcoholism, depression) especially in parents, child abuse/neglect.

3. **Community factors.** Neighborhood and media violence exposure, availability of firearms.

4. **Protective factors/patient strengths.** Strong and stable social support in home or community, child's special talents, academic success, complimentary temperament of child and parents, parental warmth and sensitivity to child.

5. **For the family.**
   • *Has there been any major change or other stress in the life of the child or family?* Lying, cheating, or stealing may manifest as a new behavior after a significant shift in the child's life and may impact the ability to cope with a new situation or event. Assess the different environments—home: parental conflict, birth of a new sibling; school: change in school or poor adjustment to new academic level, problems with friends or bullying; community: exposure to negative role model, unstable parental employment.
   • *How often does the behavior occur?* If it happens infrequently, examine the circumstances immediately preceding, during, and following the event. *Does it occur only in certain settings?* Assess patterns in the behavior, including an increased intensity or severity. If the behavior is chronic, consider depression, anxiety, conduct disorder.
   • *How do the parents respond to the behavior?*

6. **For the child.** (it may be helpful to separate the child from the parent)
   • *What happened immediately before the event?*
   • *What were you feeling when you ....?* Assess motivation and insight.
   • *How did you feel afterwards?* Regret or remorse reflects moral development. Lack of remorse may indicate a conduct disorder.
   • *How do you feel about it now?*
   • *What makes you angry? What helps you to calm down?*
   • *How do you think you could have handled the situation differently?*

D. **Behavioral observation.** Observational data in the office may be helpful in assessment. Observe the child's interactions with the parent, with you, and during self-play. Note parental warmth and sensitivity toward the child, as well as affect of the parent. Parental mental health issues or ineffective and inconsistent parenting can inhibit/contribute to a parent's ability to adequately respond to a child. For instance, disruptive behaviors are more likely in children whose primary caregiver is depressed or in parents who model aggressive conflict resolution skills. A clinical assessment of temperament as well as activity level, impulsivity, affect, cognitive functioning, and social responses should be recorded. Observed behaviors should be interpreted in the context of the child's developmental stage.

E. **Tests.** To determine the contextual aspect of the behaviors, a daily behavioral diary (following the ABC framework) is useful. For a 1–2-week period, request a recording of the antecedents to the behavior (what was going on), the behavior (what the child did or said), and the consequences (what happened after the event). Clues to specific diagnoses associated with these behaviors will surface during a comprehensive behavioral–developmental and family history. In specific situations, behavioral questionnaires or psychoeducational testing may define the problem with greater precision.

III. **Management.**

A. **Information for the family.** Educating the family is the initial step toward effective collaboration with the pediatrician. When addressing negative behavioral issues, begin the discussion by pointing out the patient's and family's strengths. Guide parents to an understanding of how these qualities support a positive outcome. Framing the behavior in context of developmental principles should lead to an understanding of the behavior and insight into the child's temperament, motivation, and responses to the environment. Discuss the child and family vulnerabilities that may be associated with the behaviors.

B. **Helpful behavioral management tips for the family.**

1. **Prevention.** Parents can be taught positive parenting strategies that focus on building a trusting relationship with the child that promotes a child's self-esteem, healthy conscience, and open parent–child communication.
   • Praise the child's efforts early and often. Remind parents to foster positive self-esteem by encouraging the child to try things and focus on the process and not the

end product. Children who receive immediate and specific praise for small steps in the right direction when learning new or complex behaviors will more likely internalize these pronouncements and feel good about their actions. They will come to readily understand parental expectations between acceptable, desired behaviors and less desired ones.

- Have realistic expectations of the child's behavior. Pediatricians can help promote an understanding of normal child development and abilities during well child visits.
- Parents can jumpstart a young child's healthy development of emotional self-regulation and empathy by commenting on the child's feelings during toddler-hood/preschool age. Children can be taught to express their emotions in verbal ways, rather than outwardly showing frustration or other negative emotions. These children will more likely be able to articulate their feelings more freely. When parents validate a child's emotions, it fosters the development of empathy and compassion.
- Role model acceptable behavior. Parents are their children's first teachers—this includes modeling appropriate verbal and nonverbal behavior.
- Reward appropriate behavior with low-cost or no-cost rewards (such as extra story at bedtime, snuggle time with a parent, going to the park) and/or social reinforcers (such as hugs, kisses and specific and immediate praise).

2. **Capitalize on teachable moments.**
   a. **Lying.** Consider the context in which it occurs and do not accuse or label the child as a "liar." The 3–4-year-old child processes experience with magical, egocentric thinking; the preschool child is in the early stage of understanding right from wrong. By 8 or 9 years of age, the conscience is more developed and becomes an internal moral guide. Help parents to use this knowledge to respond to their child. After an episode of lying, discuss the reasons for the behavior in an open manner. Reassure the child you will always love her. Reassurance can help ease a child's anxieties and help her share feelings and reasons for lying. Parents should be counseled to not set up a child for lying. If a parent wants the child to "confess" or admit to a known misbehavior, parents should be advised to bring up the issue upfront rather than start the conversation as an open-ended question. For instance, if a child misbehaved at school and the teacher contacted the parent, the parent should openly discuss this with the child, rather than leading off with a question as the child may not openly admit to any wrong-doings—leading to parental frustration.
   b. **Stealing.** A clear explanation about possessions and the concept of ownership should be given to the child. Firm limits and logical consequences should be in place. Modeling appropriate behavior and instituting consistent discipline in response, such as "let us return the toy back to Johnnie" or "let us go say sorry and pay for the candy" should be used. Do not overreact since this may frighten the child. Parents should begin to talk about ownership, sharing, and asking for what he or she wants as early as toddler age. If stealing is repetitive, seek additional help.
   c. **Cheating.** Parents can talk about how cheating hurts other people's feelings and ask the child if there is a better solution. Approach the child in a gentle manner and refrain from harsh punishment. Explain consequences in a calm, matter-of-fact way. If cheating is repetitive, closer examination into reasons for cheating should be performed (e.g., low self-esteem, learning disabilities, low impulse control) and/or seek additional help.

C. **Anticipatory guidance.**
   1. Ineffective parenting styles can be addressed in the context of helping to prevent ongoing escalations of disruptive behavior.
   2. Exposure to violence in the media should be decreased because it reduces restraints on aggressive behavior, desensitizes the response to viewing violence, and distorts a child's emerging understanding about appropriate conflict resolution.
   3. Availability of firearms, especially when in the home of a child with significant disruptive behaviors, should be discussed. Options for the removal or proper storage to ensure safety of the individual should be outlined.

D. **Treatment.** If a neurobehavioral condition is discovered, the intervention should be based on the specific diagnosis (i.e., conduct disorder depression, obsessive compulsive disorder, anxiety, ADHD).

E. **Criteria for referral.**
   1. When lying, cheating, or stealing is frequent and not responsive to education and behavior management, consider referral to a mental health professional.
   2. Domestic violence or child abuse should be reported to an appropriate agency as mandated by law.

3. Ongoing parent–child conflicts, a significant temperament mismatch, or underlying psychopathology should be managed concurrently with a mental health professional.
4. Social issues such as parental unemployment and lack of adequate childcare may be addressed by referral to a social worker or case manager involved with a community-based organization.

BIBLIOGRAPHY

For parents

Brazelton TB, Sparrow JD. *Touchpoints: Three to Six: Your Child's Emotional and Behavioral Development*. Cambridge, MA: Perseus Books, 2001.

Pruitt DB (ed). *Your Child: What Every Parent Needs to Know About Childhood Development from Birth to Preadolescence*. New York, NY: Harper Collins, 1998.

Spock B, Needlman R. *Dr. Spock's Baby and Child Care* (8th ed), New York, NY: Simon & Schuster Adult Publishing Group, Pocket Books, 2004.

Webster-Stratton C. *The Incredible Years: A Troubleshooting Guide for Parents of Children Aged 2–8 Years*. Seattle, WA: The Incredible Years, 2005.

For professionals

Dixon SD, Stein MT. *Encounters with Children: Pediatric Behavior and Development* (4th ed), Philadelphia, PA: Mosby Elsevier, 2006.

55

Masturbation

Ilgi Ozturk Ertem
John M. Leventhal

I. **Description of the problem.** The World Health Organization (WHO) defines sexual health as the "integration of the somatic, emotional, intellectual, and social aspects of sexual being, in ways that are positively enriching and that enhance personality, communication, and love." The clinician should view childhood sexuality as an integral part of child development as are physical health, growth, and other developmental domains. It is within this framework that the clinician should address parental concern with masturbation, one of the early manifestations of the sexual development of the child.

- The term *masturbation* is derived from the Latin words for "hand" (*manus*) and "defilement" (*stupratio*). It is defined as a deliberate self-stimulation that results in sexual arousal.
- At least since the time of Hippocrates (400 BC), masturbation has evoked negative attitudes within societies. For example, during the 18th century, two-thirds of all human illnesses were attributed to masturbation. Various treatment regimens, such as disciplining the patient, mechanical preventions, cautery of genitals, clitorectomy, and castration, were established and practiced until the mid-20th century. It is still true that parents' and teachers' responses to sexual behavior in children are largely influenced by cultural patterns. Some societies condone and encourage self-stimulation during childhood; others condemn it. In general, Western societies take a more restrictive view of masturbation. Childhood masturbation is not included as a specific psychiatric disorder in the *Diagnostic and Statistical Manual of Mental Disorders (4th edition)*. The WHO places excessive childhood masturbation under "Other specified behavioral and emotional disorders with onset usually occurring in childhood and adolescence" in the *International Statistical Classification System of Diseases and Related Health Problems 10th edition (ICD-10)*.

A. **Epidemiology.** Masturbation is universal and may start as early as infancy. Normative studies of sexual behavior have shown that approximately 16% of children aged 2–5 years of both sexes masturbate with their hand, and that almost all boys and 25% of girls have masturbated to the point of orgasm by age 15 years.

B. **Environmental, developmental, and transactional factors in etiology.** Masturbatory activity has been observed in the male fetus in utero. In the first months of life, infants of both sexes learn to experience the sensations associated with diapering and the cleansing of genitals. A developmental progression toward adult erotic responsiveness proceeds from these early pleasurable sensations. This includes the differentiation and appreciation of genitals, inclusion of sexual parts in the body concept, "exhibitionism" to test adult reactions, mastery of a variety of self-elicited sensations, and the integration of sexual function into the emerging self-concept.

C. **Signs and symptoms.** Masturbatory activity in older children may resemble that of adults and involves handling or rubbing of genitals, sweating, flushing, tachypnea, and muscular contractions. Masturbatory activity in infants and toddlers typically does not involve handling of the genitals and may therefore make the diagnosis difficult. More typically masturbation in infants involves: stereotyped posturing of the lower extremities; pressing and rubbing on the perineum or suprapubic area; leaning the suprapubic region on a firm edge; stiffening of the lower extremities; rocking movements in various positions; symptoms of sexual arousal including sweating, brief bouts of crying, intermittent grunting, irregular breathing, facial flushing, and diaphoresis. These episodes may last from a few seconds to several hours. At any age, there should be no alteration of consciousness; the child should stop when distracted.

II. **Making the diagnosis.**

A. **Differential diagnosis.**

1. **Masturbatory actions may be misdiagnosed as seizures** because of the abrupt onset of the episodes, the tonic posturing, facial flushing, irregular breathing, and the child's preoccupation. During masturbation, there may also be blank stares or tremulous movements. The child may resume his or her previous play or activity after the event

or may appear drowsy and fall asleep, mimicking children in the postictal phase. Tonic posturing with crossing of the thighs has been reported to occur as early as 3 months of age. Masturbatory activity in children has been associated with unnecessary investigations for organic disease such as seizures, epilepsy, paroxysmal dystonia, carcinoid syndrome, or urinary tract infections. The symptoms of masturbation also have been confused with abdominal pain or the "retentive" posturing that occurs in children who withhold stool. This is manifested as episodic tightening of the buttock and thighs, often accompanied by facial flushing and grunting.

2. **The clinician should consider the diagnosis of sexual abuse** in children with compulsive masturbation, especially if accompanied by other sexualized behaviors. The term compulsive, or excessive masturbation has not been well defined. The following uncommon sexualized behaviors should alert the clinician to the possibility of sexual abuse: obsessive masturbation with or without pleasure and with decreased interest in other activities, masturbation causing pain, using objects against own or other child's genitals/anus, attempting to make an adult touch the child's genitals or touching a child/adult's genitals using hand or mouth, inserting tongue in mouth when kissing.

B. **History: key clinical questions.** A thorough history is the key to an appropriate diagnosis and effective management. Since masturbation is not harmful, it should be considered a problem only when it causes distress to the child, parental anxiety, or social condemnation.

1. *"Tell me what you've noticed about your child's touching his or her genitals. Where does this happen? In school? At home?"* This elicits the method the child uses and the frequency and the context in which the child engages in masturbation and other sexualized behaviors.

2. Parents have different thoughts and feelings when their children touch their own genitals. *"Can you tell me how it is for you? What do you do when this happens?"* The meaning of masturbatory behavior to the parents and their responses to the behavior should be understood.

3. *"When you respond like that, how do you think he or she feels?"* The parents' perceptions of the consequences of their responses and the outcome of the behavior are important.

4. Are there any significant stressors for family and/or child, and/or developmental delays?

C. **Physical examination.** Clinical circumstances may dictate exploration of a more pathologic interpretation of the masturbatory behaviors. It should be noted that masturbation and physical illness can co-occur. Masturbation may begin with genital irritation or discomfort due to rashes, diaper dermatitis, urinary tract or parasitic infections. If the behavior is especially compulsive or of acute onset, consider the possibility of sexual abuse. A child who has been sexually abused may have physical findings suggestive of or consistent with genital trauma. Also, children may insert objects in their genitalia during sex play. Therefore, the anus, genitalia, and perineum should be examined as part of a general physical examination.

D. **Tests.** Laboratory tests are almost never required during a work-up for masturbation. However, causes of irritation such as pinworm infestations or urinary tract infections will require appropriate diagnosis and treatment. Home-video recordings have been shown to be effective in the evaluation of paroxysmal events in children. The widespread availability of home-video recordings may provide the opportunity to examine in detail the child's activity and may prevent the use of unnecessary investigations and referrals.

III. **Management.**

A. **Anticipatory guidance.** A clinician who, from the beginning of a relationship with parents, is open to discussing issues of sexuality is more likely to receive questions about sexual development, behaviors, and problems as the child grows older. Parents are less likely to be anxious, confused, or scornful of masturbatory behavior in their child if they have been told in advance that this behavior is normal, universal, and healthy. Such anticipatory guidance should be offered early in life, when infants begin to explore their bodies. During a review of developmental milestones or during a genital examination, parents can be asked in a matter-of-fact manner whether their child has discovered his or her genitals and whether he or she plays with them. Parental feelings and attitudes can then be explored and information on how they would react to the situation can be obtained.

B. **When masturbation is viewed as a problem behavior.**

• The clinician should not simply dismiss parental concerns about the issue by flatly stating that "masturbation is normal." Rather he or she should attempt to understand the level of parental discomfort and the social and psychological consequences of the behavior for the child, with the goals of alleviating parental anxiety and diminishing feelings of fear, anxiety, guilt, and shame in the child.

- A detailed history will not only establish the diagnosis but also give the parents a chance to discuss their fears and worries. Examples of parental concerns include the fear that their child has an organic disease, has been sexually abused, is experiencing conflict with a family member or teacher/caretaker, will develop promiscuity, or will be mentally handicapped. The masturbatory behavior may evoke a parent's own conflicts about sexuality, and the parent may withdraw attention and/or affection from the child. In the majority of cases, after such concerns and attitudes are explored, reassurance will be sufficient.
- Parents should be advised not to overreact to the child's behavior. It should be emphasized that punishing and scolding can be harmful to the child's self-esteem and long-term sexual development.
- Parents can tell their preschool child that masturbation is a private behavior that is best not done in public (e.g., *"There are some things that we do around other people. This is one of the things that we do in private"*).
- Behavioral modification techniques, such as positive reinforcement, have been helpful in cases of compulsive masturbation (especially in children with mental retardation).

C. Criteria for referral.
Refer to developmental–behavioral pediatric specialist if:
- When appropriate counseling by the clinician elicits complaints by the parents that the **child is in psychologic distress.**
- When **unusual manifestations or excessive masturbation impede self-esteem** and adaptive functioning of the child and/or cause social problems.
- When **other family or interpersonal pathology** is recognized by the clinician to contribute to the problem.
- When there are accompanying **developmental/behavioral or affective disturbances** in the child.

Refer to child neurology specialist if: History or physical examination indicates diagnostic work-up for seizures or paroxysmal movement disorders.
Refer to child abuse specialist if: History or physical examination indicates diagnostic work-up for child abuse.

BIBLIOGRAPHY

For parents

American Academy of Pediatrics Patient Education Online. Talking with Your Young Child About Sex. http://patiented.aap.org/content.aspx?aid=5063
University of Michigan Health System. Your Child Topics. Masturbation. http://www.med.umich.edu/yourchild/topics/masturb.htm
What Kids Want to Know about Sex and Growing Up. From Children's Television Workshop, One Lincoln Plaza, New York, NY 10023.

For professionals

Friedrich WN, Grambsch P, Broughton D, et al. Normative sexual behavior in children. *Pediatrics* 88:456–464, 1991.
Kellogg ND and the AAP Committee on Child Abuse and Neglect. Clinical report—the evaluation of sexual behaviors in children. *Pediatrics* 124:992–998, 2009.
Mallants C, Casteels K. Practical approach to childhood masturbation–a review. *Eur J Pediatr* 167:1111–1117, 2008.
Nieto JA. Children and adolescents as sexual beings: cross-cultural perspectives. *Child Adolesc Psychiatr Clin N Am* 13:461–477, 2004.
Schoentjes E, Deboutte D, Friedrich W. Child sexual behavior inventory: a Dutch-speaking normative sample. *Pediatrics* 104:885–893, 1999.
Wolf DS, Singer HS. Pediatric movement disorders: an update. *Curr Opin Neurol* 21:491–496, 2008.

Motor Delays

Peter A. Blasco

I. **Description of the problem.** Delayed motor milestones are the highest-ranked concern of parents with children between ages 6–12 months. Related complaints include vague references to tone abnormalities ("too stiff" or "too weak"), perceived structural abnormalities (most commonly the legs or feet), or an awkward/clumsy gait in the ambulating child.

   A. **Epidemiology.**
- The prevalence of significant motor delays in the general pediatric population is not established. By statistical definition, 2%–3% of infants will fall outside the range of normal motor milestone attainment. A minority of these milestone-delayed children (15%–20%) will prove to have a significant neuromotor diagnosis, most commonly cerebral palsy or a birth defect, rarely some progressive nervous system or muscle disease.
- Early motor delays in the remainder of children often represent a marker for subtle neurologic dysfunction, which manifests itself more definitively in later childhood as troublesome awkwardness (now referred to diagnostically as *developmental coordination disorder*), attention deficit syndromes, and/or specific learning disabilities.

II. **Making the diagnosis.**

   A. **Evaluation.** The clinician should organize data gathered from the history, physical examination, and neurodevelopmental examination into three domains: motor developmental milestones, the classic neurologic examination, and markers of cerebral neuromotor maturation (primitive reflexes and postural reactions).

     1. **Motor milestones** are extracted from the developmental history, as well as from observations during the neurodevelopmental examination (Tables 56-1 and 56-2). Milestone assessment is best summarized as a single (or narrow) motor age for the child. The

Table 56-1. Gross motor development timetable

Prone	
Head up	1 mo
Chest up	2 mo
Up on elbows	3 mo
Up on hands	4 mo
Rolling	
Front to back	3–5 mo
Back to front	4–5 mo
Sitting	
Sit with support ("tripod" sitting)	5 mo
Sit without support	7 mo
Get up to sit (unassisted)	8 mo
Walking	
Pull to stand	8–9 mo
Cruise	9–10 mo
Walk with 2 hands held	10 mo
Walk with 1 hand held	11 mo
Walk alone	12 mo
Run (stiff-legged)	15 mo
Walk up stairs (with rail)	21 mo
Jump in place	24 mo
Pedal tricycle	30 mo
Walk down stairs, alternating feet	3 yr

Table 56-2. Fine motor development timetable

Retain ring (rattle)	1 mo
Hands unfisted	3 mo
Reach	3–4 mo
Hands to midline	3–4 mo
Transfer	5 mo
Take 1-in. cube	5–6 mo
Take pellet (crude grasp)	6–7 mo
Immature pincer	7–8 mo
Mature pincer	10 mo
Release	12 mo

motor age can be converted to a motor quotient (MQ) giving a simple expression of deviation from the norm: MQ = motor age/chronologic age × 100.

An MQ above 70 is considered within normal limits. Those falling in the 50–70 range are suspicious and deserve further evaluation (although most of these children will turn out to be normal). An MQ below 50 is unequivocally abnormal and warrants subspecialty referral.

2. **Neurologic examination.** Motor milestones are purely measures of function and do not take into account the *quality* of a child's movement. The motor portion of the **neurologic examination** includes assessments of tone (passive resistance), strength (active resistance), deep tendon reflexes, and coordination plus observations of station and gait. The best clues often come from observation, not handling.

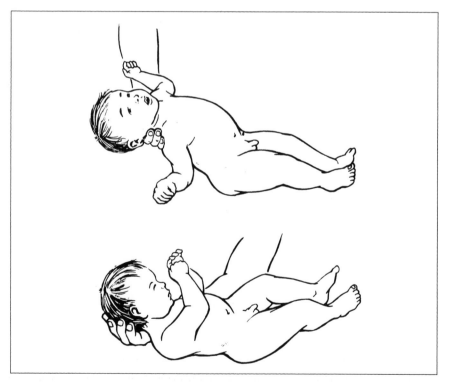

Figure 56-1. Tonic Labyrinthine Reflex. In the Supine Position, the Baby's Head is Gently Extended to About 45 Degrees Below Horizontal. This Produces Relative Shoulder Retraction and Leg Extension, Resulting in the "Surrender Posture." With Head Flexion to About +45 Degrees, the Arms Come Forward (Shoulder Protraction) and the Legs Flex. (From Blasco PA. Normal and abnormal motor development. *Pediatr Rounds* 1(2):1–6, 1992.)

    a. Tone. Spontaneous postures (e.g., frog legs seen with hypotonia or scissoring with spasticity) provide visual clues to tone abnormalities.

    b. Strength. Spontaneous or prompted motor activities (e.g., weight bearing in sitting or standing) require adequate strength. A classic example is the Gower's sign (arising from floor sitting to standing using the hands to "walk up" one's legs), which indicates pelvic girdle and quadriceps muscular weakness.

    c. Station refers to the posture assumed in sitting or standing and should be viewed from anterior, lateral, and posterior perspectives, looking for body alignment.

    d. Gait refers to walking and is examined in progress. Initially, the toddler walks on a wide base, slightly crouched, with the arms abducted and elevated a bit. Forward progression is more staccato than smooth. Movements gradually become more fluid, the base narrows, and arm swing evolves, leading to an adult pattern of walking by the age of 3 years.

3. Primitive reflexes are movement patterns that develop during the last trimester of gestation and gradually disappear between 3 and 6 months after birth. Each requires a specific sensory stimulus to generate the stereotyped motor response.

    The Moro, tonic labyrinthine, asymmetric tonic neck, and positive support reflexes are the most clinically useful (Figs. 56-1–56-3). Normal babies and infants demonstrate these postures inconsistently and transiently, whereas those with neurologic

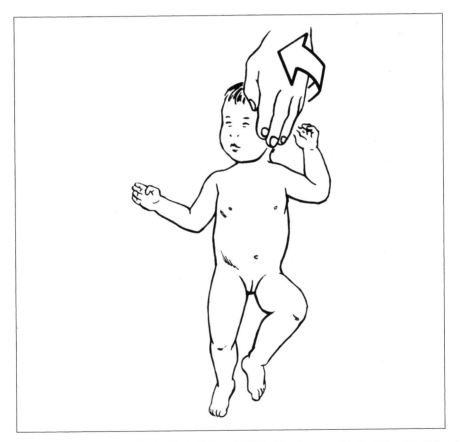

Figure 56-2. Asymmetric Tonic Neck Reflex (ATNR). The Sensory Limb of the ATNR Involves Proprioceptors in the Cervical Vertebrae. With Active or Passive Head Rotation, the Baby Extends the Arm and Leg on the Face Side and Flexes the Extremities on the Occiput Side (the "Fencer Posture"). There is also Some Mild Paraspinous Muscle Contraction on the Occiput Side Producing Subtle Trunk Curvature. (From Blasco PA. Normal and abnormal motor development. *Pediatr Rounds* 1(2):1–6, 1992.)

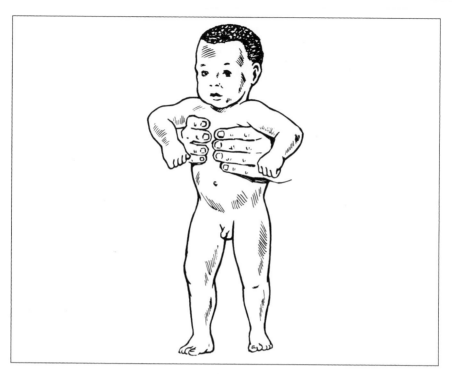

Figure 56-3. Positive Support Reflex. With Support Around the Trunk, the Infant is Suspended and Then Lowered to Pat the Feet Gently on a Flat Surface. This Stimulus Produces Reflex Extension at the Hips, Knees, and Ankles so the Subject Stands Up, Completely or Partially Bearing Weight. Children May Go Up on Their Toes Initially but Should Come Down onto Flat Feet Within 20–30 Seconds Before Sagging Back Down Toward a Sitting Position. (From Blasco PA. Normal and abnormal motor development. *Pediatr Rounds* 1(2):1–6, 1992.)

dysfunction show stronger and more sustained primitive reflex posturing. Although primitive reflexes are somewhat tricky to gauge, even in expert hands, the clinician should keep attuned to the following four factors:

    a. Some form of primitive reflex response should be clearly elicitable in the newborn through ages 2–3 months.

    b. Symmetry of response is important, especially with the Moro.

    c. An obligatory primitive reflex is abnormal at any time. This is the situation where the child remains "stuck" in the primitive reflex posture as long as the stimulus is imposed and breaks free only when the stimulus is removed.

    d. Visible primitive reflexes **should no longer be present after ages 6–8** months.

    4. Postural reactions consist of counter movements, which are much less stereotyped than the primitive reflexes and involve a complex interplay of cerebral and cerebellar cortical adjustments to a barrage of proprioceptive, visual, and vestibular sensory inputs. They are not present at birth but sequentially develop between ages 2–10 months. Postural reactions are sought in each of the three major categories: righting, protection, and equilibrium (Fig. 56-4). Although easy to elicit in the normal infant, they are markedly slower in their appearance in the baby with nervous system damage.

  B. Classification of motor impairments.

    1. Static central nervous system (CNS) disorders indicate some type of nonprogressive brain damage. The insult may have arisen during early fetal development, resulting in a CNS anomaly. Alternatively, a brain developing in a normal fashion can be damaged before, during, or after birth by a wide variety of infectious, traumatic, and other insults. When a motor impairment is due to a brain anomaly or a static lesion that occurs before cerebral maturation is complete (roughly age 16 years), the neuromotor

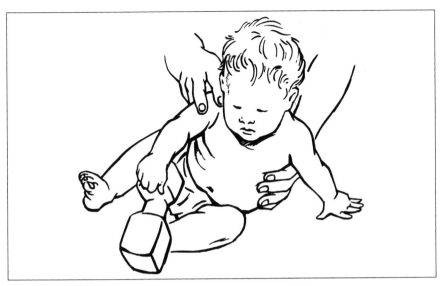

Figure 56-4. Postural Reactions. The Infant is Comfortably Seated, Supported About the Waist if Necessary. The Examiner Gently Tilts the Child to One Side Noting Righting of the Head Back Toward the Midline (Coming in at 2–3 Months), Protective Extension of the Arm Toward the Side (Coming in at 6–7 Months), and Equilibrium Counter Movements of the Arm and Leg on the Opposite Side (Appearing at 5–6 Months). (From Blasco PA. Normal and abnormal motor development. *Pediatr Rounds* 1(2):1–6, 1992.)

disorder is referred to as *cerebral palsy*. This group represents the largest number of children with disabling motor problems.

2. **Progressive diseases** of the brain, spinal cord, peripheral nerves, or muscles produce motor impairment that worsens with time (e.g., Duchenne muscular dystrophy, Werdnig-Hoffman spinal muscular atrophy, nervous system tumors). Children with progressive conditions initially experience a period of normal or near-normal development. Evidence of a progressive disease is determined by careful history and/or by repeated examinations over time. The fraction of all motor-impaired children with progressive diseases is small. Uncovering the specific diagnosis helps one anticipate the rate of progression, provides other prognostic information, and forms the basis for accurate genetic counseling.

3. **Spinal cord and peripheral nerve disorders** are almost all static conditions. The exceptions are rare instances of an intrinsic spinal cord tumor, progressive extrinsic compression syndromes, and rare neurogenetic degenerations primarily involving spinal cord tracts or peripheral nerves (e.g., the *hereditary motor and sensory neuropathies*). The largest single group in this category consists of children with myelodysplasia.

4. **Structural defects** refer to conditions in which an anatomical structure is missing or deformed (e.g., a limb deficiency) or in which the support tissues for nerves and muscles are inadequate (e.g., connective tissue defects, abnormal bones). On the mildest end of the spectrum, there exist a wide variety of fairly common orthopedic deformities, which may or may not affect early motor milestones (club feet, developmental hip dysplasia, etc.). More severe disorders in this category include osteogenesis imperfecta and some varieties of childhood arthritis.

III. **Management.** Ensuring an accurate primary diagnosis is fundamental to determining therapy. Neuroimaging, other neurodiagnostic studies, and/or metabolic and genetic tests may be needed. Direct treatment for the child with a motor disability falls into five categories: (1) counseling and support for the child and family, (2) hands-on therapy, (3) assistive devices, (4) medication, and (5) surgery. A multidisciplinary subspecialty team should be consulted to provide state-of-the-art diagnostic evaluation, treatment services, and counseling. Professionals skilled in different disciplines need to work together and *in concert with the parents*. The primary clinician's roles include seeing to the patient's general health, monitoring overall development, helping the child and family to cope with many stresses (especially at anniversary and transition times), promoting the child's self-esteem and long-term adaptation to disability, and helping parents keep the multitude of subspecialty inputs in perspective.

BIBLIOGRAPHY

For parents

Geralis E. *Children with Cerebral Palsy: A Parent's Guide* (2nd ed), Bethesda, MD: Woodbine House, 1998.

For professionals publications

Blasco PA. Normal and abnormal motor development. *Pediatr Rounds* 1(2):1–6, 1992. (Available from the author).

Shapiro BK, Gwynn H. Neurodevelopmental assessment of infants and young children. In Accardo PJ (ed), *Neurodevelopmental Disabilities of Infancy and Young Childhood: Volume 1 Neurodevelopmental Diagnosis and Treatment.* Baltimore, MD: Brookes, 2008, 367–382.

Web sites

Pathways Awareness Foundation. www.pathwaysawareness.org
Exceptional Parents. www.exceptionalparents.org/

57

Neglect

Howard Dubowitz

I. **Description of the problem.** Child neglect is usually defined as **parental omissions in care, resulting in actual or potential harm to a child**. Child Protective Services (CPS) typically requires evidence of harm, unless the risks are serious (such as when very young children are left home alone). Some states exclude situations attributed to poverty.

An alternative and broader view of neglect is from a child's perspective, defining neglect as **occurring when a child's basic needs are not adequately met**. Basic needs include adequate healthcare, food, clothing, shelter, supervision/protection, emotional support, education, and nurturance. However, it is often difficult to establish at what point any of these needs are "adequately" met and thresholds may be rather arbitrary. Usually, the "neglect" label is applied to clearly worrisome circumstances. Less serious circumstances may still require intervention, perhaps without labeling them as "neglect."

There are several advantages to this child-focused definition. It fits with the broad goal of ensuring children's health and safety. It is less blaming and more constructive. It draws attention to other contributors to the problem (discussed later) aside from parents, and encourages a broader range of interventions. Clearly, many neglect situations may require intervention (e.g., a child with failure to thrive due to an inadequate diet) but may not warrant or meet criteria for CPS involvement. Practitioners, however, need to be aware of the laws and regulations in their area and factor these into their practice.

A. **Epidemiology.** Neglect is the most common form of child maltreatment, accounting for almost two-thirds of all cases reported annually to CPS. It was a factor in approximately 70% of the estimated 1760 deaths due to child maltreatment in 2007. Because of ambiguity in diagnostic criteria and underreporting, accurate prevalence data are impossible to determine. One study in 2010 identified 30.6 cases of neglect per 1000 (or 2,251,600) children in the population, but it is likely that these are very conservative estimates, as neglect is a problem that frequently occurs "behind closed doors."

B. **Manifestations of possible neglect.** Aside from direct observation, the possibility of "neglect" should be considered in the following circumstances:
   - Noncompliance (nonadherence) with healthcare recommendations
   - Delay or failure in obtaining medical, mental health, or dental care
   - Hunger, failure to thrive, and unmanaged morbid obesity
   - Drug-exposed newborns and older children
   - Exposure to hazards in the home: ingestions, recurrent injuries, exposure of children with pulmonary disease to second-hand smoke, access to guns, and exposure to intimate partner violence
   - Exposure to hazards outside the home, failure to use car seat/belt, and not wearing bike helmet
   - Emotional concerns (e.g., excessive quietness or apathy in a toddler), behavior issues (e.g., repetitive movements), learning problems (especially if not being addressed), and extreme risk-taking behavior (*may* reflect inadequate nurturance, affection, or supervision)
   - Inadequate hygiene, contributing to medical problems
   - Inadequate clothing, contributing to medical problems
   - Educational needs not being met
   - Abandoned children
   - Homelessness

C. **Etiology.** There are often multiple *and* interacting contributors to child neglect, including the following:
   - *Child*: disability, chronic illness, prematurity, difficult behaviors, or temperament
   - *Parent*: depression, substance abuse, low IQ, limited nurturing as a child
   - *Family*: intimate partner violence, father uninvolved, many children in the family
   - *Community*: social isolation, violence, lack of treatment or support programs
   - *Society:* poverty, lack of health insurance

D. General principles for assessing possible neglect. The heterogeneity of neglect precludes specifying how to assess for the array of possible circumstances. Instead, the following general principles and questions are a guide.

- Given the complexity and possible ramifications of determining that a child is being neglected, an interdisciplinary assessment is ideal, including input from professionals involved with the family.
- Verbal children should be separately interviewed, at an appropriate developmental level. Possible questions include: *"Who do you go to if you're feeling sad? Who helps you if you have a problem? What happens when you feel sick?"*
- Do the circumstances indicate that the child's need(s) is not being adequately met? Is there evidence of actual harm? Is there evidence of potential harm and on what basis?
- What is the nature of the neglect?
- Is there a pattern of neglect? Are there indications of other forms of neglect, or abuse? Has there been prior CPS involvement?
- A child's safety is a paramount concern. What is the risk of imminent harm, and of what severity?
- What is contributing to the neglect? Consider factors listed under the section Etiology.
- What strengths/resources are there? This is as important as identifying problems.
  - Child (e.g., child wants to play sports, requiring better health)
  - Parent (e.g., parent wants to keep child out of the hospital)
  - Family (e.g., other family members willing to help)
  - Community (e.g., programs for parents, families)
- What interventions have been tried, with what results? Knowing the nature of the interventions can be useful, including from the parent's perspective. What has the pediatric clinician done to address the problem?
- Assess the possibility of other children in the household also being neglected.
- What is the prognosis? Is the family motivated to improve the circumstances and accept help, or resistant? Are suitable resources, formal and informal, available?

E. General principles for addressing child neglect.
- Convey concerns to family, kindly but forthrightly. Avoid blaming.
- Be empathic and state interest in helping, or, suggest another pediatric clinician.
- Address contributory factors, prioritizing those most important and amenable to being remedied (e.g., recommending treatment for a mother's depression). Parents may need their problems addressed to enable them to adequately care for their children. Parent training programs can be helpful.
- Begin with least intrusive approach, usually not CPS.
- Establish specific objectives (e.g., diabetes will be adequately controlled), with measurable outcomes (e.g., urine dipsticks, hemoglobin A1c). Similarly, advice should be specific and limited to a few reasonable steps. A written contract can be very helpful—a copy for the parent and one for the medical chart.
- Engage the family in developing the plan, solicit their input and agreement.
- Build on strengths; there are always some, providing a valuable hook to engage parents who may be reluctant to do so.
- Encourage positive family functioning.
- Be innovative and consider resources, such as using pots and pans for play. Encouraging reading can promote both literacy and intimacy.
- Encourage informal supports (i.e., family, friends; encourage fathers to participate in office visits). This is where most people get their support, not from professionals.
- Consider support available through a family's religious affiliation.
- Consider need for concrete services (e.g., Medical Assistance, Temporary Assistance to Needy Families (TANF), Food Stamps).
- Consider children's specific needs, given what is known about the possible outcomes of neglect. Too often, maltreated children do not receive direct services.
- Be knowledgeable about community resources, and facilitate appropriate referrals.
- Consider the need to involve CPS, particularly when moderate or serious harm is involved, and, when less intrusive interventions have failed. Present the report as a necessary effort to clarify what is occurring and what might be needed, and how to help the child and family. Most states have in recent years developed an alternative response system—especially for neglect. This approach focuses primarily on supporting families to do better, rather than on investigating what was done. It attempts to be conciliatory and constructive, rather than punitive. Most importantly, it prioritizes the crux of the issue: addressing the needs of children and families.
- Provide support, follow-up, review of progress, and adjust the plan if needed.

- Recognize that neglect often requires long-term intervention with ongoing support and monitoring.
- Try ensuring continuity of care as the primary healthcare provider.

F. **Preventing child neglect: a role for pediatric clinicians.** Instead of addressing the consequences of child neglect, it would be far preferable to help prevent the problem. There are several ways that clinicians can do so. In addition to helping prevent child neglect and abuse, these strategies can enhance family functioning; support parents; and help ensure children's health, development, and safety.

The social history offers an opportunity to learn what is happening within the family and there are brief questionnaires that can screen for specific problems, such as depression, intimate partner violence, and substance abuse. Often these problems are well masked and go undetected. Astute observation is a critical tool, noting the appearance and behavior of parent(s) and child and their interaction. In addition to noting problems (e.g., parent appears high on drugs), efforts should be made to identify strengths.

For children with chronic diseases, health education and extra support help ensure adequate care. Anticipatory guidance aims to ensure children's safety and wellbeing. Pediatricians' support, monitoring, and counseling are useful ways to help families to take adequate care of their children. Encouraging fathers to come in for routine visits and engaging them may increase their involvement in their children's lives. At times, referrals to other professionals and agencies are necessary; helping a family obtain appropriate services is another valuable role that pediatric clinicians play.

BIBLIOGRAPHY

Dubowitz H, Giardino A, Gustavson E. Child neglect: a concern for pediatricians. *Pediatr Rev* 21(4):111–116, 2000.

Dubowitz H. Tackling child neglect: a role for pediatricians. *Pediatr Clin North Am* 56:363–378, 2009.

Dubowitz H, Black M. Child neglect. In Reece RM, Christian C (eds), *Child Abuse: Medical Diagnosis and Management* (3rd ed), Elk Grove Village, IL: American Academy of Pediatrics, 2009.

58

Nightmares and Night Terrors

Barry Zuckerman

I. **Description of the problem.**

A. **Night terrors.** Children with night terrors bolt upright from their sleep to cry inconsolably for 5–20 minutes (in rare cases, even longer). They usually occur 15–60 minutes after going to sleep. Night terrors are associated with autonomic signs including a rapid pulse, increased respiratory rate, and sweating. The child has a glassy-eyed stare, which is due to the fact that the child is in rapid-eye-movement (REM) sleep and not actually awake. Following resolution, children easily return to sleep and have amnesia for the event in the morning.

   1. **Pathophysiology.** Night terrors are a *disorder of arousal*, occurring during an abrupt (rather than the usual slow) transition from stage 4 non-REM sleep to REM sleep.
   2. **Epidemiology.** Occurs in approximately 3–6% of children.

B. **Nightmares.** Nightmares are upsetting dreams that occur during REM sleep. Nightmares and night terrors are compared in Table 58-1. Nightmares are a universal occurrence in childhood and usually not due to a significant problem.

II. **Management.**

A. **Night terrors.** Because of the inconsolable crying and glassy-eyed stare, parents are usually terrified that something is wrong with their child. After the child returns to sleep, the parents may remain awake with their own terrors.

   1. The primary goal in management is to **reassure the parents** of the benign nature of these episodes. Management involves demystifying night terrors by explaining the physiologic basis of the behavior. Using an analogy like a myoclonic jerk during light sleep can help parents understand the physical nature of the night terrors. Most important, parents need to be assured that night terrors are not due to psychopathology or horrible life events. When parents know that there is nothing wrong with their child, they can usually tolerate periodic episodes.
   2. When the episodes are frequent and/or disrupt the sleep of others (especially siblings), **the child can be awakened prior to the time the episode usually occurs.** This is thought to alter the sleep cycling and prevent a night terror from occurring.
   3. **Diazepam,** which should be used only rarely, will stop the attacks by suppressing REM sleep and provide the beleaguered family with temporary relief.

B. **Nightmares.** Although night terrors are more frightening for parents to witness, nightmares are more distressing for the child. Although children may know that the nightmare is a dream, they remain frightened nevertheless.

   1. Parents need to **accept the child's fear** and not dismiss it as "just a bad dream."
   2. Parents should **comfort and stay with the child** until the child's distress has abated.
   3. Parents should **empathize with the child's fright** and tell him or her that while they cannot personally banish scary dreams, they will always come whenever the child is afraid.
   4. While dreams have magical properties, so do parents. They should assure the child that nothing will harm him or her. They can use magic of their own, like sprinkling antimonster dust around the room.
   5. **Transitional objects** (e.g., teddy bear, favorite blanket) should be at the ready; a nightlight may be comforting. Ask the child what (besides a parent) is comforting after a nightmare.
   6. In selected instances, **parents may have to remain with the child** or even take the child to their own bed.
   7. Parents should **discuss the nightmares and explain what nightmares are with the child** in the comforting light of day.
   8. Parents may consider reading a book in which the subject of the dream is resolved, with the child during the day to help increase their cognitive understanding of the fears.

Table 58-1. Comparisons of nightmares and night terrors

	Night terrors	Nightmares
Stage of sleep	Non-REM	REM
Consolability	Poor	Good
Amnesia for event	Yes	No
Interest in returning to sleep	High	Low

REM, rapid-eye-movement.

BIBLIOGRAPHY

For parents

Books

AAP eds. *Guide to Your Child's Sleep.* Chicago, IL: AAP Press, 2000.
Leuck L, Buelner M. *My Monster Mama Loves Me So.* Harper Collins, New York, NY, 1999.

Web sites

http://kidshealth.org/parent/medical/sleep/terrors.html

For professionals

Armstrong KH, Kohler WC, Lilly CM. The young and the restless: a pediatrician's guide to managing sleep problems. *Contemp Pediatr* 26:28–35, 2009.
Laberge L, Tremblay RE, Vitaro F, et al. Development of parasomnias from childhood to early adolescence. *Pediatrics* 106:67–74, 2000.

59

Oppositional/Noncompliant Behavior

Ross W. Greene

I. **Description of the problem.** Challenging behavior in children and adolescents occurs on a spectrum of severity that can include whining, pouting, crying, sulking, screaming, swearing, spitting, hitting, kicking, biting, lying, and more severe behaviors that are self-injurious or injurious to others. The degree to which one views such behaviors as "severe" is partially subjective (i.e., different adults experience various challenging behaviors to be more or less objectionable or intolerable than others) but is also clearly a function of intensity, frequency, and severity. Psychiatric diagnoses are best understood as groups of concomitant challenging behaviors that occupy points on the severity spectrum. Children meeting diagnostic criteria for oppositional defiant disorder (ODD)—generally the diagnosis of choice for oppositional/noncompliant kids—are those who exhibit "developmentally inappropriate levels of negativistic, defiant, disobedient, and hostile behavior toward authority figures," manifested in the form of many of the above behaviors.

Yet, such children do not exhibit such behaviors at all times. Rather, these behaviors occur under specific conditions; namely, *when the cognitive demands placed upon a child exceed his or her capacity to respond adaptively.* Of course, all humans behave maladaptively under exactly the same conditions, although the precise form of maladaptive behavior varies widely. The core feature of ODD—*noncompliance*—suggests that complying with adult directives requires skills that some kids lack. Thus, it is meaningful that ODD is associated with mood lability and low frustration tolerance and equally meaningful that noncompliance requires, by definition, an adult interaction partner.

A. **Epidemiology.** Prevalence rates for ODD range from 2%–16%. Research has shown that stubbornness is likely to emerge as a problem at around the age of 3 years; followed by defiance and temper outbursts at around the age of 5 years; arguing, irritability, blaming and annoying others, and anger between the ages of 6–8 years; and swearing at around the age of 9 years. ODD is thought to be somewhat more common in males, although this finding may vary with age.

B. **Compliance.** Compliance refers to a child's capacity to defer or delay his or her own goals in response to the imposed goals or standards of an authority figure. As noted above, compliance is best viewed as a *skill*, and one that is affected by a variety of other cognitive skills. Children who are frequently and/or intensely noncompliant can be viewed as lacking these cognitive skills, and noncompliant behavior can therefore be understood as a form of developmental delay.

C. **Contributing factors.** If noncompliance and its associated behaviors occur when the demands being placed upon a child exceed his or her capacity to respond adaptively, then lagging skills in the child are only part of the picture: how an adult is going about imposing goals or standards and solving adult–child problems is of equal importance. Traditionally, parents of noncompliant children have been viewed as passive, permissive, inconsistent, noncontingent disciplinarians. According to some theories, it is the tendency of such parents to capitulate to a child's wishes rather than endure tantrums that gives rise to chronic noncompliance. Thus, it's not necessarily the case that caregivers of noncompliant/oppositional kids failed to impose their will. It is possible that these caregivers learned firsthand the havoc that can ensue when one imposes will (with or without formal consequences attached) on a child who does not have the skills to handle imposition of adult will adaptively.

This mismatch between environmental demands and lagging skills could occur at any point in development, beginning in infancy (kids lacking skills at this point in development are often referred to as temperamentally difficult), the toddler years (when language development becomes increasingly crucial), and later in childhood (when demands for self-regulation increase, both at home and school). It is curious, therefore, that many popular interventions aimed at improving compliance teach parents to impose their will more firmly, consistently, and contingently. If a child's noncompliance is unsuccessfully treated and adult–child interactions remain conflictual, then the child is at significant risk for moving in the wrong direction down the spectrum of severity: almost all youth meeting diagnostic criteria for conduct disorder are diagnosed with ODD first and before that are labeled "oppositional."

II. **Making the diagnosis.** In consideration of the above information, one might rightly question whether making a formal diagnosis of oppositionality is a crucial step in the process of improving interactions between the child and his adult caregivers. Diagnoses pathologize the child, suggest that the problem resides within the child, and infer a stable (rather than situational) trait.

   A. **Identify the child's lagging skills and the conditions under which those skills are being demanded.** These conditions can be referred to as "unsolved problems," and they may include common flash points such as teeth brushing, ending screen time to come to dinner or go to bed, homework, dietary choices, and waking up in the morning, as well as (at school) situations such as riding on the school bus, recess, being at lunch, being in the hallway between classes, getting started on assignments, and interactions with certain peers or teachers. Within each child (and his or her adult caregivers), these unsolved problems are highly *predictable*, setting the stage (once they are identified) for *proactive* (rather than emergent) intervention. A brief instrument to assist in identifying lagging skills and unsolved problems called the *Assessment of Lagging Skills and Unsolved Problems* (ALSUP, see below for weblink) can be useful here.

   B. As one is assessing unsolved problems, it is important to consider the range of situations (school, church, soccer, hockey, at grandma's, with the babysitter) in which challenging episodes are occurring.

   C. And, as one is assessing a child's lagging skills, **the lagging skills of adult caregivers can also be assessed** (though more informally). Lagging skills in adult caregivers—along with stress, fatigue, marital issues, and the like—help complete the full picture of conflictual adult–child interactions. Unsolved problems, of course, are "owned" not by the child but by both interaction partners.

   D. It can also be quite useful to gather information related to the **history of the child's challenging behavior, early temperament, family history and stressors, trauma history, prior implementation of medical and psychosocial interventions, the degree to which they were effective, and why they were discontinued.**

   E. **Further, a physical and neurological screening should be conducted to rule out physical and genetic anomalies that might confer risk for lagging skills** (e.g., fetal alcohol syndrome, fragile X syndrome).

   F. **Informal and formal assessment of learning inefficiencies may also be indicated,** especially if homework and completion of classwork at school are among a child's unsolved problems.

III. **Intervention.** It is very common for pediatric clinicians to be the first to hear about a child's oppositional behavior. Explanations related to gender or the possibility that the behavior is a passing phase that will be outgrown tend to be unhelpful. Naturally, the popular culture has significant bearing on caregiver explanations for a child's noncompliant/oppositional behavior thus it is not unusual for caregivers to interpret this behavior as indicative of attention-seeking, manipulation, poor motivation, limit-testing, and coercion. The clinician can be helpful in a variety of ways:

   A. **Initial screening-assessment as intervention.** It is crucial for the clinician to present information to help caregivers begin the journey toward understanding children's oppositional/noncompliant behavior as a form of developmental delay and helping caregivers appreciate that such behavior is rarely as simple as it may seem. The ALSUP is best used as a discussion guide rather than as a free-standing checklist.

   B. **Find suitable resources (books, Web sites, etc.) for the family.**

   C. Referral to a psychologist or other mental health professional may be necessary if noncompliant/oppositional "episodes" are causing significant and frequently escalating conflict in the life of the child and family. Psychosocial intervention can take a variety of forms, ranging from individual therapy to parent management training to Collaborative Problem Solving (CPS). These are described below.

   - Individual Therapy: Although individual therapy is commonly employed in cases of oppositional and noncompliant children—and provides an opportunity for children to process issues that may be contributing to episodes of challenging behavior—this form of therapy typically does not directly address issues related to parent–child interactions or help children and adult caregivers learn how to solve problems together.

   - Parent Management Training: This form of therapy typically focuses on altering patterns of parental discipline that contribute to the development of oppositional behavior and problematic parent–child exchanges and relies heavily on the use of incentives to motivate the performance of desirable behaviors and decrease the likelihood of undesirable behaviors. Skills typically taught to parents in such models include attending to positive behaviors; use of appropriate commands; contingent attention and reinforcement; and use of a time-out procedure. In general, research has documented the efficacy of these procedures.

- CPS: In this model, adults are helped to conceptualize oppositional behavior as the byproduct of a "developmental delay" in the global domains of flexibility/adaptability, frustration tolerance, and problem solving. The CPS model is intended to help adults proactively solve problems collaboratively with children as a means of reducing challenging episodes and indirectly teaching lagging cognitive skills. The CPS also aims to help adults respond to oppositional behavior in a less personalized, less reactive, and more empathic manner. The specific goals of the CPS approach are to help adults to (1) identify the lagging cognitive skills contributing to a child's challenging episodes; (2) understand that these lagging skills are especially problematic in the specific conditions in which they are demanded (unsolved problems); (3) understand that imposition of adult will (unilateral problem solving) is a common precipitant to challenging behavior; and (4) begin using CPS instead. CPS consists of three "ingredients": the first, historically referred to as the empathy step, involves achieving an understanding of a child's concern or perspective on a given unsolved. The second, called the define the problem step, is where adult caregivers enter their concern or perspective on the same unsolved problem into consideration. The third ingredient, called the invitation, is where adult and child brainstorm solutions that will address the concerns of both parties, with an eye toward solutions that are realistic and mutually satisfactory.
  - **D.** There are some contributing factors—hyperactivity, poor impulse control, inattention, obsessiveness, irritability, mood instability—for which pharmacologic intervention may be indicated.

BIBLIOGRAPHY

For parents and educators

Web sites

Lives in the Balance. A nonprofit organization founded by Dr. Greene to disseminate the Collaborative Problem Solving Approach. www.livesinthebalance.org

Books

Greene RW. *The Explosive Child: A New Approach for Understanding and Helping Easily Frustrated, "Chronically Inflexible" Children* (4th ed), New York, NY: HarperCollins, 2010.
Greene RW. *Lost at School: Why Our Kids with Behavioral Challenges are Falling Through the Cracks and How We Can Help Them* (2nd ed), New York, NY: Scribner, 2009.

For professionals

Books and other references

Greene RW. Conduct disorder and oppositional defiant disorder. In Thomas J, Hersen M (eds), *Handbook of Clinical Psychology Competencies*. New York, NY: Springer Publishing, 2010, 1329–1350.
Greene RW, Ablon S, Miller KJ. Effectiveness of Collaborative Problem Solving in affectively dysregulated youth with oppositional defiant disorder: initial findings. *J Consult Clin Psychol* 72:1157–1164, 2004.
Assessment of lagging skills and unsolved problems. http://www.lostatschool.org/pdf/ALSUP.pdf

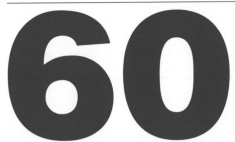

Oppositional Defiant Disorder

Heather Walter
Phillip Hernandez
Krista Kircanski

I. **Description of the problem.** Many children go through oppositional stages including angry outbursts, arguing, vindictiveness, and disobedience, generally directed at authority figures (such as parents and teachers) (see Chapter 59). Their behaviors will normally present in all children and adolescents from time to time, particularly during the toddler and early teenage periods, when autonomy and independence are developmental tasks. Reports suggest that most oppositional symptoms peak between 8 and 11 years of age and then decline in frequency.

Oppositional behavior becomes a concern when it is intense, persistent, and pervasive, and when it affects the child's family, social, and academic functioning to a significant degree. The pediatric clinicians' role is to differentiate children whose oppositional behaviors are more severe and persistent so that they can refer them to a mental health clinician.

Estimates of the prevalence of oppositional defiant disorder (ODD) vary depending upon the methodologic characteristics of the study. Recent surveys using *Diagnostic and Statistical Manual of Mental Disorders, Fourth Edition (DSM-IV)* criteria suggest a point prevalence approximating 3% of children aged 6–18 years, and a lifetime prevalence approximating 10%.

II. **Making the diagnosis.**
   A. **Signs and symptoms.** The *DSM-IV-TR* describes specific criteria for this diagnosis listed in Table 60-1. Disruptive behavior disorder, not otherwise specified (subsyndromal disruptive behavior) is diagnosed when some symptoms of ODD are present, but not enough to meet full diagnostic criteria.
   B. **Differential diagnosis.** Although ODD shares a number of characteristics with conduct disorder (CD), ODD can be distinguished from CD by the absence of severe forms of antisocial behavior, such as physical assault, destruction of property, theft, and other serious violations of societal norms. When the youth's pattern of behavior meets the criteria for both ODD and CD, the diagnosis of CD takes precedence. Other diagnoses to consider in the differential include attention-deficit/hyperactivity disorder (ADHD), bipolar, pervasive developmental, anxiety, mood, psychotic, and communication disorders, in which anger and disruptive behavior can be associated symptoms.
   C. **Comorbidity.** The most frequent comorbidities with ODD are ADHD (about 10 times more often than expected), major depression (about seven times), and substance abuse (in adolescents, about four times). Other less commonly co-occurring disorders are bipolar, anxiety, posttraumatic stress, impulse control, somatoform, adjustment, learning, and communication disorders. Comorbidities can exacerbate the symptoms of ODD by increasing negative parent–child interactions.
   D. **History: key clinical questions.**
   - *Does your child have trouble controlling his anger or behavior?*
   - *Why is this child not completing schoolwork? Is the work too difficult (always a possibility), or is the child too difficult?* Ruling out a potential comorbid learning problem is an important facet of the work-up.
   - *Does your child have friends?*
   - *How does your child respond to correction from adults?*
   - *How often does your child lose his or her temper, argue with adults, act defying or refuse to follow rules, deliberately annoy others, blame others for his or her mistakes, is easily annoyed, get angry and resentful, and be spiteful and vindictive?*

III. **Management.**
   A. **Refer for diagnostic evaluation to a pediatric mental health clinician.** Your role involves supporting parenting capacities. Key points of information are as follows:
   - Children learn to control their feelings and behavior when appropriate expression of feelings and behavior are modeled by parents in the context of a warm, loving, and respectful relationship.

Table 60-1. *DSM-IV-TR* diagnostic criteria for oppositional defiant disorder

A. A pattern of negativistic, hostile, and defiant behavior lasting at least 6 months, during which four (or more) of the following are present:
   (1) Often loses temper.
   (2) Often argues with adults.
   (3) Often actively defies or refuses to comply with adults' requests or rules.
   (4) Often deliberately annoys people.
   (5) Often blames others for his or her mistakes or misbehavior.
   (6) Is often touchy or easily annoyed by others.
   (7) Is often angry and resentful.
   (8) Is often spiteful or vindictive.
B. The disturbance in behavior causes clinically significant impairment in social, academic, or occupational functioning.
C. The behaviors do not occur exclusively during the course of a psychotic or mood disorder.
D. Criteria are not met for conduct disorder, and, if the individual is 18 years or older, criteria are not met for antisocial personality disorder.

American Psychiatric Association. *Diagnostic and Statistical Manual of Mental Disorders* (4th ed, text rev), Washington, DC: American Psychiatric Association, 2000. Used with permission.
Note: Consider a criterion met only if the behavior occurs more frequently than is typically observed in individuals of comparable age and developmental level.

- If children feel loved and respected by their parents, they will naturally want to please their parents by behaving in accordance with their parents' wishes. Rules and discipline do not work without a good parent–child relationship.
- Although they may complain when they are imposed, children thrive on structure and consistency. It will be very difficult, if not impossible, for children to learn to control their feelings and behavior in the absence of these two elements.
- Children who have more difficult temperamental characteristics are not "bad"; rather, they should be seen as having inherited a tendency for a different set of behaviors than children who inherited easy temperamental characteristics. Children inheriting a difficult temperament can be thought of as similar to children who inherit a vulnerability to a medical illness; in both situations, extra help is needed to prevent the vulnerabilities from escalating into problems.

B. **Refer to parent management training.** Parents should be referred to parent management training because of its evidence of effectiveness for the treatment of ODD. This intervention is targeted at the parents of young children (preschool to early elementary school age) and typically is delivered in 12–16 group or individual settings by specially trained interventionists. The goal of parent management training is to strengthen the parent–child attachment and to interrupt the dysfunctional parent–child interactions that are characterized by mutual and escalating aversive behaviors resulting from the attempts of both the parent and child to control the actions of the other. Accordingly, in parent management training the first goal is to strengthen the parent–child attachment.

Once the attachment is strengthened through child-directed play, parent management training teaches specific behavior management techniques based upon social learning theory. Parents must change their behavior to incorporate clear limit setting in the context of an authoritative relationship. Such parental "scaffolding" is necessary, given that children do not yet have the cognitive ability to reflect on and change their behavior without external support.

C. **Anger management/social skills training.** A second type of intervention with evidence of effectiveness for the treatment of ODD is anger management/problem-solving skills training, which are grounded in social learning theory, which postulates that behavior change occurs through a systematic process of behavioral modeling, rehearsal, practice, feedback, and reinforcement. Children learn strategies to increase their awareness of feelings (particularly anger) and techniques to express anger in socially appropriate ways. In problem-solving skills training, children are taught problem-solving strategies, including identifying the problem, generating solutions, weighing positive and negative elements of each solutions, making a decision based upon this analysis, and evaluating the outcome.

D. **Medication.** At present, no evidence exists to support an indication for specific medications in the treatment of ODD. As such, clinical practice guidelines recommend that psychotherapeutic interventions for the child and family are the first-line treatments for ODD. However, there are reports of reduction in oppositional behaviors with indicated pharmacologic treatment of comorbid disorders, such as ADHD. Thus, medications for ADHD, including stimulants (e.g., methylphenidate and amphetamine formulations) and alpha adrenergic agonists (e.g., clonidine and guanfacine) have been noted to reduce comorbid oppositional behaviors along with the primary symptoms of inattention, hyperactivity, and impulsivity.

E. Natural history. Approximately two-thirds of children with a diagnosis of ODD exit from the diagnosis after a 3-year follow-up. Earlier age at onset of oppositional symptoms conveys a poorer prognosis, and preschool children with oppositionality are at heightened risk for the development of other psychiatric disorders several years later. An estimated one-third of children with ODD progress to CD; the risk of progression is higher with comorbid ADHD.

If diagnosis persists, children develop a wide range of psychiatric disorders in adulthood (e.g., substance abuse, major depression, antisocial personality disorder) as well as many other adverse outcomes such as suicidal behavior, delinquency, educational difficulties, unemployment, and teenage pregnancy. The disruptive disorders often trigger a chain of adverse events (e.g., parental hostility, peer rejection) that heighten the risk for additional adverse events (e.g., conflict with authority, deviant peers) extending through adolescence and into adulthood.

BIBLIOGRAPHY

American Academy of Child and Adolescent Psychiatry. Practice parameter for the assessment and treatment of children and adolescents with oppositional defiant disorder. *J Am Acad Child Adolesc Psychiatry* 46:126–141, 2007.

Eyberg SM, Nelson MM, Boggs SR. Evidence-based psychosocial treatments for children and adolescents with disruptive behavior. *J Clin Child Adolesc Psychol* 37(1):215–237, 2008.

Ipser J, Stein DJ. Systematic review of pharmacotherapy of disruptive behavior disorders in children and adolescents. *Psychopharmacology* 191:127–140, 2007.

Parent management training programs

Helping the Noncompliant Child; Incredible Years. http://www.incredibleyears.com
Triple P-Positive Parenting Program. http://www.triplep.net
Parent–Child Interaction Therapy. http://www.pcit.org

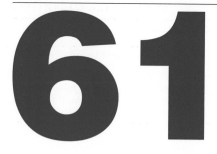

Pediatric Overweight and Obesity

Carine Lenders
Lauren Oliver
Shaheen Lakhani
Catherine Logan
Margaret Marino
Alan Meyers
Hannah Milch
Vivien Morris

I. **Description.**
   A. **A definition of obesity is useful only if it predicts morbidity or mortality. Body mass index (BMI)** is defined as the weight of an individual divided by his/her height (kg/m^2). Since most complications of obesity are associated with body fat and not muscle mass, obesity defined on the basis of BMI represents an attempt to estimate the adipose compartment. Overweight (BMI >25) and obese (BMI >30) adults are at increased risk for morbidity and mortality.

   Childhood weight status is classified on the basis of the BMI percentiles for age and gender, unlike the absolute values of BMI in adulthood (Table 61-1). There is increasing evidence that BMI ≥95th percentile in childhood predicts adult obesity, adiposity, and mortality; however, more tracking (longitudinal) data are needed, especially on clinical risks associated with obesity. Although BMI is an adequate screening method for older children and at a group level, its strength as an indicator of adiposity decreases at younger ages (<13 years) and may vary by ethnicity/race. There is no current valid measure for children with severe obesity or children younger than 2 years. However, there is emerging evidence that rapid weight gain, or the crossing of several major weight-for-age percentiles, may be a risk factor for obesity especially in the first year of life.
   B. **Prevalence.** Since the 1960s, the prevalence of childhood obesity in the United States has more than tripled. The 2005–2006 national survey estimates that nearly 32% of children aged 2–19 years are overweight or obese, with disproportionately higher rates among minority populations.
   C. **Etiology.**
      1. **Heritability and imprinting.** Adoption studies tend to generate the lowest heritability estimates (30%), whereas twin studies provide the highest heritability estimates (70%). These observations are consistent with the "thrifty genotype hypothesis," in which genes predisposing to energy conservation were preserved as a survival characteristic in former times of famine but become a liability in environments with plentiful food and low physical activity. There is also evidence that exposure to environmental factors early in life may affect metabolism, as described in the "thrifty phenotype theory."
      2. **Most causes of obesity are described as idiopathic or exogenous,** which consist of a combination of hereditary traits and a "toxic" environment. In addition to an environment where high-energy processed foods are abundant and sedentary behaviors are favored, parental feeding practices and restrained feeding may contribute to rapid weight gain especially in young children. Less than 5% of causes of obesity are defined as endogenous causes, due to human genetic syndromes displaying mendelian patterns of transmission or endocrinopathies (e.g., hypothyroidism, Cushing syndrome). However, emerging evidence from neuroimaging studies suggest that food intake may affect neurological pathways involved in substance abuse (e.g., cocaine, alcohol) and thus lead to compulsive eating behaviors.
II. **Clinical evaluation. Pediatric weight management is ultimately about behavior change.** The first step, therefore, is to identify families who would benefit from behavioral health services *prior to starting* a behavioral weight management intervention. Screen for history and symptoms of trauma, psychiatric disorders, weight teasing, and disordered eating and sleeping. Evaluate family functioning and lifestyles, as well as current stressors to further determine to what extent the family will be able to carry out treatment goals. The identification of medical and psychosocial complications related to obesity as well as family readiness and motivation to change will allow the clinician to make an informed decision on how to further approach treatment. In addition to the key questions below, specific motivational interviewing techniques may be helpful in guiding families toward behavior changes (Table 61-2).

Table 61-1. BMI classifications for children and adults

Weight status	BMI-adults (kg/m^2)	BMI-children 2–18 years
Underweight	<18.5	<5th percentile for age and gender
Normal weight	18.5–24.9	5–84.9th percentile
Overweight	25–29.9	85–94.9th percentile
Obese	≥30	≥95th percentile for age and gender

A. History: key questions.
  1. **Family lifestyle assessment. For toddlers and preschoolers** who are gaining weight rapidly, parenting skills and parent style may either be supportive of or undermine positive feeding and activity level. Start by asking the parent (or guardian) if they have any concerns about the child's eating behaviors or growth. Ask parents about feeding and activity dynamics. Assess to what extent the family is in agreement with Ellyn Satter's division of responsibility in feeding.
     "Parents are responsible for the what, when, and where of feeding. Children are responsible for the how much and whether of eating."
     • *"Tell me about how you feed your child."* Evaluate whether the parent provides meals and snacks at about the same times everyday or if patterns of feeding are unpredictable. Assess how often the parent allows caloric drinks or grazing on food between meals.
     • *"Who eats together for meals?"* Ask to what extent members of the family eat together, with the child, on a regular basis. Assess to what extent the parent determines what food will be offered (versus letting the child choose). Also inquire about the extent to which the parent determines that the child has eaten enough (by forcing or limiting) and how the child behaves at the table while eating. Determine whether the child is "picky" or a "great" eater.
     • Ask to what extent the parent uses food for non-nutritive purposes, such as rewards, bribes, or punishment.
     Among older children and teens. Assess both past and present feeding dynamics, but also begin to ask the 5Ws "When, where, what, why, with whom." Address the older child directly as he or she becomes the agent of change. Separate the parent and child to ask some questions.
     • *"When do you usually eat meals and snacks?"* Determine reasons why the child may skip meals, especially breakfast, or have an inconsistent meal schedule.
     • *"Tell me about a typical meal (e.g., lunch or dinner)?"* Ask where (home, restaurant, etc.) and with whom the child eats. Ask what is offered, at what time, and what location (in the car, at a kitchen table, in front of the TV, etc.). Ask who serves the food, if it is served family style, and if the child is allowed second servings. Find how often the family offers fruits/vegetables and whether the child usually eats them.
     • *"What type of beverages do you like to drink (especially juice/milk/soda) and how often?"*
     • *"What does the family/child eat for snacks/desserts and how often?"*
     • *"How often does the family/child get fast food or order take-out?"* Ask questions about types and amounts of fast food items eaten during school time, at home, and at other restaurants.

Table 61-2. Techniques for eliciting self-motivational statements in adolescents or parents

Themes	Sample questions
Ask open-ended questions	Tell me the ways in which your ... (e.g. child's excess weight) has caused you or your child problems.
Explore pros/cons of change	What are the good/not so good aspects of you or your child ... (e.g., not drinking sodas)?
Ask for elaboration	Please tell me more about how...
Imagine extremes	If you/your child continue(s) to ... (e.g., eat fast food two to three times a week), where do you think you/your child will be in 5 years?
Looking back	Tell me what life was like before you/your child ... (e.g., were not able to play football).
Looking forward	Where would you/your child like to be in five years and where does your weight fit in with these goals?

In addition, identify who is in charge of buying, cooking, and serving food, and who "shares the refrigerator." Assess food access by asking questions regarding the availability of grocery store(s) in the neighborhood, density of fast food restaurants in the area, funds for food, utilities and cooking facilities at home, and school meals assistance. Determine whether the family has to make difficult choices such as "heat or eat."

2. **Key physical activity/activity questions.**
   Questions to ask the parent of a young child include the following:
   - *What kind of games/activities does your child play?"*
   - *"How long does s/he usually spend playing alone, with other children, or with you or another adult each day?"* Also ask about activities at childcare and about TV watching.
   Questions for parents and/or the older child/teen include the following:
   - *"What physical activities or sports, including school gym and chores at home, does your child participate in? For how long? How many days per week? What setting?"*
   - *"Has there been a recent increase or decrease in the intensity, frequency, or duration of your child's activity? Can you point to a reason for this change?"*
   - *"How much time does your child spend in front of a 'screen' after school each day, including the computer, hand-held device, and the television? Does your child have access to any of them in the bedroom?"*
   - Inquire about physical activity access such as availability of space for physical activity at home, school physical education, before- and after-school program participation, recreational programs (YMCA, etc.), safe play spaces, and areas designed for walking or biking in the community.

3. **Cultural history.** Culture and country of origin may shape health beliefs about weight gain. Some cultures may value a more full-bodied appearance, which may be seen as a sign of good health and not a problem. Avoid "correcting" the belief and instead focus the discussion on risks, not appearances. Some cultural norms may value limited questioning of clinicians (i.e., sign of disrespect) or expect clinicians to do most of the talking during a consult (i.e., a sign of expertise). Modify key elements of your approach when motivational interviewing technique is used (Table 61-2). For example, limit the handing over of some of the decision-making responsibility to the family and focus on building self-efficacy to change behavior. Be aware that minimal eye contact and limited questioning by the family may not be a sign of poor motivation. Finally, raising awareness and concern about obesity may render people in communities of color less satisfied with themselves and less able to cope with one more thing for which a good solution cannot yet be offered.

B. **Physical examination.** The initial step for the medical assessment of the child with obesity is to exclude potential associated rare syndromes or endocrinopathies and to diagnose possible associated complications. Table 61-3 includes red flags for syndromes and endocrinopathies, Table 61-4 gives key elements of the physical examination, and Table 61-5 provides relevant information on complications. Of note, height velocity is typically accelerated in early stages of obesity, but children tend to reach similar height potential as their nonobese peers.

C. **Laboratory tests.** Current recommendations from an Obesity Expert Committee (EC, 2007) are summarized below:
   - First fasting lipid profile screening is recommended after 2 years of age but not later than 10 years of age. Screening before 2 years of age is not recommended.
   - A fasting glucose level for children with obesity with additional risk factors, which according to the American Diabetes Association (2000) include age below 10 years with Tanner Stage 2–5 or above 10 years regardless of Tanner Stage, along with two of the

Table 61-3. Red flags for organic causes of obesity

	Endocrine	Syndromic	Exogenous
Bone age	Decreased	Increased	Appropriate
Development delay	No	Yes	No
Dysmorphic features	No	Yes	No
Early obesity onset	No	Yes	No
Hypogonadism	Yes	Yes	No
Kidney condition	No	Yes	No
Muscle strength	Decreased	Normal	Normal
Short stature	Yes	Yes	No
Tone	Normal	Decreased	Normal

Note: These are typical red flags. However, being tall for stature does not necessarily exclude the presence of a syndrome.

Table 61-4. Key elements of the physical examination

Vitals: weight, height, BMI, patterns of *weight gain over time*, percentile status, shortness of stature, height potential, blood pressure, and pulse

General appearance: body habitus, central fat, hyperactivity status, concentration, cognitive delays, mood, and affect

Skin: acanthosis nigricans (can be found in folds, joints, and areas of pressure), severe acne and hirsutism, violaceous striae, infectious lesions, peripheral edema, and excessive bruising

Eyes: evaluate if eye contact is appropriate, assess for papilledema especially if there is a history of headaches and blurred vision

ENT: signs of allergies (eye shiners, enlarged and inflamed turbinates, sinus tenderness, and mouth breathing) dental damage (carries, enamel punched out by vomiting), and enlarged tonsils

Chest: evaluate for wheezing, rhonchi, anatomical anomalies, breast size (fat pad vs. breast bud including size and symmetry), Tanner stage

Heart: rule out murmur, gallop, and arythmia

Abdomen: evaluate for bowel sounds, tenderness, and organomegaly

Pelvic: Tanner stage, clitoris enlargement if hirsute girl, as well as penile and testicle size in boys.

Skeletal–muscular: posture, obvious deformities, tenderness, limitation of movements, and flat feet

Neurology: reflexes, gait, and central tone

three following factors: (1) type 2 diabetes mellitus (T2DM) in first- or second-degree relative; (2) minority (Native-, African-, Latino-, Asian American, or Pacific Islander); and (3) at least acanthosis nigricans, hypertension, dyslipidemia, or polycystic ovary syndrome.

- Aspartate aminotransferase/alanine aminotranferease (AST/ALT) biannually beginning at 10 years of age.

Of note, the Endocrine Society (2008) does not recommend routine laboratory evaluation for endocrine causes of obesity in children or early to mid-pubertal obese adolescents except when height velocity is attenuated given pubertal stage and mid-parental height potential. In practice, many clinicians obtain a nonfasting lipid assay as a screening test and substitute hemoglobin A1C for fasting glucose determination. In fact, hemoglobin A1C and nonfasting lipids appear to be on the threshold for official recognition as the preferred diagnostic tests for T2DM and cardiovascular risk. There is a need for further evidence-based recommendations about frequency of testing.

III. Management.

A. The primary goal of obesity treatment is improvement of long-term physical health through lifestyle changes. As a result, the Expert Committee (2007) suggests a four-staged approach to obesity treatment, with each stage lasting 3–6 months before progressing to the next, more intensive stage. Patients begin with office-based interventions that increase in intensity based on need and access to the clinical office, the motivation of the family, and degree of child obesity. If a family and/or teen initially presents as resistant or ambivalent to lifestyle changes, a referral to a mental health clinician or dietitian with experience in client-centered motivational interviewing techniques may be more useful. Although raising awareness and acknowledging ambivalence or barriers to change may be helpful, recommending changes before a patient is ready for change may prove counterproductive. Those who begin changes in early stage interventions with less than expected progress may be candidates for more aggressive treatment. In cases of significant psychosocial contributors, family therapy may be needed before or along with nutrition counseling.

B. Suggested weight goals by weight categories. Although weight goals are recommended by age group, they may be difficult to achieve. Therefore, consider focusing on behavioral progress and metabolic health markers instead of weight changes with families, especially if the child may be vulnerable to poor self-esteem or body image. Weight goals suggested by the EC 2007 include the following:

- 2–5 years: weight maintenance, slowing of weight gain, or gradual weight loss up to 1 lb/mo for BMI >21–22 kg/m^2.
- 5–11 years: weight maintenance, slowing of weight gain, or gradual weight loss (up to 1 lb/mo for BMI >95th percentile, 2 lb/wk for BMI >99th percentile).
- 12–18 years: weight maintenance, slowing of weight gain, or gradual weight loss up to 2 lb/wk for BMI >95th percentile.

Table 61-5. Complications associated with obesity in children and youth

Body system	Relevant history and examination	Diagnostic tests
Cardiovascular		
Dyslipidemia	Family Hx; xanthomas	Fasting or nonfasting lipid profile
Hypertension	Family Hx; 14% children with persistent HBP have LVH	SBP and/or BP >90th percentile
Endocrine		
Impaired OGTT	Red Flag of T2DM; typically asymptomatic or fatigue	Elevated fasting, 2 hr-OGTT glucose, A1c
T2DM	High thirst, urination, appetite, fatigue, acanthosis, blurred vision, skin/GU infections, family history	Elevated fasting glucose or OGTT
PCOS	Amenorrhea, acne, hirsutism, acanthosis	Testosterone (total, free), TSH, PRL, 17-OH progesterone; Option: ovaries US, FH/FSH
Gastroenterology		
Constipation	Scybalous, pebble-like, hard stools most of the time; or firm stools two or more times/week; abdominal/rib pain	Rectal examination, abdominal x-ray; no evidence of structural, endocrine, or metabolic disease
Fecal soiling	At least 12 wk: large BM < 2X/wk and retentive posturing	Rectal examination, abdominal x-ray
GERD	Overfeeding, vomiting, chest pain/burning, asthma	PH probe if treatment trial fails
High ALT	Abdominal pain, nausea, vomiting, asymptomatic	ALT/AST ≥2–3Xnl, repeat, referral to GI
Orthopedic		
Blount's disease	One/both knees; deformity; intra-articular instability	X-ray, orthopedic referral
Flat feet	With pain	Orthopedic referral
SCFE	Often painless limp; knee pain; flexed hip in external rotation	X-ray, rapid orthopedic referral
Neuropsychiatric		
Pseudotumor cerebrei	Blurred vision; headaches	Fundi examination, LP
Sleep disturbances	Difficult to focus, to learn, or to perform daily activities, excessive daytime sleepiness, irritability, easy frustration, and difficulty with impulses and emotions (sometimes attributed to hyperactivity or behavior disorders)	Sleep hygiene
Sleep apnea	Snoring; witnessed apnea; cyanosis; concern with child's breathing, restless sleep; daytime somnolence; enuresis; can lead to RVH and RVF	High RBC count, metabolic alkalosis; polysomnography; ENT evaluation
Binge eating	Large amount of food in discrete time period (e.g., 2 hr); lack of control, distressed by binging; sneaking/hoarding food; excessive concern with body shape and weight; persists for at least 3 months, no compensatory behaviors	Eating Attitudes Test–Child Version (chEAT) Eating Disorder Inventory–C (preteens and teens), QEWP-A (adolescent version), Eating Disorder Examination (ChEDE)–interview. Use ChEDE-Q self-report

(continued)

Table 61-5. (*Continued*)

Body system	Relevant history and examination	Diagnostic tests
Compulsive overeating	Characterized by episodic binge eating; may also include uses of purging or restrictive eating; fear of not being able to stop eating; depressed mood, food can become 1° mood regulator	See above
Night eating syndrome	Little/no appetite for breakfast; most caloric intake at night; leaves bed to snack at night; anxious; sleep disturbance; persists at least 2 months	N/A for children or adolescents, screen for symptoms present
Depression	Depressed mood, low self-esteem, anhedonia, irritability, hopelessness, hx of suicide ideation, sleep disturbance, fatigue, diminished concentration	Child Depression Inventory (CDI)
Anxiety	Excessive worry; sleep disturbance; tantrums/crying; obsessive thoughts, fatigue, low self-esteem; avoidance; hx of trauma; r/o social phobia and separation anxiety	Child Behavior Checklist (CBCL)
Weight Teasing	Target of name-calling, ridicule, put-downs, verbal insults; can occur at home and at school	Teasing and Bullying Survey (TABS-C)–Bodin (2004) (still in research stage)
Dermatology		
Acanthosis nigricans	Elevated skin texture at pressure points	Physical examination
Cutaneous candidiasis	Signs of candidiasis	Fasting glucose, HbA1C

HBP, high blood pressure; LVH, left ventricular hypertrophy; ALT/AST, alanine aminotranferease/aspartate aminotransferase; SBP, systolic blood pressure; OGTT, oral glucose tolerance test; T2DM, type 2 diabetes mellitus; GU, genitourinary; PCOS, polycystic ovary syndrome; TSH, thyroid-stimulating hormone; PRL, prolactine; FSH, follicle-stimulating hormone; GERD, gastroesophageal reflux disease; SCFE, slipped capital femoral epiphysis; LP, light perception; RVH, right ventricular hypertrophy; RVF, right ventricular failure; RBC, red blood cell.
Adapted from Apovian C, Lenders C (eds). *A Clinical Guide for Management of Overweight and Obese Children and Adults.* Boca Raton, FL: CRC Press, 2006.

C. **Behavioral goals.** Work with families around two to three specific goals at each visit.
   1. **With parents of young children.** Work to restore the appropriate division of responsibility of feeding to allow the child to revert to internal regulation of food intake. Address meal patterns, parent versus child roles, and food quality. Focus on *how* the child is being fed before *what* the child is being fed.
   • Encourage family-style meals where parents decide the menu.
   • Encourage structured snacks, with only water offered between meals/snacks.
   • Encourage parents to role model for children; parents may need to change their own habits to set a good example.
   • Encourage increased activity, both free play and adult-led activities.
   • If a family is food insecure, refer them to appropriate resources such as the Supplemental Nutrition Assistance Program (SNAP-formerly Food Stamps), Supplemental Nutrition Program for Women, Infants and Children (WIC), or food pantries and/or soup kitchens.
   2. **For older children (6–12 years) and teenagers.** Consider the family's/teen's readiness to change for individual behavior changes; do not push recommendations or set goals if the family/teen is not currently interested or able to make such changes. For families who seem ready to make behavior changes, suggest one/some of the options below, and ask which the family would like to work toward first, if any. Involvement of the entire family is important for achieving and maintaining lifestyle changes.

The Expert Committee (Barlow et al., 2007) target behaviors include the following:
- Family meals—sit with others in a pleasant mealtime environment on a regular basis, not watching TV; avoid overly restricting intake.
- Breakfast—eat everyday, stop skipping meals.
- Food preparation—prepare more meals at home instead of eating at fast food or restaurants.
- Sugary beverages—gradually decrease (goal <8 oz/day 100% juice).
- Fruits and vegetables—gradually increase servings/day.
- Television/screen time—decrease to ≤2 hours/day (no TV <2 years old).
- Physical activity—increase gradually to goal of ≥1 hour/day.

It is critical to find physical activity options that each child/teen finds fun. Overweight teens may feel more successful by beginning with activities like weight lifting and/or swimming due to their increased body size. Some teens may need considerably more than 1 hour/day of activity to see weight change.

If feeding problems and weight gain continue despite these suggestions, or in complicated cases, consider addressing readiness to change and/or move to stage 2, "structured weight management": referral to a registered dietitian who can assess the child's diet and make specific recommendations for change. Failure to make progress after 3–6 months would prompt stage 3, "comprehensive multidisciplinary intervention" in a subspecialty program, if available. Stage 4 comprises tertiary care interventions, including meal replacement and weight loss surgery.

D. **Medications and weight loss surgery.** There is currently not enough evidence for long-term safety and efficacy of medications for weight management among children and adolescents. Weight loss surgery has been recommended for adolescents aged 12–18 years with more severe obesity using specific eligibility criteria but is rarely reimbursed by third payers.

ACKNOWLEDGEMENTS

This chapter is the result of collaboration between multidisciplinary staff and consultants of the Nutrition and Fitness for Life program at Boston Medical Center.

CL and LO are the chapter primary authors and coauthors are listed by alphabetic order. Support is provided in part by the New Balance foundation and the Loomis and Sayles Charitable Fund.

BIBLIOGRAPHY

For parents

Satter E. *Your Child's Weight: Helping Without Harming.* Madison, WI: Kelcy Press, 2005.

For professionals

Apovian C, Lenders C (eds). *A Clinical Guide for Management of Overweight and Obese Children and Adults.* Boca Raton, FL: CRC Press, 2006.

Barlow SE, Expert Committee. Expert committee recommendations regarding the prevention, assessment, and treatment of child and adolescent overweight and obesity. *Pediatrics* 120 S4:S164–S192, 2007.

Daniels SR, Greer FR, Committee on Nutrition. Lipid screening and cardiovascular health in childhood. *Pediatrics* 122(1):198–208, 2008.

Pratt J, Lenders C, Dionne E, et al. Best practice updates for pediatric/adolescent weight loss surgery. *Obesity (Silver Spring)* 17(5):901–910, 2009.

Web sites

www.ellynsatter.com.

CDC tips for children and adult nutrition, physical activity, and BMI calculator. http://www.cdc.gov/healthyweight/.

USDA guidelines, tips and resources in nutrition and physical activity. http://www.mypyramid.gov/.

Community Food Security Coalition. Resources, publications, policy information and organizing activities regarding food security at the local, regional and national levels. http://www.foodsecurity.org.

A newsletter and other information for teachers on obesity treatment and prevention in K-12 settings. http://www.impactchildhoodobesity.org.

National Association of Sports and Physical Education: activity guidelines for young children. http://www.aahperd.org/Naspe/.

62 Child Physical Abuse

Christine E. Barron
Carole Jenny

I. **Description of the problem.** Child physical abuse is defined as **acts of commission involving physical violence that results in injuries.** These injuries include fractures, bruises, burns, head trauma, and internal injuries. When making the diagnosis of child physical abuse, one needs to consider the age of the child, the plausibility of the history, alterations in the history, delays in seeking medical care, possible mechanisms of injury, potential eyewitnesses, and other possible causes within the differential diagnosis.

A. **Epidemiology.** Despite almost certain underreporting, physical abuse accounts for approximately 10.8% of substantiated cases of child maltreatment in the United States. Although certain social and demographic factors have been identified as risk factors, children can be victims of physical abuse regardless of their age, gender, and ethnic and socioeconomic backgrounds. In fact, cases without these identified risk factors are more likely to be misdiagnosed.

B. **Etiology/contributing factors.** There are many identified risk factors for child physical abuse, including the following:

1. **Unrealistic expectations.** Often the lack of understanding a child's developmental abilities and needs results in caregivers establishing unrealistic developmental and social expectations. These unrealistic expectations can lead to frustration and anger, which can result in abuse.

2. **Social isolation.** Lack of parenting skills often combine with inadequate parenting models and additional life stressors, and limited resources from family, friends, and community, to increase the risk of abuse.

3. **Domestic violence.** Children who live in homes where domestic violence is present are more likely to be victims of physical abuse (up to 15 times the national average).

4. **Substance abuse.** The most frequently reported cause for neglect and abuse of children is parental substance abuse.

II. **Making the diagnosis.**

A. **Signs and symptoms.** Child physical abuse has variable presentations and should be considered when

1. A child presents with unexplained injury or pattern injuries.
2. A nonmobile child present with injuries.
3. Illogical or changing explanations are offered by a caregiver to account for an injury.
4. A child presents with multiple injuries with different stages of healing.
5. There is a delay in seeking medical care.

B. **Differential diagnosis.** The history and physical examination are helpful in excluding many competing diagnostic possibilities that can mimic child physical abuse. Table 62-1 identifies possible differential diagnoses but is not an exhaustive list.

C. **History: interviewing guidelines.** Interviews should be conducted in a nonjudgmental manner, acknowledging that everyone's goal is to simply ensure the safety of the child. Open-ended questions should be asked to determine how an injury occurred. Specific notations should be made for changing histories or if the injury is blamed on the child or the siblings.

1. **Interviewing the parents.** All caregivers should be interviewed separately. The interview should obtain information regarding the following:

a. The sequence of events that resulted in the injury.
b. Identification of all caregivers during the time of the injury.
c. Any other potential witnesses to the injury, including verbal children.
d. Information regarding past medical history, developmental history, and social history should be obtained.
e. Social history including questions that identify any potential risk factors such as domestic violence, substance abuse, and limited support system.

Record parents information using exact quotes when possible.

Table 62-1. Diagnostic possibilities to consider when evaluating children for possible physical abuse

Findings	Diagnostic possibilities
Bruising	Accidental bruising in mobile children
	Blood disorders—hemophilia, idiopathic thrombocytopenic purpura, von Willebrand's disease, vitamin K deficiency, leukemia
	Dye or ink
	Birth marks—dermal melanocytosis, café au lait spots
	Phytophotodermatitis
	Ehlers–Danlos syndrome
	Infectious diseases—meningococcemia, Henoch–Schönlein purpura
	Folk remedies—Cao gao, cupping
	Contact dermatitis
Burns-	Accidental burns
	Car seat or seat belt burns
	Infections—impetigo, Staphylococcal scalded skin syndrome
	Folk medicine—cupping, moxibustion
	Fixed drug eruptions
	Phytophotodermatitis
Fractures-	Birth trauma
	Congenital syphilis
	Accidental trauma
	Osteogenesis imperfecta
	Leukemia
	Infections—osteomyelitis, septic arthritis
	Scurvy
	Rickets
	Menkes syndrome
Intracranial bleeding	Motor vehicle accidents
	Aneurysms
	Accidental head injuries
	Glutaric aciduria type I

2. **Interviewing the child.**
   a. Verbal children should be interviewed separately.
   b. It is important to ask open-ended questions and to completely avoid asking direct or leading questions such as, *"Your father hits you doesn't he?"*
   c. Children should be interviewed at eye level, using age-appropriate language. If a child makes a disclosure, ask further questions such as, *"Can you tell me more about that?"*
   d. Record child's disclosures using exact quotes.
   e. Further detailed interviews should be completed by trained professionals in response to a report of suspicious injuries to the child welfare agency.
D. **Physical examination.** The physical examination should be completed in a child-friendly examination room with adequate lighting and with the goal of putting the child at ease.
   1. An entire examination should be completed, *not* simply focus on areas of obvious injury.
   2. All children should be examined in a gown, with inspection of the entire skin surface.
   3. Clear documentation of any injuries should be completed using photographs and drawings to describe location, size, and pattern of injuries.
      Table 62-2 covers specific area of detail to be noted.
E. **Other testing: imaging studies.**
   1. Skeletal imaging
      a. Children younger than 2 years with suspected physical abuse require a complete skeletal survey to identify occult osseous trauma.
      b. Children with acute injuries should receive a second skeletal survey 2 weeks after the first.

Table 62-2. Parameters of the physical examination in cases of suspected abuse

Examination	Important physical examination findings
Growth parameters	Obtain and plot growth parameters
General	Altered level of consciousness
	Distress or discomfort
	Behavior during examination
Head Ears Eyes Nose Throat (HEENT)	Traction alopecia
	Subgaleal hemorrhages
	Facial bruising
	Subconjunctival hemorrhages
	Retinal hemorrhages (consider ophthalmological examination)
	Pinnae injuries
	Hemotympanium
	Nasal–septal injuries
	Frenum injuries
	Dental injuries
	Dental impressions on mucosal surface of upper lip
Chest/back	Crepitus from rib fractures
	Bruises
Abdomen	Bruises (lack of bruising on the abdominal wall does not rule out abdominal trauma)
	Distension, tenderness (consider pediatric surgery consult)
Genital	Bruising
	Bite marks
Extremities	Soft tissue swelling
	Tenderness to palpation
	Bruising
	Deformities
Skin	Location of injuries
	Recognizable patterns
	Bilateral injuries
	Circumferential injuries
	Multiple injuries in different stages of healing

    2. Central nervous system (CNS) imaging
      a. Computed tomography (CT) to identify acute CNS injuries.
      b. Magnetic resonance imaging better identifies parenchymal injuries and helps determine the age of injuries.
    3. Intra-abdominal imaging.
      a. Abdominal CT
      b. Upper gastrointestinal study
      c. Ultrasound
III. Management.
    A. Primary goals. The goal for the clinician addressing possible child abuse is to make the diagnosis, provide needed treatment, report suspicious injuries to child welfare agencies, and ensure the safety of the patient and other children within the same environment. In all states, clinicians are responsible by law for reporting suspicion for abuse to child welfare agencies. These cases require a multidisciplinary approach from medical personnel, child welfare authorities, and law enforcement officials.
IV. Clinical pearls and pitfalls.
    • Obtain all information in a nonjudgmental manner.
    • Nonmobile children with unexplained bruising should have a workup completed for possible child physical abuse.
    • Rely on history and physical examination findings to narrow the differential diagnosis.

BIBLIOGRAPHY

For parents

Parents Anonymous©. http://www.parentsanonymous.org/pahtml/progNet.html
Childhelp USA. http://www.childhelp.org/1-800-4-A-CHILD

For professionals

U.S. Department of Health and Human Services, Administration on Children, Youth and Families. *Child Maltreatment 2007*. Washington, DC: U.S. Government Printing Office, 2009.
Kleinman PK. *Diagnostic Imaging of Child Abuse* (2nd ed), St. Louis, MO: Mosby, 1998.
Jenny C (ed). *Child Abuse and Neglect: Diagnosis, Treatment, and Evidence*. Philadelphia, PA: Elsevier Saunders, 2010.
Kellog ND, Jenny C, Christian CW, et al. Evaluation of child physical abuse. *Pediatrics* 119:1232–1241, 2007.

Organizations

AAP. www.aap.org
American Professional Society on the Abuse of Children (APSAC). www.apsac.org

63

Picky Eating

Julie Lumeng

I. **Description of the problem.** Picky eating occurs on a continuum and there is no clear cutoff for when it becomes problematic. Parental perception that their child's unwillingness to eat familiar foods or sample new foods is outside the range of normal is probably the major reason for seeking medical advice. Therefore, the best definition of picky eating incorporates parental concern: *an unwillingness to eat familiar foods or try new foods, severe enough to interfere with daily routines to an extent that is problematic to the parent, child, or parent–child relationship.*

A. **Epidemiology.**
   - Although prevalence is hard to pin down because there is no strict definition, normative data tell us that about 36% of toddlers are described as "picky eaters." In addition, 54% are not always hungry at mealtime, 33% do not seem to enjoy mealtimes, 34% have strong food preferences, 26% frequently refuse to eat, 21% request specific foods and then refuse them, and 42% try to end a meal after a few bites. Nearly two-thirds of parents report one or more problems in eating with their toddler.
   - Children who are picky eaters more often have negative temperamental traits and are more often behaviorally inhibited (shy) and anxious. Their parents report more difficulties in the parent–child relationship.
   - The most commonly rejected foods are vegetables, and picky eaters have lower dietary variety, but no significant difference in overall nutrient intake.
   - Picky eating in childhood has been associated with higher socioeconomic status, fewer children in the family, and being thinner. Having been breastfed and having a mother who eats more fruits and vegetables have been linked with being less picky. Being picky has not been associated with race, gender, having medical problems, food allergies, or maternal age. Picky eating is linked with more behavior problems in general but not eating disorders in particular.
   - The prevalence of picky eating increases over infancy and toddlerhood, from 19% at 4–6 months of age to 50% at 19–24 of age months. There is significant continuity in pickiness during this age range. Pickiness seems to continue to increase to 3 years of age, but thereafter seems to decline to about 20% by 8 years of age. If children are still described as picky after about 8–9 years of age, they are likely to be picky for the rest of their lives.
   - There seems to be a critical period during which children will expand the repertoire of liked foods in their diet that closes around 4 years of age. After 4 years of age, parents continue to introduce new foods, but the number of new foods children try that they learn to like does not continue to increase in the same way it did before 4 years of age.

B. **Evolutionary framework.** Picky eating seems to increase as children gain mobility. Some theorize that children are "wired" for pickiness to protect them from eating potentially poisonous substances in the environment. Children who are inherently reluctant to eat an unfamiliar food, or to eat a variety of foods, will not "wander into the bush and eat a poison berry."

C. **Etiology.**
   - People reject foods because they (1) dislike the sensory characteristics (flavor and appearance); (2) have a fear of negative consequences (e.g., it causes stomach upset upon eating); or (3) are disgusted by the food (due to contamination or the thought of where it came from), which does not begin until 7–8 years of age.
   - Pickiness runs in families: about two-thirds of the variability in pickiness is explained by genetics. However, "nurture" (child caregiving practices) can modify "nature."

II. **Making the diagnosis.**

A. **History: key clinical questions.**
   1. *"Tell me which foods she won't eat."* A pattern of refusal, such as only refusing milk products or certain textures, raises the question of food allergies/intolerances or oral hypersensitivity.

2. *"Tell me what she ate yesterday, starting with breakfast."* A diet history can give a flavor to how picky the child is and opens a discussion about what foods are presented to the child, how, and what is done when the child rejects them.

3. *"What do you do when she rejects a food at dinner? What sort of rules do you have in your house around eating?"* Obtaining a history that the child is required to remain at the table until his plate is clean, or that the child is coerced to eat a particular food, is important. Neither of these methods has been shown to result in a long-term improvement in picky eating, and both likely simply add stress and negativity to the family mealtime.

4. *"What worries you the most about your child's eating?"* Frequently, parents are concerned the child has a growth or vitamin deficiency. Reassurance that the child is growing adequately (try showing the parent a growth chart) is often helpful, as is demystifying the behavior by describing how common it is (see prevalence data above) and the theories as to why it is present (see evolutionary framework). Explaining that a multivitamin with iron (and supplemental fiber if needed) can replace vegetables in the diet often assuages a great deal of parental concern. Today, the risk of obesity is greater than the risk of malnutrition and in some studies, less pickiness is linked with higher weight status. Therefore, some degree of pickiness, within reason, may have benefits.

5. *"Is there anyone else in your family who is a picky eater?"* This question (to which the answer is nearly universally "yes") often opens the door to talking about the natural course of picky eating and may provide some insight into why the parent views the behavior as so problematic.

B. **Physical examination and laboratory testing.** Careful measurement of weight and height, with plotting on the appropriate growth chart, is important. If growth deficiency is present, a different approach should be taken, which includes an exhaustive history with directed laboratory testing. If the child's diet is particularly restricted in iron-rich foods, testing for iron deficiency anemia is warranted. Children should also be screened by history and physical examination for constipation. The picky eater's diet is often low in fiber, and constipation can result in abdominal discomfort that only worsens the eating behavior.

C. **Differential diagnosis.**
 • Lactose intolerance or food allergies can present with refusal of specific types of foods.
 • Gastroesophageal reflux disease, as evidenced by frequent vomiting or pain after eating, can result in problematic eating behavior.
 • Children can present with oral hypersensitivity, the etiology of which is not always clear. These children respond negatively to oral stimuli and have particular difficulty with textured foods.
 • Escalating negative affect in the mother and child, or an unusually strong focus on the issue may signal an interactional problem. Picky eating may be the presenting complaint of a larger relationship problem that may benefit from an appropriate mental health referral.
 • Unrealistic parental expectations about the quantity and range of food that a child will eat may be present. Expecting the child to eat every food presented at the dinner table every evening (including spicy or bitter flavors) may be a goal that cannot be met by all children.
 • Limitation of resources. The family may not have adequate financial resources to supply a range of palatable foods at each meal. Parents may be concerned that the child's picky eating, in combination with limited choice, is affecting the child's health.
 • Children with autistic spectrum disorders are commonly picky eaters.

III. **Management.** A thorough history is essential to clearly define the problem. The mainstay of management is to demystify for parents that picky eating is, in most cases, a behavior that worsens during the toddler and preschool years, and then begins to improve through the early elementary years. In other cases, it can be seen as a personality trait. Either way, there is rarely a medical indication for intervention. Behavioral interventions should be recommended only when parents are eager to put effort into modifying the behavior. Interventions must be benign and simple, and should never be continued if they result in increased stress or discord at mealtimes. Some strategies that could be suggested to parents to reduce picky eating are listed in Table 63-1.

IV. **Clinical pearls and pitfalls.** Parents who are concerned about a child's picky eating may be articulating the eating as the problem, when it is really a discrete symptom of an overarching concern: a difficult temperament. Although picky eating occurs on a continuum and is a "normal" behavior, parental concerns should not be minimized. Helping the parent to understand the child's temperamental qualities, and how the picky eating is a symptom of them, will likely be most helpful in the long term in the parent–child relationship.

Table 63-1. Strategies to suggest to parents to reduce picky eating

Strategy	Comments
Functional analysis. What are the properties of the foods the child likes?	If child likes food with a particular temperature or texture, try expanding the repertoire of foods with similar kind of foods first.
Mealtime atmosphere. Calm, pleasant meals can improve willingness to try new foods. Food tastes better when it is eaten in a positive social context.	Children who are prone to anxiety or overstimulation may benefit from a calm eating atmosphere.
Social cues. Modeling eating a food by a parent is helpful, but peers are more powerful.	If child has the opportunity to eat meals with other children (such as in preschool), this may be an opportunity to expand the child's repertoire of foods.
Positive reinforcement. Parents should not provide material, verbal, or food rewards for eating, and children should never be punished for refusal to try a new food.	When children are given a reward (dessert) for eating a food (a vegetable), they eventually learn to like the food they were rewarded for eating (the vegetable) less over time (not the desired goal).
Repeated exposure. Increased familiarity results in increased liking, and foods typically must be introduced 10 times before they are accepted. Less than 10% of parents offer a food to a child this many times before giving up based on the impression that the child does not like it.	If the family wishes for the child to accept a vegetable, choose a generally mild, palatable vegetable to be served at dinner repeatedly.
Forced exposure. The "try one bite" rule has been shown to result in an increased willingness to try other new foods over time. It may be due to decreasing the expectation of disliking the target food.	If the child has a difficult temperament, however, and requiring the child to take a bite is disruptive to mealtime, this method should be abandoned.
Providing information. For older children, providing information about a food's flavor will increase willingness to try the food.	If younger children do not grasp the meaning of "flavor words" (i.e., sweet, salty, sour), or have not yet developed a vocabulary of "food words," this method may not be effective.
Combining foods. Combining a nonpreferred food (a meat) with a preferred food (ketchup) may be helpful—even in seemingly illogical combinations.	If a child wants to dip carrot sticks in soup, and this increases his willingness to eat the carrots, this should be accepted (in lieu of disallowing it because it is "bad manners").

BIBLIOGRAPHY

For parents

Your Child: Development and Behavior Resources, University of Michigan Health System. http://www.med.umich.edu/1libr/yourchild/

Ellyn Satter has published several books for parents and professionals about childhood eating and feeding behavior, and maintains a Web site. http://www.ellynsatter.com/

LA Jana, Shu J. *Food Fights: Winning the Nutritional Challenges of Parenthood Armed with Insight, Humor, and a Bottle of Ketchup.* Elk Grove Village, IL: American Academy of Pediatrics, 2008.

For professionals

Dovey TM, Staples PA, Gibson EL, et al. Food neophobia and 'picky/fussy' eating in children: A review. *Appetite* 50(2–3):181–193, 2008.

Dietz W, Birch LL. *Eating Behaviors of the Young Child: Prenatal and Postnatal Influences for Healthy Eating.* Elk Grove Village, IL: American Academy of Pediatrics, 2007.

64
Posttraumatic Stress Disorder in Children

Glenn Saxe

I. **Description of the problem.** Trauma exposure is an international public health problem. Large-scale epidemiologic studies have reported extraordinarily high percentages of exposure to trauma. A national representative study found that up to 40% of children have experienced a traumatic event. This rate is much higher among inner-city children. Studies of the prevalence of posttraumatic stress disorder (PTSD) have varied widely depending on the type of trauma and the child's proximity to it. In addition, the likelihood of a child getting PTSD if traumatized depends on many factors independent of the trauma itself. Consequently, the research literature has increasingly focused on constitutional factors within the child that determine resiliency or vulnerability to trauma.

A. **Epidemiology.** Prevalence studies suggest between 5%–70% of traumatized children qualify for a diagnosis of PTSD. Depending on the study, exposure to sexual assault or abuse yields a prevalence of PTSD between 40%–60%, disasters between 5%–70%, injuries 10%–30%, and war 20%–70%.

B. **Etiology/contributing factors.**
   1. **Genetic.** Studies using twin registries of Vietnam veterans have found higher concordance rates in monozygotic twins. There is no doubt, however, of a complex polygenetic vulnerability to the effects of environmental trauma. Recent research has focused on a series of candidate genes. Our group found that variance on the *FKPB5* gene was associated with traumatic stress responses in children hospitalized with injuries.
   2. **Environmental.** Children with PTSD frequently grow up in environments saturated with ongoing stressors, including parental mental health and substance abuse problems, marital stress, and exposure to ongoing community and family violence. Each of these appears to increase the risk for contracting PTSD. Treatment must address both the child's traumatic stress symptoms and the ongoing social environmental problems, which may perpetuate these symptoms.
   3. **Organic.** A number of biochemical and neuroanatomical correlates to PTSD have been identified. For each, the research does not always distinguish which may be a *cause* of PTSD versus a *consequence* of PTSD. For example, a number of studies have found smaller hippocampal sizes in adults with PTSD. It remains undetermined whether this smaller hippocampal size is preexisting and predisposes an individual who is traumatized to get PTSD or whether this smaller hippocampal size is a consequence of PTSD (and some of the biochemical changes that occur with it). This *cause* or *consequence* problem is found in the other organic correlates of PTSD, such as lower levels of cortisol, hypersupression of cortisol with dexamethasone, and higher noradrenergic levels. Some of the emerging neurodevelopmental findings are particularly worrisome, such as studies reporting smaller brain sizes and larger ventricles in children with PTSD.
   4. **Developmental.** PTSD has been diagnosed in children as young as 1 year. An alternative criteria set for PTSD has been developed for preschool children, which relies far less on verbal report of the child and more on report from the parent and on behavioral observations of the child. Younger children's reactivity to traumatic reminders is much more likely to be observed in their behavior. School-aged children will begin to talk about their fears and anxiety. Adolescents will begin to focus on the meanings of the trauma for themselves, their world, and their future.

II. **Making the diagnosis.** Symptoms can look different depending on the developmental age of the child. See Table 64-1 for *Diagnostic and Statistical Manual of Mental Disorders, Fourth Edition (DSM-IV)* criteria.

A. **Signs, symptoms, and behavioral observations.**
   1. **Infant/toddler.** Infants and preschool children are often unable to describe internal states or to know how or why they are responding to the environment. Accordingly, PTSD is assessed by observing behaviors in infants and toddlers. Very young children with PTSD will become **aggressive, withdrawn, or very distressed at reminders**

Table 64-1. *DSM-IV* criterion for PTSD

A. The person has been exposed to a traumatic event in which both of the following were present:
   (1) The person experienced, witnessed, or was confronted with an event or events that involved actual or threatened death or serious injury, or a threat to the physical integrity of self or others.
   (2) The person's response involved intense fear, helplessness, or horror.
B. The traumatic event is persistently reexperienced in one (or more) of the following ways:
   (1) Recurrent and intrusive distressing recollections of the event, including images, thoughts, or perceptions.
   (2) Recurrent distressing dreams of the event.
   (3) Acting or feeling as if the traumatic event were recurring (includes a sense of reliving the experience, illusions, hallucinations, and dissociative flashback episodes, including those that occur on awakening or when intoxicated).
   (4) Intense psychological distress at exposure to internal or external cues that symbolize or resemble an aspect of the traumatic event.
   (5) Physiological reactivity on exposure to internal or external cues that symbolize or resemble an aspect of the traumatic event.
C. Persistent avoidance of stimuli associated with the trauma and numbing of general responsiveness (not present before the trauma), as indicated by three (or more) of the following:
   (1) Efforts to avoid thoughts, feelings, or conversations associated with the trauma.
   (2) Efforts to avoid activities, places, or people that arouse recollections of the trauma.
   (3) Inability to recall an important aspect of the trauma.
   (4) Markedly diminished interest or participation in significant activities.
   (5) Feeling of detachment or estrangement from others.
   (6) Restricted range of affect (e.g., unable to have loving feelings).
   (7) Sense of a foreshortened future (e.g., does not expect to have a career, marriage, children, or a normal life span).
D. Persistent symptoms of increased arousal (not present before the trauma), as indicated by two (or more) of the following:
   (1) Difficulty falling or staying asleep.
   (2) Irritability or outbursts of anger.
   (3) Difficulty concentrating.
   (4) Hypervigilance.
   (5) Exaggerated startle response.

From American Psychiatric Association. *Diagnostic and Statistical Manual of Mental Disorders* (4th ed, text rev), Washington, DC: American Psychiatric Association, 2000.

of the trauma. Frequently, children will repeatedly play about the trauma (**posttraumatic play**). There may be **significant sleep disruption** including nightmares (which may or may not be about the trauma).
   2. **School age.** School-aged children may more easily talk about the trauma and its impact on them. Children of this age group are particularly vulnerable to the **feelings of helplessness** often elicited by experiencing a trauma and becoming overwhelmed with traumatic stress symptoms. Often school-aged children respond to memories of the trauma with behavioral reactions (e.g., **aggression, withdrawal, avoidance**).
   3. **Adolescence.** Adolescents are better able to describe their internal states and properly attribute these states to the traumatic event, which helps facilitate treatment. Adolescents are often highly focused on the **social stigma of the trauma**, particularly sexual trauma. Adolescents can also be very focused on the **interpersonal, societal, or spiritual meanings** of the traumatic event and being a victim of it. The impact of trauma on self-concept is particularly important to adolescents as they consolidate a sense of their own identity. Guilt and shame may emerge prominently in adolescence. Related to the impact of trauma on self-concept, the transition into puberty may be particularly difficult.
B. **Comorbid and differential diagnoses in children with PTSD.**
   1. It is clear that PTSD is not the only diagnosis related to trauma. Other psychiatric diagnoses that have been associated with trauma include mood disorders, conduct disorders, attention deficit disorders, dissociative disorders, somatoform disorders, eating disorders, and substance abuse. In addition, exposure to trauma has been

associated with chronic health problems, educational problems, and youth violence. Regarding psychiatric diagnoses, the issue of what is comorbidity and what is differential diagnosis is a complex clinical problem as there is diagnostic overlap between symptoms of PTSD and other disorders.

C. **History: key clinical questions.** Our group has found that the affirmative answers to at least two of the following questions suggest that the child is at high risk for PTSD. If these questions are asked in the days after the child is exposed to a trauma, they predict the eventual development of PTSD.

   1. *"Does your child have **physical** symptoms (headaches, stomach aches, sick feelings, etc.) when reminded of the trauma?"*
   2. *"Does your child avoid **talking** about the trauma?"*
   3. *"Does your child have a **startle** reaction when he hears a loud noise or see something suddenly?"*
   4. *"Does your child get **distressed** when he is reminded of the trauma?"*

   The mnemonic for remembering these screening questions is PTSD:

   • **P—Physical** symptoms
   • **T—Talking** avoidance
   • **S—Startle** reactions
   • **D—Distress** on reminders

D. **Physical examination.** Physical examination is useful to rule out medical illness as a cause of the symptoms. The clinician must be very mindful that physical examinations may be powerful "triggering" stimuli in children with sexual abuse histories.

E. **Tests.** Screening laboratory tests should be performed only when suggested by the history and physical examination.

III. **Management.** Children with PTSD require treatment that **focuses on safety.** Children will need to develop skills that will help them to manage emotional states, to talk about the trauma in a safe way, and to be less consumed by the past and more focused on the future. There are a number of different models of intervention. Most help by addressing the aforementioned goals. This treatment usually requires a trained mental health professional and can be conducted in an outpatient setting. **Family involvement** is usually required to help the family support the child's emotional regulation capacities and work toward limiting stresses and reminders in the environment. When families are unable to do this, home-based intervention is often helpful. Treatment frequently will involve some case management and integration of mental healthcare with other service systems such as school, social services, and medical system.

The primary care clinician can be extremely helpful to monitor treatment progress and to facilitate the families' engagement in care across the service system. Urgent psychiatric consultation is indicated whenever the child or adolescent is thought to be psychotic or engaging in violent or self-destructive behaviors. Psychopharmacology will occasionally be required to help the child manage emotional states. Currently, selective serotonin reuptake inhibitors are considered first line. Psychopharmacology should always be conducted in coordination with psychosocial interventions.

BIBLIOGRAPHY

For parents

National Child Traumatic Stress Network has handouts and other literature for families that can be downloaded at www.nctsnet.org

For professionals

American Academy of Child and Adolescent Psychiatry. Practice parameters for the assessment and treatment of children and adolescents with posttraumatic stress disorder. *J Am Acad Child Adolesc Psychiatry* 37(10 Suppl):4S–26S, 1998.

Cicchetti D, Lynch M. Toward an ecological/transactional model of community violence and child maltreatment: consequences for children's development. *Psychiatry* 56:96–118, 1993.

DeBellis MD, Keshava MS, Clark DB, et al. Developmental traumatology, part 2: brain development. *Biol Psychiatry* 45:1259–1270, 1999.

Saxe GN, Ellis BH, Kaplow J. *Collaborative Treatment of Traumatized Children and Teens: The Trauma Systems Therapy Approach.* New York, NY: Guilford, 2006.

Bosquet Enlow M, Kassam-Adams N, Saxe GN. The Child Stress Disorders Checklist–Short Form: a four-item scale of traumatic stress symptoms in children. *Gen Hosp Psychiatry* 32(3):321–327, 2010.

Prematurity: Follow-Up

James A. Blackman
Robert J. Boyle

I. **Description of the problem.** Infants born before the 37th week of gestation are at risk for chronic medical, neurodevelopmental, and behavioral problems. The shorter the gestation and greater the number of associated medical and psychosocial complications, the higher the risk and need for close primary care surveillance.

A. **Epidemiology.**
- Approximately 13% of all births are less than 37 weeks' gestation; 2% less than 32 weeks.
- Survival rate for infants born at 23–25 weeks gestation has improved.
- The incidence of prematurity has increased over the last decade but mortality and morbidity risk for this group has declined dramatically (Table 65-1).
- The births, often premature, of multiples due to popularity of in vitro fertilization have increased.

B. **Risk factors for developmental and behavioral problems.** Risk factors mandating especially close developmental surveillance include the following:
- Very low birth weight (<1500 g)
- Gestational age <28 weeks
- Intrauterine growth restriction
- Neonatal seizures
- Persistent head ultrasound/computed tomography/magnetic resonance imaging (MRI) abnormalities, including ventricular dilatation or asymmetry, periventricular leukomalacia, diffuse white matter injury, or porencephalic cysts
- Chronic lung disease
- Persistent feeding problems (e.g., need to gavage feed beyond 34 weeks postconceptual age)

Biological risk alone does not determine outcome. Rather, it is the interaction of those risks with social and environmental factors that best predicts long-term functioning. In the first 2 years, biological factors are strong predictors of developmental function, especially in the motor domain. However, after 2 years of age, socioenvironmental factors assume a far more prominent role in determining cognitive outcome and school success. The primary care clinician is not able to change the preexisting organic insults but can alter and improve a child's developmental and behavioral functioning by supporting the social environment.

II. **Evaluation.**

A. **Common health problems of the premature infant.** Since chronic medical problems and developmental and behavioral difficulties are inextricably linked, meticulous management of these problems will enhance the likelihood of good outcomes.

1. **Neurologic.** Maintain good seizure control through judicious use of anticonvulsant medications. Anticonvulsants for neonatal seizures often are weaned during the first year of life.

2. **Ophthalmologic.** Many premature infants leave the neonatal intensive care unit (NICU) with retinopathy of prematurity that is not fully resolved. Strabismus and myopia are more common among premature infants. Ensure follow-up by a pediatric ophthalmologist.

3. **Audiologic.** Newborn hearing screening is mandatory in most states. Be certain that hearing has been tested or that screening failures are followed-up. Infants with a history of prematurity or neonatal intensive care, or other risk factors should be retested at least once in the first 3 years of life. Infants with syndromes associated with hearing loss, hyperbilirubinemia requiring exchange transfusion, or congenital infection should be screened more frequently (see Chapter 50).

4. **Respiratory.** Pulmonary symptoms can impede developmental progress. In concert with specialists in chronic lung disease, optimize pulmonary function. Annual

Table 65-1. Risk by birth weight

Birth weight (g)	Mortality (%)	Major morbidity of survivors[a] (%)	Minor morbidity of survivors[b] (%)
<800	20–50	20–30	20–30
800–1000	10–20	15–20	15–20
>1000–1500	5–10	10–15	10–15

[a]Includes developmental quotient below 70, severe cerebral palsy, deafness, and blindness.
[b]Includes learning disabilities, borderline cognitive function, attention deficits, and poor school achievement (5%–10% in the general population) among children without major morbidity.

influenza vaccine and respiratory syncytial virus prophylaxis for eligible infants will decrease respiratory morbidity.

B. Growth and feeding. Premature infants may come home from the hospital with continuing feeding problems: tube dependency, inadequate caloric intake, or volume intolerance due to cardiopulmonary or gastrointestinal disease. Good nutrition provides the necessary substrate for optimal developmental gain. Premature infants should remain on special care formulas for 9–12 months. Key questions to ask include the following:

- Is weight gain appropriate?
- What is the caloric density of the formula?
- What is the daily caloric intake?
- How long does it take to feed the child?
- Does the child have difficulty sucking or swallowing?
- Are the feeding techniques appropriate, given the child's development and capabilities?

Growth patterns should be interpreted from a longitudinal perspective using standard growth charts. For premature infants, measurements can be plotted on special growth charts for premature infants, or, after age adjustment (chronological age in weeks minus number of weeks premature), they can be plotted on a regular growth chart. Beyond 18–24 months of age, continued age adjustment is unnecessary.

1. Growth trends.

a. Dropping growth percentiles or moving further below the fifth percentile. This may be secondary to medical, nutritional, environmental, or neurologic factors. Further investigation is warranted.

b. Catch-up growth or forward movement across percentiles. Catch-up growth may begin slowly and continue over the first 2 years of life.

c. Growth parallel to fifth percentile. The child may continue to be small or catch up in future years. This pattern is often seen following extreme low birth weight and/or intrauterine growth restriction.

d. Rapid head growth. Catch-up head growth is a good sign. However, when head circumference crosses percentiles more rapidly than length or weight, head ultrasound evaluation for hydrocephalus should be considered. Benign enlargement of the subarachnoid space is usually a benign and transient condition. Babies with grade III–IV intraventricular hemorrhage may have late onset hydrocephalus requiring a shunt.

e. Head growth lagging behind other parameters. This is a concerning sign, often associated with intellectual disability.

C. Behavior and development.

1. History: key clinical questions.

a. *"Are you concerned that your baby is too passive or overly irritable?"* Premature babies may be especially passive or irritable due to central nervous system (CNS) injury or the prolonged hospital experience. Infants with CNS injury manifest the same problems as all other infants (e.g., colic, night wakening, temper tantrums), but they tend to be more intense or prolonged.

b. *"Do you see your child as especially fragile or vulnerable?"* It is sometimes difficult for parents to modify their perception of the child from "fragile" to "healthy." Although it may take months (or years) for the child to achieve medical stability, it may take parents even longer to accept this reality. Common pediatric illnesses may be overinterpreted as evidence of continuing vulnerability (see Chapter 107).

c. *"Does your child seem either stiff or floppy?"* Hypotonia is fairly common among premature infants and usually resolves. Persistent hypertonia may be a sign of cerebral palsy. Initial hypotonia may evolve over several months into hypertonia.

d. *"Does your child have any unusual movement patterns?"* Dragging the legs along in crawling, body rolling (instead of crawling), or seat scooting may be manifestations of neuromotor abnormalities. Early hand preference is abnormal and may indicate injury to subcortical white matter or the corticospinal tract contralateral to the less used upper extremity. In such a case, a head imaging (MRI) study is indicated.

2. **Assessment.** Although developmental surveillance is recommended for all children, careful and regular assessment is even more important for premature children (see Chapter 12).

The exact timing, frequency, instrumentation, and venue for formal developmental screening and/or assessment for premature infants are debatable, but the following checkpoints have been recommended by a national panel of experts (Follow-up care of high-risk infants. *Pediatrics* 114:1377–1397, 2004.):

- 6–8 months: Identification of eligibility for early intervention services.
- 12 months: Biomedical issues resolved; emerging cognitive and language processes accessible.
- 18–24 months: Environmental factors exert stronger influence on test results. Cognitive and motor abilities diverge; language skills are developing and can be assessed.
- 3–4 years: "Intelligence" can be first assessed as well as concept development and pre-academic skills.
- 6 years: Variety of tests and procedures can be used; attention and school achievement can be assessed.
- 8 years: IQ, neuropsychological function, school performance, and behavioral adjustment can be adequately assessed.

As with growth, premature infants tend to catch-up to their like-aged peers over the first years of life. Most screening and assessment tests recommend full correction until 2 years of age. If the child is not achieving age-appropriate skills for corrected age, an in-depth assessment by a developmental specialist or early intervention program is warranted.

D. **Psychosocial issues.**
   1. **Family dynamics and stress.** Shortened gestation interrupts the normal psychological preparation for life with a newborn. The long, uncertain intensive care experience can drain the family's physical and emotional stamina. Parents take home a normal but fragile, slow-starting, or clearly abnormal infant. The clinician should schedule an early "decompression visit" for the parents to discuss the NICU experience and to give vent to their frustrations and fears. Counseling or family support groups may be helpful.
   2. **Child care issues.** Because of the increased morbidity from respiratory tract infection in premature infants with a history of chronic lung disease, day care settings with extensive exposure to other children with respiratory illnesses should be avoided. Families may need assistance and guidance with appropriate child care arrangements.

III. **Management.** Each infant should have an identified medical home where primary care and regular developmental surveillance occurs, usually in coordination with an NICU follow-up clinic. The clinician must be aware of the infant's and family's needs and assist the family in obtaining and coordinating other necessary services. Ideal follow-along should be viewed as a multidisciplinary team function, with the primary care clinician coordinating medical specialists, early intervention and nutritional services, and other therapies (occupational or physical) participating as needed.

IV. **Clinical pearls and pitfalls.**
   - Beware of overwhelming the family with services or appointments. Simplification and coordination of services as well as family involvement in the process will decrease family stress and ensure better overall compliance and satisfaction.
   - Do not assume that an infant will outgrow any identified problems. Appropriate evaluation and correction for the degree of prematurity should allow the clinician to make an informed judgment about the infant's status.

BIBLIOGRAPHY

For parents

Web sites

American Association for Premature Infants. www.aapi-online.org
Premature Baby/Premature Child. www.prematurity.org
Parents of Premature Babies, Inc. www.preemie-l.org
Premature Baby. kidshealth.org/parent/growth/growing/preemies.html
March of Dimes. www.marchofdimes.com/prematurity

Publications

Bradford N. *Your Premature Baby: The First Five Years*. Toronto, ON: Firefly Books, 2003.

Davis DL, Stein MT. *Parenting Your Premature Baby*. Golden, CO: Fulcrum Publishing, 2004.

Madden SL. *The Preemie Parents' Companion: The Essential Guide to Caring for Your Premature Baby in the Hospital, at Home, and Through the First Years*. Boston, MA: Harvard Common Press, 2000.

Sears W, Sears R, Sears J, et al. *The Premature Baby Book: Everything You Need to Know about your Premature Infant from Birth to Age One*. New York, NY: Little Brown and Company, 2004.

Zaichkin J. *Newborn Intensive Care: What Every Parent Needs to Know*. Elk Grove Village, IL: American Academy of Pediatrics, 2010.

For professionals

Brodsky D, Ouellette MA. *Primary Care of the Premature Infant*. Philadelphia, PA: Saunders, 2008.

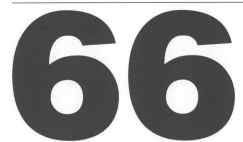

School Refusal

Jan Harold D. Sia
Barton D. Schmitt
Carol C. Weitzman

I. Background

A. Description of the problem. School refusal is defined as "child-motivated refusal to attend school or difficulties remaining in school for an entire day." It is a heterogenous, complex, and multicausal syndrome. Children with school refusal repeatedly stay home from school or are sent home from school for physical symptoms of emotional origin. School refusal is not a formal psychiatric diagnosis but, rather, a sign or symptom that leads to many possible diagnoses including social/school problems. Identified children and adolescents may suffer from significant emotional distress, especially anxiety and depression. Hersov described a common pattern of school refusal behavior that "often starts with vague complaints about school or reluctance to attend progressing to total refusal to go to school or to remain in school (Fig. 66-1) in the face of persuasion, entreaty, and punishment by parents and pressure from teachers, physicians, and education welfare officers." The behavior may be accompanied by overt signs of anxiety or even panic when the time comes to go to school and although these children desire to attend school, many children cannot leave home to set out for school. The terms *school refusal*, *school avoidance*, and *school phobia* are often used interchangeably. School refusal is the preferred term because of its descriptive and comprehensive nature. Children with school refusal have different characteristics from children who are truant (Table 66-1). Truancy is defined as any unexcused, intentional, and unauthorized absence from compulsory schooling.

B. Epidemiology.

1. School refusal is the most common cause of vague physical symptoms in school-aged children. It is also the most common presentation of separation anxiety.
2. Approximately 5% of elementary school children and 2% of middle school children have this disorder. It is equally common in boys and girls.
3. It occurs across all socioeconomic groups.
4. School refusal has a bimodal peak: at 5–7 years of age and at 10–11 years of age.
5. The incidence of school refusal may be decreasing because of the increasing numbers of working mothers, which requires most children to master their separation fears long before entering kindergarten.
6. The homeschooling movement shelters many of these children.

C. Etiology. Many of these children have a shy and sensitive temperament. In general, affected youths are good to excellent students with no behavioral problems in the classroom. Approximately 20% of these children also have an acute precipitating event (e.g., being teased by someone at school).

1. Clinical studies have suggested three types of school refusers:
   - **Separation-anxious school refusers.** School refusal associated with *separation anxiety disorder* often begins following a period at home with a parent, such as a summer vacation, holiday break, or physical illness. It is more common in the younger children. Affects girls more than boys. Onset is usually seen when entering kindergarten. Mothers of these affected children were more likely to have experienced anxiety-based school refusal themselves compared with mothers of children who are phobic or anxious/depressed school refusers.
   - **Phobic school refusers.** These children have more severe and pervasive school refusal behavior. Later age of onset. Phobic stimuli include the school environment (school phobia), examinations, crowds, and animals
   - **Anxious/depressed refusers.** Often affect older children and adolescents. Affected adolescents frequently report moderate to severe somatic complaints of the autonomic (e.g., dizziness, diaphoresis, palpitations, shakiness) or gastrointestinal type (e.g., abdominal pain, nausea, diarrhea).

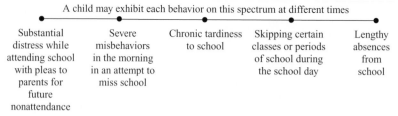

A child may exhibit each behavior on this spectrum at different times

| Substantial distress while attending school with pleas to parents for future nonattendance | Severe misbehaviors in the morning in an attempt to miss school | Chronic tardiness to school | Skipping certain classes or periods of school during the school day | Lengthy absences from school |

Figure 66-1. Spectrum of School Refusal Behavior.

2. Other causes.
   a. Family functioning. Few studies have systematically evaluated and measured these problems. Family interactions that are associated with school refusal include the following:
   - **Enmeshed parent–child dyads**—characterized by dependency and overindulgence.
   - **Conflictive families**—characterized by high rates of coercion, noncompliance, and aggression.
   - **Detached families**—characterized by diffusion of activity and minimal intrafamilial interaction.
   - **Isolated families**—characterized by minimal extrafamilial contact.
   - **Healthy families characterized by having an individual child with a behavioral problem.** Most families of children with school refusal behavior show adaptive or healthy daily functioning.
   b. Learning and language difficulties. This has not been extensively investigated. However, academic and communicative difficulties may have a significant contribution in the etiology of school refusal.
   c. School-based stressors.
   - **Environmental.** May include-bathroom restrictions for children; unsupervised toilets, changing areas, and public areas causing the child to feel unsafe and vulnerable.
   - **Academic.** May include change of school or syllabus, excessive academic pressure, an impending test, a requirement to recite in class, a poor report card.
   - **Interpersonal.** May include discordant/adverse relationship with peers (e.g., bullying, teasing on the school grounds), loss of a school friend, teachers/supervisors unjustly blaming the child for their deficiencies, impersonal or hostile teacher–student relationships, physical fitness requirements for overweight or clumsy children.

Table 66-1. Criteria for differential diagnosis of school refusal and truancy

School refusal	Truancy
Severe emotional distress about attending school; may include anxiety, temper tantrums, depression, or somatic symptoms.	Lack of excessive anxiety or fear about attending school.
Parents are aware of absence; child often tries to persuade parents to allow him or her to stay home.	Child often attempts to conceal absence from parents.
Absence of significant antisocial behaviors such as juvenile delinquency.	Frequent antisocial behavior, including delinquent and disruptive acts (e.g., lying, stealing), often in the company of peers.
During school hours, child usually stays home because it is considered a safe and secure environment.	During school hours, child frequently does not stay home.
Child expresses willingness to do schoolwork and complies with completing work at home.	Lack of interest in schoolwork and unwillingness to conform to academic and behavior expectations.

Adapted from Fremont WP. School refusal in children and adolescents. *Am Fam Physician* 68(8):1555–1560, 2003.

Table 66-2. Presenting physical symptoms for school refusal

1. General—**insomnia,** excessive sleeping, fatigue, "always tired," "fever," "always sick" temper tantrums
2. Skin—**pallor**
3. Eye—blurred vision
4. ENT—recurrent sore throats, recurrent sinus problems, constant colds, dysphagia
5. Respiratory—**hyperventilation,** coughing tics, **vocal cord dysfunction**
6. Cardiovascular—**palpitations,**[a] chest pains[a]
7. Gastrointestinal—**recurrent abdominal pains, anorexia, nausea, recurrent vomiting, diarrhea**
8. Renal/genital—**frequency-urgency syndrome**
9. Skeletal—bone pain, joint pain, back pain, "fibromyalgia"
10. Neuromuscular—**headaches,**[a] dizziness,[a] syncope,[a] "weakness," "always tired"
11. Pervasive symptoms—acute anxiety attack or **panic reaction**[a]

The **symptoms** are physiological manifestations of anxiety. The other symptoms may be fabricated or exaggerated.
[a]More common in older children.

 D. Sequelae of school refusal. School refusal has very significant consequences.
- Short-term consequences—poor academic performance, family difficulties and conflict, peer relationship problems, financial and legal consequences.
- Long-term consequences—academic underachievement, fewer opportunities to attend institutions of higher education, employment difficulties, social difficulties, increased risk of psychiatric illness.

II. Making the diagnosis.
 A. Signs and symptoms. Tables 66-2 and 66-3 review common presenting symptoms. Most children with school refusal complain of anxiety-related physical symptoms at the time of departure for school. When the child is permitted to stay home from or is sent home from school, these symptoms quickly improve and completely disappear.
 B. Confirming the diagnosis. School refusal is a diagnosis of inclusion that can be confirmed by documenting these common features.
1. Severe difficulty in attending school, often resulting in prolonged absence.
2. Severe emotional upset, which may involve such symptoms as excessive fearfulness, temper tantrums, misery, or complaints of feeling ill when faced with the prospect of going to school.
3. The child complains of recurrent and vague physical symptoms predominantly in the morning. These become accentuated when the family tries to send the child to school and often improves and disappears by midmorning. No organic cause is found on careful evaluation, including a physical examination and appropriate laboratory tests. *The discrepancy between how sick the child sounds and how well the child looks is a hallmark of this disorder.*
4. During school hours the child remains at home with the knowledge of the parents.
5. Absence of significant antisocial disorders such as juvenile delinquency, disruptiveness, and sexual activity.
 C. Differential diagnosis. Each physical symptom listed in Table 66-2 has a specific and lengthy differential diagnosis.
1. The primary care clinician should attempt to rule out within reason physical disease as a cause of the school refuser's symptoms. Excessive or chronic school refusal also can have other causes (Table 66-4).

Table 66-3. Common behavioral symptoms of school refusal behavior

Internalizing/covert symptoms	Externalizing/overt symptoms
Depression	Aggression
Fatigue/tiredness	Clinging to an adult
Fear and panic	Excessive reassurance-seeking behavior
General and social anxiety	Noncompliance and defiance
Self-consciousness	Refusal to move in the morning
Somatization	Temper tantrums and crying
Worry	

Adapted from Kearney CA. Dealing with school refusal behavior: a primer for family physicians. *J Fam Pract* 55(8):685–692, 2006.

Table 66-4. Chronic school refusal: a differential diagnosis

School refusal
   Separation anxiety
   Phobia
   Anxiety/depression
School stressors
Truancy
Family dysfunction
Learning problems
   Learning disability with poor adaptation
   Language disorders
Medical causes
   Overresponse to minor illnesses
   Chronic physical disease with poor adaptation
Other mental health disorders
   Psychosis
   Adjustment disorder
   Disruptive behavior disorders
Vulnerable child syndrome
Substance abuse
Teenage pregnancy

2. Some parents keep a child at home for a prolonged period of time because of misconceptions regarding the need for bed rest or isolation. Children with chronic physical disease or learning disabilities may become reluctant to attend school because they are unable to adapt well to the academic environment or to the other children.

D. Assessment. It is important that a multimethod and multi-informant approach be utilized in the evaluation of youth with school refusal owing to their differing clinical presentation, family dynamics, and school situation. The evaluation should include interviews with the family and individual interviews with the child and parents as well as the school staff. Assessment should include a complete medical history and physical examination, history of the onset and development of school refusal symptoms, associated stressors, school history, peer relationships, family functioning, psychiatric history, substance abuse history, and a mental status examination. Identification of specific factors responsible for school refusal behaviors is important.

E. Key clinical questions.
1. *"How is your child doing in school?"* Do not assume that parents will bring up poor school attendance to the clinician during office visits.
2. *"How much school has your child missed because of these symptoms?"* Some parents may underestimate their child's school absences until a direct question such as this is posed.
3. *"How many days of school did your child miss last year?"* This information is needed when parents blame the problem on some illness or stress that began during the current school year.
4. *"When did your child's school refusal behavior develop?"* This pertains to the acuteness or chronicity of the problem.
5. *"What is your child's academic and social status?"* This should include a review of academic records, report cards, attendance records, and individualized education plans or 504 plans as applicable.
6. *"When are the symptoms worse?"* In school refusal, the symptoms are usually worse on Sunday nights, early mornings, Mondays, during the start of the school year, and following holidays. The onset of symptoms often dates to entering kindergarten or first grade.
7. *"What do you think is causing the symptoms?"* or *"What is the worst diagnosis your child could have?"* The parents may fear a specific disease that the child does not harbor.
8. *"Have any major changes occurred in your family?"* This question may help the family acknowledge stressors they may have initially overlooked, denied, or not linked to the child's school refusal.

9. *"Does your child ever stay overnight with friends at their homes?"* or *"How does your child do with activities away from home (e.g., camps)?"* An inability to be away from parents supports separation issues.

10. *"What is the worst possible thing that could happen if you sent your child to school with these symptoms?"* This addresses the parents' fear that their child will emotionally decompensate at school, have embarrassing symptoms, or be teased.

11. The function of the behavior should also be explored with the child. Is he avoiding school because of fears provoked by the school environment (e.g., examinations, recitation), separation anxiety, to escape from aversive social situations (e.g., bullying), or to seek attention (e.g., somatic complaints or crying spells)?

F. **Clinical measures.** Standardized parent and teacher behavior checklists, child self-report measures, and mental health scales help delineate problems and compare severity of behaviors at home and at school.

1. Generalized scales—used to identify areas of difficulties. The utility of these measures in developing effective treatment strategies have not been demonstrated. Examples include the following:
   a. Child Behavior Checklist
   b. Teacher's Report Form
   c. Behavior Assessment System for Children, Second Edition

2. Specific scales—used to assess symptoms and severity of mental health problems including anxiety and depression. Examples include the following:
   a. Screen for Child Anxiety-Related Disorders
   b. Spence Children's Anxiety Scale
   c. School refusal–specific scale—School Refusal Assessment Scale (See Kearney reference). Provides a functional and symptomatic assessment of refusal behaviors

G. **Physical examination.** The physical examination of these children should be **completely normal**. The performance of a meticulous examination is often reassuring to parents.

H. **Laboratory tests.** Each specific physical symptom will determine which laboratory studies (if any) are appropriate.

III. Management.
A. Principles of treatment.

1. Return the child to full-time school attendance.
   a. Gradual return
   b. Forced return
      • highly controversial
      • **may be useful for acute cases** where onset is rapid and there has been no prior history of similar problems
      • highly stressful for both the child and the parents

2. Removal from school (e.g., hospitalization, homeschooling) is avoided whenever possible

3. Supportive parental involvement

4. Close communication between physician and school regarding support for the child in school

5. Individualized treatment plan according to the underlying motivation for school refusal

6. Monitoring of child's progress and prevention of relapse upon successful reintegration

B. Strategies.
A collaborative team approach that involves the primary care clinician, the child, family, school staff, and mental health professional should be utilized.

1. **Education for the family and the child.** The main barrier to successful treatment is changing the family's focus from an organic to a nonorganic etiology for the behavior.
   a. **Explain what school refusal is and that many things can cause real physical symptoms.** No matter the etiology, reassure the parents and the child that you recognize that the symptom described is real.
   b. **Partner with parents.** Once the primary care clinician has reassured the family that the child is well, he or she should work with the parents to institute an immediate return to school. Being in school is intrinsically therapeutic and breaks the negative cycle that occurs when a child gets out of step with schoolwork and friendships. Parents and pediatric clinician may need to collaborate intensively to ensure the child's daily attendance to school. The pediatric clinician should support parents in their efforts and reassure them that the child's symptoms are not due to poor parenting.
   c. **Engage the child by acknowledging the reality of feelings,** working together to plan return to school and dealing with anxieties through problem solving, relaxation training, breathing retraining, and social skills training.

    d. Be specific with the parents as to why you believe the symptom is not the result of physical disease. Explain the diagnosis by pointing to the timing of the symptoms, the age of onset that coincides with school entry, the presence of the symptoms during previous school years, the normal physical examination and normal laboratory tests (if done).

    e. Clarify that the child is in excellent physical health. Pronounce the child *unequivocally* physically well. Do not leave the parents hanging with statements such as, "He *probably* has school refusal, but we cannot be certain."

    f. Use appropriate diagnoses. If the child meets criteria for a specific anxiety or mood disorder, pediatricians should inform parents and explain the diagnostic criteria that the child fulfilled.

    g. Reassure parents that you can effectively treat this condition. The primary care clinician can promise to provide a treatment plan that will reduce the symptoms in the majority of cases. The minimal goal of this discussion should be to get the parents to agree to regular school attendance pending additional observations, even if they cling to the idea that their child may have some rare disease.

2. Behavior interventions. These techniques focus on the child's behaviors and emphasize treatment in the context of the family and school.

    a. These are primarily exposure-based treatments.

    b. Examples include systematic desensitization (i.e., graded exposure to school environment) and relaxation training. This is the recommended intervention where the refusal is considered to be primarily the result of a strong phobic reaction to being in school.

    c. Cognitive behavior therapy (CBT) as a behavior intervention is a highly structured approach where children learn specific techniques on how to confront their fears and modify negative thoughts. CBT, modeling, and role playing are recommended techniques for school refusal behavior that is largely based on avoidance of social and/or evaluative situations.

    d. Educational-support therapy is another form of behavior intervention. This involves a combination of educational presentations; supportive psychotherapy; and a daily diary for the child to record his or her fears, thoughts, coping strategies, and feelings associated with the fears. In comparison to CBT, no specific instructions are given to the child on how to handle his or her anxiety.

3. Parent–teacher interventions and contingency management are suggested interventions for school refusal behavior that results from a desire to obtain caregiver attention.

For the parents:

    a. Plan calm morning routines.

    b. Escort the child to school.

    c. Allow the child to stay in contact with parents by phone.

    d. Provide positive reinforcement for school attendance.

    e. Decrease positive reinforcement for staying home (e.g., allowing child to watch television while home from school).

    f. Provide attention-based consequences for school nonattendance (e.g., early bedtime, limited time with parent at night).

    g. Cognitive training to help reduce their own anxiety and understand their role in helping their child makes effective changes.

For the teacher:

    a. Use of positive reinforcement—access to school garden, special lunchtime activities, privileges, and rewards.

    b. Making academic, social, emotional, and environmental accommodations for the child.

        • Gradual reintegration to school and classes, which may include initial attendance at lunchtime, one or two favorite classes or in an alternative classroom setting such as a guidance counselor's office or the library.

        • Modified curriculum for the child.

        • Reduced homework.

    c. Communication between the primary care clinician and the school nurse is essential. The clinician should be called if the child's attendance remains poor or if the child is in the nurse's office and wants to go home. The clinician and school nurse can then work together to decide whether the child should stay in school.

4. Family therapy.

    a. Effectiveness is unclear.

    b. Rarely used in isolation.

  c. Tends to focus on parent training and contingency management.
  d. Nature of the family dynamic should be assessed.
  e. Suggested approach for school refusal behavior that may result from pursuit of tangible reinforcers outside of school.
5. **Pharmacotherapy.**
  a. Rarely used but may be particularly useful in school refusal behavior that is based on anxiety and/or depression. Data are inconclusive as to the effectiveness of pharmacologic agents in the treatment of school refusal. Selective serotonin reuptake inhibitors—research has shown that these agents can be effective and safe in the treatment of childhood anxiety and depression.
  b. Should be used in conjunction with behavioral and psychotherapeutic interventions, not as a first-line or sole treatment.
6. **Follow-up visits** are essential for monitoring attendance. Children with school refusal should have return visits in approximately 1 week, 1 month, and again approximately 2 weeks into the following school year. Parents also need to call their clinician on the first day of acute illnesses to help decide whether the child needs to stay home.
C. **Criteria for referral.** The primary care clinician needs to refer the child with more severe, intractable emotional problems or chronic school refusal to a developmental–behavioral pediatrician, child psychiatrist, psychologist, or social worker. Most children who have been on prolonged bed rest should also be referred. Most of all, patients who are unresponsive to pediatric counseling need referral.
IV. **Prognosis.** Most early school refusal situation will improve spontaneously or with consistent and firm parental input and support. School refusal for longer than 2 years (child most likely being homeschooled), occurrence in adolescence, associated with depression, lower IQ, and having a comorbid mental health disorder correlate with a poor prognosis (e.g., severe emotional and social difficulties into adulthood).
V. **Clinical pearls and pitfalls.**
  - Suspect school refusal by the symptom's pattern because no organic disease has this profile or keeps this timetable.
  - Ask about school attendance and academic performance whenever you evaluate a child for recurrent or persistent symptoms.
  - Do not be misled because the child "likes school," is a good student or "wants to go back."
  - Protect these children from unwarranted laboratory tests, procedures, prescriptions, hospitalization, and surgery.
  - Request that children return to school, even while the evaluation is ongoing. The response will be either diagnostic or therapeutic.
  - Primary care clinicians should avoid writing excuse letters for children to stay out of school unless there is a medical condition that necessitates them to stay home.
  - Comorbid psychiatric disorders, family dysfunction, and other contributing problems should always be considered in the evaluation and treatment.

BIBLIOGRAPHY

For parents

Kearny CA. *Getting Your Child to Say "Yes" to School: A Guide for Parents of Youth with School Refusal Behavior*. New York, NY: Oxford University Press, 2007.
Schmitt BD. When your child has school phobia (a parent information sheet). *Contemp Pediatr* 7(8):41–42, 1990.

Web sites

American Family Physician. http://www.aafp.org/afp/20031015/1563ph.html
American Academy of Child and Adolescent Psychiatry. http://www.aacap.org/publications/factsfam/noschool.htm
Children's Hospital Boston. http://www.childrenshospital.org/az/Site1562/mainpageS1562P0.html

For professionals

Egger HL, Costello EJ, Angold A. School refusal and psychiatric disorders: a community study. *J Am Acad Child Adolesc Psychiatry* 42:797, 2003.
Fremont WP. School refusal in children and adolescents. *Am Fam Physician* 68(8):1555–1560, 2003.
Hanna GL, Fischer DJ, Fluent TE. Separation anxiety disorder and school refusal in children and adolescents. *Pediatr Rev* 27:56–63, 2006.

Kearney CA. Identifying the function of school refusal behavior: a revision of the school refusal assessment scale. *J Psychopathol Behav Assess* 24:235–245, 2002.

Kearney CA. Dealing with school refusal behavior: a primer for family physicians. *J Fam Pract* 55(8):685–692, 2006.

King NJ. School refusal in children and adolescents: a review of the past 10 years. *J Am Acad Child Adolesc Psychiatry* 40:107–205, 2001.

Web sites

American Academy of Family Physicians. http://www.aafp.org/afp/20031015/1555.html

NYU Child Study Center. http://www.aboutourkids.org/articles/understanding_school_refusal

67

School Failure

Paul H. Dworkin

I. **Description of the problem.** More than 10% of schoolchildren in the United States are receiving special education and other services because of difficulties with school performance. School failure is a complex issue that defies traditional methods of pediatric evaluation and management. Although learning problems are of obvious multidisciplinary concern, the primary care clinician plays a vital role in clarifying the reasons for school failure and facilitating appropriate evaluation and intervention.

A. **Reasons for school failure.** A wide variety of causes may contribute to a child's failure in school. A simple classification scheme identifies **intrinsic** or child-related causes (e.g., specific learning disabilities (LDs), attention deficits) and **extrinsic** or environmental-related causes relating to either the home (e.g., parental separation or divorce) or the school setting (e.g., poor instruction). In most cases, school failure is not due to a single factor but rather the result of a **complex interaction of child-, family-, and school-related variables**.

B. **Specific causes.**

1. **Learning disabilities.** As defined by federal legislation: *Specific learning disability means a disorder in one or more of the basic psychological processes involved in understanding or in using language, spoken or written, which may manifest itself in an imperfect ability to listen, think, speak, read, write, spell, or to do mathematical calculations.*

   The term includes such conditions as perceptual handicaps, brain injury, minimal brain dysfunction, dyslexia, and developmental aphasia. The term does not include children who have problems that are primarily the result of visual, hearing, or motor disabilities; intellectual disability; emotional disturbance; or environmental, cultural, or economic disadvantage. Family, genetic, cognitive, and neuroanatomical factors are all implicated as etiologies for LDs.

   LDs are traditionally characterized by a **discrepancy between ability (as measured by intelligence tests) and actual academic achievement**. Federal guidelines also ask whether a child could achieve at a level commensurate with age and ability if provided with appropriate learning experiences. Their prevalence is estimated **at 3%–5% of schoolchildren**. Although most children with LDs have underlying weaknesses in language function, weaknesses in other higher-order cognitive functions (so-called metacognitive skills) have been increasingly recognized among children with nonverbal LDs. Such children may have difficulties with reasoning, memory, or focusing their attention and have been described as "passive learners" because of their difficulties with selecting strategies for problem solving.

2. **Attention deficits** (see Chapter 25). There exists significant overlap between children with LD and attention-deficit/hyperactivity disorder (ADHD). From a clinical standpoint, distinguishing between children with an intrinsic deficit of attention and those with attention deficits secondary to other developmental and behavioral dysfunctions (e.g., language impairment, depression) is often difficult.

3. **Intellectual disability** (see Chapters 51 and 52). Mild disability (i.e., IQ in the 50–70 range) is often not identified until children are confronted with the cognitive demands of school. At that time, a slow learning rate and ultimate acquisition of academic skills up to the fifth- or sixth-grade level is typically seen.

4. **Sensory impairment.** Hearing loss results in a significant educational handicap because language acquisition and communication skills are impaired. Such students typically experience difficulties in reading, arithmetic reasoning, and problem solving. They may exhibit classroom maladjustment, behavioral problems, and social immaturity. The prognosis directly relates to the age at which identification occurs. In comparison, blind children usually fare better within the classroom. Visually impaired children who experience school failure tend to have additional handicaps.

317

5. **Emotional illness.** From 30%–80% of emotionally disturbed students have problems with academic achievement and classroom behavior. Emotional problems such as low self-esteem and poor self-image often exacerbate school failure brought on by other causes, such as LD or ADHD.

6. **Chronic illness.** From 25%–33% of chronically ill students have problems with academic achievement (see Chapter 36). Possible adverse influences on school performance include limited alertness or stamina, chronic pain, medication side effects, absenteeism, emotional maladjustment, low intelligence (primarily children with certain neurologic disorders), the inferior quality of alternative classroom placement, and inappropriate or unrealistic expectations by teachers and parents. In addition, certain chronic diseases (e.g., epilepsy, cerebral palsy, myelomeningocele) are associated with an increased incidence of LD.

7. **Temperamental dysfunction** (see Chapter 81). The temperamentally "difficult" student may become easily frustrated and angry when confronted with material not easily mastered. The initial reluctance to participate and tendency to withdraw of the "slow-to-warm-up" child may be misinterpreted as anxiety or as a limited capacity for learning. Although the temperamentally "easy" student usually fares well, problems may arise when expectations for behavior markedly differ between home and school. For example, a student's mild intensity of reaction to situations or stimuli may be misinterpreted within the classroom as a lack of interest or motivation.

8. **Family dysfunction and social problems.** Family issues that contribute to school failure include parental separation and divorce, child abuse and neglect, the illness or death of an immediate family member, parental psychopathology, early parenthood, substance abuse, and poverty.

9. **Ineffective schooling.** School *processes* are more important determinants of students' performance than such features as whether schools are public or private, class size, the age and spaciousness of school buildings, and student teacher ratio. Rather, the school's academic emphasis, expectations for attainment, amount of homework, teachers' actions during lessons, use of group instruction, and the use of rewards and praise have major influences on students' performance. Aspects of the school's social environment (such as the amount of praise offered to children) may be particularly important for children from disadvantaged homes in which less emphasis is placed on academic attainment and standards for classroom behavior. Knowledge of the relationships between school effectiveness and school achievement has important implications for assessing and promoting both individual student performance and public policy.

II. **Making the diagnosis.** If psychoeducational evaluation has already identified the reasons for a student's school failure (e.g., LD or mild intellectual disability), the goal of pediatric evaluation is to exclude medical problems as contributors to poor classroom performance. In addition, the primary care clinician's familiarity with the child and family may be helpful in identifying social or emotional factors that further impair school performance. For the child with newly recognized school failure, the pediatric clinician must identify such conditions as sensory impairment or chronic illness, while searching for medical, neurophysiologic, and psychological correlates of such other conditions as LD, intellectual disability, and emotional illness. Possible components of the evaluation of children with school failure include the following:

A. **History.** Important historic information should be sought from parents, teachers, and the child. Review of the student's perinatal and past medical history, developmental milestones, past and present behavior, and family and social history may yield findings with possible implications for school failure (Table 67-1).

B. **Key clinical questions.**
1. *"Which subjects are particularly difficult for the child?"* The pattern of delays may suggest a specific etiology; for example, children with an LD typically have discrete difficulties in selected subjects, whereas students with mild cognitive impairment have more pervasive academic delays.

2. *"How does the child behave in the classroom?"* Classroom behavior may suggest ADHD, poor self-image, or conduct disorder.

3. *"How many days has the child missed school?"* Poor school attendance may be due to chronic illness, school phobia, or poor motivation due to LD.

4. *"Has past testing been performed?"* Past educational or psychological testing may have identified causes of a child's school failure.

5. *"What special services has the child received?"* Responses to different instructional techniques ("diagnostic teaching") may suggest reasons for school failure.

Table 67-1. The role of history in the evaluation of school learning problems

Aspect	Findings suggestive of learning disorders
School functioning	
Academic achievement	Discrete delays in select subject (e.g., language)
	Adequate early performance, with difficulties emerging later (e.g., mathematics, writing)
Classroom behavior	Long-standing, pervasive problems with inattention, impulsivity, overactivity
	Disorganization and poor strategy formation
	Depression, moodiness
Attendance	Excessive absenteeism
	School avoidance
Past psychoeducational testing	Discrepancy between cognitive abilities and academic achievement
Special required school services	Response to "diagnostic teaching"
Perinatal history	Clusters of adverse events
	Maternal alcohol or drug intake
Medical history	Recurrent and/or persistent otitis media
	Iron deficiency anemia
	Lead poisoning
	Seizures
	Frequent injuries
	Chronic medication use
Development	Delayed or disordered language acquisition and communication skills
	Subtle delays in select milestones
	Uneven pattern of skills and interests
Behavioral history	Long-standing, pervasive problems with attention span, impulsivity, acting out, overactivity
	Sadness
	Poor self-esteem
Family history	Learning problems
	School failure among first-degree relatives
Social history	Child abuse or neglect
	Other stressors

From Dworkin PH. School learning problems and developmental differences. In McInerny TK, Adam HM, Campbell DE, et al. (eds), *Textbook of Pediatric Care* (1st ed), Elk Grove Village, IL: American Academy of Pediatrics, 2009, 1149–1155.

C. Physical examination. The physical examination has a limited, but important, role in the evaluation of children with school failure. Certain specific aspects deserve special emphasis (Table 67-2).

D. Mental status examination. Simple projective techniques may suggest emotional issues such as depression, anxiety, or poor self-image as the cause or, even more likely, the consequence of school failure. Examples include the following:

1. *"If you had three wishes, what would they be?"*
2. *"If you could make three changes in your life, what would they be?"* The sad or anxious child may be unwilling to offer wishes or hope for changes in family or school circumstances.
3. *"Draw a picture of your family"* may suggest concerns with family composition or reveal anxiety or uncertainty regarding the child's status within the family.

E. Neurodevelopmental assessment. Surveying the child's abilities in different areas of development may help to identify weaknesses contributing to school failure. For example, the developmental profile of a child with an LD is typically characterized by an uneven pattern, with discrete areas of relative strength and weakness. The significance of minor neurologic indicators ("soft neurologic signs") is controversial; such findings should not serve as a basis for diagnosing an LD.

F. Laboratory studies. No laboratory studies are routinely indicated in the assessment of school failure (except perhaps screening for lead poisoning). Rather, tests should be performed on the basis of specific indications.

Table 67-2. The physical examination and evaluation of school learning problems

Aspect	Findings suggestive of learning disorders
General observations	Sadness, anxiety
	Short attention span, impulsivity, overactivity
	Tics
Phenotypic features	Stigmata of genetic syndromes (e.g., sex chromosome abnormalities, fetal alcohol syndrome)
	Minor congenital anomalies
Skin	Multiple cafe au lait spots
	"Ash-leaf" spots, adenoma sebaceum
Tympanic membranes	Signs of recurrent or chronic otitis media
Genitalia	Delayed sexual maturation in boys
Growth measurements	Short stature
	Microcephaly and macrocephaly
Sensory screening	Poor hearing or vision

From Dworkin PH. School learning problems and developmental differences. In McInerny TK, Adam HM, Campbell DE, et al. (eds), *Textbook of Pediatric Care* (1st ed), Elk Grove Village, IL: American Academy of Pediatrics, 2009, 1149–1155.

G. **Further investigations and referrals.** Psychoeducational evaluation is critically important in the evaluation of children with school failure.
  1. **Goals.** The goals of such evaluations include the following:
    a. **To examine the student's academic strengths and weaknesses.**
    b. **To determine the child's cognitive ability,** including such higher-order functions as abstract reasoning, problem solving, and learning style.
    c. **To assess perceptual strengths and weaknesses.**
    d. **To examine communicative ability.**
    e. **To assess social and emotional adaptation.**
  2. **Performance.** Ideally, such evaluations are performed by the child's school system, in accordance with state and federal mandates. There is no one standardized evaluation appropriate for all children, and the specific tests used depend on the preference and expertise of the examiner and the child's needs. Examples include intelligence tests; tests of general learning abilities; academic achievement tests; diagnostic reading, math, and writing tests; tests of perceptual and motor function; and such informal techniques as diagnostic teaching. School personnel performing such evaluations may include psychologists, special educators, LD specialists, speech-language pathologists, and social workers.
III. **Management.** For LDs, mild cognitive impairment, and other common causes of school failure, educational intervention is the most crucial. Nonetheless, a variety of important primary care roles are both feasible and important in the management of school failure.
  A. **Specific medical intervention** is the most traditional of pediatric roles. Examples include the following:
    1. **The treatment of underlying medical conditions,** such as asthma or a seizure disorder, that influence school performance.
    2. **Pharmacologic management** of ADHD.
  B. **Counseling** is a traditional mode of pediatric intervention. Aspects may include the following:
    1. **Clarification of a student's strengths and weaknesses and demystification of any diagnosis such as LD and cognitive impairment.**
    2. **Anticipatory guidance regarding commonly encountered school difficulties** and the consequences of school failure (e.g., low self-esteem).
    3. **Alleviation of guilt and anxiety.**
    4. **Explaining the legal rights of students and families.**
    5. **Guidance regarding the lack of effectiveness of nontraditional treatment strategies** (e.g., dietary manipulation, optometric training).
    6. **Offering advice regarding specific behavior management strategies,** such as timeout and positive reinforcement.
    7. **Recommending educational and advocacy organizations to families** such as the International Dyslexia Society (www.interdys.org), the Learning Disabilities Association of America (www.ldaamerica.org), the National Center for Learning Disabilities (www.ncld.org), and the National Institute of Neurological Disorders and Stroke (www.ninds.nih.gov).

C. The primary care clinician can assume an active role in monitoring the progress of children with learning problems. Office visits provide important opportunities to monitor self-esteem, search for signs of depression, and offer encouragement and praise for progress.

BIBLIOGRAPHY

For parents

Organizations

Council for Exceptional Children (CEC) Division for Learning Disabilities (DLD). www.dldcec.org
Council for Learning Disabilities (CLD). www.cldinternational.org
Learning Disabilities Association of America. www.ldanatl.org
Great Schools. www.greatschools.org

Books

Levine M. *A Mind at a Time.* New York, NY: Simon & Schuster, 2002.

For professionals

American Academy of Child and Adolescent Psychiatry. Practice parameters for the assessment and treatment of children and adolescents with language and learning disorders. *J Am Acad Child Adolesc Psychiatry* 37(10 Suppl):46S–62S, 1998.
Barnes MA, Fuchs LS. Learning disabilities. In Wolraich ML, Drotar DD, Dworkin PH, et al. (eds), *Developmental-Behavioral Pediatrics*. Philadelphia, PA: Mosby Elsevier, 2008.
Capin DM. Developmental learning disorders: clues to their diagnosis and management. *Pediatr Rev* 17:284, 1996.
Dworkin PH. School failure. *Pediatr Rev* 10:301–312, 1989.
Lindsay RL. School failure/disorders of learning. In Bergman AB (ed), *Common Problems in Pediatrics*. New York, NY: McGraw-Hill, 2001.

68

School Readiness

Margot Kaplan-Sanoff

I. **Description of the problem.** *School readiness* is the term used to describe those characteristics, which are considered prerequisites for a child to be ready to succeed in a school setting. Table 68-1 lists the criteria most often identified as necessary for academic success in kindergarten or first grade. The question of school readiness also raises emotional concerns for both parents ("unfamiliar people will be judging my child and, by extension, my parenting") and children ("can I meet the challenges of the BIG school?"). There are a number of social, emotional, motoric, and cognitive factors to consider when assessing school readiness:

A. **Ability to master new experiences.** The ability to grapple with and master new experiences defines the initial task of school success. Children are asked to listen and relate to unfamiliar adults, to follow specific rules, to interact with a large group of children, and to manage daily tasks by themselves. Children who can build on familiar experiences and who can pick out the novel features of a new experience and compare the "new" with the known will quickly gain mastery of the new situations required by school, such as getting your lunch in the cafeteria. On the other hand, children who are easily overwhelmed, who panic at new experiences, and who are unable to bring knowledge of the familiar to bear on new demands may have a difficult time assimilating new knowledge in to a coherent context. Each new piece of learning disorients them, and they are unable to understand how to manage successfully in school.

B. **Lack of experience.** Some children simply lack the experience of being in a group of children of their own age. Others may lack access to books and learning materials in their homes. Because of the enormous burdens of poverty, family trauma and stress, domestic violence, inappropriately low expectations for preacademic development, or diverse cultural backgrounds, these children are unfamiliar with the tasks required for success in school (such as waiting in line, sharing materials, taking turns, or following verbal directions).

C. **Ability to tolerate separations from primary caregivers.** The relationships that children develop with teachers are different from their relationships with parents and extended family. Children are expected to establish and maintain the teacher's attention in a large group through such socially acceptable ways (e.g., waiting to be called on, or holding up their hands to answer a question or make a request).

D. **Independence in most activities of daily living.** Separated from primary caregivers, children are required to be independent in such caregiving functions as eating, toileting, napping, dressing, and taking care of their possessions.

E. **Executive function and the ability to control impulses.** Executive function refers to the skills that children develop to help them order and coordinate their thoughts and behavior, process information in a coherent way, hold relevant details in their short-term memory, avoid distractions, and focus on the task at hand. These skills include decision making, selective attention by filtering out unimportant information, and inhibiting impulses. To succeed in school, young children also need strong self-regulation skills, including organization and planning, attention, and working memory. Children should have the self-control to sit in a circle without bothering other children, to attend to adults for a limited amount of time (5–10 minutes), and to listen to and follow adult directions, some of which might be delivered from the other side of a busy room. Children are required to regulate their impulses to delay their own needs, urges, and feelings; to defer snack when they are hungry; to modify their wishes or accept alternatives to the plans they want to pursue; and to tolerate the feelings of others without resorting to inappropriate outbursts. Finally, they should be able to persist and follow through on a difficult task. Self-regulation skills have been linked to mental health, social competence, and academic achievement, more adaptive and healthy coping mechanisms and have been shown to predict academic success more reliably than IQ tests.

Table 68-1. School readiness skills

Kindergarten
Listens to stories without interrupting
Recognizes rhyming sounds
Pays attention for short periods of time to adult-directed tasks
Understand actions have both causes and effects
Show understanding of general times of day
Draws a person
Prints name
Cuts with scissors
Traces basic shapes
Begins to share with others
Plays cooperative with peers
Starts to follow rules
Able to recognize authority
Manages bathroom needs
Buttons shirts, pants, coats, and zip up zippers
Begins to control oneself
Separates from parents without being upset
Speaks understandably
Talks in complete sentences of five to six words
Looks at pictures and then tells stories
Identifies rhyming words
Identifies some alphabet letters
Recognizes some common sight words like "stop"
Sorts and labels similar objects by color, size, and shape
Recognizes groups of one, two, three, four, and five objects
Counts to 10

First grade
Identifies upper and lower case letters
Identifies numerals to 10
Copies letters and numerals
Demonstrates conservation of mass, length, and volume
Knows address and birth date
Reads simple sight words
Works cooperatively with groups of children

F. **Appropriate play skills.** Early school success is dependent, in part, on the child's ability to get along with peers, to manage in a group, and to engage in developmentally appropriate play. Children should be able to play with other children without resorting to hitting, biting, or yelling to resolve conflicts. They should be able to manage the give and take of peer relationships, both within a structured play activity like a board game and in fantasy play. Children should also be able to differentiate fantasy play and stories from reality. Opportunities to engage in sustained, mature play can foster strong executive function and self-regulation skills.

G. **Mental health concerns**. There is growing awareness of mental health concerns in young children. From 9.5%–14.2% of children younger than 6 years have emotional problems serious enough to hurt their ability to function, including anxiety or behavioral disorders and depression. Early stresses, including child abuse or neglect, domestic or community violence, extreme poverty and food insufficiency, and parental mental health concerns and/or substance abuse, can prime neurobiological stress systems to become hyperresponsive to adversity. Known as "toxic stress," these early stressors interfere with developing brain circuits and pose a serious threat to young children not only by undermining their emotional well-being but by impairing early learning, exploration and curiosity, and school readiness.

H. **Developmental delays.** Specific cognitive or learning problems, receptive or expressive language delays, and visual motor or sensory integration problems may make it difficult for a child to succeed in a regular school classroom. Yet these are the very children who benefit most from a more formal learning environment. They should be evaluated by the school department and placed in the least restrictive learning environment within the school, perhaps in a transitional classroom or a resource room program with a significant portion of their school day spent in a regular classroom. Children who do not possess sufficient school readiness skills due to developmental delays will not benefit from "another year" at home or in childcare waiting to be ready for school. At 3 years of age, they are legally eligible for public school services and should be provided with specific educational placements, which maximize their strengths and address their problems.

II. **Making the diagnosis.** The skills listed in Table 68-1 constitute the "how" of school readiness. Such specific cognitive and motor tasks (e.g., knowing the ABCs, printing one's name, using a computer mouse, or cutting with scissors) are highly idiosyncratic milestones and do not automatically correlate to the actual tasks of school learning. For example, knowing the alphabet by singing the ABC song is a far less powerful predictor of reading success than is the child's understanding of the power and function of the written word.

A. **History taking.** Involving both parents and child in a developmental history taking can provide the clinician with a great deal of information pertinent to the issue of school readiness. This activity can have particular significance when considering the 3- or 4-year-old well child visit as a "transition/school readiness" check to determine how well the child is acquiring the skills needed to succeed in kindergarten. Input from the childcare provider can add an additional perspective to the diagnosis. The following clinical inquiries can be used to guide the discussion and trigger the need for additional information:

1. *"Has the child followed an age-appropriate developmental trajectory in language, cognitive, social, and motor development?"*
2. *"How does the child respond to unusual events at home or in childcare such as a substitute provider or a change in the daily routine?"*
3. *"Has the child had any preschool or group care experience? How has he done in these settings?"*
4. *"Were there any developmental or behavioral concerns during those experiences in group care?"*
5. *"Does the child play well with peers? Or does the child consistently choose to play with younger children?"*
6. *"Does the child cling to behaviors more appropriate for a younger child (e.g., continual thumb sucking, frequent toileting accidents, tantrums)?"*
7. *"Can the child identify colors, shapes, letters, and numbers?"*
8. *"Is the child's speech understandable and can he converse with the clinician about everyday topics of interest?"*
9. *"Does the child sit and listen to stories and look at picture books by him/her self?"*
10. *"Has the child developed a dominant hand?"*

B. **Issues within the family.** In some situations, children's behavior and development might be hampered by patterns within the family such as domestic conflict, alcohol or substance abuse, parental depression, financial concerns and food insecurity, crisis within the extended families, and loss and grief. In other families, developmental expectations might be based on gender, birth order, or learning problems within the family. Inappropriate family expectations for school success or differences between family members about school readiness should be discussed. Questions assessing the level of family functioning and the support systems, which are available to the family can be helpful to a diagnosis of school readiness:

1. *"Have there been any changes within the family such as a move, change in employment, unemployment, illness or death within extended family or friends? Have you noticed any changes in your child's behavior as a result?"*
2. *"All couples have their ups and downs. Would you say that currently your relationship is up, down, or in the middle? How do you and your partner resolve conflicts?"*
3. *"How is your health and the health of family members? Has that changed recently?"*
4. *"What was your experience in school? Were you happy and successful in school or was it a difficult experience for you? For the child's father/mother?"*
5. *"Are you getting any pressure from family members to send or not to send your child to school?"*
6. *"What are your expectations for this child in school?"*
7. *"What schools have you considered?"*
8. *"With whom have you discussed these decisions?"*

C. **Physical examination.** During the routine physical examination, place emphasis on handedness, coordination of gross, visual motor and fine motor activities, and the presence or absence of excessive overflow movements. Examine the child's vision, hearing, neurologic status, sensory integration, and neurodevelopmental maturation.

D. Developmental assessment. Unfortunately, there are currently few good developmental screening tests that are predictive of school success. Most instruments available to the pediatric clinician are not equipped to detect subtle learning disabilities or a more complicated diagnosis. If assessment is warranted because of parental, school, or pediatric concern, a referral should be made, either to the school district for an evaluation, or to an independent specialist such as a developmental and behavioral pediatrician, neuropsychologist, or learning disabilities specialist.

III. Management.

A. Children with specific learning or developmental problems. Children with identified learning problems should be referred for a complete evaluation by the school department or by an independent evaluator. Under federal law, children with special learning needs are required to receive appropriate services within "the least restrictive environment." Parents may opt to provide additional independent services such as speech or sensory integration therapy if these are not provided in the child's individual education plan. Clinicians should monitor the child's progress carefully to determine the accessibility and effectiveness of the particular therapy or educational plan. For children with identified problems or global delays (such as intellectual disability or attention-deficit/hyperactivity disorder), school entry can be a particularly challenging time for parents who may have been able to deny the extent of their child's learning problems during the preschool period. Parents often look to clinicians for projections about their child's future, thus it is important to provide realistic, but hopeful, parameters for families.

B. Behavioral issues. School placement for children who present with either acting out, impulsive behaviors, or extremely shy, inhibited behaviors should be carefully considered. Parents and clinicians must be vigilant in addressing the issues behind the labeling so that the label does not become a self-fulfilling prophecy for the child. Some school settings are a bad fit for these children. Because of overcrowding, inadequate teaching, or the overwhelming needs of the larger school population, withdrawn or inhibited children who cause no trouble can be ignored as attention goes to more aggressive or demanding children. Similarly, disruptive children or those with impulse control problems can be quickly identified as difficult students even if they are quite bright. Not surprisingly, kindergarten teachers report that it is easiest to help children to develop their academic skills and hardest to make an impact in developing their self-regulation skills.

C. Is the school ready for the child? Current kindergarten curriculum, driven by a focus on accountability and testing, focuses primarily on academic skills such as letter, number, and shape recognition. Yet few gains have been reported from this academic approach; in fact, recent research indicates that incorporating pretend play into classroom settings improves children's executive function and self-regulation skills. Used in this context, pretend play refers to "mature dramatic play" that is complex, involving multiple children in child-led extended make-believe scenarios, and lasting for hours.

Perhaps the most challenging task for clinicians is to help families negotiate school entrance when the school does not have appropriate options for children with particular special needs. Although schools are required to educate all children within the least restrictive environment, they are often unable to provide carefully planned learning experiences for children with significant emotional or technological needs. Some schools cannot provide the developmentally appropriate experiences needed by children who have experienced such trauma as extreme poverty, child abuse, domestic violence, or parental depression and substance abuse. Finally, many schools do not have the resources to cope with the increasing linguistic demands of children who have recently immigrated to this country. Clinicians have tremendous untapped power to advocate on behalf of these children. They need to join voices with the families to persuade schools to provide appropriate educational experiences for all children.

D. Waiting another year. School entrance deadlines are arbitrarily set, based as much on demographics and finances (how many young children are in the upcoming kindergarten cohort and does the school have the space and teaching resources to provide for them if the cutoff date is June or November?) as they are on best practice. There is no magic age when all children are optimally ready for school. It is important to support parents of babies born in late summer or early fall as they think through the options available to them and their child, by exploring whether to keep their child in preschool for another year:

1. *"Will there be appropriate social and learning peers in the preschool for the child?"*
2. *"Will there be adequate new challenges in the preschool for the child?"*
3. *"Are the child's physical appearance and social skills in line with the proposed preschool placement? This may differ for boys and girls."*
4. *"Do both parents agree with the decision to retain the child in preschool?"*

5. *"Does the preschool program agree with the parents' decision to retain the child for another year?"*
6. *"What is the community norm? Do many parents hold back their 'fall' children?"*
7. *"What does the child expect to happen? Will the child perceive staying in preschool as a failure if everyone else goes on the kindergarten?"*
8. *"If needed, will supplemental interventions and extra support such as speech therapy by provided?"*

If the parents decide to send the child on to elementary school:
1. *"What options might be available now for preparing the child for school entry?"*
2. Parents can ask for the upcoming class list and arrange for their child to spend time with a few children who will be in the same class. Seeing familiar faces when entering a new school can be extremely reassuring, especially to shy or slow-to-warm-up children.
3. *"Does the school have options for additional support for the child such as a transitional classroom, a second year of kindergarten if warranted, resource room support or after school programming?"*

If the child begins to have serious problems in school, it is important to acknowledge the placement mistake early on, rather than continuing to push the child ahead in the hope that he or she will catch up. It is much easier to retain a child for a second year in kindergarten or first grade than it is to repeat the fourth grade where serious learning problems may prevent the child from keeping up. Many parents report that their young or immature children do all right in the first half of the school year when much of the work is reviewed, but that they encounter significant and disheartening failure during the second half of the school year as teachers push children to master the required curriculum. Because school learning and success are so closely related to lifelong self-esteem, initial placement decisions should be taken seriously and careful thought given to possible retention if the child is struggling in kindergarten or first grade.

BIBLIOGRAPHY

For parents

Pianta R, Kraft-Sayre M. *Successful Kindergarten Transition: Your Guide to Connecting Children, Families, & Schools.* Baltimore, MD: Paul H. Brookes Pub Co, 2003.
Ryan B. *Helping Your Child Start School: A Practical Guide for Parents.* New York, NY: Citadel Trade, 1996.
Walmsley BB, Walmsley SA. *Kindergarten: Ready or Not?: A Parent's Guide.* Portsmouth, NH: Heinemann Publishing, 1996.

For children

Davis K. *Kindergarten Rocks!* New York, NY: Harcourt Children's Books, 2005.
McGhee A. *Countdown to Kindergarten.* New York, NY: Harcourt Children's Books, 2002.
Cohen M, Hoban L. *Will I Have a Friend?* New York, NY: Aladin Paperbacks, 1986.
Wing N, Durrell J. *The Night Before Kindergarten.* New York, NY: Grosset & Dunlap, 2001.

For professionals

National Scientific Council on the Developing Child. Mental health problems in early childhood can impair learning and behavior for life: Working paper #6. http://www.developingchild.net, 2008.
Miller E, Alomon J. *Crisis in the kindergarten: Why children need to play in school.* College Park, MD: Alliance for Childhood, 2009.
Pianta R, Cox M, Snow L. *School Readiness and the Transition to Kindergarten in the Era of Accountability.* Baltimore, MD: Paul H. Brookes Pub Co, 2007.
American Academy of Pediatrics Policy. The inappropriate use of School Readiness Tests. http://www.aap.org/policy/00694.html
Palfrey JS, Rappaport LR. School placement. *Pediatr Rev* 8:261–270, 1987. Ready Web http://readyweb.crc.uiuc.edu/library.html

69

Selective Mutism

Naomi Steiner

I. **Description of the problem.** Selective mutism is an **anxiety-related condition** and can be seen as the symptomatic expression of social anxiety in an **extremely shy child**. It is characterized by:
- A child's inability to speak in certain social settings (such as childcare, school) where speaking is expected, despite speaking in other, usually more familiar settings (such as at home). This disturbance affects the child's daily function.
- Onset **usually before age 5 years**, although it may not come to clinical attention until school entry.
- **Lasting for at least 1 month** (not including the first month of school or child care, during which many children may be shy or reluctant to speak).

A. **Epidemiology.**
- Limited research reports a **prevalence of 0.1%–0.7%** children in the general population and 1% of children in mental health centers
- At least **90% of these children also have social phobia** (social anxiety disorder)
- Girls outnumber boys 2 to 1
- Although selective mutism usually lasts for only a few months, it may persist longer and may even continue for several years.

B. **Etiology/contributing factors.**
1. **Genetic predisposition.** There is often a first-degree family history of social phobia (70%) and selective mutism (37%).
2. **Speech and language delays** are present in 20%–30% (most commonly language and articulation disorders).
3. **Bilingualism.** Immigrant children who are unfamiliar with or uncomfortable in a new language may refuse to speak to strangers in their new environment; this behavior should not be misdiagnosed as selective mutism. However, a prolonged silent phase should be seen as a potential red flag when selective mutism and language delay are being considered.
4. Contrary to popular belief, **no research has associated selective mutism with abuse, neglect, or trauma**.

II. **Making the diagnosis.** Initial screenings are simple, involving some observation and a few questions. The classic sign of selective mutism is that the child talks well within the home but not outside in social settings.

A. **Behavioral observations.**
- Symptoms of withdrawal in unfamiliar situations are, difficulty with eye contact, avoidance of social interaction, stiff body language, blank facial expression, using only gestures to communicate in the office.
- Marked contrast between selected environments and **the home situation,** where parents often report a very chatty child. Clinicians may want to view a videotape of the child at home to be reassured that the child's language in a comfortable environment is normal.
- Shy children will "button up" and not speak for a few hours or days but will eventually start speaking. A shy child can function. Those with selected mutism will not speak for a prolonged period of time, causing significant and prolonged social dysfunction.

B. **History: key clinical questions.**
- *"How was your child as an infant or toddler?"*
- *"How is he at school? Or birthday parties?"*
- *"How is he at home?"*
- *"Is there anybody in your family with selective mutism, anxiety, panic attacks, extreme shyness, or other emotional issues?"*

C. **Differential diagnosis.** In the past, selective mutism was sometimes misunderstood as a strong-willed and manipulative child *refusing* to speak (as in oppositional defiant disorder), as opposed to a child conditioned by a true fear of speaking. This misconception was reinforced by the former name "elective mutism." Selective mutism should be distinguished from speech disturbances that are **better accounted for by a communication disorder such as phonological disorder** or developmental language disorder. Individuals with pervasive developmental disorder or intellectual disability may have problems in social communication and be unable to speak appropriately in social situations. However, in contrast, in selective mutism the child has an established capacity to speak in some social situations, for example, typically at home.

   D. Tests.
   1. **Audiogram**—as with any speech and language disorder, it is always prudent to assure normal hearing.
   2. **Speech and language evaluation** is often indicated as 20%–30% of children with selective mutism also have some speech and language delay. This may be very difficult to obtain as the stress of the testing situation may preclude optimal testing in which case a videotape may suffice.

III. Management.
   A. Early diagnosis and rapid referral is essential for the child with selective mutism. Children with selective mutism do not necessarily outgrow their disability. Many may start to speak a little, whereas others spend years growing up without speaking. If these children do not learn to cope, they may remain significantly impaired compared to their unaffected peers. The overall goal is to treat the anxiety rather than force the child to speak.
   1. **Team approach.** The family, school, and therapist should work together to develop an individualized plan to **reduce anxiety, reduce pressure to speak, and increase self-esteem**. Consistent, supportive relationships outside the home are the mainstay of achieving these goals.
   2. **Cognitive behavioral therapy** is increasingly recognized as the first-line approach for treatment of selective mutism. It is extremely important that the child be referred to an experienced clinician who will work closely with the family and the school. Often weekly appointments will be necessary with "homework" to achieve progress. Group therapy can be very effective.

   The therapist will use techniques such as contingency and stimulus fading (where the child requires less and less prompting to speak out loud in a given situation), positive reinforcement, systematic desensitization (or gradual exposure therapy, offers situations where the child is able to practice speaking), extinction (where refusing to speak is ignored), modeling (even using videotapes), and social problem solving.
   3. **Other psychological approaches** such as relaxation training (e.g., learning breathing techniques) and social skills groups can also be helpful in adjunct to the cognitive behavioral approach.
   4. **Medication in combination with therapy** is used in the most chronic cases. Selective serotonin reuptake inhibitors (SSRIs), most commonly fluoxetine, have been shown to have a positive effect as they lower the anxiety threshold. They are usually given for 9 to 12 months.

BIBLIOGRAPHY

For parents

Selective Mutism www.selectivemutism.org
Anxiety Network www.anxietynetwork.com

For professionals

Black B, Uhde TW. Psychiatric characteristics of children with selective mutism: a pilot study. *J Am Acad Child Adolesc Psychiatry* 34:847–856, 1995.
Dow SP, Sonies BC, Scheib D, et al. Practical guidelines for the assessment and treatment of selective mutism. *J Am Acad Child Adolesc Psychairty* 34:836–846, 1995.
Dummit ES III, Klein RG, Trancer NK, et al. Systematic assessment of 50 children with selective mutism. *J Am Acad Child Adolesc Psychiatry* 36:653–660, 1997.
Stein M (ed). Selective mutism. *J Dev Behav Pediatr* 22(Suppl 2): S123–S126, 2001.

70

Self-Esteem and Resilience

Robert B. Brooks

I. **Description of the problem.** Self-esteem plays a significant role in virtually every sphere of a child's development and functioning. Performance in school, the quality of peer relationships, the ease and effectiveness of dealing with mistakes and failure, the motivation to persevere at tasks, and the abuse of drugs and alcohol are behaviors influenced by a child's self-esteem.

Self-esteem is also implicated strongly in whether or not a child is resilient. Resilience may be understood as **the capacity of a child to deal effectively with stress and pressure, to cope with everyday challenges, to rebound from disappointments, mistakes, trauma, and adversity, to develop clear and realistic goals, to solve problems, to interact comfortably with others, and to treat oneself and others with respect and dignity**. Given the importance of self-esteem and resilience and the number of children who are burdened by low self-esteem, it is a worthwhile goal of the primary care clinician to become knowledgeable about effective strategies to foster a child's sense of self-worth, competence, hope, and resilience.

Some clinicians have proposed that self-esteem is a product of the difference between our "ideal self," or how we would like to be and what we would like to accomplish, and how we actually see ourselves—the larger the difference, the lower our self-esteem. A broader definition was offered by the California Task Force to Promote Self-Esteem and Personal and Social Responsibility, which envisioned self-esteem not only in terms of "appreciating my own worth and importance" but also "having the character to be accountable for myself and to act responsibly toward others." This definition incorporates the respect and caring we show toward others as a basic feature of self-esteem, thereby lessening the possibility that self-esteem will be confused with conceit or self-centeredness.

A. **Etiology/contributing factors.**

1. **Parent–child "goodness-of-fit".** The development of self-esteem and resilience is a complex process that can best be understood as occurring within the dynamic interaction between a child's inborn temperament and the environmental forces that affect the child. "Mismatches" between the style and temperament of caregivers and children may trigger anger and disappointment in both parties. In such a situation children may come to believe that they have disappointed others, that they are failures, or that others are unfair and unkind. Low self-esteem and a sense of pessimism are common outcomes unless parents are able to lessen the impact of these mismatches by understanding and appreciating their child's unique make-up and by modifying their own expectations and reactions so that they are more in concert with their child's temperament.

2. **Attribution theory.** Attribution theory is one promising framework for articulating the components of self-esteem by looking at the reasons that people offer for why they think they succeeded or failed at a task or situation. The explanations given are directly linked to an individual's self-esteem and resilience. It appears that children with high self-esteem perceive their successes as determined in a large part by their own efforts, resources, and abilities (internal locus of control). These children assume realistic credit for their achievements and possess a sense of personal control over what is occurring in their lives. This feeling of personal control is one of the foundations of a resilient mindset and lifestyle.

In contrast, children with low self-esteem often believe that their successes are the result of luck or chance and factors outside their control. Such a view lessens their confidence in being successful in the future.

Self-esteem also plays a role in how children understand mistakes and failures in their lives. Children with high self-esteem typically believe that mistakes are experiences to learn from rather than to feel defeated by. Mistakes are attributed to factors within their power to change, such as a lack of effort on a realistically attainable goal. Children who possess this view are better equipped to deal with setbacks and, thus, are more resilient.

On the other hand, children with low self-esteem, when faced with failure, tend to believe that they cannot remedy the situation. They believe that mistakes result from situations that are not modifiable, such as a lack of ability, and this belief generates a feeling of helplessness and hopelessness. This profound sense of inadequacy makes future success less likely because these children expect to fail and begin to retreat from age-expected demands, relying instead on self-defeating coping strategies. Resilience is noticeably absent when a child's life is dominated by feelings of resignation and hopelessness.

Attribution theory has significant implications for designing interventions for reinforcing self-esteem, optimism, and resilience in children. It serves as a blueprint for asking the following questions:

- "How do we create an environment in homes and schools that maximizes the opportunity for children not only to succeed but to believe that their accomplishments are predicated in great measure on their own abilities and efforts?"
- "How do we create an environment that reinforces the belief in children that mistakes and failure often form the very foundation for learning and growth—that mistakes are not only *accepted* but *expected*?"

These are important questions to address since a feeling of being in control of and taking responsibility for one's life and dealing effectively with mistakes and setbacks are significant features of resilience.

II. **Making the diagnosis.** The signs of low self-esteem and limited resilience vary considerably. Children may display low self-esteem in situations in which they feel less than competent but not in those in which they are more successful. For instance, children with a learning disability may feel "dumb" in the classroom but may engage in sports with confidence. For some children, a sense of low self-esteem is so pervasive that there are few, if any, situations in which low self-esteem is not manifested.

With some children there is little question that their self-esteem is low or that they are not very resilient. They say such things as, "I'm dumb," "I hate how I look," "I never do anything right," "I always fail," "I'm a born loser," "I'll always be stupid."

Other children do not directly express their low self-esteem. Rather, it can be inferred from the coping strategies they use to handle stress and pressure. Children with high self-esteem use strategies for coping that are adaptive and promote growth (such as a child having difficulty mastering long division who asks for additional help from a teacher). They demonstrate a feeling of hope.

In contrast, children with low self-esteem often rely on coping behaviors that are counterproductive and intensify the child's difficulties. These self-defeating behaviors typically signal that the child is feeling vulnerable and is desperately attempting to escape from the problematic situations. Commonly used self-defeating coping behaviors are listed in Table 70-1. Although all children at some time engage in some of these behaviors, it is when these behaviors appear with regularity that a significant problem with self-esteem is suggested.

III. **Management.**

A. **Primary goals.** The strategies that follow have the greatest chance of being effective if adults convey to the child a sense of hope, caring, and support. It is well established that a basic foundation of resilience in children is the **presence of at least one adult (hopefully, several) who believes in the worth and goodness of the child.** The late psychologist, Julius Seagull referred to that person as a "charismatic adult," an adult from whom a child "gathers strength." Primary care clinicians, even in brief encounters with a child, can become charismatic adults for that child.

Table 70-1. Counterproductive coping strategies: signs of low self-esteem

Behavior	Example
Quitting	Ending a game before it is over to avoid losing
Avoiding	Not even trying something for fear of failure
Cheating	Copying answers from someone else on a test
Clowning around	Acting silly to minimize feeling like a failure
Controlling	Telling others what to do
Bullying	Putting others down to hide feelings of inadequacy
Denying	Minimizing the importance of a task
Rationalizing or making excuses	Blaming the teacher for failing a test

Strategies to nurture self-esteem and resilience should take into consideration the child's *islands of competence*, that is, areas that are (or have the potential to be) sources of pride and accomplishment. Caregivers have the responsibility to identify and build on these islands of competence, and, in so doing, a ripple effect may occur that prompts children to be more willing to venture forth and confront the tasks that have been problematic for them.

B. **Selected strategies for fostering self-esteem and resilience.**

1. **Developing responsibility and making a contribution.** If children are to develop a sense of ownership and commitment, it is important to provide them with opportunities for assuming responsibilities, especially those that involve helping them to feel that they are capable and are contributing in some way to their world and that they are truly making a difference. For example:

   - Asking an 8-year-old child to set the table at dinner or a 4-year-old child to place his clothes in the laundry bag at the end of each day—requests framed as ways of helping the family.
   - Encouraging and helping a child to write a story about his learning disability to be used to increase the understanding of others about the challenges faced by children with learning problems.
   - Asking a sixth grader with low self-esteem, who enjoyed interacting with younger children, to tutor first and second graders in the school or to be a babysitter.
   - Enlisting children to participate in a "Walk for Hunger" charity drive.

2. **Providing opportunities for making choices and decisions and solving problems.** An essential ingredient of high self-esteem and resilience is the belief that one has some control over the events of one's life. To reinforce this belief, adults must provide children with opportunities to make choices and decisions, and to solve problems that have an impact on their lives. These kinds of choices promote a sense of personal control and ownership. For example:

   - A clinician allowing a fearful child the choice of having his eyes or ears examined first so that the child is provided a sense of control.
   - Parents permitting a finicky eater to select (and eventually help prepare) the dinner meal at least once a week.
   - Having a group of elementary school students interview a town selectman, a police officer, and a lawyer as part of the process to decide whether skateboards should be allowed on school grounds, especially given the possible liability issues.
   - Parents asking their children whether they wanted to be reminded 10 or 15 minutes before bedtime that soon it would be time to get ready to go to bed.
   - A teenager deciding at what time parents may remind him to take medication, should he or she forget to do so.

3. **Offering encouragement and positive feedback and helping children to feel special.** Self-esteem and resilience are reinforced when adults communicate appreciation and encouragement to children. Words and actions conveying encouragement and thanks are always welcome and energizing. They are especially important for children burdened by self-doubt. Even a seemingly small gesture of appreciation can trigger a long-lasting, positive effect. For example:

   - Parents setting up a "special" 15-minute time in the evening with each of their two young children. The time can occur before each child goes to bed. The parents can highlight the importance of this time by calling it "special" and by saying that even if the telephone rings they will not respond to the call but instead will let the answering machine do so.
   - A primary care clinician sending a postcard to a child after an examination, saying how much he or she enjoyed seeing the child (as long as this is an honest sentiment).
   - Parents writing a brief note to their child commending the child for a particular accomplishment.
   - A recognition assembly in school in which student achievements and contributions are highlighted.

4. **Establishing self-discipline.** If children are to develop high self-esteem, they must also possess a comfortable sense of self-discipline, which involves the ability **to reason and to reflect on one's behavior and its impact on others**. The goal of discipline is to teach children, not to ridicule or humiliate them. If children are to take ownership for their actions and become resilient, they must be increasingly involved in the process of understanding and even contribute to the rules, guidelines, limits, and consequences that are established. Adults must maintain a delicate balance between being too rigid and too permissive. They must strive to blend warmth, nurturance, and acceptance with realistic expectations, clear-cut rules, and logical consequences. In addition, if

children are continuously misbehaving, the adults in their lives should attempt to understand why and focus on ways to prevent misbehavior from occurring in the first place. Examples of the effective use of discipline—including those that emphasize a preventive approach—are:

- Parents having difficulty getting a preschool child to bed; they yelled, but this only made matters worse. A consultation with a clinician revealed that the child was having nightmares and was frightened about going to bed. Greater empathy on the part of the parents and the use of a nightlight, as well as placing a photo of the parents next to the child's bed, significantly lessened his anxiety and misbehavior.
- Parents not permitting their child to use the bike for several days after he had taken a bike ride on a dangerous street that he was not allowed to ride on (an example of the use of logical consequences).
- Parents asking a child who bounced a ball that broke a window in the house to help pay for the repairs.

5. **Teaching children to deal with mistakes and failure.** The fear of making mistakes and feeling embarrassed is a potent obstacle to meeting challenges, taking appropriate risks, and therefore, to the achievement of positive self-esteem and resilience. Caregivers should find ways to communicate to children that mistakes go hand in glove with growing and learning. Examples of helping children to deal more effectively with mistakes include:

- Parents who avoid overreacting to their children's mistakes and who avoid remarks such as "Why don't you use your brain?" or "What a stupid thing to do!"
- Adults who share what they personally learned from mistakes and failures during their own childhood.
- A teacher who on the first day of the new school year asks students, "Who thinks they will probably make a mistake or not understand something in class this year?" Then, before any of the children can respond, the teacher raises his own hand. Acknowledging openly the fear of failure renders it less potent and less destructive and increases the child's courage to face new tasks. This courage is a major characteristic of resilient children.

BIBLIOGRAPHY

For parents

Books

Brooks R, Goldstein S. *Raising Resilient Children: Fostering Strength, Hope, and Optimism in Your Child*. New York: Contemporary Books, 2001.
Brooks R, Goldstein S. *Nurturing Resilience in Our Children: Answers to the Most Important Parenting Questions*. New York: Contemporary Books, 2003.
Samalin N. *Loving without Spoiling and 100 Other Timeless Tips for Raising Terrific Kids*. New York: Contemporary Books, 2003.

Web sites for parents and professionals

National PTA http://www.pta.org/topic_parent_involvement.asp. Accessed June 1, 2010.
Community Learning Network http://www.cln.org/themes_index.html. Accessed June 2, 2010.
http://www.drrobertbrooks.com. Accessed June 2, 2010.

For professionals

Brooks R. *The Self-Esteem Teacher*. Circle Pines, MN: American Guidance Service, 1991.
Katz M. *On Playing a Poor Hand Well*. New York: Norton, 1997.
Shure M. *Raising a Thinking Child*. New York: Holt, 1994.

Sensory Processing Disorder

Marie E. Anzalone

I. **Description of the problem.** Sensory processing refers to the way the nervous system receives messages from the senses and turns these messages into appropriate motor and behavioral responses. **Sensory processing disorder** (SPD, formerly referred to as **sensory integration disorder**, or SID) refers to problems in organizing and using sensory information from both the environment and the child's own body, specifically impairments in detecting, modulating, interpreting, or responding to sensory stimuli. The ability to integrate or process sensory information is a temperament-related process that varies in children and, if problematic, may interfere with the child's ability to participate in activities and relationships and affect learning capacities.

II. **Epidemiology.** Estimates place the prevalence as high as 1 in every 20 children who may experience symptoms significant enough to impact their daily life. The only study thus far conducted on prevalence of sensory integration found the incidence of SPD to be 13.9% in kindergarteners. Clinicians report higher incidence of SPD disorders in boys than girls. Families often report similar untreated traits in parents of identified children, but again, no genetic studies have been conducted. In addition, SPD may be present in children with varying diagnoses including autism spectrum disorders, nonverbal learning disabilities, attention deficit hyperactivity disorder (ADHD), and developmental coordination disorder.

III. **Etiology/contributing factors.** The etiology of SPD is not known. Some evidence has been found that children with sensory modulation disorder, specifically those with over responsivity (see preceding text) have heightened sympathetic arousal. It is hypothesized that children with SPD have atypical autonomic (both sympathetic and parasympathetic) responses to sensory challenges. The evidence supporting parasympathetic and cortisol differences in children with SPD and no co-occurring diagnoses is not convincing. It is hypothesized, but not verified, that the underlying processes contributing to SPD are temperamentally related differences in the way sensory input is processed in the central nervous system. While individual temperamental differences are considered the basis of SPD, the ultimate expression of that challenge is often dependent upon the children's interaction with their environments. Social environments that are responsive to the child's cues and thereby provide an optimal goodness-of-fit with the child's sensory needs and motor capacities can decrease behavioral disorganization, thus forming the theoretical basis of intervention.

IV. **Classifications of SPD.**

  A. **Sensory modulation disorder (SMD).** Sensory modulation is the process of grading and regulating one's response to sensory input. Sensory modulation disorder is an impairment in regulating the degree, intensity, and nature of responses to sensory input, resulting in considerable problems with daily roles and routines. One way to think of SMD is to consider that the magnitude of the child's response is in line with the magnitude of the perceived stimulus (so the over-responsive child perceives even a light affectionate touch as threatening while the under-responsive child does not even register typical ambient stimuli). There are four types of SMD:

   1. **Sensory over-responsivity**
   2. **Sensory under-responsivity**
   3. **Sensory avoidance**
   4. **Sensory seeking**

   Table 71-1 outlines the behavioral manifestation of this self-regulation in these different types of sensory modulation disorders.

  B. **Sensory discrimination disorder** is characterized by a **deficit in perception or discrimination** in one or more sensory modalities (including vision, tactile, proprioception/kinesthesia). Poor discrimination can be best understood within the literature of neurocognition and will not be discussed fully here. One unique aspect of sensory discrimination as understood within this model is the inclusion of proprioceptive discrimination. This sensory modality, not usually considered in cognitive models of discrimination is

Table 71-1. Behavioral regulation in children with different types of sensory modulation disorder

	Sensory over-responsivity (SOR)	Sensory avoidant (a subgroup of SOR)	Sensory under-responsivity (SUR)	Sensory seeking
Arousal	Usually high arousal	Attempts to modulate arousal, so often (not always) appears calm	Usually decreased arousal	Arousal may be heightened, but labile
Attention	Inability to focus attention, distractible	Hypervigilant, since need to "scan" for sensory threats	Inattentive, has a latency to attend, lack of awareness of novelty	Poorly modulated attention
Affect	Predominantly negative affect—often in "fight or flight" state	Fearful or anxious—when older may be demanding	Restricted or flat affect—may appear sad or emotionally unavailable	Affect is variable, but may become overexcited with excess sensory input
Action	Impulsive reaction—may seem aggressive	Constrained, and often avoids developmentally appropriate exploration	Passive—may observe other children, but not engage in active peer play	Action is geared primarily to gaining sensation, may be impulsive and take excess risks

essential to motor control and contributes to the sensory-based motor disorders described later.

C. **Sensory-based motor disorders.** There are two different types of sensory-based motor disorders: **dyspraxia** and **postural**. Both of these disorders are characterized by motor impairment, but while expressed in terms of motor impairment (either clumsiness, or poor balance and equilibrium), the underlying etiology for the motor impairment is a hypothesized deficit in sensory processing.

   1. *Dyspraxia* is an **inability to formulate, plan, and execute unfamiliar complex motor acts.** Children with dyspraxia may have problems in one or more of the steps involved in praxis: ideation (figuring out what to do), motor planning (figuring out how to move based on a sensory feed-forward), and execution (actually doing the action). All children with dyspraxia appear **clumsy** or **accident-prone,** and tend to avoid unfamiliar gross and fine motor actions while inflexibly relying on the "over learned" activities. Children may also have difficulty initiating age-appropriate action or play schemes and prefer familiar to novel situations. When motor planning is involved, children may have poor timing, grading, and accuracy of movement; poor handwriting, inability to imitate static or dynamic postures; or exhibit general sloppiness in schoolwork. Motor planning problems may result in difficulty in learning new motor tasks or generalizing a learned skill to new situations. Children with dyspraxia, often aware of their difficulty in learning and performing motor actions, may have low self-esteem, a low frustration tolerance, engage in controlling behaviors, prefer sedentary or language-based activities, and prefer to play with children significantly younger or older than they are.

   2. **Postural disorders** are characterized by difficulty in moving, stabilizing, and adjusting posture. It is often associated with neurological soft signs such as mild hypotonia, poor bilateral coordination, and poor equilibrium reactions. These disorders are thought to be associated with poor processing of vestibular and proprioceptive input. Postural disorders often occur in combination with sensory modulation and discrimination disorders or dyspraxia.

V. **Making the diagnosis.**

A. **Signs and symptoms.** Underlying problems in sensory processing are often expressed clinically as **poor self-regulation of arousal, attention, affect, and/or action**. These symptoms may then contribute to functional difficulties in play, peer relationships, and school performance.

B. **Differential diagnosis.** SPD is not a discrete medical diagnosis, but it can be seen in isolation. It is more often seen as a dimension of other diagnoses such as learning disabilities, autism, or ADHD. SPD, as described in this chapter, is consistent with, and does not need to be differentiated from, a regulatory disorder of sensory processing [as outlined in the Diagnostic Classification of Mental Health and Developmental Disorders of Infancy and Early Childhood—Revised (DC:0–3-R)]. Sensory-based motor disorders are considered to be subtypes of developmental coordination disorder (DCD) as described in DSM-IV. Sensory modulation disorders should be differentiated from purely behavioral patterns in which children exhibit undesired behaviors (e.g., hand flapping).

   SPD should be considered when behavior management techniques result in one behavior being extinguished, only to be replaced by another undesired behavior that provides similar sensory input. It should also be noted that a diagnosis of SPD should only be made when sensory preferences **interfere with the child's function**; not all stylistic differences in sensory processing are indicative of dysfunction. Finally, parents are frequently confused because different professionals label/diagnose these behaviors differently.

C. **History: key clinical questions.**

   1. **Developmental history.** Parents of children with SPD usually report development skill acquisition that is within low normal limits. If present, delays are most often seen in gross motor area with decreased tolerance of prone positioning, late onset walking, and limited flexibility in the generalization of new skills.

   2. **Sensory history.** The historian often reports **unusual sensory avoidances** or **craving** and concomitant behavioral disorganization in children with SPD. In infancy, these children often do not cuddle and are fussy, with problematic sleep patterns. These tendencies are often longstanding, even though they may not be problematic until the children reach school age or are in other group settings. Problematic behaviors may be inconsistent (i.e., present in the evening, but not in the morning; or present when touched, but not when the child touches) and also may not be associated with sensory processing (e.g., fussy eating, or sleep problems).

3. **Key clinical questions.**
  - *"Does the child have sensory preferences or avoidances in attention and learning? Are these preferences inconsistent?"*
  - *"Does the child over-react (or under-react) to input in particular modalities? Does the child express and appropriate range of affect in response to sensory input?"*
  - *"Was the child unusually fussy, difficult to console, or easily startled as an infant?"*
  - *"Is the child over- or underaware of clothing (e.g., refusal to wear certain fabrics or types of clothes; not notice wearing shoes on the wrong foot)?"*
  - *"Did the child have difficulty regulating sleep/wake cycle—settling for sleep, staying asleep, and waking without irritability or strongly dislike baths, haircuts, or nail cutting?"*
  - *"Does the child use an inappropriate amount of force when handling objects, coloring, writing, or touching with siblings or pets?"*
  - *"How does the child manage transitions and changes in daily routines? Is there a predictable time of day or type of activity when the child is most and least organized? What type of experiences proceeded these periods of disorganization?"*
  - *"Does the child need more practice than other children to learn new skills, and then do them the same way each time?"*
  - *"Is the child clumsy, fall frequently, bump into furniture or people, or have trouble judging position of body in relation to surrounding space?"*

VI. **Management.**
  A. **Evaluation.** If sensory processing problems are suspected, an occupational therapy evaluation should be performed. The evaluation should include both standardized testing, as well as informal observation by a qualified specialist. Since children with SPD often have concomitant learning or behavioral disorders, a multidisciplinary team evaluation and treatment plan may be indicated.
  B. **Parent education.** Parents of children with SPD need help understanding the problematic behaviors. There should be three goals for this education:
  - To help parents understand their child's unique sensory profile
  - To help them create a better goodness-of-fit between their child's needs and the sensory–motor challenges in their environment
  - To encourage parents to support the child's self-esteem and social participation
    Parents may need help to **understand their child's affective response to sensation** (e.g., pulling back from hugs may be due to hypersensitivity but may be interpreted as withdrawing from social contact). It is also important to share information with parents about what types of behaviors to observe after changes in routines or environment (e.g., autonomic signs, increased arousal, and more disorganization during holiday chaos).
    While structure and predictability are important for some children, a sense of novelty is essential for others to encourage sensory-based exploration. The pediatric clinician, in addition to the occupational therapist, is essential in developing parental understanding and enhancing their ability to advocate for their child across contexts.
  C. **Intervention.** Direct and indirect strategies for SPD are usually provided by specially trained occupational therapists. The goals of the intervention should be individualized based on each child's unique sensory and motor profile. Direct intervention usually requires a specialized treatment environment (with suspended equipment and many opportunities to enrich sensory input) to enable flexible enhancements of sensory and motor challenges, and it works toward integrating improved sensory-based self-regulatory abilities into social and functional participation. Indirect strategies and consultation should be implemented to improve goodness-of-fit in school or other environments.

BIBLIOGRAPHY

For parents

Books

Dunn W. *Living Sensationally: Understanding Your Senses.* Philadelphia, PA: Kingsley Publishers, 2008.
Miller LG, Fuller DA. *Sensational Kids: Hope and Help for Children with SPD.* New York, NY: Perigee, 2007.
Kranowitz CS. *The Out of Sync Child: Recognizing and Coping with Sensory Integrative Dysfunction: The Revised Edition.* New York, NY: Perigee, 2006.
Kranowitz CS. *The Out of Sync Child Has Fun, The Revised Edition: Activities for Kids with SPD.* New York, NY: Perigee, 2006.

Web sites

The Sensory Processing Disorder Resource Center. http://www.sensory-processing-disorder.com/
Sensory Processing Disorder Foundation. http://www.spdfoundation.net/

For professionals

Bundy AC, Lane SJ, Murray, EA (eds). *Sensory Integration: Theory and Practice*. (2nd ed). Philadelphia: FA Davis Co., (2002).

Cermak SA, Larkin D. *Developmental Coordination Disorder*. Albany, NY: Delmar, 2002.

Reynolds S, Lane SJ. Diagnostic validity of sensory over-responsivity: a review of the literature and case reports. *J Autism Dev Disord* 38(3):516–529, 2008.

Schoen SA, Miller LJ, Brett-Green BA, et al. Physiological and behavioral differences in sensory processing: a comparison of children with autism spectrum disorder and sensory modulation disorder. *Front Integr Neurosci* 3:29, 2009.

Smith-Roley S, Blanche EI, Schaaf RC (eds). *Understanding the Nature of Sensory Integration With Diverse Populations*. San Antonio, TX: Harcourt, 2001.

Williamson GG, Anzalone ME. *Sensory integration and self-regulation in infants and toddlers: Helping young children to interact with their environments*. Washington, DC: Zero-to-Three, 2001.

72

Sex and the Adolescent

Linda Grant

I. **Description of the problem.** The expression of human sexuality is the result of a complex interplay of biologic, psychological, interpersonal, and social factors—each with varying importance as the child grows up. In adolescence, the newly discovered ability to engage in sexual activity implies neither the cognitive and emotional maturity to deal with intimacy nor an understanding of its negative consequences (such as premature pregnancy and sexually transmitted diseases). It is the role of the primary care clinician to: (1) prepare the family to guide their adolescent through puberty, and (2) guide the adolescent in *responsible sexual decision-making*.

A. **Epidemiology.**

1. **Sexual experience.**
   - There is no one profile of adolescent sexuality. Trends in coital initiation and continuation of sexual activity reflect differing ethnic, cultural, and sex-specific rates. There are also few methodically sound scientific investigations of teen sexuality, due to the controversial nature of interviewing adolescents about their sexual behavior.
   - In general, the majority of adolescents are virginal at the age of 15; by the senior year in high school, approximately 60% are coitally experienced.
   - Males consistently report earlier coital initiation than females.
   - Sixty percent of sexually active high school seniors report using a condom at the last intercourse.
   - Noncoital sexual behaviors are prevalent. Over half of adolescent males and females aged 15 to 19 report engaging in oral sex with someone of the opposite sex; 11% of 15- to 19-year-olds of both sexes had engaged in anal sex with the opposite sex.
   - Gay, lesbian, bisexual, and transgender (GLBT) adolescents have higher rates of attempted and completed suicide, violence victimization, substance abuse, and human immunodeficiency virus (HIV) risk. Most have an awareness of their orientation by the age of 9 or 10.
   - Drugs and alcohol were involved in 23% of high school students before their last intercourse.
   - Although the rate of negative sexual outcomes has been declining over the last decade, there is evidence that this trend may be slowing.

2. **Teenage pregnancy.**
   - The United States has one of the highest rates of teenage pregnancy of any industrialized country.
   - Of the 2.4 million pregnancies occurring in US females under 25 years of age, 30% are to 15- to 19-year-old adolescents. Of these adolescent pregnancies, 57% are carried to term; the other half is therapeutically or spontaneously terminated.

3. **Sexually transmitted diseases.**
   - The 15 to 24-year-old age group acquires half of all sexually transmitted diseases (STD's) although they represent only 25% of the sexually active population, with Chlamydia the most frequently reported.
   - Each year approximately 14% of all newly reported AIDS diagnoses are of 13- to 24-year-olds.
     - Nearly a quarter of females aged 15 to 19 years had HPV infection in a one-year study

4. **Sexual aggression.**
   - About one in three high school students report that they have been hit, slapped, or physically hurt by someone they were dating. Dating violence includes psychological and emotional abuse, physical abuse, and sexual abuse.
   - Children with disabilities are sexually abused at a rate that is 2.2 times higher than that for children without disabilities.
   - In a magazine survey of teenagers and young adults of both sexes, 20% of teens (13–19) and 33% of young adults (20–26) report sending nude or semi-nude photographs

of themselves electronically. Additionally, 39% of teens and 59% of young adults had sent sexually explicit text messages.

B. Developmental considerations.
   1. **Dealing with body changes.** Adolescents must learn to be comfortable with their new physical identity. Puberty is a time when they come to terms with a changing body and bewildering emotions fueled by hormonal surges. The reproductive capacity, however, is present well before emotional and cognitive maturity have developed.
   2. **Developing a separate identity.** The adolescent must develop an identity that is separate from the family. Sexual behavior is often viewed as a rite of passage into adulthood and as a way to become a distinct entity from the family. As adolescents separate from the family, they develop replacement relationships with their peers. Technology has contributed new venues for social networking, expanding risk-taking options such as "sexting," the act of sending sexually explicit messages or photographs.
   3. **Developing intimate relationships.** Another task of adolescence is to achieve the capacity to develop intimate and meaningful mutual relationships. Early relationships may involve physical intimacy as a means of comparison and experimentation. Later, with the addition of formal operational thinking, emotional intimacy and reciprocity can be incorporated into relationships.
   4. **Developing the ability to think abstractly.** Concrete operational thinking dominates early and mid adolescence. Therefore, young adolescents are incapable of fully understanding the ramifications of their actions. This, coupled with a sense of infallibility and invulnerability, heightens the risk for sexual activity. Formal operational thinking, which develops around the age of 15, allows the adolescent to generate a more appropriate decision-making tree and to develop abstract thinking on moral values.
   5. **Personality characteristics.** The degree of any risk-taking behavior in adolescence is mitigated by the individual's personality profile. In general those with low self-esteem, a tolerance for deviant behavior, and a propensity for sensation seeking are at highest risk. Those who place a high value on achievement and future orientation and who have strong religious beliefs are generally in lower risk categories.
   6. **Sexual orientation.** Children have a sense of their sexual orientation at an early age. Gay teens have the same developmental tasks as heterosexual teens but may not have access to positive support systems that allow for fine-tuning the learning tasks of dating and loving (see Chapter 46).
   7. **Special needs.** Children with cognitive and physical disabilities have the same sexual feelings and sexual developmental needs as their nondisabled peers. Discussions and/or planning for these needs are an integral part of medical home management.

II. Making the diagnosis.
   A. History. The key to engaging adolescents is providing a trusting, confidential, nonjudgmental, and honest atmosphere. In order for adolescents to talk about their risk behaviors and sexual orientation with the primary care clinician, they must be assured that disclosure will not compromise their relationships with their family, their friends, or the community. Adolescents often resist medical visits because they fear that the information will be shared with the parent. **It is important to establish with them that what is said will be confidential and equally important is to inform them of any qualifying parameters.** For example, when an adolescent's or another's safety is jeopardized (as in suicidal or homicidal ideation, physical or sexual abuse, and life-threatening illnesses), confidentiality may need to be breached. Informing the adolescent and his or her parent of these guidelines at the initial visit allows for a clarifying discussion of safety, communication, and trust. Clinicians should be aware of their state's statutes regarding mature and emancipated minors.

   The sexual history should be part of a larger sociologic history that screens for all risk behaviors. The goal of a sexual history is to determine if there has been sexual activity and if so, the degree of health and emotional risk involved. Questioning needs to be direct and comprehensive. The clinician should make no a priori assumptions about the sexual activity, practices, or sexual orientation of any adolescent.

   B. Key clinical questions.
   1. *"Are you currently in a relationship?"*
   2. *"Does this relationship include having sex?"*
   3. *"What kind of protection do you use to avoid pregnancy and sexually transmitted diseases?"*
   4. *"Have you ever had any sexually transmitted disease?"*
   5. *"How many partners have you had?"*
   6. *"How old were you when you first had intercourse?"*
   7. *"What made you decide to have sex?"*

8. *"Has anyone ever forced you to have sex?"*
9. *"Have you ever been pregnant? What happened to the pregnancy?"* or *"Have you ever fathered a child?"*
10. *"Have you ever had sex with someone of the same sex?"*
11. *"Have you ever had rectal or oral sex?"*
12. *"Is sex an enjoyable experience for you?"*
13. *"Tell me what you know about AIDS."*
14. *"What do you know about the different methods of birth control?"*
15. *"How do you feel about not being sexually active?"*
16. *"Have you ever 'sexted'?"*

C. **Physical examination.**
When the examiner is of the opposite sex from the patient, it is prudent to ask about the patient's comfort level and request for a chaperone.

1. **Pelvic examination.** Sexually active adolescents should seek preventative healthcare to address risks and screen for STDs. However, new guidelines suggest that adolescents do not need cervical cancer screening until the age of 21. Before that time, the need to perform a pelvic exam will depend on the gynecological symptoms, history, and the availability of newer urine tests for STDs.

    • There continues to be some debate as to when to initiate a pelvic examination in an adolescent who is *not* sexually active. Variables to consider include the patient's request, the nature of the gynecologic complaint, and the gynecologic versus chronologic age of the adolescent. For the young, virginal adolescent with a gynecologic complaint, external visualization and bimanual rectal palpation and/or pelvic ultrasound may be adequate.
    • The development of a positive attitude toward pelvic examinations begins with the first. It is helpful to have the adolescent as involved as possible so that she feels in control of the process. For example, she can be asked if she wants to look at her cervix and external genitalia in a hand-held mirror. She should also be told that the examination will be stopped if she feels pain and she should describe any discomfort. Each step should be anticipated so that there are no surprises.
    • As the examination proceeds, the clinician might continue a relaxing and empowering dialogue.

2. **Male genitalia examination.** The adolescent male examination may also be anxiety provoking. Explanations and demonstrations of testicular self-examination as well as reassurance of normality help to relieve the anxiety. The male should be examined while standing, and it is helpful and educational to describe anatomic findings as a diversion during the examination. It is not necessary to comment on an erection unless the adolescent seems particularly embarrassed by it. The normality of the examination should always be stressed.

D. **Tests.** If an adolescent is sexually active, there should be routine screening for STDs. In females this means at least yearly testing for gonorrhea and chlamydia. (However, screening intervals should take into account the epidemiology of the community.) Rectal and pharyngeal gonococcal cultures should be considered if there is a history of oral or rectal sex, and rectal chlamydia screening should be considered in males who have receptive intercourse. A pap smear is currently recommended starting at age 21. Women often think that the "pap smear" and "pelvic exam" are interchangeable, when a pap smear is just a test performed occasionally during a pelvic exam. It is important to stress the distinction. Males can be screened for asymptomatic STDs using urine dipstick testing for leukocyte esterase in areas of high STD prevalence. Both males and females should be offered syphilis and Hepatitis C serology testing if they have had unprotected sex. Adolescents should be aware of and have access to confidential and anonymous HIV testing.

III. **Management.**

A. **Anticipatory guidance.** Anticipatory guidance about sexual issues should be a part of routine healthcare maintenance throughout childhood (Table 72-1) and adolescence (Table 72-2). Thoughtful, knowledgeable, and developmentally appropriate parental guidance as well as preparation of young children allow for a more natural dialogue about sexual issues at puberty.

B. **Addressing adolescent sexuality.**

1. **Primary goals.** The primary goals are to promote a healthy sexual attitude, to decrease sexual risk behaviors, and to assist parents in dealing with their child's sexuality.

2. **Developmental level.** Throughout adolescence, the progression of cognitive and emotional development influences sexual practices. A 13-year-old deals with sexuality in a different way than does a 19-year-old. The older teenager may better understand

Table 72-1. Preadolescent sexuality anticipatory guidance

Age	Sexuality issues and development	Parental concerns	Areas of anticipatory guidance
Prenatal	Fetuses have been shown to suck their fingers in utero	"I don't care if it's a boy or girl as long as it's healthy"	Sex stereotyping: expectations for male–female differences in behavior are present even before birth. Awareness of this allows for later dialogue about expressions of individuality.
		"If it's a boy, what about circumcision?"	Discussing circumcision provides an introduction to discussing sexually related topics.
		"Should I breast feed?"	Breast-feeding discussions help emphasize importance of body contact. It is also important to stress importance of paternal body contact, cuddling, stroking.
2 wk	Temperament	"When I change the baby, his wee-wee stands up. Am I stimulating him too much?"	Use appropriate genitalia names (penis, vagina, clitoris) during the examination. This facilitates discussions as child ages. Infants and children enjoy and respond to touch but not with the same sexual/erotic context as adults. It is unlikely that normal touching is ever overstimulating at this age.
2 mo	Bonding	"I feel sexually aroused when I nurse."	Parents (both father and mother) may have erotic sensations and dreams about their child, especially in the first few months. This is normal. (Acting on one's fantasies with a child is not.)
		"My wife and I don't have a relationship like we used to."	The postpartum period is often a stressful time in a previously happy relationship. The clinician may be the only medical provider involved with the family at this point and can help the parents recognize and deal with the changes a new baby brings, including changes in sexual activity.
4–6 mo	Genital play initiation; body exploration	"My son plays with his penis when I change his diaper."	Exploration of the body (toes, fingers, genitalia) is a normal aspect of human development. Self-pleasuring (thumb sucking, genital manipulation) is a natural extension of this. Masturbation continues throughout life. Start discussions early.
9–12 mo	Avoidance of stigmatization	"I'm afraid to let my daughter go without a diaper at the beach because she plays with herself."	As with other social behaviors (e.g., eating, play), sexuality and its expression must be shaped into a social context. This is a process that starts at this age and proceeds gradually to ages 3–4 yr. Shame, doubt, and confusion result from inappropriate expectations.

(continued)

Table 72-1. (Continued)

Age	Sexuality issues and development	Parental concerns	Areas of anticipatory guidance
12–15 mo	Sex-stereotyped play	"I bought my son a doll, but he only wants to play with trucks."	Most parents would like their daughters to achieve to their abilities and sons to be empathetic and caring. Responding to the child's individuality rather than trying to alter sex-specific behaviors is the appropriate path to this goal.
18 mo	Toilet training	"I want her out of diapers before this baby is born."	Toilet training should be initiated on the child's schedule of readiness, not the parents'.
2–3 yr	Anatomical comparisons	"He's asking questions. What should I say?"	Simple but accurate explanations are best. If a child wants to know more and if the answer is straightforward, he will generally ask more. Pregnancy is a fascination; sibling births provide opportunities to discuss reproduction as well as feelings. Toddlers are very much aware of the anatomical similarities with the same-sex parent and the contrasts with the opposite-sex parent. They identify their concept of gender role in this manner.
	Relationships	"My son saw my husband and I having sex. Is that bad for him?"	If intercourse is explained as a way that mothers and fathers have of showing affection and love, there is no psychological trauma for the child who interrupts his parents *in flagrante delicto.* Parents should initiate discussions of privacy and closed doors.
3–4 yr	Family flirtation	"My daughter flirts with my husband. Is this normal?"	Family members are the child's source of learning about human relationships. This is a time of magical thinking when children imagine marrying their opposite-sex parent. At this time children can begin to understand parental love for each other as different from a parent's love for a child.
	Sex play with peers	"I found my 4-year-old daughter with the 4-year-old neighbor boy without any clothes."	Sex play between children of the same or opposite sexes continues through childhood without harm, as long as adults remain calm when they discover their children in these games. Children at this age can begin to understand the difference between such play with same-age children and such play with adults or older children.
4–6 yr	Sexual appropriateness	"When can I teach my child about good and bad touching?"	Children at this age can understand that their bodies are their own, that sex play between adults and children is not appropriate, that children have a right to say "no" to an adult's touching if it makes them feel funny or uncomfortable or if they don't understand what's happening.

342

6–10 yr	Modesty	"My son and daughter share a room. Is this a problem?"	The beginnings of privacy were taught with early body exploration. No matter how relaxed a child's family has been about bodies, the child's natural modesty at this age should be respected.
	Intimacy	"I've taken showers with my daughter since she was an infant. Should I stop this?"	Each family needs to decide what they are comfortable with and to discuss it. As long as feelings can be discussed openly, there should be no conflict or feelings of rejection if parent–child bathing is discontinued. There are many other comfortable ways for families to show affection.
			Children and parents sometimes find it comfortable to acknowledge that fantasies are common and are not a problem unless acted upon.
	Fantasy versus reality	"My 9-year-old son seems to have a crush on a 14-year-old neighbor boy. I'm concerned he might be gay."	Same-sex crushes are a normal part of development for both males and females and help consolidate gender identity. Discussion helps both child and parent appreciate normal development. Most who will continue with same-sex experiences recognize their homosexuality at this age.
	Out-of-home influences increase	"I won't let him watch the Playboy channel on cable so he goes next door and watches it."	Media influences are so pervasive that isolated censorship generally does not work. Open discussion of sexual themes in movies, magazines, and songs can help parents open conversations about attitudes that they are not comfortable with and this allows their children to express their viewpoints.
	Sex education	"When should I be having the 'birds and the bees' talk?" I am concerned about internet safety"	Puberty is occurring at an earlier age. The average 8-year-old is developmentally able to understand simple explanations about sexual activity. Parents should be encouraged to initiate this discussion.

New technologies supporting networking have broadened sexual risk taking. It is important to begin discussions of the risks of cyber sharing of personal information |

Table 72-2. Anticipatory guidance for adolescent sexuality

Age	Sexual areas of concern	Risk factors	Anticipatory guidance
Early adolescence, early puberty: 10–12 yr	Pubertal changes	Self-image	Gynecomastia is normal in adolescent males as is breast asynchrony in females. Such body disproportions distort adolescents' image of themselves.
		Hormonal influences	Early maturers, particularly females, need special guidance to avoid low self-esteem and premature sexual advances.
			Masturbation is a normal behavior that relieves sexual tension. Fantasies are normal while masturbating. Masturbation is a choice—teens can choose to do it or not.
	Children with developmental disabilities		Issues of sexuality are as important to children and adolescents with disabilities as they are to other children and adolescents. Providing clinical supervision to children and adolescents with disabilities includes helping them understand their changing, maturing bodies and the choices available to them.
Late puberty: 12–14 yr	Initiation of sexual activity without intimacy	Concrete thought. Cannot perceive long-range implications of current actions	Discussions of sexual choices should emphasize that it is all right to say "no"; discussions regarding contraceptive use need to emphasize more immediate as well as long-term benefits (e.g., in addition to pregnancy prevention, oral contraceptives may relieve dysmenorrhea).
Mid-adolescence: 14–17 yr	Intimacy related to sexual romanticism rather than genuine commitment	Looks to peer group for support as he separates from family	Parents should be encouraged to continue sexual dialogue begun in latency. They should know their own values (what sex is for; who it is for; what makes it enjoyable; what makes it exploitive). Parental values should be shared with opinions, rather than judgments. Parents should respect teens' decisions. Discussions about sexting and cyber relationships are especially important at this age.
	Sporadic or absent use of birth control; sexual experimentation	Formal operational thinking, variably applied	Teens begin to understand future implications of current actions; they know that use of birth control will protect from unwanted pregnancy, condoms will protect from STDs. Adolescents at this age may believe that oral sex is not as big a deal as sexual intercourse and is safe.
		Risk taking and sense of omnipotence	Risk taking should be discussed. Once a young woman risks unprotected intercourse without becoming pregnant, she is likely to risk it again. Other risk behaviors such as drunk driving and drug use may have a negative interactive effect on sexual decision-making.
Late adolescence: 17–21 yr	Intimacy involves commitment	Family conflicts resolving as independence established	Teen begins to plan for future, including marriage and family.
		Comfort with bodies and gender identity	Relationships involve a mutual reciprocity. Counseling involves understanding of female sexual response, couple's discussions of feelings.

Adapted from Grant L, Efstratios D. Adolescent sexuality. *Pediatr Clin North Am* 35(6):1271–1289, 1988.

the repercussions of unprotected sex, be less dominated by the need for romantic spontaneity, and may begin to examine differential benefits and risks of various birth control methods. The younger teenager tends to be dominated more by immediate gratification, spontaneity, and peer approval. Oral and anal sex may be utilized to avoid heterosexual vaginal intercourse. Male-oriented methods of contraception (e.g., withdrawal and condoms) tend to be more popular with the younger age group, while middle adolescents opt for pharmacologic management, whether oral, transdermal, or injectable. As adolescents mature, they develop comfort with their own bodies and a better ability to assess a situation and employ methods such as the vaginal ring.

Adolescents at this age are also better able to understand the implications of "sexting" and other noncoital risk taking.

It is important to appreciate that GLBT youth have to negotiate the same sexual developmental issues as heterosexual youth but may be in a social climate that does not allow them the same openness as their heterosexual peers.

3. **Empowerment.** Whether it is "saying no" or requesting that a partner use a condom, all adolescents need to hear that it is their right with whom, when, and how they express their sexuality. The clinician should help them understand that sex should never be something that is "done" to them. The practitioner can role-play situations to assist these concepts. For example, he or she can strategize empowered constructive responses to typical lines, such as "It doesn't feel as good with a rubber" or "If you really loved me you'd do it with me" or "What? You're still a virgin! I can't believe it!"

4. **Sexuality and a partner.** Involving a partner in the visit can help to facilitate joint sexual decision-making and may improve compliance with safer sexual practices. Males often have no understanding of the nature of a pelvic examination. Observation of the examination can be a powerful reinforcer of mutual sexual responsibility.

5. **Promoting condoms.** If an adolescent is sexually active, condom use should be promoted at every opportunity, no matter what the nature of the office visit.

6. **Abstinence as a healthy choice.** An adolescent needs to hear that abstaining from sexual activity is normal and is becoming increasingly common, and that masturbation and noncoital petting are acceptable ways to relieve sexual tensions safely. Oral and anal sex, with its risk of STDs, is not abstinence.

7. **Contraceptive choices.** What might work for one adolescent may not work for another, irrespective of developmental level. The best contraceptive is one that will be used; the adolescent is often the best judge of which method will work best for him or her.

8. **"Teachable moments" in daily life.** Broadcast and written media offer frequent examples of sexual subject matter. News events cover stories on sexual assault and controversies over gay and lesbian issues. Rock stars use explicit language in their lyrics, and actors have explicit love scenes. Parents and clinicians should be encouraged to use these examples to initiate conversations with their children and patients around these experiences.

9. **Advertising in the waiting room.** Adolescents may need an impetus to begin discussions of sexual issues. Availability of factual sexual information in the waiting room (e.g., posters, pamphlets, books, or fact sheets) will alert the adolescent that it is acceptable to raise these issues.

10. **School-based teaching.** School systems have become increasingly active in dealing with many adolescent behavioral issues, including sexuality. Condom availability and distribution programs, for example, have been incorporated into some health programs and have been shown to support sexual responsibility. The pediatric practitioner is in an ideal position to advocate for these services in his or her school system and help dispel the myths that open discussions of sexuality contribute to sexual risk taking.

IV. **Clinical pearls and pitfalls.**
- A clinician must come to terms with his or her own sexuality. A clinician who is uncomfortable with gender issues or explicit sexual questions cannot effectively counsel. A practitioner who is unwilling to discuss sexuality issues objectively should have appropriate referral sources so that patients are not denied information. Alternatively, this practitioner should not see adolescent patients.
- Teenagers need guidance, not directives. A practitioner should express his or her opinions in a nonjudgmental way and allow adolescents the legitimacy of their own opinions. *"I don't judge and I won't be disappointed. My job is to listen and give you honest feedback about safety."*

- Do not assume that all sexual relationships are heterosexual. Providing literature in the waiting room on gay, lesbian, and bisexual health issues signals that the practitioner is comfortable in discussing same-sex experiences.
- The parent–practitioner relationship needs to be renegotiated prior to puberty so that parents understand confidentiality issues. Practitioners and parents should be partners in educating about sexuality. Values belong in the family and parents can be reassured that the adolescent/practitioner relationship is value-neutral. Safety is the main concern of the practitioner.
- Sexuality is not a joking matter. Too often, adults deal with their own discomfort about sex by making jokes. Discussions with adolescents should always be serious but not somber.

BIBLIOGRAPHY

For parents and adolescents

Books

Bell R. *Changing Bodies, Changing Lives. Expanded Third Edition. A Book for Teens on Sex and Relationships.* New York: Random House, 1998. For 8th grade and up.

Harris R. *It's Perfectly Normal: Changing Bodies, Growing Up, Sex and Sexual Health.* Cambridge, MA: Candlewick Press, 2009. For 9–12 year olds with chapter on Internet safety.

Web sites

SIECUS (Sexuality, information and education council of the United States), excellent resources for accurate information for both parents and teens; includes numerous Web sites. www.siecus.org. Accessed June 4, 2010.

For professionals

Gavin L, MacKay A, Brown K, et al. Sexual and reproductive health of persons aged 10–24 years - United States, 2002–2007. *MMWR Surveill Summ* 58(SS-6):1–58, 2009.

Hoff T, Greene L, Davis J. *National Survey of Adolescents and Young Adults: Sexual Health, Knowledge, Attitudes and Experiences.* Menlo Park, CA: Henry Kaiser Family Foundation, 2003.

Murphy NA, Elias ER. Sexuality of children and adolescents with developmental disabilities. *Pediatrics* 118(1):398–403, 2006.

73

Sexual Abuse

Deborah Madansky
Christine E. Barron
Carole Jenny

I. Description of the problem.

Sexual abuse is defined as the **engagement of a child in sexual contact or activities that the child cannot comprehend, for which the child is developmentally unprepared and cannot give informed consent, and/or that violate societal, legal, and social taboos**. The activity occurs for the **gratification of the older individual** and can include forms of anal, genital, and oral contact to or by the child, exhibitionism, voyeurism, or using the child for the production of pornography. Force is not always involved, but coercion or threats are commonly used by the perpetrator.

A. Epidemiology.

The true prevalence of sexual abuse is unknown since many cases go unreported. In retrospective surveys of adults, about **25% of women and 15% of men** report sexual contact with an adult during childhood or adolescence.

1. 7.6% of reported cases of child abuse and neglect involve sexual abuse.
2. 75% of reported victims are female, but there is evidence that male victims are less likely to report.
3. Men are more commonly perpetrators.
4. The vast majority of perpetrators are known to the child.
5. Sexual abuse crosses all socioeconomic, ethnic, and racial lines.

B. Contributing factors.

Children at higher risk are those with a diminished capacity to resist or disclose, such as preverbal, developmentally delayed, or physically handicapped children, and children in dysfunctional or reconstituted families.

II. Making the diagnosis.

A. Presentations of child sexual abuse.

1. **Acute assault.** A child presenting within 72 hours of an assault should be referred to an emergency room, or to child protection programs when available, where forensic specimens may be collected.
2. **In the pediatric office.**
   a. The child is **referred by protective services or law enforcement** for a medical evaluation as part of an investigation.
   b. The child is **referred by a family member** who is aware of or suspects sexual abuse.
   c. The child is **seen for a routine examination** or medical and behavioral complaint where the differential diagnosis includes sexual abuse.

B. Signs and symptoms.

1. **Specific indicators.**
   a. Genital or rectal pain, bleeding, trauma, or infection
   b. Sexually transmitted diseases (Table 73-1)
   c. Developmentally inappropriate sexual behavior in young children, such as engagement in intercourse, oral sex, or sexual coercion.
2. **Behavioral indicators** are nonspecific and similar to symptoms due to other stressors. They are not indicative of specifically sexual abuse:
   a. Fears and phobias, especially of circumstances similar to the abuse
   b. Nightmares and other sleep disturbances
   c. Appetite disturbance or eating disorders
   d. Enuresis or encopresis
   e. Change in behavior, attitude, or school performance
   f. Depression, withdrawal, or suicidality
   g. Excessive anger, aggression, or running away
   h. Promiscuous behavior or substance abuse
3. Some sexually abused children develop **post-traumatic stress disorder** (see Chapter 64)

Table 73-1. Implications of commonly encountered sexually transmitted diseases for the diagnosis and reporting of sexual abuse of prepubertal infants and children

	Likelihood of sexual abuse	Suggested action
Gonorrhea[a]	Certain	Report[b]
Syphilis[a]	Certain	Report
Chlamydia[a]	Probable	Report
Condylomata acuminatum[a]	Possible	Evaluate. Report if sexual abuse is suspected based on history and physical exam
Trichomonas vaginalis[c]	Probable	Report
Herpes simplex type 1 (genital)	Possible	Evaluate. Report if sexual abuse is suspected based on history and physical exam.
Herpes simplex type 2	Probable	Evaluate. Report if sexual abuse is suspected based on history and physical exam.
Bacterial vaginosis	Uncertain	Medical follow-up
Candida albicans	Unlikely	Medical follow-up

[a]If not perinatally acquired.
[b]To agency mandated in community to receive reports of suspected sexual abuse.
[c]Differentiate from *Trichomonas hominis*.

C. History.

1. The **parent or guardian** should be interviewed alone regarding his or her concerns, the child's disclosures or complaints, and a review of the child's medical, developmental, emotional, and behavioral status. The clinician should ask specifically about the following:
   a. The child's disclosures
   b. Content of sexual play with peers, adults, or dolls
   c. Masturbation or genital fondling
   d. Genital complaints or symptoms
   e. Toileting difficulties
   f. Sleep disturbances (difficulty falling asleep, night waking, nightmares)
   g. Behavioral difficulties or changes
   h. School performance
2. The **child** should be interviewed by trained interviewers. At times medical clinicians may need to interview a child for possible sexual abuse and should follow this sequence:
   a. **Interview the child alone,** and record the child's statements. (Children often are uncomfortable speaking about abuse in front of a parent, or the parent might try to influence the child's disclosure.)
   b. **Sit at eye level and take time to establish rapport** with neutral topics (e.g., ask about the child's living situation, pets, school, favorite activities).
   c. **Gear the discussion to the child's developmental level,** and use his or her own terms for body parts. (For young children line drawings can be helpful.) Anatomical drawings and dolls should not be used.
   d. **Introduce the topic of possible sexual abuse in a general way,** such as,
      "Do you know why you are here today?"
      "Is there anything that you feel uncomfortable about that you would like to talk about?"
      If these opening questions do not result in a spontaneous account, inquire more specifically, *"Has anyone touched you or bothered you in a way that made you feel uncomfortable?"* If the child says, *"Yes,"* then ask, *"Tell me about that."*
   e. **Use nonleading questions,** such as what, who, where, and when. Avoid any demonstration of emotion, pressure, or correction of the child. Have a "then-what-happened/tell-me-more" approach.
   f. Be aware that **disclosures may take place during the physical examination** as the affected body parts are examined.

g. **Document what the child says verbatim** in the record. Videotaped interviews are usually conducted by protective services or law enforcement and are unnecessary in the pediatric office.

h. **Reassure the child** that it was okay to tell you, and whatever happened was not his or her fault.

i. Do not make promises to the child, such as they will only have to tell you and not tell anyone else.

D. Physical examination.

Do a complete physical examination. This allows a familiar context for the child, opportunities for further rapport, and screening for other problems. Confirm positive findings with a clinician experienced in examining children for sexual abuse.

1. **Genital examination.**
   a. **Be aware of examination positions** (supine frogleg, prone knee-chest, lithotomy) and techniques (labial separation, labial traction).
   b. **Use a good light source with magnification,** such as an otoscope head, hand-held or headpiece lens, magnifying fluorescent light, or colposcope.
   c. **Be aware of genital anatomy and normal developmental variations:**
      (1) All girls are born with a hymen
      (2) Newborn hymens are fleshy and redundant secondary to maternal estrogen effect
      (3) Prepubertal hymens have thinner tissue
      (4) Pubertal hymens are thickened and redundant from renewal of the estrogen effect
   d. **Be aware of normal anatomic variations**
      (1) Most hymens fit into one of five categories: crescentic (posterior rim), circumferential (annular), fimbriated (redundant), sleeve-like, or septate.
      (2) Nontraumatic variations include periurethral and perihymenal bands, small hymenal mounds adjacent to vaginal ridges, perineal midline raphe, and hymenal tags.
   e. **Be aware of abnormal findings not due to sexual abuse** (straddle injuries, genital hemangiomas, lichen sclerosis, urethral prolapse)
   f. **Prepare the child** prior to the examination with an explanation of the examination
   g. **Boys** should receive a careful inspection of the penis, urethral meatus, scrotum, and surrounding skin
   h. Prepubertal **girls** require a careful inspection of the vulva, unless internal trauma is suspected (which requires a pelvic exam under anesthesia)
   i. **Genital findings consistent with sexual abuse include:**
      (1) **Acute:** lacerations, abrasions, ecchymoses, edema
      (2) **Chronic:** scarring of hymen or other genital structures; absent or markedly diminished hymenal tissue

2. **Anal examination.**
   a. Be aware of **normal anal anatomy and variations,** including smooth areas at 6 and 12 o'clock (diastasis ani), erythema, midline skin tags, increased pigmentation, venous congestion, anal dilation with feces in the rectum.
   b. **Findings consistent with sexual abuse include:**
      (1) **Acute:** lacerations, edema, abrasions, ecchymoses, fissures that come out past the anal verge
      (2) **Chronic:** scars, persistent dilation without feces in the rectum

E. Laboratory tests.

1. When indicated by the history or physical findings, test **gonorrhea** in the throat, anus, and vagina/urethra, and for **Chlamydia** in the vagina and anus.
2. **Serologic tests for syphilis and human immunodeficiency virus (HIV)** should be performed if warranted by the history (taking into account the incubation periods: up to 3 months for syphilis; up to 6 months for HIV).
3. **Symptomatic children** should be investigated for other genital infections, such as *trichomonas*, herpes, condyloma acuminata, *Gardnerella vaginalis, Streptococcus pyogenes,* and *Candida.*
4. Consider a **urinalysis** and **urine culture.**
5. Perform a **pregnancy test** for pubertal girls.

III. Management.

A. **Primary goals.** The goals of management are to provide medical treatment for injuries or infections, arrange for psychosocial support for the child and family, and protect the child from further abuse by reporting to child protective services (Table 73-2).

Table 73-2. Guidelines for making the decision to report sexual abuse of children

| Data available | | | Response | |
History	Physical	Laboratory	Level of concern about sexual abuse	Action
None	Normal examination	None	None	None
Behavioral changes	Normal examination	None	Low (worry)	± Report[a]; follow closely (possible mental health referral)
None	Nonspecific findings	None	Low (worry)	± Report[a]; follow closely
Nonspecific history by child or history by parent only	Nonspecific findings	None	Possible (suspect)	± Report[a]; follow closely
None	Specific findings	None	Probable	Report
Clear statement	Normal examination	None	Probable	Report
Clear statement	Specific findings	None	Probable	Report
None	Normal examination, nonspecific or specific findings	Positive culture for gonorrhea: positive serologic test for syphilis: presence of semen, sperm, acid phosphatase	Definite	Report
Behavioral changes	Nonspecific changes	Other sexually transmitted diseases	Probable	Report

[a]A report may or may not be indicated. The decision to report should be based on discussion with local or regional experts and/or child protective services/agencies.
Reprinted with permission from the American Academy of Pediatrics Committee on Child Abuse and Neglect. Guidelines for the evaluation of sexual abuse of children. *Pediatrics* 87(2):254–260, 1991.

B. Ongoing role of the practitioner.
  1. Help guide the family toward healing.
   a. Provide or arrange crisis intervention counseling.
   b. Alert the family to their possible behavioral and emotional reactions, especially if the family constellation is disrupted.
   c. Encourage a sense of physical security for the child after the disclosure; reassure children who were threatened with harm that there is no danger.
   d. Parents should neither try to make children forget nor pry into details, but rather be open to children's negative or positive expressions about the experience.
   e. Help parents avoid overprotection and maintain normal routines, physical affection, and limit setting whenever possible.
   f. Help parents remember the needs of the rest of the family and themselves.
  2. Monitor the child and family adjustments over time. As the victim enters each succeeding developmental stage, new questions and feelings often arise.
  3. Be aware of local resources, such as parent groups, offender treatment, victim witness advocates, and children's groups available to the family.
C. Criteria for referral.
  1. A clinician who does not have sufficient evidence to report to child protective services but is still concerned should refer the child to an experienced mental health clinician for a full sexual abuse evaluation.
  2. A clinician who cannot conduct a complete medical evaluation (or if the initial evaluation raises questions) should refer to a Child Abuse Pediatrician.
  3. In most cases, sexually abused children should be referred to an experienced mental health clinician to evaluate the need for ongoing treatment. Even children without overt symptoms can harbor negative or confused feelings that might be revealed only in the context of a full evaluation.
IV. Clinical pearls and pitfalls.
Rely on the history for the diagnosis; most sexually abused children have no physical findings. This is because they were fondled, engaged in oral sex, or had minor injuries that healed quickly. Even hymenal tears can heal without a trace. A normal examination neither rules out nor confirms the possibility of sexual abuse or prior penetration.

Take the child's statements and behavior seriously. The incidence of genital complaints is higher than the incidence of genital findings in sexually abused children.

Children who imitate adult sex acts or molest other children should be evaluated for possible sexual abuse. (Normal sex play among peers is, "You show me yours, and I'll show you mine.") Children who demonstrate overt behaviors might also be exposed to age-inappropriate media and information.

Make sure the parent(s) have adequate support; the child's adjustment is related to family adjustment.

Sexually abused children need reassurance that their bodies are healthy and fine.

BIBLIOGRAPHY

For parents

Doty SW, Fent T (eds). *Keeping Them Safe*. Tulsa, OK: Argessias, LLC & MMDK, 2009.
Tobin P, Levenson MSS. *Keeping Kids Safe: A Child Sexual Abuse Prevention Manual*. Aladema, CA: Hunter House, 2002.

For children

Gurard LW. My *Body is Private*. Park Ridge, IL: Albert Whitman & Co., 1992.
Kleven S. *The Right Touch: A Read-Aloud Story to Help Prevent Child Sexual Abuse*. Kirkland, WA: Illumination Arts Publishing, 1998.
Voelkel-Haugen R, Fortune MM. *Sexual Abuse Prevention: A Course of Study for Teenagers*. San Francisco, CA: Pilgrim Press, 1996.

For professionals

Block RW, Hibbard RA, Jenny C, et al. The evaluation of sexual abuse in childhood. *Pediatrics* 116:506–512, 2005.
Jenny C (ed). *Child Abuse and Neglect: Diagnosis, Treatment, and Evaluation*. Philadelphia, PA: Elsevier Saunders, 2010.
Heger AM, Emans SJ, Muram D (eds). *Evaluation of the Sexually Abused Child: A Medical Textbook and Photographic Atlas*. London: Oxford University Press, 2000.

74

Shyness

Jonathan M. Cheek

I. **Description of the problem.** Shyness is the tendency to feel tense, worried, or awkward during social interactions, especially with unfamiliar people. This definition reflects three categories of shyness symptoms: somatic anxiety, cognitive anxiety, and observable behavior.

A. **Epidemiology.**

Although transient situational shyness is virtually universal, about 33% to 45% of school-aged children and adults in the United States label themselves as shy.

There is a developmental peak for shyness during adolescence, when 60% of the girls and 50% of the boys in seventh and eighth grades identify themselves as shy.

Less than 50% of the children who first became shy during later childhood and early adolescence still consider themselves to be shy by age 21.

75% of college students who say they were shy in early childhood continue to identify themselves as shy persons.

B. **Clinical features.** In early childhood, shyness is usually manifested as the relative absence or inhibition of normally expected social behaviors. The child appears excessively quiet, with diminished social participation. For shy children, the normal peaks of stranger anxiety (9 months) and separation anxiety (18 months) do not fade away. In later childhood and early adolescence, the cognitive symptoms of shyness, such as painful self-consciousness and anxious self-preoccupation, begin to become a significant component of this personality syndrome.

Longitudinal research indicates that shyness that continues into adulthood can create significant barriers to satisfaction in love, work, recreation, and friendship. Shy adults tend to be more lonely and less happy than those who are not shy. Childhood shyness does not, however, predict psychopathology in adulthood and should be considered part of the normal range of individual differences in personality and social behavior. At times it may be difficult to differentiate shyness from a communication disorder such as an autism spectrum disorder. A thorough history may help tease out the core characteristics of autism—that is social communication and behavioral concerns—versus symptoms of shyness alone.

C. **Etiology.**

1. **Temperament.** Shyness is one of the few temperamental traits whose precursors in infancy are often clear. About 15% to 20% of infants typically respond to a new situation or stimulus (e.g., an unfamiliar toy, person, or place) by withdrawing and becoming either emotionally subdued or upset (crying, fussing, and fretting). It has been speculated that this pattern of inhibition to novelty is related to a lower threshold for arousal in sites in the amygdala. Infants with this highly reactive temperament in the first year of life are more likely to be wary or fearful of strangers at the end of the second year and are also more likely to be described as shy by their kindergarten teachers.

2. **Transactional model.** Behavioral inhibition in infancy does not lead invariably to childhood shyness. Parents who are sensitive to the nature of their inhibited child's temperament, who take an active role in helping the child to develop relationships with playmates, and who facilitate involvement in school activities appear to ameliorate the impact of shyness on the child's subsequent social adjustment. Childhood shyness is a joint product of temperament and socialization experiences within and outside the family.

3. **Late-onset shyness.** Many of the children who first become troubled by shyness between the ages of 8 and 14 do not have the temperamental predisposition for behavioral inhibition. Late-developing shyness is usually caused by adjustment problems in adolescent social development. The bodily changes of puberty, the newly acquired cognitive ability to think abstractly about the self and the environment, and the new demands and opportunities resulting from changing social roles combine to make adolescents feel intensely self-conscious and socially awkward.

The inability of some adolescents to outgrow late-developing shyness has been linked to several factors. Research on the timing of puberty indicates that early-maturing girls and late-maturing boys suffer more severe social adjustment problems with their peers. Moving to a new neighborhood or school can disrupt the development of social skills, which are most easily practiced in safe and familiar surroundings. Shy adolescents need to experience positive social relationships in order to develop a healthy level of self-esteem. If parents, siblings, teachers, or peers tease and embarrass the shy adolescent, he or she may develop the self-image of being an unworthy and unlikable person.

Sex role socialization puts different pressures on adolescent girls and boys. Teenage girls experience more symptoms of self-conscious shyness, such as doubts about their attractiveness and worries about what others think of them, whereas teenage boys tend to be more troubled by behavioral symptoms of shyness because the traditional male role requires initiative and assertiveness in social life.

II. Recognizing the issue.

A. Signs and symptoms. The child's visit to a primary care clinician is itself a prototypical shyness-eliciting situation, so signs of fearfulness and inhibition should be easily detectable.

B. Differential diagnosis. Some people prefer to spend time alone rather than with others, but they also feel comfortable when they are in social settings. Such people are nonanxious introverts, who may be unsociable but not shy. The opposite of shyness is social self-confidence, not extroversion. The problem for truly shy people is that their anxiety prevents them from participating in social life when they want to or need to.

C. History: key clinical questions.

   1. *"Is your child usually shy and withdrawn in new situations and when meeting new people?"* An affirmative answer rules out the possibilities that the child is just nervous about the visit or is just in a sensitive mood on that particular day.

   2. *"Are you worried that your child is too shy to make friends or to do well in school?"* Answers that indicate severe anxiety reactions, phobias, or withdrawal similar to mild forms of autism are red flags for more severe pathology. Some parents, particularly those who are somewhat shy yet have adapted well themselves, will label their child as shy but not see it as a problem. They are often sufficiently sensitive to the issue that no further intervention may be necessary.

   3. *"Do you feel disappointed or embarrassed that your child can't seem to be more outgoing or adventuresome?"* Research suggests that an affirmative answer indicates the potential for significant long-term adjustment problems for shy children. For example, the feelings of disappointment in some fathers that their shy sons are not "masculine" enough can be a particularly painful problem. It is important for the parents of a shy child to understand the nature of the temperament and to help their child develop on his or her individual pathway, rather than attempting to enforce a personal or cultural ideal that will never be a good fit for the shy child.

III. Management.

A. Advice to parents. The goals of intervention in this case are essentially proactive and preventative in nature: helping the shy child to achieve better adjustment in his or her current and future social life. It is worth noting that retrospective interviews with painfully shy adults frequently contain complaints that doctors and teachers had ignored their childhood shyness. They expressed the wish that some adult had become an ally or advocate by validating their problem and persuading their parents to help them deal more effectively with their shyness at an early age.

   1. Do not overprotect or overindulge. Allow the shy child to experience moderate amounts of challenge, frustration, and stress rather than rushing to soothe away every sign of anxiety. With emotional support from parents and gradual exposure to new objects, people, and places, the child will learn to cope with his or her own special sensitivity to novelty. Gently and consistently nudge (but do not push) the child to continue gaining experience with new things.

   2. Respect the shy temperament. Talk with the child about feeling nervous or afraid. Once the reality of these negative feelings has been acknowledged, encourage the child to talk about what can be gained from trying a new experience in spite of being afraid (an example from the parent's own childhood might be particularly helpful). Progress is usually slow because shy feelings may remain even after a particular shy behavior has been overcome. Sympathy, patience, and persistence are needed.

   3. Help the child deal with teasing about being shy. Shy children are highly sensitive to embarrassment and need extra comfort when they have been the victim of teasing.

They also need more support and encouragement to develop positive self-esteem than do children who are not shy.

4. **Help the child to build friendships.** Inviting one or two playmates over to the house lets the child experience the security of being on home territory. Sometimes a shy child will do better when playing with children who are slightly younger.

5. **Talk to teachers.** The child's teacher can be an important ally, but teachers sometimes overlook the shy child or incorrectly assume that excessive quietness indicates lack of interest or lack of intelligence.

6. **Prepare the child for new experiences.** Take the child to visit a new school or classroom before school starts. Help the child rehearse (e.g., by practicing for show-and-tell or an oral book report). Role-play anticipated anxieties, such as what a party or the first day of summer camp will be like.

7. **Find appropriate activities.** Help the child get involved in a club or after-school activity that can expand social contacts with others who share similar interests and enthusiasms. Be careful not to impose what you would like, or wish you had done as a child, onto a child who has different likes and dislikes.

B. **Advice to the shy child.** Shy children usually appreciate being made to feel that their problems of social anxiety are understood sympathetically by an adult and that they are not alone in experiencing these feelings. It is important not to minimize the significance of shyness but rather to emphasize to the child the increased enjoyment of social rewards that can be obtained if he or she begins to participate more actively in social life. Acknowledge that the shy child may always feel a bit anxious inside but emphasize that the anxiety is not nearly as visible to other children or adults as the child thinks it is. By focusing on what others are saying or doing a shy child can practice being less self-focused and self-critical.

IV. **When to refer.** If the parents of a child troubled by shyness appear to lack confidence in their ability to implement the advice, it may be appropriate to suggest a referral to a mental health professional. Children who appear particularly silent or withdrawn should be screened for social phobia, selective mutism, and an autism spectrum disorder.

BIBLIOGRAPHY

For parents

Web sites

The Shyness Institute. www.shyness.com
www.shykids.com
www.theintrovertadvantage.com
Selective Mutism Group/Childhood Anxiety Network. www.selectivemutism.org

Books

Carducci BJ. *The Shyness Breakthrough: A No-Stress Plan to Help Your Shy Child Warm Up, Open Up, and Join the Fun.* Emmaus, PA: Rodale, 2003.
Laney MO. *The Hidden Gifts of the Introverted Child.* New York, NY: Workman Publishing, 2005.
Markway BG, Markway GP. *Nurturing the Shy Child.* New York, NY: Thomas Dunne Books of St. Martin's Press, 2006.

For professionals

Beidel DC, Turner SM. *Shy Children, Phobic Adults: Nature and Treatment of Social Phobia.* Washington, DC: American Psychological Association, 1998.
Cheek JM, Krasnoperova EN. Varieties of shyness in adolescence and adulthood. In: Schmidt LA, Schulkin J (eds), *Extreme Fear, Shyness, and Social Phobia: Origins, Biological Mechanisms, and Clinical Outcomes.* New York, NY: Oxford University Press, 1999.
Crozier WR (ed). *Shyness: Development, Consolidation, and Change.* London: Routledge, 2001.

75

Sleep Problems

Judith A. Owens

I. Description of the problem.

A. Sleep problems constitute one of the most frequent parental complaints in pediatric practice.

- Childhood *sleeplessness,* insufficient or disturbed sleep, in its many forms, clearly is a common parental concern.
- In contrast, the relationship between **sleepiness** and its many manifestations is less frequently recognized by parents, but is nonetheless a significant clinical concern. A wealth of empirical evidence from several lines of research clearly indicates that children and adolescents experience significant daytime sleepiness as a result of inadequate or disturbed sleep, and that significant performance impairments and mood dysfunction, as well as behavior, academic, and health problems in childhood, are associated with that daytime sleepiness.

B. Epidemiology.

1. 25% of all children experience a sleep problem at some point during childhood, ranging from short-term situational difficulties in falling asleep, to night wakings, to more chronic and persistent sleep disorders.

2. Although many sleep problems in infants and children are transient and self-limited, the common wisdom that children "grow out of" sleep problems is not an accurate perception. Certain intrinsic and extrinsic risk factors (e.g., difficult temperament, maternal depression, family stress) may predispose a given child to develop a more chronic sleep disturbance.

3. Sleep problems are a **significant source of distress** for families. There may be, for example, a primary reason for caregiver stress in families with children who have chronic medical illnesses or severe neurodevelopment delays.

4. The impact of childhood sleep problems is intensified by their direct relationship to **the quality and quantity of parents' sleep**, particularly if disrupted sleep results in parental daytime fatigue and mood disturbances, which impact negatively on the quality of parenting.

5. Vulnerable populations, such as children who are at high risk for developmental and behavioral problems because of poverty, parental substance abuse and mental illness, or violence in the home, may be even more likely to experience "double jeopardy" as a result of sleep problems.

C. Etiology/contributing factors.

1. **Child variables** include temperament and behavioral style, individual variations in circadian preference, cognitive and language **delays**, and the presence of comorbid medical and psychiatric conditions.

2. **Parental variables** include parenting and discipline styles, parents' education level and knowledge of child development, mental health issues such as maternal depression, family stress, and quality and quantity of parents' sleep.

3. **Environmental variables** include the physical environment (space, noise, perceived environmental threats to safety, room and bed sharing, televisions in the bedroom), family composition (number, ages, and health status of siblings and extended family members), and lifestyle issues (parental work status, competing priorities for time).

4. **Cultural and family context,** for example, co-sleeping of infants and parents is a common and accepted practice in many ethnic groups (including African Americans, Hispanics, and Southeast Asians) both in their countries of origin and in the United States. Therefore, the developmental goal of independent "self-soothing" in infants at bedtime and after night wakings may not be shared by all families.

5. **Specific medical conditions** that may have an increased risk of sleep problems include the following:
   - Asthma and allergies
   - Headaches

- Neurologic disorders and rheumatologic conditions
- Children with anxiety and affective disorders are particularly vulnerable to sleep problems. Studies of children with major depressive disorder, for example, have reported a prevalence of insomnia of up to 75%, and sleep onset delay in one-third of depressed adolescents. Use of psychotropic medications in these children may have significant negative effects on sleep.
- Significant sleep problems occur in 30% to 80% of children with severe mental retardation and in at least 50% of children with less severe cognitive impairment. Similar estimates in children with autism/pervasive developmental delay are in the 50% to 70% range.

II. **Making the diagnosis.**

A. **Sleep physiology.**

1. **The framework or architecture of sleep** is based upon recognition of two distinct sleep stages. These stages are defined by distinct polysomnographic (or "overnight sleep study") features of EEG patterns, eye movement, and muscle tone.
   - **REM sleep** (rapid eye movement or "dream" sleep). REM sleep (20%–25% of total) is characterized by high levels of cortical activity and low or absent muscle tone.
   - **Non-REM sleep** (75%–80% of sleep in healthy young adults). Non-REM sleep is further divided into:
     - **Stage 1** sleep (2%–5%) which occurs at the sleep–wake transition and is often referred to as "light sleep"
     - **Stage 2** sleep (45%–55%) which is usually considered the initiation of "true" sleep and is characterized by bursts of rhythmic rapid EEG activity and high amplitude slow wave spikes
     - **Stages 3 and 4** sleep (3%–23%) which are otherwise known as "deep" sleep, "slow wave sleep," or "delta sleep," during which the highest arousal threshold (most difficult to awaken) also occurs

2. **Cycling of stages.**
   - Non-REM and REM sleep alternate throughout the night in cycles of about 90 to 110 minutes in adults (50 minutes in infancy and gradually lengthening through childhood to adult levels).
   - Brief arousals normally followed by a rapid return to sleep often occur at the end of each sleep cycle (4–6 times per night in adults; 7–10 times per night in infants).
   - The relative proportion of REM and non-REM sleep per cycle changes across the night, such that slow wave sleep predominates in the first third of the night and REM sleep in the last third.

3. **Two-process sleep system.** Sleep and wakefulness are regulated by two basic highly coupled processes operating simultaneously:
   - The **homeostatic process,** which primarily regulates the length and depth of sleep. The homeostatic "pressure" for sleep builds as time awake increases in duration.
   - **Endogenous circadian rhythms** ("biological time clocks"), which influence the internal organization of sleep and the timing and duration of daily sleep–wake cycles.
   - **Circadian rhythms** (which govern many other physiologic systems in addition to sleep–wake cycles) are also synchronized to the 24-hour-day cycle by environmental cues, the most powerful of which is the light–dark cycle which influences melatonin secretion by the pineal gland.

4. **Duration of sleep.**

   a. **Newborns.**
   - Newborns sleep approximately 16 to 20 hours per day, in 1- to 4-hour sleep periods, followed by 1- to 2-hour awake periods.
   - Sleep–wake cycles are largely dependent upon hunger and satiety. Sleep amounts during the day approximately equal the amount of nighttime sleep.

   b. **Infants (0–12 months).**
   - Infants generally sleep a total of about 14 to 15 hours at 4 months and a total of 13 to 14 hours at 6 months.
   - Sleep periods last about 3 to 4 hours during the first 3 months, and extend to 6 to 8 hours at 4 to 6 months.
   - By 9 months, 70% to 80% infants **"sleep through the night"** (*sleep consolidation*).
   - **Day/night differentiation** develops between 6 to 12 weeks and nocturnal sleep periods become increasingly longer.
   - The ability to **regulate sleep or control internal states of arousal in order to fall asleep** at bedtime and to fall back asleep during the night, begins to develop in the first 12 weeks of life.

- Most infants nap between 2 and 4 hours divided as 2 naps per day.
- Issues of attachment and social interaction also play an important role in shaping sleep behaviors in infants. Transitional objects such as a pacifier or a blanket and bedtime routines become more important as infancy progresses.
  c. **Toddlers (12–36 months).**
  - Toddlers sleep about 12 hours per 24 hours.
  - Most give up a second nap by 18 months and generally nap 1.5 to 3.5 hours as 1 nap per day.
  - The peak of separation anxiety at 9 to 18 months is often associated with increased night wakings.
  d. **Preschoolers (3–5 years).**
  - Total sleep duration is about 11 to 12 hours per night.
  - Most children give up napping by 5 years.
  - Difficulties falling asleep and night wakings (15%–30%) are still common in this age group, in many cases coexisting in the same child.
  e. **Middle childhood (6–12 years).**
  - Total sleep duration is approximately 10–11 hours per night.
  - Although it was previously believed that sleep problems are rare in middle childhood, recent studies have reported a high prevalence of significant parent-reported sleep problems in this age group.
  f. **Adolescents (12–18 years).**
  - Adolescents require just over 9 hours of sleep per night. However, a number of studies have suggested that the average adolescent actually *gets* about 7 hours of sleep.

B. **Etiology.**
- **Behavioral insomnia of childhood (difficulty initiating and/or maintaining sleep).** "Insomnia" is a symptom and not a diagnosis. The causes of insomnia are varied, and range from the medical (i.e., drug-related, pain-induced, associated with primary sleep disorders such as obstructive sleep apnea) to the behavioral (i.e., associated with poor sleep hygiene or sleep-onset association disorder) and are often a combination of these factors. The most common causes of adolescent insomnia are listed next.
  1. **Sleep-onset association disorder.** The child has learned to fall asleep only under certain conditions or associations, such as being rocked or fed, and does not develop the ability to self-soothe. During the night, when the child experiences the type of brief arousal that normally occurs at the end of a sleep cycle (7–10 times per night) or awakens for other reasons, he is not able to get back to sleep without those same conditions being present. Thus, the problem is one of prolonged night waking resulting in insufficient sleep.
  2. **Limit-setting sleep disorder. Characterized by difficulty falling asleep and bedtime resistance ("curtain calls") rather than night wakings.** Most commonly, this disorder develops from a parent's inability or unwillingness to set consistent bedtime rules and enforce a regular bedtime, often exacerbated by the child's oppositional behavior. In some cases, however, the child's resistance at bedtime is due to an underlying problem in falling asleep caused by other factors (e.g., medical conditions such as asthma or medication use, a sleep disorder such as restless legs, or anxiety) or a mismatch between the child's intrinsic circadian rhythm ("night owl") and parental expectations.
  3. **Psychophysiologic insomnia** (difficulty initiating and/or maintaining sleep) is more common in older children and adolescents. In this disorder, the individual develops conditioned anxiety around falling or staying asleep, usually in combination with poor sleep habits, which leads to heightened arousal and which further compromises the ability to sleep.
  4. **Sleep anxiety.** Nighttime fears are common, and typically both normal and benign. Parental anxiety and family conflict may also play a role in exacerbating nighttime fears in children by increasing the level of emotional arousal in the child. Anxiety around sleep is characterized by fearful behaviors, such as crying, clinging, and leaving the bedroom to seek parental reassurance (at bedtime or in the middle of the night), and bedtime resistance, including refusal to go to bed, frequent "curtain calls," or requiring a parent to be present at bedtime. Some children may also experience frequent nightmares as part of the anxiety picture.

C. **Differential diagnosis.**
  1. **Insufficient sleep and inadequate sleep hygiene.** The resulting chronic sleep deprivation impacts on daytime functioning and causes excessive daytime sleepiness, which can be manifested in a number of ways in children and adolescents: falling asleep

at unintended times, overactivity, and behavior problems. Inadequate sleep hygiene includes practices that increase arousal and practices that are inconsistent with sleep organization.

    a. Practices that increase arousal include caffeine intake, evening television viewing, and bright light in the bedroom during the night or in the early morning.

    b. Practices that are inconsistent with sleep organization include napping late in the day, a disorganized sleep–wake cycle, and excessive time in bed in comparison to time asleep.

  2. Circadian issues may also play a role in some cases of bedtime struggles. When a relatively early bedtime coincides with the normal late-day circadian-mediated surge in alertness ("circadian nadir"), a child may have significantly more difficulty settling and this can result in bedtime resistance. Children with an "owl" circadian preference for later sleep onset and wake times also tend to have a later circadian nadir and are thus particularly likely to have a settling problem if bedtime is set too early.

  3. Bedtime struggles may be the result of a more global problem with **noncompliance,** including **oppositional defiant disorder (ODD)** or may be a feature of a more pervasive psychiatric problem.

  4. Primarily medically based sleep problems such as **obstructive sleep apnea and restless legs/periodic limb movements** may present with bedtime resistance and/or night wakings and disturbed sleep.

D. History: key clinical questions. The clinical evaluation of a child presenting with a sleep problem involves a **careful medical and developmental history** to assess for potential medical causes of sleep disturbances, such as allergies, concomitant medications, and acute or chronic pain conditions.

  1. Current **sleep patterns,** including usual sleep duration and sleep–wake schedule, are often best assessed with a sleep diary, in which parents record daily sleep behaviors for an extended period.

  2. A review of **sleep habits,** such as bedtime routines, daily caffeine intake, and the sleeping environment (temperature, noise level, etc.) may reveal environmental factors that contribute to the sleep problems.

  3. Use of additional diagnostic tools such as **polysomnographic evaluation** are seldom warranted for routine evaluation of pediatric insomnia, but may be appropriate if organic sleep disorders, such as obstructive sleep apnea or periodic limb movements, are suspected.

III. Management. Successful treatment of pediatric sleep problems is highly dependent upon identification of parental concerns, clarification of mutually acceptable treatment goals, active exploration of opportunities and obstacles, and ongoing communication of issues and concerns. Hypnotic medications are rarely needed.

A. Sleep-onset association disorder. The treatment approach to sleep-onset association disorder typically involves a program of withdrawal of parental assistance at sleep onset and during the night (**systematic ignoring**).

  1. In older infants, the introduction of more appropriate sleep associations which will be readily available to the child during the night (**transitional objects** such as a blanket or toy) in addition to **positive reinforcement** (e.g., stickers for remaining in bed) are often beneficial. The goal is to allow the infant or child to develop skills in self-soothing during the night, as well as at bedtime.

  2. Graduated extinction is a more gradual process of weaning the child from dependence upon parental presence that utilizes periodic "checks" by the parents at successively longer time intervals during the sleep–wake transition. Parents must be consistent in applying behavioral programs to avoid inadvertent intermittent reinforcement of night wakings; they should also be forewarned that crying behavior frequently temporarily escalates at the beginning of treatment (**"post-extinction burst"**).

B. Limit-setting sleep disorder. Successful treatment of limit-setting sleep disorder generally involves a combination of the following:

- Decreased parental attention for bedtime-delaying behavior.
- Establishment of bedtime routines.
- Positive reinforcement (e.g., sticker charts) for appropriate behavior at bedtime.
- Older children may benefit from being taught relaxation techniques to help themselves fall asleep more readily.

C. Psychophysiologic insomnia. Treatment usually involves educating the adolescent about **principles of sleep hygiene** (e.g., regular sleep–wake schedule, avoidance of stimulants like caffeine and nicotine, bedtime routine), instructing them to **use the bed for sleep only** and to get out of bed if unable to fall asleep (**stimulus control**), restricting time-in-bed to the actual time asleep (sleep restriction), and teaching **relaxation techniques to reduce anxiety**.

D. Sleep anxiety. In general, strategies aimed at younger children more often involve parental reassurance, while older children typically benefit from an approach that includes teaching and positive reinforcement for independent coping skills.

- Use of security objects should be encouraged, as they can be comforting to the child.
- Television shows and movies that may be frightening or overstimulating, particularly just before bedtime, should be avoided. Also, televisions should be kept out of the bedroom.
- Many children may benefit from learning relaxation strategies, such as deep breathing or visual imagery, which can help a child relax at bedtime and fall asleep more easily.

IV. Clinical pearls and pitfalls.

- Because multiple sleep problems may co-exist in the same child, it is always important to assess for additional nocturnal symptoms that may be indicative of a medically based sleep disorder, such as obstructive sleep apnea (loud snoring, choking/gasping, sweating) or periodic limb movements (restless sleep, repetitive kicking movements), even if the presenting complaint appears behaviorally based.
- All children presenting to pediatric clinicians with learning, attention, behavioral, or emotional concerns, especially attention deficit hyperactivity disorder (ADHD), should be carefully assessed for underlying or comorbid sleep disorders as part of the routine evaluation. There is considerable overlap between the diagnostic features of ADHD (inattention, hyperactivity, impulsivity) and neurobehavioral deficits associated with any significant sleep problems in children. A number of primary sleep disorders, including Obstructive Sleep Apnea (OSA) and Restless Legs/Periodic Limb Movements (RLS/PLMD), frequently include ADHD-like symptoms as part of their clinical presentation.
- Because parents of older children and adolescents, in particular, may not be aware of any existing sleep difficulties, it is also important to directly question the patient about sleep issues as well.

V. When to refer. Referral to a sleep specialist for diagnosis and/or treatment should be considered under circumstances in which children or adolescents with persistent or severe bedtime issues do not respond to simple behavioral measures or for whom the sleep problems are extremely disruptive.

BIBLIOGRAPHY

For parents

Books

Cohen G, ed. *American Academy of Pediatrics Guide to Your Child's Sleep.* New York, NY: Villard, 1999.

Ferber R. *Solve Your Child's Sleep Problems.* New York, NY: Simon & Schuster, 1985.

Mindell J. *Sleeping Through the Night: How Infants, Toddlers, and Their Parents Can Get a Good Night's Sleep.* New York, NY: Harper Collins, 1997.

Web sites

National Sleep Foundation www.sleepfoundation.org. Accessed June 4, 2010.

American Academy of Sleep Medicine www.aasmnet.org. Accessed June 4, 2010.

For professionals

Giannotti F, Cortesi F. Family and cultural influences on sleep development. *Child Adolesc Psychiatr Clin N Am* 18(4):849–61, 2009.

Kryger M, Roth T, Dement W. *Principles and Practices of Sleep Medicine.* Philadelphia, PA: Saunders, 2000.

Mindell J, Owens J. *A Clinical Guide to Pediatric Sleep: Diagnosis and Management of Sleep Problems in Children and Adolescents.* Philadelphia, PA: Lippincott Williams & Wilkins, 2003.

Owens J. Classification and epidemiology of childhood sleep disorders. *Prim Care* 35(3):533–546, 2008.

76

Speech-Sound Disorders

Rebecca McCauley

I. **Description of the problem.** Speech-sound system disorders consist of a *delay or difference in speech-sound acquisition, resulting in speech that is difficult to understand or that sounds immature.* Many children with these disorders are at risk for social–emotional and learning difficulties because of their poor speech or because of associated oral and written language problems. Historically, these disorders were referred to as articulation or phonological disorders. When severe, these disorders may be identified as "developmental apraxia of speech," "developmental verbal dyspraxia," or most recently "childhood apraxia of speech."

A. **Epidemiology.** Speech-sound disorders have a prevalence of 5% in the school-aged population and 10% in younger children, making them one of the most frequently identified communication disorders.
- Increased risk in boys.
- Increased risk in children with cognitive impairment.
- A significant number of children with a history of unintelligibility will experience academic difficulties through high school. Some will have negative academic and job prospects thereafter, especially those who also have identified oral and written language problems.
- Whereas almost all children will outgrow the speech differences characteristic of this disorder by adolescence, its academic and social–emotional consequences nonetheless make identification and treatment an important goal. In addition, a small number of these children will exhibit distortion errors that will affect their speech into adulthood.

B. **Familial transmission/genetics.** A genetic basis for severe forms of speech-sound disorder (especially childhood apraxia of speech) has recently been suggested. Family histories of children with this disorder are often positive for other speech and language disorders and for written language problems.

C. **Etiology/contributing factors.**
1. **Organic.** Early recurrent periods of otitis media with effusion are an important risk factor in about one-third of children with speech-sound disorders. There is little evidence that an abnormally short lingual frenulum ("tongue-tied") affects articulation and ambiguous evidence for the role of infantile swallow (tongue thrust) in the disorder. Childhood apraxia of speech is now seen as occurring in three contexts: idiopathically, as a result of known neurologic impairment, or as part of a complex neurobehavioral disorder of known or unknown etiology (e.g., Down syndrome, autism spectrum disorder).
2. **Developmental.** Diagnosis before age 3 is difficult because young children are highly variable in their speech-sound productions and in their cooperation with structured tasks. However, infrequent vocalizations or feeding or swallowing problems may indicate oromotor problems that can predispose the child to speech-sound disorders.

II. **Making the diagnosis.**
A. **Signs and symptoms.** (See Table 76-1.)
B. **Differential diagnosis.** Conditions resulting in delayed speech-sound development include oral anomalies (e.g., submucous cleft palate), hearing impairment, frank neurologic conditions associated with dyspraxia or dysarthria, and cognitive impairment. Co-occurrence with language disorders is quite common and the frequency of co-occurrence with voice disorders and with stuttering also appears to be elevated.
C. **History: key clinical questions.**
1. *"How well do you and others understand your child's speech, compared to the speech of other children his or her age?"* Reduced intelligibility compared to peers is a strong indicator of a speech-sound disorder.
2. *"Has your child's speech changed much during the past 6 months?"* For children up to age 5 years, any response suggesting little change over time is a cause for concern.
3. *"How do you and others respond to your child's poor speech? How does your child respond to any negative reactions?"* Teasing, frequent corrections, or requests to repeat

Table 76-1. Signs and symptoms of speech-sound disorders

Any age	Speech is more difficult to understand than that of peers
	Teasing by others about speech (e.g., about a lisp)
	Shyness about speaking or excessive frustration when not understood
2 years or older	Intelligibility less than 50%
	Use of only 4–5 consonants (e.g., sounds represented by the letters *p, b, w, y, m*) and a limited number of vowels
	Consistent errors in the use of the sounds represented by the letters *p, b, m, n, h, w,* or any vowel sounds
	Consonants at the beginning of words are omitted (e.g., "ow" for "cow")
	One sound is used in the place of many others (e.g., *p* is used when *f, v, t, or k* is expected)
	The sounds *k* or *g* are used when *t* or *d* is expected (e.g., "ko" for "toe")
3 years or older	Intelligibility less than 75%
3½ years or older	Consistent errors in the use of the sounds *f, v, k, g,* or *y* (e.g., "wu" for "you")
	Consistent errors that assume the following patterns:
	Consonants at the ends of words are omitted
	The sounds *t* or *d* are used when *k* or *g* is expected
4 years or older	Intelligibility less than 100%
5½ years or older	Errors on two or more speech-sounds that are obvious enough to call attention to the child's speech

can make the child frustrated or shy and withdrawn. Spontaneous and frequent use of informal signs and gestures by the child is facilitative, but may suggest compensation for speech motor planning difficulties.

4. *"Does your child have a history of problems with feeding or swallowing?"* This question addresses the possibility of developmental dysarthria as part of differential diagnosis.

5. *"Do you ever think your child has day-to-day fluctuations or problems in hearing?"* This question addresses the potential for chronic hearing impairment, as well as the issue of fluctuating hearing loss related to otitis media.

D. **Physical examination.** The physical examination can help rule out significant oral anomalies and screen for frank neurologic abnormalities, as well as provide information about the child's middle ear status.

E. **Tests.** A certified speech-language pathologist can perform testing necessary for confirmation of speech-sound disorder.

III. **Management.**

A. **Primary goals.** The primary care clinician's principal goals in speech-sound disorders are appropriate referral as well as management of middle ear status.

B. **Criteria for referral.** Refer to a speech-language pathologist if the child's speech demonstrates any of the signs or symptoms mentioned in Table 76-1. Speech-language pathologists in public school systems assess and treat children with communication disorders—regardless of age. Even very young children at risk for speech-sound system disorders may benefit from early efforts to stimulate vocal production and language development.

IV. **Clinical pearls and pitfalls.**

- Remember the guidelines regarding intelligibility (Table 76-1): A stranger should be able to understand about 50% of what a 2-year-old says, 75% of what a 3-year-old says, and 100% of what a 4-year-old says.
- Tantrums or indications of extreme frustration from a child over the age of 3 years because of the parent's inability to understand the child's speech, suggest a significant problem in speech or language development.
- To avoid judging the child in terms of their own speech dialect, clinicians should ask parents to gauge how well the child is understood compared to peers.
- Delays in referral not only can deprive the child of early treatment but can also result in increased parent–child conflict.

BIBLIOGRAPHY

For professionals

Caruso A, Strand E. *Clinical Management of Motor Speech Disorders in Children*. New York: Thieme, 1999.

Williams L, MacLeod S, McCauley RJ, eds. *Interventions for Speech Sound Disorders in Children.* Baltimore: Brookes Publishers, 2010.

Web sites

Apraxia, for parents and professionals on severe speech sound system disorders in children, including childhood apraxia of speech. www.apraxia-kids.org

American Speech-Language-Hearing Association, an information page prepared by the organization responsible for credentializing speech-language pathologists. www.asha.org/public/speech/disorders/childsandL.htm

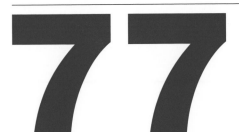

Stuttering

Barry Guitar

I. **Description of the problem.** Stuttering is a disruption of speech, characterized by repetitions, prolongations, and/or blockages. These may be accompanied by physical struggle, frustration, and fear of speech. The term *disfluency* is often used synonymously with *stuttering*, but it also may refer to the hesitations common in the speech of typical children learning to talk.

A. **Epidemiology.**
- The prevalence of stuttering is 1% among school-aged children, slightly lower in adults, and slightly higher in preschool children. The incidence is 5%.
- The difference between prevalence and incidence figures reflects the tendency for children who stutter to recover, usually before puberty.
- The male–female ratio among children younger than 6 is about 2:1 and rises to 4:1 in adulthood, suggesting that females are more likely to recover.

B. **Familial transmission/genetics.** Parents who stutter are more likely to have children who stutter; this is especially so for women who stutter. A multifactorial (polygenic) model has been suggested to account for the transmission.

C. **Etiology/contributing factors**
1. **Environmental.** A home or school environment that places high demands on a child's performance can contribute to stuttering. Examples of demands include a communication environment that pressures the child to speak more rapidly, articulately, or with more advanced language than the child is easily able to. Stuttering may also be exacerbated by stressful but normal life events such as the birth of a sibling, separation from a parent, or a family move.
2. **Organic/transactional.** Predispositions to stuttering include an inherited or acquired difficulty in speech motor coordination and a temperament, which reacts to stress with excess muscular tension and effort. Brain imaging studies of children who stutter suggest reduced gray matter volume in speech areas and abnormal white matter tracts in speech planning and speech motor areas.
3. **Developmental.** Stuttering usually appears between the ages of 18 months and 5 years. In 70% of children who begin to stutter, early symptoms will resolve. Early onset of stuttering (between years 2–3) is associated with more likely natural recovery than later onset. In children who do not recover naturally, the signs and symptoms may worsen from (1) easy repetitions with minimal awareness to (2) rapid and physically tense repetitions with evidence of frustration to (3) blockages of speech, accompanying struggle behaviors, and avoidance of words and speaking situations.

II. **Making the diagnosis.**

A. **Signs and symptoms/differential diagnosis.** (See Table 77-1.)

B. **History: key clinical questions.**
1. *"How long have you been aware of your child's stuttering?"* If the child has stuttered for more than 6 months, suspect a potential chronic problem, particularly if it has not decreased in frequency or severity since onset.
2. *"How has the stuttering changed since it began?"* If there has been an increase in effort, emotion, or avoidance associated with stuttering, it is worsening.
3. *"What is your child's stuttering like at its worst?"* Many children who stutter will not stutter in the clinician's office; it is important to have the parents describe the signs and symptoms that have caused them concern.
4. *"Is the child bothered by their stuttering?"* If so, the child may soon react to his stuttering with physical tension and struggle and should be referred.

C. **Tests.** Ask the child several direct questions (e.g., name, age, address) that must be answered without substitution or circumlocution. This is likely to elicit stuttering or avoidance if child is a stutterer.

Table 77-1. Signs and symptoms of normal disfluency and stuttering

	Normal disfluency	Mild stuttering	Severe stuttering
Speech behavior	Occasional brief repetitions of sounds, syllables, or short words (li-like this)	Frequent long repetitions of sounds, syllables, or short words (li-li-li-like this). Occasional prolongations of sounds	Very frequent and often very long repetitions of sounds, syllables, or short words. Frequent sound prolongations and blockages
Other behavior	Occasional pauses, hesitations or fillers. Changing of words or thoughts	Repetitions and prolongations associated with blinking, looking away, and physical tension around mouth	More evidence of struggle, including pitch rise in voice. Extra words used as "starters"
When most noticeable	Comes and goes when child is excited, tired, sick, talking to inattentive listeners	Comes and goes in similar situations but is more often present than absent	Present in most speaking situations. More consistent
Child's reaction	Usually none apparent	May show a little concern or some frustration and embarrassment	Embarrassment, shame, and fear of speaking. Lack of eye contact when speaking
Parents' reaction	None to a great deal	Some concern, but not a great deal	Considerable degree of concern
Referral decision	Refer only if parents quite concerned and are convinced their child is stuttering	Refer if continues for 6–8 weeks or if parental concern justifies it	Refer as soon as possible

III. Management.

A. Primary goals. The family must understand that the child is doing the best that they can with their speech and will only get worse if the family criticizes. Rather, the family should find ways to reduce stress and to verbalize their acceptance to the child.

B. Information for family.

1. It should be emphasized to the parents that **they did not cause the problem.**
2. The etiology may be a slight difference in brain organization, which favors some skills (e.g., drawing or music) but creates more hesitancy in speech, especially during childhood.
3. The onset of stuttering may be associated with a spurt in speech and language development or an increased stress, but most frequently onset occurs in normal circumstances.
4. Parents should know that if the child is frustrated by their stuttering, **the parents should occasionally acknowledge it, in an accepting, encouraging way.** They can also assure the child that if she or he would like help with it, there are professionals who can help.

C. Initial treatment strategies.

1. As much as possible, **parents should talk with their child in a slow, relaxed manner,** using short sentences and frequent pauses to promote fluency. The speaking style of television's Mr. Rogers is an excellent model.
2. **A brief period should be set aside each day at a regular time when one parent can interact alone with child.** The parent should use a slow speech rate and follow the child's lead in choosing topics of conversation and play activities. The aim is to give the child a sense of being the center of attention for this time.
3. **Family should institute turn-taking in competitive speaking situations,** such as dinner table conversations, especially if these are times when the child stutters more.

4. **Parents should occasionally make a comment expressing empathy,** such as "Lots of kids get stuck on their words sometimes. I know it makes talking hard, but it's ok and you can take as long as you like."

5. **Attempts should be made to slow down the pace of life in the home,** including the pace of conversations. After the child says something, parents should pause for a second or two, before responding.

D. Criteria for referral.

1. The child is stuttering with physical tension and is showing concern or frustration. The child should be referred immediately.

2. If initial strategies have been tried for a month without appreciable lessening of the stuttering, referral should be made.

3. Referral should be made to a speech-language pathologist certified by the American Speech-Language-Hearing Association, preferably one who specializes in stuttering. (The Stuttering Foundation Web site contains a referral list of clinicians experienced in the treatment of stuttering.)

IV. Clinical pearls and pitfalls.

● Most parents blame themselves. Reassure them that they didn't cause their child's stuttering, but they can play a big part in their child's ability to cope with it.

● Most children will outgrow stuttering, especially if parents can reduce psychosocial pressures and increase acceptance of the child as he is now.

● Parental attitudes that put a high premium on completely fluent speech probably interfere with recovery.

● Effective programs for preschool children who stutter are intensive, involve the parents, and focus on natural, fluent speech. Intervention in the preschool years can eliminate stuttering.

● Effective treatments for school age children help the child speak more fluently and become confident about talking, but do not aim for perfection.

● Transient stuttering is sometimes associated with the use of medications for allergies, attention deficit disorders, and other childhood disorders.

BIBLIOGRAPHY

Web sites

Stuttering Foundation. www.stutteringhelp.org (This site contains a streaming video for parents of children who may be stuttering, a list of 7 things parents can do to help their child, a referral list of experienced clinicians for every state and many other countries, as well as an online store containing many inexpensive books and videos for parents and children who stutter.)

Stuttering Home Page. www.mnsu.edu/comdis/kuster/stutter.html (This site contains excellent resources for parents, children, and teens. There are support and discussion groups and a wealth of written material and links to other useful Web sites.)

National Stuttering Association. www.nsastutter.org (This site is run by an organization of people who stutter and has information about support groups around the world and about NSA's annual conference.)

For parents

Conture E, Fraser J. *If Your Child Stutters: A Guide for Parents*. Memphis, TN: Stuttering Foundation, 2002.

For professionals

Bloodstein O, Ratner N. *A Handbook on Stuttering*. Chicago, IL: National Easter Seal Society for Crippled Children and Adults, 2008.

Guitar B. *Stuttering: An Integrated Approach to Its Nature and Treatment*. Baltimore, MD: Lippincott, Williams & Wilkins, 2006.

Guitar B, McCauley R. *Treatment of Stuttering*. Baltimore, MD: Lippincott, Williams & Wilkins, 2009.

Yairi E, Ambrose N. *Early Childhood Stuttering*. Austin, TX: Pro-Ed, 2005.

78

Substance Use in Adolescence

Anna Maria S. Ocampo
John R. Knight

I. **Description of the problem.** Use of alcohol and drugs by adolescents is a major national problem. Alcohol use is associated with the leading causes of death among U.S. teenagers; including unintentional injuries (e.g., motor vehicle crashes), homicides, and suicides. Greater than 30% of all deaths from injuries can be directly linked to alcohol, and substance use is also associated with a wide range of serious problems, including school failure, respiratory diseases, high-risk sexual behaviors, transmission of HIV, gang membership, use of firearms, and other illegal activities. Early age of first use increases the risk of developing a substance use disorder during later life, and the age of onset of use among U.S. teens is falling.

A. **Epidemiology.**
   1. According to the Monitoring the Future Study (2008), 72% of adolescents have begun to drink, 55% have gotten drunk, 47% have tried an illicit drug, and 25% have tried an illicit drug other than cannabis by the time they reach senior year in high school. Because of relatively high prevalence, experimentation with alcohol or cannabis, or getting drunk once, can arguably be considered developmental variations. However, health care clinicians should always consider recurrent drunkenness, recurrent cannabis use, or any use of other drugs as serious risks.
   2. Alcohol is the most commonly used psychoactive substance among youth, more than tobacco and illicit drugs. Marijuana continues to be the most widely used illicit drug. Cigarette use among adolescents is declining and has reached its lowest level in many years. Perhaps antismoking campaigns have resulted in an increased perception of risk and disapproval. During recent years, adolescents have increasingly reported misuse of anabolic steroids, prescription medications (e.g., narcotic analgesics, stimulants, and sedatives), and over-the-counter drugs (e.g., cough and cold remedies). Adolescents may perceive pharmaceutical products as inherently less risky. The preponderance of advertisements directed at consumers gives the impression of "a pill for every ailment." Some adolescents take these medications from parents' medicine cabinets or homes of relatives and friends, some misuse their own prescription, and others obtain them from acquaintances or drug dealers.
   3. Misuse of alcohol is found among all demographic subgroups, with higher risk associated with being male, white, and from middle to upper socio-economic status families. Despite common stereotypes, drug use may be less prevalent among inner city minority students compared to their white suburban counterparts. Rises in usage of specific illicit drugs are positively associated with the perceived availability of the drug and negatively associated with the perceived risk of harm associated with use of the drug.

B. **Etiology/contributing factors.**
   1. Substance use during adolescence is associated with a variety of risk and protective factors, which may be characteristics of the individual, family, or community.
      a. Individual risk factors include male gender, school failure, attention-deficit/hyperactivity disorder (ADHD) and learning disabilities, other co-occurring mental disorders (e.g., anxiety and mood disorders, conduct disorder), poor coping skills, nonconformity, and low religiousness. Family factors include genetic risks, a family member who is actively abusing alcohol or drugs, parent–child conflict, permissive or authoritarian parenting style, and unstable parent relationships or parental divorce. Community risks include widespread alcohol advertising, density of alcohol outlets, availability of other drugs, and substance using peers.
      b. Individual protective factors include high self-esteem, internal locus of control, emotional well-being, resilient temperament, and school achievement. Family protective factors include frequent communication about alcohol and drug use, good parental modeling, involvement and monitoring, and eating meals together regularly as a family. Community protective factors include use of evidence-based prevention programs, availability of after school programs and mentoring, and monitoring of alcohol outlets.

2. Substance use disorders (SUDs) are diagnosed based on the following DSM-IV criteria: Substance *abuse* is defined by one or more of four criteria occurring *repeatedly* over the course of the past 12 months, but not meeting criteria for diagnosis of dependence:
   a. Substance-related problems at school, work, or home
   b. Use of substance in hazardous situations (e.g., driving a car)
   c. Substance-related legal problems
   d. Continued use despite problems or harm
   Substance *dependence* is defined by meeting any three of seven criteria during the past twelve months:
   a. Tolerance
   b. Withdrawal (may be either physiological or psychological)
   c. Using more of substance for longer periods of time than intended
   d. Unsuccessful attempts to quit or cut down use of substance
   e. Spending a great deal of time obtaining, using, or recovering from effects of the substance
   f. Giving up important activities because of substance use
   g. Continued use of substance despite medical or social problems caused by the substance
   SUDs have a multi-factorial etiology, including interaction between genetic predisposition, environmental exposures during childhood, and personal choice. Twin and adoption studies have shown that alcoholism has strong genetic determinants, and recent genomic studies have shown that a number of specific genes are likely involved. Exposure to parental heavy drinking, especially during adolescence, is also associated with higher risk of substance abuse. Animal studies suggest that early nicotine use may independently increase the risk of a SUD by altering the dopaminergic pathways within the brain's reward system.

C. ADHD and SUD.
1. Given the risk-taking tendency and impulsivity of adolescents with ADHD, they may begin experimenting with tobacco, alcohol, and drugs at an earlier age compared to those without the disorder. Furthermore, children with ADHD are at elevated risk of developing a substance use disorder later in life, and the presence of other co-occurring mental disorders raise the risk even higher. In adults, there is an overrepresentation of ADHD among those with substance use disorders (i.e., one in five adults with a SUD also has ADHD). SUDs in individuals with ADHD tend to emerge at an earlier age, follow a more severe and aggressive course, and are associated with higher rates of substance-related motor vehicle crashes and injuries.
2. Misuse and diversion of prescribed stimulants may occur among adolescents with ADHD and their peers. This is especially true among college students who are male, white, have a grade point average less than 3.5, belong to social fraternities, reside off campus, and attend the most competitive colleges. Greater than half of college students being treated with stimulant medication for ADHD are approached by their peers and asked to divert their medication. Long-acting stimulants are less likely to be misused or diverted, compared to short-acting forms.
3. Although adolescents with ADHD are at higher risk for SUD, appropriate treatment does not increase that risk. Psychostimulant therapy initiated during childhood reduces the risk of future SUD.

II. Making the diagnosis.
A. Signs and symptoms. The signs of substance use during adolescence are largely non-specific and include: declining school performance, change in dress and friends; sudden mood swings (either depression or euphoria); drug or drug paraphernalia found in room, car or clothes; diluted or missing alcohol from parent's home supply; stealing, lying, or missing money, including unexplained withdrawals from a bank account. Physical signs include as dilated pupils (stimulants, cocaine); constricted pupils (alcohol, opioids, sedatives); odor of alcohol on breath or appearance of obvious intoxication, or volatile odor on person or clothes (inhalants).
B. Differential diagnosis. Considerations include metabolic disorder, neurological disease, accidental poisoning, ADHD, depression, anxiety, bipolar disorder, post-traumatic stress disorder, oppositional defiant disorder, schizophrenia, bulimia nervosa, and social phobia. All of these may also co-occur with substance abuse.
C. History.
1. Screening. As part of a routine history, every adolescent should be asked about use of alcohol and drugs. *"During the past 12 months, did you drink any alcohol, smoke any marijuana or hashish, or use anything else to get high"?* A yes answer to any of these questions should be followed by a structured substance abuse screening tool. One

Begin: **"I'm going to ask you a few questions that I ask all my patients. Please be honest. I will keep your answers confidential."**

Part A

During the PAST 12 MONTHS, did you:	No	Yes
1. Drink any <u>alcohol</u> (more than a few sips)? (Do not count sips of alcohol taken during family or religious events.)	☐	☐
2. Smoke any <u>marijuana or hashish</u>?	☐	☐
3. Use <u>anything else</u> to <u>get high</u>? ("anything else" includes illegal drugs, over-the-counter and prescription drugs, and things that you sniff or "huff")	☐	☐

For clinic use only: Did the patient answer "yes" to any questions in Part A?

No ☐   Yes ☐

↓   ↓

Ask CAR question only, then stop.   **Ask all 6 CRAFFT questions.**

Part B	No	Yes
1. Have you ever ridden in a **CAR** driven by someone (including yourself) who was "high" or had been using alcohol or drugs?	☐	☐
2. Do you ever use alcohol or drugs to **RELAX**, feel better about yourself, or fit in?	☐	☐
3. Do you ever use alcohol or drugs while you are by yourself, or **ALONE**?	☐	☐
4. Do you ever **FORGET** things you did while using alcohol or drugs?	☐	☐
5. Do your **FAMILY** or **FRIENDS** ever tell you that you should cut down on your drinking or drug use?	☐	☐
6. Have you ever gotten into **TROUBLE** while you were using alcohol or drugs?	☐	☐

CONFIDENTIALITY NOTICE:
The information recorded on this page may be protected by special federal confidentiality rules (42 CFR Part 2), which prohibit disclosure of this information unless authorized by specific written consent. A general authorization for release of medical information is NOT sufficient for this purpose.

Figure 78-1. The CRAFFT Screening Interview.

such screen is the CRAFFT test, which consists of six yes/no questions that are easy to score (each "yes" answer = 1). Key words in the test's six items form its mnemonic ("CRAFFT"). (Fig. 78-1)

A CRAFFT total score of two or higher indicates 50% probability of a SUD diagnosis; this probability reaches 100% for a CRAFFT total score of six.

2. Assessment. A positive CRAFFT should be followed by additional alcohol and drug use history, including age of first use, current pattern of use (quantity and frequency), and impact on physical and emotional health, school and family, and other negative consequences from use (e.g., legal problems). Taking a good substance use history begins the process of therapeutic intervention. Other helpful questions:

a. *"What is the worst thing that ever happened to you while you were using alcohol or drugs?"*

b. *"Have you ever regretted something that happened when you were drinking (using drugs)?"*

c. *"Do your parents know about your alcohol and drug use? If so, how do they feel about it? If not, how do you think they would feel about it?"*

d. *"Do you have any younger brothers or sisters? What do (or would) they think about your alcohol and drug use?"*

The assessment should also include a screening for co-occurring mental disorders and parent/sibling alcohol and drug use.

D. Other diagnostic procedures.

1. Physical findings. A targeted physical examination is indicated, but is unlikely to yield significant findings in the absence of acute intoxication. Check vital signs and pupil size. Hypertension, tachycardia, and dilated pupils may suggest either acute intoxication (amphetamines, cocaine, MDMA) or withdrawal (opioids). Inflammation or erosions of the nasal septum may suggest insufflation ("snorting") of drugs, but can also result from common upper respiratory infections or digital excoriation. Auscultation of the lungs may reveal wheezing in those who smoke tobacco, marijuana, or other drugs. Abdominal tenderness associated with gastritis, hepatitis, or pancreatitis may occasionally be found in heavy drinkers. Examination of the skin rarely reveals venous scarring from intravenous drug use in adolescents.

2. Drug testing. The American Academy of Pediatrics endorses that laboratory testing for alcohol or drugs of abuse should not be performed on a conscious adolescent without his/her knowledge and consent. Clinicians should consult with a toxicologist before ordering drug screens, to minimize the risks of false negatives. The window of detection for most drugs of abuse is less than 72 hours, with the notable exception of tetrahydrocannabinol (THC), which for heavy users may be detectable in the urine up to several weeks after the last episode of marijuana use. Specimens must be collected using the federal protocol, or by direct observation of urine flow from the urethra into the specimen container. Always include urine specific gravity and creatinine level as markers of validity. Positive screening immunoassays must always be confirmed with gas chromatography and mass spectrometry. Taking a good history, with reasonable assurance of confidentiality, is often more informative than laboratory testing. However, properly conducted laboratory testing may be a useful therapeutic adjunct for drug-using adolescents who are receiving treatment and are motivated to stop using.

III. Management.

A. Assess the level of severity of use (Fig. 78-2).

1. Experimentation. First use of psychoactive substance, most commonly alcohol, marijuana, prescription medications, or inhalants
2. Nonproblematic use. Regular pattern of use, regardless of frequency, usually with peers and without serious consequences
3. Problem use. Adverse consequences first appear (e.g., decline in school performance, suspension, accident, injury, arguments with parents, or peers)
4. Abuse
5. Dependence

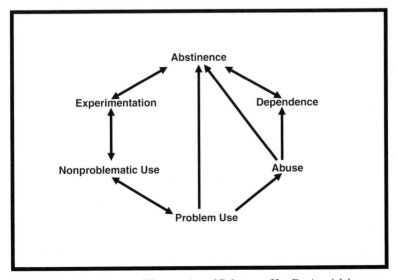

Figure 78-2. Developmental Progression of Substance Use During Adolescence.

Table 78-1. Stage appropriate therapeutic goals

Stage	Intervention goal
Abstinence	Positive reinforcement, anticipatory guidance
Experimentation	Education regarding risks
Nonproblematic use	Risk reduction advice (e.g., driving/riding while impaired)
Problem use	Brief intervention (BI)
Abuse	BI, Outpatient counseling, follow-up
Dependence	Referral to intensive treatment
Secondary abstinence	Positive reinforcement, support, follow-up

B. Deliver a therapeutic intervention. Stage specific goals are presented in Table 78-1. Provide positive reinforcement for those who are abstinent. For those at the stages of experimentation and nonproblematic use, clinicians should explain the health risks of alcohol and drugs (e.g., the potential harm on developing brain), give clear advice not to use, and focus on risk reduction. For example, the clinician should mention the serious risks associated with drinking and driving, or riding with an intoxicated driver, and suggest strategies for safe transportation home following events where alcohol or drugs are present. For those at the stages of problematic use or abuse, office-based brief interventions have been shown to be effective among adults, and emerging evidence suggests brief advice based on health risks works well among adolescents. Most brief interventions include six key steps:

1. Feedback. Deliver feedback on the risks and/or negative consequences of substance use. Use the information gathered during screening and assessment, and repeat the consequences whenever possible in the adolescent's own words, beginning with *"You told me that ... "*

2. Education. Explain the health risks of alcohol and drugs, for example, *"the latest science shows that alcohol and drugs cause greater damage to the adolescent brain, because it is still developing, and brain development continues well into your twenties. Alcohol causes greater impairment and places you in greater danger, compared to adults, and marijuana smoking during the teen years places you at greater risk for developing a serious mental disorder later in life."*

3. Recommendation. Recommend that your patient use no alcohol and drugs for a specified time period (e.g., three weeks).

4. Negotiation. If the patient refuses, attempt to elicit any commitment to change. For example, try to have your patient commit to stopping drugs (if s/he refuses to stop drinking), or confining use to weekends, etc.

5. Agreement. Ask for a brief written agreement that both of you will sign that specifies the change and the time period. This can be done on your letterhead or office notepad (be sure to keep these private).

6. Follow-up. Make an appointment for a follow-up meeting to monitor success (or need for more intensive intervention). Consider use of laboratory testing to verify abstinence only if you are adequately trained and experienced in proper collection and handling, validity checks (specific gravity and creatinine), and understand the variations in screening assays and confirmatory testing.

C. Some adolescents, such as those with alcohol/drug dependence or co-occurring mental disorders, will require more directive intervention, parental involvement, and referral to intensive treatment. Healthcare clinicians should be familiar with treatment resources in their own communities. Whenever possible, refer to adolescent-only programs that have staff specifically trained in counseling adolescents with SUDs. However, adolescent specific treatment is uncommon in many communities. Effective treatment programs should offer treatment for co-occurring disorders and include the family as part of treatment.

1. Outpatient treatment.

   a. Behavioral therapies. Individual, group, or family counseling. Cognitive behavioral therapy, multi-dimensional family therapy, and motivational enhancement therapy and contingencies (incentives) appear promising.

   b. Pharmacotherapies. Three medications have been FDA-approved for treating alcohol dependence: naltrexone, acamprosate, and disulfiram. We have had limited experience with naltrexone long-acting (by injection), none with acamprosate, and do not recommend disulfiram, which causes an adverse reaction if the individual drinks, because adolescents tend to be more impulsive than adults. Nicotine replacements (patch, inhaler, nasal spray, gum, lozenges) are available over-the-counter and two prescription medications: bupropion and varenicline are FDA-approved for treating tobacco addiction. Methadone is restricted to specially licensed programs, and most do not accept minors. Buprenorphine, which is available in combination with naloxone in a sublingual tablet, is a safe and effective replacement therapy for opioid dependence. One study to date showed it more effective than detoxification in the short term. Longer clinical trials among youth are needed. However, interested physicians can receive a waiver from the DEA after completing 8 hours of training, and prescribe it to opioid-dependent youth as a maintenance therapy.

    c. 12-step fellowships (e.g., Alcoholics Anonymous). Adolescents need an adult guide or temporary sponsor to make attendance at AA groups meaningful. Adolescents who attend these meetings have higher rates of successful recovery than those who do not.

  2. Inpatient treatment.

    a. Detoxification. 2 to 3 days of medical treatment for physiological withdrawal symptoms, indicated only for acute management of alcohol, sedative-hypnotic, benzodiazepine, or opioid dependence.

    b. Rehabilitation. 2 to 3 weeks of intensive behavioral therapy, usually including individual and group counseling, psychoeducational sessions, family therapy, and introduction to 12-step fellowships.

    c. Long-term residential treatment. These include residential schools, therapeutic communities, and halfway houses. Most offer 3 to 12 months closely supervised aftercare (i.e., following completion of a detoxification and/or rehabilitation program), which includes weekly counseling and group therapy, behavioral management strategies, and required attendance at school and/or work.

    d. Unproven programs. Some families may choose to send their teenaged children to wilderness programs or so-called "boot camps," which have not been scientifically evaluated.

IV. Clinical pearls and pitfalls.

  1. Many adolescents who abuse substances are also depressed. Provide treatment for both substance abuse and depression *simultaneously* when they co-occur. Treatment of either one alone is unlikely to be successful.

  2. Caution is advised when first diagnosing ADHD in an adolescent with substance use. Recurrent use of alcohol or drugs may cause inattentiveness and cognitive impairment. It is best to revisit the diagnosis of ADHD after a period of abstinence from substance use. For patients with both ADHD and SUD, it is important to treat both conditions. To prevent diversion or nonmedical use, we recommend that parents retain control of the prescription bottle.

  3. Treatment of chronic severe pain with opioid analgesics seldom causes addiction in individuals who do not have a pre-existing SUD or some other mental disorder. Chronic use of opioid analgesics leads to development of physiological tolerance and withdrawal, but these two alone do not define an addictive disorder. *Physiological dependence* on opioid analgesics should not be confused with a *drug dependence* diagnosis.

BIBLIOGRAPHY

Parents

Web sites

A Family Guide To Keeping Youth Mentally Healthy and Drug Free: http://family.samhsa.gov/. Accessed June 2, 2010.

Parents: The Anti-Drug: http://www.theantidrug.com/. Accessed June 2, 2010.

Partnership for a Drug Free America: http://www.drugfree.org/. Accessed June 2, 2010.

Mothers Against Drunk Driving: http://www.madd.org. Accessed June 2, 2010.

Books

7 ways to protect your teen from alcohol and other drugs [educational brochure]. Boston, MA: Bureau of Substance Abuse Services, Massachusetts Department of Public Health. 2004: may be ordered on-line at: http://www.maclearinghouse.com/PDFs/SubstanceAbuse/SA1037.pdf. Accessed June 2, 2010.

Substance Abuse and Mental Health Services Administration. *Keeping Youth Drug Free*. Center for Substance Abuse Prevention. Rockville, MD: DHHS, 2002.

Drug Strategies. *Treating Teens: A Guide to Adolescent Drug Programs*. Washington, DC: Drug Strategies, 2003.

Teens

Web sites

Students Against Destructive Decisions: http://www.sadd.org/. Accessed June 2, 2010.
Check Yourself: http://www.checkyourself.com/. Accessed June 2, 2010.
NIDA for Teens (National Institute on Drug Abuse): http://www.teens.drugabuse.gov/. Accessed June 2, 2010.
What's Driving You? http://www.whatsdrivingyou.org/. Accessed June 2, 2010.
Above the Influence: http://www.abovetheinfluence.com/. Accessed June 2, 2010.

Professionals

Web sites

National Clearinghouse for Alcohol and Drug Information: http://ncadi.samhsa.gov/. Accessed June 2, 2010 (includes a special section for health professionals)
National Institute on Drug Abuse: http://www.nida.nih.gov. Accessed June 2, 2010.
National Institute on Alcohol Abuse and Alcoholism: http://www.niaaa.nih.gov/. Accessed June 2, 2010.
Substance Abuse and Mental Health Services Administration: www.samhsa.gov. Accessed June 2, 2010.
Monitoring the Future: www.monitoringthefuture.org. Accessed June 2, 2010.
Youth Risk Behavior Surveillance: http://www.cdc.gov/HealthyYouth/yrbs/index.htm. Accessed June 2, 2010.
National Survey on Drug Use and Health: http://oas.samhsa.gov/nhsda.htm. Accessed June 2, 2010.
Office of National Drug Control Policy: http://www.whitehousedrugpolicy.gov/streetterms/default.asp. Accessed June 2, 2010.

Tools

Contract for Life: http://www.sadd.org/contract.htm
Clinical guidelines for use of buprenorphine in the treatment of opioid addiction: http://buprenorphine.samhsa.gov/Bup_Guidelines.pdf. Accessed June 2, 2010.

Publications

Kulig JW. Tobacco, alcohol, and other drugs: the role of the pediatrician in prevention, identification, and management of substance abuse. *Pediatrics* 115(3):816–821, 2005.
Levy S, Knight J. Screening, brief intervention, and referral to treatment for adolescents. *J Addict Med* 2(4):215–221, 2008.
Knight JR. Substance use, abuse, and dependence and other risk taking (chapter). In Carey WB, Crocker AC, Coleman WL, Elias ER, Feldman HM, (eds). *Developmental-Behavioral Pediatrics* (4th ed), Philadelphia, PA: WB Saunders Co, 2009.
American Academy of Pediatrics. Testing for Drugs of Abuse in Children and Adolescents: Addendum – Testing in Schools and at Home. *Pediatrics* 119(3):627–630, 2007.
Knight JR, Shrier LA, Bravender TD, et al. A new brief screen for adolescent substance abuse. *Arch Pediatr Adolesc Med* 153(6):591–596, 1999.
American Psychiatric Association. *Diagostic and Statistical Manual of Mental Disorders* (4th ed), text revision. Washington DC: American Psychiatric Association, 2000.

79

Suicide

Heather Walter
Phillip Hernandez
Joanna Cole

I. **Description of the problem.** Suicide ranks as the third and fourth leading cause of death among young people aged 15 to 24 and 10 to 14 years, respectively. Each year, there are approximately 10 suicides for every 100,000 youngsters less than age 19, an estimated 12 suicides every day. Research implicates a number of psychological, biological, environmental, social, and cultural risk factors for suicide, and knowledge of these risk factors can facilitate pediatric clinicians' identification and management of youths at highest risk.

Suicidality presents on a dimensional spectrum ranging from thoughts about causing intentional self-injury or death (suicidal ideation) to acts that cause intentional self-injury (suicide attempt) or death (completed suicide). The intent to harm oneself, which may be explicit and strong or ambiguous and vague, is the defining characteristic of suicidal behavior. Intentionality is complicated by developmental variations among children and adolescents.

A. **Epidemiology.** Suicide is rare before puberty. Rates of completed suicide increase steadily across the teen years, rising from 1.3 per 100,000 in 10- to 14-year-olds to 8.2 per 100,000 in 15- to 19-year-olds. Teenage/young adult males complete suicide at a rate four times that of females and represent nearly 80% of all suicides. Suicide rates are highest among American Indian/Alaska Native youths (15.1 per 100,000) and non-Hispanic whites (13.9 per 100,000). Rates are lowest among Asia/Pacific youths (5.7 per 100,000), non-Hispanic blacks (5.0 per 100,000), and Hispanics (4.9 per 100,000). From 1950 to 1990, the suicide rate for adolescents aged 15 to 19 years increased by 300%. Firearms remain the most commonly utilized method of completing suicide for males, whereas females are more likely to complete suicide by poisoning. Hanging/suffocation is gaining prominence as a common method, especially among children and among females. Firearms in the home, regardless of whether they are kept unloaded or locked, are associated with a higher risk of completed adolescent suicide.

Although reliable data for suicide attempts is difficult to obtain, it is estimated that for every completed youth suicide, as many as 200 attempts are made. Ingestion of medication is the most common method of attempted suicide. Attempts are more common in girls than boys (approximately 3:1), and in Hispanic girls and gay, lesbian, and bisexual youths. Attempters who have made prior suicide attempts, who used a method other than ingestion, and who still want to die are at increased risk of completed suicide.

On the basis of the 2007 Youth Risk Behavior Survey, 14.5% of students in grades 9 through 12 reported that they had seriously considered attempting suicide in the 12 months preceding the survey (18.7% of females and 10.3% of males). Nearly 7% of students reported that they had actually attempted suicide one or more times during the same period.

B. **Developmental considerations.** Young children do not know that death is final. Comprehension of the finality of death may fluctuate throughout early childhood and is not fully realized until adolescence. Similarly, intentionality may be difficult to ascertain in pre-adolescents. As such, children who commit self-injurious acts should be considered potentially suicidal even in the absence of clearly stated intent. Young children are more susceptible to accidental suicide through imitation or suggestion.

C. **Risk factors.**

1. Psychiatric disorders.

A prior history of a suicide attempt increased the risk of suicide nearly 90-fold. Approximately 90% of these youths who completed suicide had a psychiatric disorder at the time of death, and more than 70% had multiple disorders. A large proportion of youths with psychiatric disorders at the time of suicide had not sought or been provided with treatment. The most common disorders, found in 60% to 75% of youths who completed suicide, were mood disorders, which together increased the likelihood of committing suicide 8- to 13-fold. Rates of major depressive disorder ranged from 30% to 50% among suicide victims, and the likelihood of committing suicide was increased 27-fold by the presence of a current episode of major depression. Approximately one-fifth of youth suicide victims were diagnosed with bipolar disorder, which increased the likelihood of completed suicide nine-fold.

The second most common group of psychiatric disorders was any substance abuse disorder, which occurred in approximately 30% to 60% of youth suicide victims and increased the likelihood of committing suicide nearly nine-fold. Studies of nonfatal suicidal behavior suggest that rates and types of psychiatric disorders are similar as for suicide victims.

2. Neurobiological factors.

In adults, positive correlations have been found between suicidal behavior and dysregulation of neurotransmitter systems, especially serotonergic systems. While not adequately studied, similar findings related hypothalamic–pituitary–adrenal axis, has been shown to be dysregulated among suicidal youths.

3. Psychosocial stressors.

Youths who report suicidal ideation or attempts experience high rates of cumulative stressors, including family losses, family discord and dysfunction, and parental incapacity. Approximately two-thirds of suicide victims had parents or adult relatives with suicidal acts, emotional problems, absence from the home, or abusive behavior. Physical or sexual abuse is a strong risk factor for youth suicidal behavior, associated with an estimated 12% of suicide attempts—an eight-fold greater risk of completed suicide among adolescents. Other psychosocial stressors related to suicidality include living outside the home, neither working nor attending school, and having difficulties in school. For males, but not females, sexual orientation has been associated with suicidal intent and attempts. Media coverage of an adolescent's suicide may lead to cluster suicides, with the magnitude of additional deaths proportional to the amount, duration, and prominence of the media coverage.

II. Assessing the risk.

Assessment of suicidal ideation should be a regular part of patient visits with youths. When not specifically asked, youth are less likely to disclose depression, suicidal thoughts, or patterns of drug use. Specific questions include the following:

- *"Did you ever feel so sad or upset that you wished you were not alive or wanted to die?"*
- *"Did you ever do something that you knew was so dangerous that you could get hurt or killed by doing it?"*
- *"Did you ever hurt yourself or try to hurt yourself on purpose?"*
- *"Did you ever try to kill yourself?"*

If suicidal ideation or behavior has occurred, a thorough assessment must ensue. Evaluating the presence and degree of suicidality and underlying risk factors is complex. For pediatric clinicians who are less well trained in mental health, this type of clinical assessment is best conducted by a qualified mental health professional. In areas where the resources necessary to make a timely mental health referral are lacking, pediatric clinicians are strongly encouraged to obtain additional training in assessment of suicidality. Older children and adolescents should be evaluated with and without the presence of the primary caregiver; the limits of confidentiality should be explained at the outset (i.e., clinicians must inform caregivers if risk of suicide is present).

For suicidal ideation, the key assessment issues pertain to identifying underlying psychiatric disorders known to be associated with suicidality. For suicidal behavior, the key assessment issues pertain to precipitating, predisposing, perpetuating, and protective factors related to the behavior, including the following:

- Circumstances leading to the act
- Extent of planning for and the intention associated with the act
- Potential lethality of the act and the likelihood of rescue
- Presence of risk factors known to be associated with suicidality
- Presence of protective factors, including the absence of a firearm and other means of suicide in the hone; a close relationship with a responsible and empathic caregiver who can supervise the youth and ensure adherence to recommended follow-up care; the absence of an altered mental status; and a problem-solving coping style.

Suicide attempters at highest risk for completed suicide are those that are:

- Male
- Have made a prior suicide attempt
- Have current suicidal ideation, intent, or plan
- Have a current mental status altered by depression, mania, anxiety, intoxication, psychosis, hopelessness, rage, humiliation, or impulsivity
- Lack supportive family members who can provide supervision, safeguard the home, and ensure adherence to treatment recommendations.

III. **Management.**

Because suicidal behavior is an episodic phenomenon that cannot be foreseen or prevented, management is based upon the magnitude of risk associated with the current situation. Youths who are at moderate to high risk of completed suicide should immediately be assessed by a qualified mental health professional. Options for assessment include mental health consultation during pediatric hospitalization, transfer to an emergency department for mental health assessment, or an outpatient assessment appointment on the same day with a mental health professional. Most youths who are examined in emergency departments and referred to outpatient mental health facilities fail to keep their appointments. Pediatric clinicians can enhance continuity of care by maintaining contact with the suicidal youth even after referrals are made. Youths judged to be at low risk of suicide should nonetheless receive referral for a mental health assessment to rule out underlying untreated psychiatric disorders.

Interventions should be tailored to the youth's needs. Some youths with a responsive and intact family, good peer relationships and social support, hope for the future, and a desire to solve problems may require only brief crisis-oriented intervention. In contrast, youths deemed to be at moderate to high risk for completed suicide might require psychiatric hospitalization and long-term psychiatric treatment.

To date, there are no empirically supported individual psychotherapies for youths shown to be effective through randomized controlled trials in reducing suicidal behavior. Individual dialectical behavioral therapy, family therapy, group therapy, and brief adjunctive psychosocial interventions have been tested in suicidal adolescents and all have shown some promise, but none have been definitively efficacious.

IV. **Prevention.**

One of the most important suicide prevention strategies is the early identification and treatment of psychiatric disorders known to be associated with increased risk for suicidality. Pediatric clinicians can play a key role in this strategy by systematically inquiring about symptoms of psychiatric disorders, especially depression, mania, and substance use, particularly in their post-pubertal patients. Because treatment of depressed youths with antidepressant medication increases the risk of suicidal thoughts, such youths require close monitoring, particularly in the first weeks following medication initiation.

At present, there is insufficient evidence to either support or refute universal suicide prevention programs, which typically are implemented in school settings. Screening for suicidality is fraught with problems related to low specificity of the screening instrument, poor acceptability among school administrators, and paucity of referral sites. "Gatekeeper" (e.g., student support personnel) training is effective in improving skills among school personnel and is highly acceptable to administrators, but has not been shown to prevent suicide.

BIBLIOGRAPHY

American Academy of Child and Adolescent Psychiatry. Practice parameter for the assessment and treatment of children and adolescents with suicidal behavior. *J Am Acad Child Adolesc Psychiatry* 40(Suppl):24S–51S, 2001.

Kuchar PS, DiGuiseept C. Screening for suicide risk. In: *Guide to Clinical Preventive Services, Second Edition: Mental Disorders and Substance Abuse.* U.S. Preventive Services Task Force, 2003. Available at http://cpmcnet.columbia.edu/texts/gcps.gcps0060m. Accessed February 28, 2009.

National Institute of Mental Health. *Suicide in the U.S.: Statistics and Prevention.* Available from http://www.nimh.nih.gov/health/publications/suicide-in-the-us-statistics-and-prevention/index.shtml. Accessed February 28, 2009.

Shain BN, Committee on Adolescence. Suicide and suicide attempts in adolescents. *Pediatrics* 120(3):669–676, 2007.

80

Temper Tantrums

Robert Needlman

I. Description of the problem. Behaviors comprising temper tantrums include crying, yelling, stamping, stiffening, attacking self and others, throwing things, dropping to the floor, and running away. Tantrums typically begin with anger (e.g., yelling or hitting) and then progress to distress or sadness (e.g., crying and attempts to gain proximity to the parent). Most tantrums last less than five minutes; the briefest ones tend to begin with stamping or dropping to the ground. Typical tantrums are normative; those predicting disruptive disorders are longer, more frequent, more violent, and persist past age four.

A. Epidemiology.
- 50% to 80% of 2- to 3-year-old children have tantrums at least weekly.
- 20% have at least daily tantrums.
- 60% of 2-year-olds with frequent tantrums will continue to have them at 3 years. Of these, 60% will continue at 4 years.
- The prevalence of explosive "tempers" remains approximately 5% throughout childhood.
- Severe tantrums are often accompanied by other significant behavioral problems, such as disturbed sleep or overactivity.
- Tantrum frequency is variably related to gender or social class; severe tantrums are more common in low-SES boys.

B. Etiology/contributing factors.
1. **Normal development.** Tantrums reflect frustration when normal drives for autonomy conflict with parental prohibitions and limited competence, especially under stress (e.g., hunger, tiredness), in the presence of limited emotional self-regulation (e.g., through self-directed speech).
2. **Medical problems.** Consider (among others) recurrent URIs or otitis; respiratory or GI allergies; eczema; endocrine disorders (particularly androgen excess); obstructive sleep apnea and other sleep disturbance; hospitalization or invasive medical procedures; certain medications (e.g., most anticonvulsants, many antihistamines).
3. **Disabilities.** Consider autism spectrum disorders; cognitive disability; attention deficit hyperactivity disorder; traumatic brain injury (especially frontal lobe); unrecognized deafness or visual impairment.
4. **Temperament.** Predisposing traits include high intensity and activity; persistence; predominantly negative mood; low sensory threshold; and high sensitivity to novel stimuli. Irregular timing of sleep and hunger make it difficult for parents to anticipate the child's needs.
5. **Environment.** Physical factors include overcrowding; limited access to outdoor play; and nonchildproofed homes that make frequent parental prohibitions necessary. Social factors include martial stress and verbal or physical violence; tensions arising from siblings or grandparents with behavioral problems or medical illness; parental depression, and alcohol and/or drug abuse.
6. **Parenting.** Tantrums may be reinforced either by parental compliance or, paradoxically, by the intense negative attention they elicit. Contributing factors include corporal punishment or abuse; inconsistent limit setting; over-permissiveness; intrusiveness; failure to recognize stressors (e.g., frightening movies or even the TV news); and unrealistic expectations for self-control or delay of gratification, particularly in children who look older and older children with cognitive delay.
7. **Interacting factors.** Tantrum persistence is predicted by either (a) high tendency to frustration plus high parental intrusiveness; or (b) low emotional self-regulation plus low parental control.

C. Recognizing the issue.
1. **Signs and symptoms.** Concerning features include the following:
   a. A high degree of parental concern, anger, guilt, or sadness. Tantrums are a problem if parents think they are.

    b. Parents are unable to identify positive things about the child, seeing the child as antagonistic and controlling. Such complaints may signal a toxic parent–child relationship, often associated with domestic violence and maternal depression.

    c. Aggression (hitting, biting) with self (associated with depression) or others (associated with disruptive disorders).

    d. Children aged less than 12 months or greater than 48. Tantrums, if present, tend to be mild and infrequent in these age ranges.

    e. Tantrums occur more than three times a day and last 15 minutes or longer. Frequent, prolonged tantrums are associated with multiple behavior problems, for example, problems with sleeping, eating, or peer interactions.

    f. Tantrums in school. Children typically "pull it together" in front of peers; tantrums in school may be due to social, academic, or emotional problems.

2. History: key clinical questions.

    a. *"What exactly happened the last time your child had a tantrum? What set it off? What did your child do first? How did you respond? Was that a typical episode?"* Try to get a play-by-play account of a recent episode. Focus on the ABCs: antecedents, behaviors, and consequences. Look for triggers (hunger, tiredness, sources of frustration); unintentional reinforcement (e.g., increased attention); and delayed consequences, such as special treats the parents may offer to atone for their own feelings of anger.

    b. *"What feelings do your child's tantrums bring out in you?"* If parents report extreme anger, shame, or guilt, these feelings need to be addressed.

    c. *"How often do tantrums result in your child's getting what he or she wants?"* Behaviors maintained by intermittent reinforcement (i.e., child gets what he wants or escapes unwanted task) are particularly resistant to extinction.

    d. *"What do other adults in the family say about the tantrums? How do they respond? How do they say you should respond?"* Family dynamics often plays a role in maintaining tantrums. If tantrums occur more frequently with, say, the mother, it may be that she is more ambivalent about limit setting; or the other parent may be subtly undercutting her authority, for example, by acting overly solicitous to the child after a tantrum.

    e. *"Does your child have other behavior problems, such as overactivity, aggressiveness, food refusal, clinginess, or sleep problems?"* A pattern of multiple behavior problems suggests the need for a more comprehensive psychological evaluation. Consider developmental delay as well.

    f. *"When your child is happy, how does she show it? Are all emotions expressed intensely? Does she tend to stick with a challenge until she masters it?"* In the absence of other concerning features, long and loud tantrums in an intense, persistent child may be normal.

    g. *"How was your pregnancy with this child? What about the delivery, newborn period, first year of life, etc? Any significant illnesses or injury?"* A special pregnancy (e.g., unplanned, or long-awaited) may fuel parental guilt and poor limit-setting. A past life-threatening event and continued perceived vulnerability suggests vulnerable child syndrome (see Chapter 107).

3. Office evaluation.

    a. Physical examination. Look for signs of allergies, recurrent otitis, dental caries (a source of pain), scars suggestive of abuse, evidence of endocrinopathy (e.g., genital enlargement, striae).

    b. Observations. Crayons and paper may elicit themes of anger or threat (e.g., a burning house, a shark that eats everything up), indicating that the child understands that gaining some control over such feelings is the purpose of the visit. Provision of a few age-appropriate toys allows observation of the child's play skills, an indication of cognitive development, and the child's response to the request to clean up.

    c. Written data and tests. A tantrum log, listing the antecedents, behaviors, and consequences of each tantrum, as well as the times of onset and resolution, can help you identify patterns and document improvement with therapy. A standardized parent-report instrument (e.g., the Pediatric Symptom Checklist) can detect relevant patterns of behavior and may suggest the presence of more significant problems.

D. Management.

1. Primary goals.

    a. Clarify the diagnosis. Differentiate between tantrums due to developmentally appropriate stresses or challenges of temperament (parents' and/or child's), and tantrums due to underlying delays, disorders, or familial dysfunction.

     b. Address contributing factors. For example, refer for speech and language therapy; adjust medications for asthma or allergies; advocate for improved housing; refer parents for marital counseling or treatment of depression.

     c. Educate parents. Reduce parental distress by correcting unrealistic expectations and fears, and explaining the developmental forces driving the tantrums; help parents to problem solve (e.g., providing a small snack before going to the grocery store).

2. **Specific strategies.** Tantrums respond well to parent counseling/training individually and in groups.

     a. Child-proof the home. Reducing hazards and temptations minimizes how often the child must hear "no;" nonetheless, there will be plenty of opportunities for the child to learn to accept limits.

     b. Allow limited choices. Children comply better when they feel in control. For a young child, it is best to offer two alternatives, both acceptable (e.g., red shirt or blue shirt.) Small children need to make small choices.

     c. Provide routines. Predictability increases a small child's sense of control, reducing frustrations; for example, before going to the store, make a list of what you will buy.

     d. Adjust to temperament. A very active child needs space to run around; a slow-to-warm-up child needs time to adjust to new situations and people; a highly persistent child may need five- and one-minute warnings to prepare to end a pleasurable activity.

     e. Pick battles and win them. Parents often say "no" when they really mean, "I'd rather you didn't." If the issue really isn't worth a fight, the parents are apt to reverse themselves in the face of a tantrum. For such issues, it's better for parents to state their preference ("I'd rather you didn't have a cookie right now"), offer alternatives ("How about a carrot stick?), or simply say "yes" right off the bat. When parents do say "no," they should mean it and stick to their guns. "No" needs to be absolute and nonnegotiable.

     f. Ignore when possible. Specific instructions for ignoring may include, "Stand five feet away. Keep doing whatever you were doing. Do not speak to your child, or speak in a neutral tone of voice." When ignoring is first instituted, tantrums may get worse for several days. With young children, parents may need to stay in the same room so the child does not become scared, in addition to being upset.

     g. Prevent harm. The parent may have to move the child to a rug or away from hard furniture. A child intent on hurting himself or anyone else needs to be stopped, even if that means physical restraint. Parents should not allow a child to hit, pinch, or bite them.

     h. Use helpful language. How parents talk about a child's tantrums matters. Tantrums are about "losing control" rather than "being bad." It is not helpful to dwell in detail on tantrums past, but it may help to remind a child to, "Tell me when you're mad; use your words." Parents can make up stories about children who are furious but triumph by controlling themselves, or stories about how they (the parents) have needed to take three deep breaths to avoid "losing it."

     i. Celebrate successes. Parents need to pay attention whenever their child uses words to express frustration or to protest a perceived injustice. A warm "good job!" and a hug powerfully reinforce the child's accomplishment.

3. **Criteria for referral.** The following features should suggest referral for sub-specialist care for tantrums.

     a. Developmental disability. Severe tantrums arising in the context of cognitive disability, autism spectrum disorders, deafness, or other developmental disabilities may benefit from intensive behavioral approaches.

     b. Emotional disturbance. Consider among others: parental depression or other mental illness; traumatic separations or recurrent hospitalizations; presence of a sibling with special healthcare needs; domestic violence; associated internalizing or externalizing behaviors.

     c. Failure to improve. In the absence of anymore specific indications, failure for tantrums to show improvement after two or three visits may trigger referral for more extensive evaluation and protracted management.

BIBLIOGRAPHY

For parents

Ginott H. *Between Parent and Child.* New York: Macmillan, 1965. (Still one of the best guides for talking with children, giving clear messages and effective feedback.)

Lieberman A. *The Emotional Life of the Toddler*. New York: Free Press, 1993. (A remarkably clear, insightful, readable explanation of toddlers and their feelings.)

Turecki S, Tonner L. *The Difficult Child*. New York: Bantam Doubleday, 1989. (Practical and sensitive advice, with an emphasis on temperament as a major determinant of children's behavior.)

Web sites

KidsHealth http://kidshealth.org/parent/emotions/behavior/tantrums.html (Conversational, solid information.) Accessed June 2, 2010.

Iowa State University Extension—www.extension.iastate.edu/publications/PM1529J.pdf (Clear, low literacy, includes a helpful worksheet.) Accessed June 2, 2010.

For professionals

Belden AC, Thomson NR, Luby JL. Temper tantrums in healthy versus depressed and disruptive preschoolers: defining tantrum behaviors associated with clinical problems. *J Pediatr* 152(1):117–122, 2008. (Describes tantrums associated with behavioral disorders.)

Degnan KA, Calkins SD, Keane SP, et al. Profiles of disruptive behavior across early childhood: contributions of frustration reactivity, physiological regulation, and maternal behavior. *Child Dev* 79(5):1357–1376, 2008. (A developmental psychopathology analysis explaining tantrums that persist past the toddler years.)

Goodenough F. *Anger in Young Children*. Minneapolis, MD: University of Minnesota Press, 1931. (A classic monograph.)

Needlman R, Stevenson J, Zuckerman B. Psychosocial correlates of severe temper tantrums. *J Dev Behav Pediatr* 12:77–83, 1991. (An analysis of a large, community-based sample.)

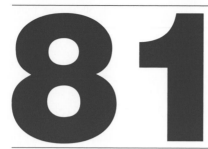

Temperamentally Difficult Children

Stanley Turecki

I. **Description of the problem.** A "difficult child" is a normal young child whose innate temperament makes them hard to raise. Inherent in this definition is a view of normality that is broad: children are different and do not have to be average in order to be normal. For a child to be considered temperamentally difficult, a basic criterion has to be met: the child's constitutionally determined personality traits—their very nature—must cause significant problems in child rearing.

A. **Epidemiology.**
   - About 15% of young children are temperamentally difficult according to this definition.
   - Difficult children are not all alike. Some are impulsive, distractible, and highly active; others are shy and clingy. Some throw loud tantrums; others whine and complain. Some can hit, kick, or even bite; others are verbally defiant. Some are unpredictable in their eating or sleeping habits; others are sensitive to noise, textures, or tastes. Most difficult children have trouble dealing with transition and change, and almost all are strong-willed and extremely stubborn.
   - Highly active, impulsive, difficult children are more likely to be boys. All other temperamentally difficult traits are as likely to be seen in girls as in boys.
   - There is no correlation with birth order, intelligence, or socioeconomic status.

B. **Etiology.**
   - Temperament refers to dimensions of personality that are largely constitutional in origin. Genetic factors definitely contribute. Pregnancy and delivery complications may be somewhat more common in the histories of difficult children. Some of these children are allergic, with a propensity to develop ear infections. Uneven language and development of learning skills are not uncommon. Many difficult children are intelligent but socially immature. All of these factors suggest a biologic basis for a difficult temperament.

C. **The concept of temperament.** Temperament is the *how* of behavior, rather than the *why* (motivation) or the *what* (ability). For example, three equally motivated and able children may approach a homework assignment quite differently, depending on their behavioral style. One will begin on time and work steadily to completion, the second will delay and procrastinate but then work very persistently, and the third will jump in immediately and quickly lose patience. Inherent in the temperamental perspective is a broad view of normality and a bias toward seeing atypical behavior as different rather than abnormal.

Temperament may also be defined as the behavioral expression, evident early in life, of those dimensions of personality that are constitutional in origin. Family, twin and adoption studies point to a 50% multigenetic heritability. The stability of temperament is detectable at 18 months, substantial at 3 years, and most evident in middle childhood. As development proceeds, temperamental qualities are neither rigidly fixed nor completely malleable—like cartilage rather than bone or muscle. A range exists for each category. Table 81-1 lists the categories of temperament.

1. **The child and the environment: A transactional model.** The concept of a difficult temperament should always be combined with that of ***goodness of fit***—the match or compatibility between a child and their environment. Behavior that presents a problem to one family may be readily accepted by another. For example, a child's idiosyncratic and strongly held tastes in clothing and food would only trouble a fashion- and nutrition-conscious parent. The context of the behavior is always important. A highly active boy who has some problems with self-control and concentration, if placed in a class of 25 children (of whom another 5 are "challenging") with one somewhat inexperienced teacher, would undoubtedly meet all the criteria for attention deficit hyperactivity disorder (ADHD). However, if the following year he is in a class of 15 children with a high ratio of girls to boys and the teacher has an assistant, the child would still be a handful but a clinical diagnosis of disorder would be inappropriate.

2. Difficult children are, above all, **hard to understand.** Their behavior confuses and upsets the most experienced parent or teacher. The tried-and-true methods of child

Table 81-1. Categories of temperament

Trait	Description	Easy	Difficult
Activity level	General statement about level of motor activity; actual amount of physical motion during play, eating, sleep etc.	Low to moderate	Very active, restless, fidgety; always into things; makes you tired; "ran before they walked"; easily overstimulated; gets wild or "revved up"; impulsive, loses control, can be aggressive, hates to be confined
Self-control	Ability to delay action or demands	Good, patient	Poor, impulsive
Concentration	Ability to maintain focus in the face of distractions	Good, stays with task	Poor, distractible, has trouble concentrating and paying attention especially if not really interested; doesn't listen, tunes you out; daydreams, forgets instructions
Intensity	Energy level of responses; how forcefully or loudly reactions are expressed, whether positive or negative	Low, mild, low-keyed	High, loud, forceful whether miserable, angry, or happy
Regularity	Predictability of physical functions such as appetite, sleep–wake cycle, and elimination	Regular, predictable	Irregular, erratic, can't tell when they'll be hungry or tired; has conflicts over meals and bedtime; wakes up at night; moods are changeable; has good or bad days for no obvious reason
Persistence	Single-mindedness, "stick-to-itiveness"; may be positive (focused when involved) or negative (stubborn and doesn't give up	Low, easily diverted	High, stubborn, won't give up, goes on and on nagging, whining, or negotiating if wants something; gets "locked in"; has long tantrums
Sensory threshold	Sensitivity to physical stimuli—sound, light, smell, taste, touch, pain, temperature	High, unbothered	Low, physically sensitive, "sensitive"—physically not emotionally; highly aware of color, light, appearance, texture, sound, smell, taste or temperature; "creative" but with strong and unusual preferences that can be embarrassing; clothes have to feel and look right; picky eater; refuses to dress warmly when weather is cold
Initial response	Characteristic initial reaction to new persons or new situations	Approach, goes forward	Withdrawal, holds back, doesn't like new situations; may tantrum if forced to go forward
Adaptability	Tolerance of change; ease with which gets used to new or altered situations	Good, flexible	Poor, rigid, has trouble with change of activity or routine; inflexible, very particular, notices minor changes; can want the same food or clothes over and over
Predominant mood	General quality of mood; basic disposition	Positive, cheerful	Negative, serious, or cranky; doesn't show pleasure openly; not a "sunny" disposition

381

rearing simply do not work, so that effective discipline is replaced by inconsistency, power struggles, excessive punishment, or overindulgence. Parents will say that "nothing works" or that the child controls the family. A vicious cycle develops wherein the child's trying behavior and the erratic overreactions of the parent augment each other.

The primary caregiver of such a difficult child (usually the mother) may also be bewildered, overinvolved, and exhausted. She may feel guilty, inadequate, and victimized. Often such children are somewhat easier with their fathers, who may become increasingly critical of the mothers. Marital strain is common. A fragile but potentially viable marriage may be ruptured by the stress of a difficult child. In addition, individual vulnerabilities of adult personality may be accentuated, resulting in parental syndromes of anxiety, depression, or substance abuse. The siblings are often expected to behave in an excessively adult manner and their needs can be neglected as the household increasingly revolves around the difficult child. The child is also affected by the vicious cycle. Behavior problems are accentuated and secondary manifestations, such as fears and feelings of being "bad" are quite often evident.

II. **Making the diagnosis.** A pathology-oriented model is limiting and often counterproductive. There is no "difficult child syndrome," just as there is not a definitive "test for ADHD." Much more valid in dealing with problem behaviors in young children is a **model that focuses on individual differences and goodness of fit.** The aim is to describe the child's behavior, temperamental profile, and strengths, as well as areas of vulnerability.

  A. **History.** Questioning the parent about the manifestations of a child's difficult temperament and its impact on the family is the key to identification. The clinician should inquire about the parents' approach to discipline, the child's school functioning, and the presence of secondary manifestations, such as fearfulness, nightmares, excessive anger, and emotional oversensitivity. Impaired self-image is seen in poorly managed difficult children.

  B. **Temperamental questionnaire.** These may be used as part of well-child examinations or to determine areas of difficulty with a view to temperament-based parent guidance. Research-based questionnaires tend to be lengthy with 75 to 100 parent responses. It is often acceptable for a busy primary care clinician to devise their own brief questionnaire, provided it is used as an aid in conjunction with other information and not as a "diagnostic instrument."

  C. **Behavioral observations.** Some problem behaviors are readily apparent in the office visit: impulsivity, hyperactivity, disruptiveness, clinging and withdrawal, tantrums, aggressiveness, or undue sensitivity to pain. However, a child may be stubborn, irregular, negative and cranky, intense, sensitive to light and taste, or poorly adaptable. When a parent reports such "nonvisible" difficult behavior that is not apparent during the office visit, the clinician should not assume that the parent is inventing or causing the problem.

  D. **Differential diagnosis.** A difficult temperament is evident from an early age and is relatively stable and consistent over time. A child, 3 years or older, whose behavior has become difficult may be going through a developmental stage or reacting to stress. An example is a youngster who begins to misbehave after parents separate. When does the clinical picture go beyond a very difficult temperament and become indicative of a psychiatric disorder? The distinction is not only problematic but it is actually often irrelevant to treatment decisions. A "brain disorder," such as ADHD, is essentially a behavioral syndrome based on descriptive criteria subject to some extent of observer bias. There is no "test" for ADHD. While it is now generally accepted that ADHD is neurobiologically based, the same can be said for temperament. Adopting a continuum-based, rather than a categorical approach to diagnosis allows a clinician much greater flexibility.

III. **Management: The role of the pediatric clinician—helping the child and family.** The difficult child's adjustment can be greatly enhanced by the ongoing involvement of the primary care clinician. The central therapeutic goals are to improve the compatibility between a child and the significant persons in their life, relieve the child's suffering, and improve adaptation.

  A. **General issues.**
    1. **Erroneous perceptions can be corrected.** The parents of very difficult children invariably feel victimized and often assume that the child's behavior is intentional. Parents need to understand that their children are not enemies who are "out to get them." Seeing the problem behavior as temperamentally determined rather than willful disobedience allows the parent to deal with it far more neutrally. Many parents are confused and made anxious by pressures to have their child "diagnosed" and placed on medication.
    2. **The caregivers need support and understanding.** Especially so when the child's behavior is very difficult at home but unremarkable at school or in the clinician's office.

3. **Practical advice can be offered.** Parents can be guided on issues such as school selection and communication with teachers. The parents may need guidance on how to share responsibility more evenly, how to deal with other family members, and how to respond to the often plentiful advice offered from several quarters that tends to make parents (particularly single parents) feel defensive and inadequate.

B. **Principles of adult authority.** The fundamental goal for the parents of a difficult child is to replace the power struggles, frustration, and wear-and-tear of an ineffective disciplinary system with an educated, rational, kind, accepting, yet firm attitude of adult authority. Inevitably, habitual patterns of negative interaction have developed. It is the parents' job to initiate the necessary changes to improve the fit between their child-rearing style and expectations and their child's temperament. In order to begin the process, a key shift in attitude is needed. It should be clear to everyone that the parents are in charge. Certainly the child's opinion should be solicited when appropriate, but the ultimate decision lies with the parents. The model is that of the excellent supervisor at work: approachable, supportive, clear in expectations, and very much in charge. Key ingredients of this model are:

1. **Strategic planning and planned discussions.** The automatic, often excessively punitive reactions to the child's behavior must be replaced with a system that emphasizes structure and predictability. Decisions about rules, new procedures or routines, and consequences should be made privately by the adults and then presented to the child. Such a planned discussion always takes place away from the heat of the moment. The child is calmly, clearly, and deliberately told what will be expected from now on. Both parents, if possible, should be present at such a meeting. The attitude is kind but serious. The parents should be concise and avoid moralizing, lest they lose the child's attention. The child should be viewed to some extent as a junior collaborator in the planning to improve the family atmosphere and input elicited. At the end of a planned discussion, the child needs to repeat the key points to make sure they understood them and is then encouraged to "do your best." Asking a young child, at a calm time, to try hard to meet a specific and reasonable expectation is a very powerful statement. Generally planned discussions can be used with children as young as age 3 years.

2. **Active acceptance.** The parent makes the deliberate choice, based on understanding their child and the child's temperament, to accept the youngster for the person they truly are, vulnerabilities as well as strengths. The practical consequence of this conscious decision is that parental expectations become more consistent with the genuine capacities of the child.

3. **Rational punishment.** Going hand in hand with planned discussions is the clear and firm enforcement of consequences for unacceptable behaviors that are within the child's control and important enough to warrant taking a stand. In a typical vicious cycle, a mother may find herself punishing and saying "no" repeatedly, but no parent can possibly be effective in such circumstances. Most difficult children need less punishment, rather than more, and this can be achieved through consistency, structure, and routines in everyday life.

   The important first step for parents is to recognize and address major unacceptable behaviors and ignore the myriad minor irritations that take place every day with a very difficult child. Whenever possible, punishment should contain a natural consequence. For example, a child who continues to act too roughly with the family pet should be prohibited contact for a day, rather than being given a time-out. Ideally, a punishment should be administered briefly and without anger. Its main objective is to show the child that the parents are serious about stopping the behavior. Simplicity and predictability are important; a variety of punishments are unnecessary. With a younger child, parents can show seriousness by facial expression, direct action, and tone of voice.

C. **Management strategies.** Management, as distinct from punishment, is used when the adult decides that the misbehavior is temperamentally based; the child, in effect, "can't help it." The parent's attitude, while still firm, is much more sympathetic and kind. The basic message is, "I understand what's happening. I know you can't really control yourself, and I am going to help you with this." Sometimes behavior falls into a gray area, where it is not clear whether it is deliberate. In such instances, it is best for the parent to make the emotionally generous decision and help rather than punish the child.

   Management suggestions designed to promote the child's success can be geared to particular temperamental characteristics. Strategies should be explained to the youngster during a planned discussion.

1. **The impulsive child.** A child who is easily excited can lose control in an overly stimulating environment and misbehave or become aggressive. The most common mistake parents and teachers make is to wait for the youngster to strike out and then lecture or punish, instead of intervening early.

   If the child is easily excited, it is important to recognize the signs of escalation—for example, moving more rapidly, talking in a louder voice, or laughing excessively. The adult should try to step in before the child gets out of hand. This technique is called **early intervention.** Some youngsters can be distracted. Others need a **time-out** (not as punishment, but as a cool-down period away from the action). A parent can say, "You're getting too excited. Let's do something quiet until you calm down."

2. **The highly active child.** High-energy children can become restless when they are confined to the dinner table or a classroom seat. They may begin to fidget or have difficulty paying attention. This behavior can be managed once the adults in charge **recognize the signs.** A restless youngster can be permitted to leave the dinner table and walk around between courses; a sympathetic teacher could ask the child to run an errand. Building vigorous physical activity into their daily routine is also helpful.

3. **The irregular child.** Most people fall easily into a regular rhythm of sleeping and eating, but some are naturally irregular. Battles can result when parents insist that a child who is not hungry must eat or that a youngster who is not tired must sleep. One strategy is to **differentiate between bedtime and sleep time, mealtime and eating time.** It is reasonable to require a child to be in bed by a certain hour or to join parents and siblings at dinner. However, parents should not force a youngster to sleep when he is not tired or to eat when he is not hungry. To avoid overburdening the family chef, a child with an irregular appetite can be taught to fix simple snacks, such as fruit, cold cereal, or yogurt.

4. **The poorly focused child.** Some children are easily distracted by their environment or even by their own thoughts. As a result, they appear to not "listen" or, if they miss instructions, to be willfully disobedient. Parents and teachers can manage the problem by **making eye contact** in a friendly way before giving such a child directions. Instructions should be kept brief and simple. Set up, with the child, a system of reminders. Begin to teach organizational skills early.

5. **The child who resists change.** Some youngsters have difficulty with transitions. A poorly adaptable or shy child may be distressed by anything new. Other children focus so intently that they are locked into one activity and refuse to move to another. When they are asked to shift gears, they may cling, have a tantrum, or otherwise react negatively. If the issue is poor adaptability, parents can help by **preparing the child for change.** Even a simple warning, such as, "Finish playing with your trains, because we have to go shopping in 10 minutes," can be effective.

6. **The shy child.** Shy children require time and sympathetic understanding. A parent might say, "I know it's hard for you to get accustomed to new things, so I won't leave until you're used to being here." At the same time encourage a time-limited trial of an activity the youngster has previously shown he enjoys.

7. **The stubborn child.** Persistent, stubborn children can be extremely frustrating for parents and teachers. With these children, adults can take a stand early and terminate the confrontation. This technique is called **bringing it to an end.** A parent should not try to reason with a stubborn expert negotiator. Instead, the discussion should be ended. However, it is common for parents of a stubborn child to engage in a constant battle of wills and say "no" all the time. They should be encouraged to say "yes" more often, especially when the issue at hand is not really important.

8. **The finicky child.** Certain children are particular because they have heightened sensitivity to touch, taste, smell, sound, temperature, and colors (not necessarily all of these). Parents may get into arguments because a youngster insists on wearing the same comfortable green corduroy pants day after day or refuses to eat the inexpensive brand of frozen pizza that the rest of the family enjoys. Parents should be advised to **respect a child's preferences** when possible and to seek compromises that avoid unnecessary power struggles.

9. **The cranky child.** Parents can be distressed and angered by a child who is generally negative, somber, or pessimistic. Treats that would delight most children scarcely rate a smile from this youngster. The harder the parent tries (and fails) to make the child happy, the greater the tension becomes. A suggestion for parents is to **accept the child's nature** and not to expect a level of enthusiasm that they cannot give. The parent should not feel guilty; the child's negative mood is not the parent's fault.

D. **The use of medication.** If one aims for the relief of suffering rather than the cure of illness, target symptoms can be greatly reduced by the judicious and often temporary use of psychotropic medications. According to this view, the use of a stimulant would be completely appropriate for the balance of the school year in the child described earlier who was in an unfortunate but unavoidable classroom situation. A referral to the parent's clinician may be appropriate for the parent who is tense and caught up in the "vicious cycle."

E. **Criteria for referral.** The decision to refer to a mental health professional is often determined by the primary care clinician's interest in behavioral issues, expertise in parent guidance, and time availability. Assuming the presence of all these, a referral would still be needed in the case of an extremely difficult child, when the vicious cycle of ineffective discipline is longstanding, or when a clinical syndrome is suspected or can be identified in the child or other family members.

BIBLIOGRAPHY

For parents

Books

Brazelton T. *Touchpoints: Emotional and Behavioral Development.* Reading, MA: Addison-Wesley, 1992.
Carey WB. *Understanding Your Child's Temperament.* New York: MacMillan, 1997.
Chess S, Thomas A. *Know Your Child.* New York: Basic Books, 1987.
Turecki S. *The Difficult Child.* New York: Bantam, 1989.

Web sites

NYU Child Study Center. http://www.aboutourkids.org/articles/parenting_styleschildren039s_temperaments_match

For professionals

Carey WB, McDevitt S. *Coping with Children's Temperament.* New York: Basic Books, 1995.
Chess S, Thomas A. *Temperament in Clinical Practice.* New York: The Guilford Press, 1986.
Kagan J. *The Nature of the Child.* New York: Basic Books, 1984.
Najmi S, Bureau JF, Chen D, et al. Maternal attitudinal inflexibility: longitudinal relations with mother-infant disrupted interaction and childhood hostile-aggressive behavior problems. *Child Abuse Negl* 33(12):924–932, 2009.
Thomas A, Chess S. *Temperament and Development.* New York: Brunner-Mazel, 1977.
Turecki S. *The Emotional Problems of Normal Children.* New York: Bantam, 1994.

82

Thumb Sucking

Stephanie Blenner

I. **Description of the problem.** Most infants engage in nonnutritive sucking. They may use fingers, toes, a pacifier, or other object as a means of self-soothing. In some children, this behavior persists into early or middle childhood.

A. **Epidemiology.**
- Seen in the fetus on ultrasound as early as 16 to 18 weeks.
- Infants commonly suck their fingers or toes.
- Thirty percent to forty-five percent of preschool children and 5% to 15% of children over age 5 continue to engage in thumb sucking.
- Thirty percent to fifty-five percent of children who suck their thumb or fingers also use an attachment object, blanket, or twirl or caress their own hair when thumb sucking.

B. **Etiology.** Historically, psychoanalysts conceptualized thumb sucking as an expression of infantile drives and felt it could reflect emotional disturbance if it persisted beyond infancy. Some believe thumb sucking is a learned habit. Most view thumb sucking as a means of self-comforting. It may help relieve stress and calm a child in the face of environmental challenges. Thumb sucking is often seen when a child is falling asleep, tired, bored, hungry, or anxious. It is not associated with emotional disturbance in most cases.

C. **Negative sequelae.**
1. **Dental.** The most common consequences of thumb sucking are dental, in particular, malocclusion of both primary and permanent dentition. It may also lead to temporomandibular problems, anterior overbite, posterior cross bite, atypical root resorption, mucosal trauma, narrowing of the maxillary arch, and abnormal facial growth. The risk is highest among children who suck continuously and persist beyond age 4.
2. **Digit abnormalities.** With chronic thumb sucking, a digital hyperextension deformity can occur that may require surgical correction. Callous formation, paronychia, irritant eczema, and herpetic whitlow are also seen.
3. **Psychological effects.** Thumb sucking can contribute to impaired parental and peer relationships. It is often viewed as immature and socially undesirable. Parents and peers may criticize, tease, or punish the child for engaging in thumb sucking. These reactions may, in turn, adversely affect a child's self-esteem.
4. **Accidental poisoning.** Children who thumb suck are at increased risk of accidental poisoning (e.g., lead poisoning).

II. **Making the diagnosis.** Thumb sucking becomes a problem at any age when it interferes with normal developmental achievements, physical health, social interactions, or self-esteem.
- **Physical examination.** Examination may reveal a wrinkled, red digit with or without callous formation. Oral examination should be performed looking for malocclusion or other dental complications.

III. **Management.**
A. **Primary goals.** The goals of treating thumb sucking are to prevent dental complications and potential adverse effects on the child's social interactions and self-esteem. In general, targeted intervention is not necessary until after age 4, when adverse sequelae become more common. Most children will spontaneously stop thumb sucking as they develop other self-regulatory strategies.

B. **Treatment strategies.**
1. **Identify triggers and reinforcers.** Emotional and situational triggers should be identified. Thumb sucking often occurs at particular times of day, during certain activities, or accompanying specific emotional states. Some children only thumb suck while twirling their hair or holding a blanket. As a child gets older, thumb sucking may provide secondary gain through attention paid to the behavior. Intervention should not be considered during a time of unusual stress for the child. For example, it would not be ideal to begin an intervention program at the start of school or during a family move.

2. **Empower the child.** For successful treatment, the child must be actively involved, cooperative, and motivated to stop. Parents should be counseled not to use threats or punishment as these may increase resistance, paradoxically prolonging the behavior. Parents should remain patient and provide support without criticism. They need to realize it is the child's, not their, task to overcome the habit.

3. **Interventions.**

   a. **Prior to age 4 years.** Thumb sucking is normal if it does not interfere with social or developmental functioning. The behavior should be ignored and given no special attention lest it accrue secondary gain. When thumb sucking is noted, the child should be distracted without mentioning the behavior. The child should be praised when not sucking their thumb.

   b. **After age 4 years.** Infrequent thumb sucking is still not usually a significant issue. If thumb sucking is persistent and problematic, however, several behavior modification and habit reversal techniques can be used:

      (1) **Gentle reminders** such as a chart or calendar the child uses to keep track of progress.

      (2) **Rewards** such as stickers, treats, extra story time, or special outings with parents for specified periods without thumb sucking.

      (3) **Praise,** given when the child is not thumb sucking.

      (4) **Modifying associations** by changing the bedtime routine for a child who sucks while falling asleep or encouraging giving up attachment objects, such as a blanket used while sucking.

      (5) **Replacing** thumb sucking with a socially acceptable habit that occupies the thumb, such as squeezing a foam ball or holding the thumb with the other hand.

      (6) **A bitter tasting, nontoxic liquid** (available over the counter) is consistently applied to the thumb, morning, night, and each time the child is known to thumb suck. If after 1 week, the child does not thumb suck, the morning application is discontinued. After another week passes with no thumb sucking, the nighttime application is stopped. Should thumb sucking recur, the full application schedule is resumed. This approach is useful with children who want to stop but put their thumb in their mouth without thinking. It should be emphasized the liquid is a reminder to help the child stop, not a punishment.

      (7) If thumb sucking occurs at night, **thumb splints, gloves, or socks** can be tried. Thumb splints specifically designed for children who thumb suck are available for purchase (see below). An elastic bandage can also be wrapped around a straightened elbow. When the child raises hand to mouth, gentle pressure is exerted reminding the child not to thumb suck. The child should be responsible for putting on the splint or bandage at bedtime and should not be reminded.

      (8) **Referral to a pediatric dentist** for placement of an intraoral device may be considered with an older motivated child who has been unsuccessful using other measures and is developing malocclusion as a consequence of thumb sucking. A palatal bar or crib interferes with placement of the thumb in the palatal vault and often can be removed once the habit has extinguished.

IV. **Clinical pearls and pitfalls.**
   * Do not worry about thumb sucking until a child is over age 4 years.
   * Keep the child actively involved in management and treatment choice.
   * Ensure the solution is not worse than the problem and doesn't become the focus of parent–child interactions.

BIBLIOGRAPHY

For clinicians

Davidson L. Thumb and finger sucking. *Pediatrics in Review* 29:207–208, 2008.

For parents

Mayer CA. *My Thumb and I: A Proven Approach to Stop a Thumb or Finger Sucking Habit, For Ages 6–10.* Chicago: Chicago Spectrum Press, 1997.
Van Norman RM. *Helping the Thumb-Sucking Child: A Practical Guide for Parents.* Vonore, TN: Avery Publishing Group, 1999.

For children

Ages 4 to 8

Dionne W. *Little Thumb.* Grenta, LA: Pelican Pub Co, 2001.

Heitler S. *David Decides About Thumbsucking.* Denver, CO: Reading Matters, 1996.

Sonnenschein H. *Harold's Hideaway Thumb.* New York: Simon & Schuster Books for Young Readers, 1991.

Wulfing Van Ness A. *Thumbuddy to Love: Fireman Fred.* (or *Ballerina Sue* version for girls), Denver, CO: LLC, 2008.

Ages 6 to 10

Mayer CA. *My Thumb and I: A Proven Approach to Stop a Thumb or Finger Sucking Habit, For Ages 6–10.* Chicago: Chicago Spectrum Press, 1997.

83

Tic Disorders and Tourette Syndrome

Adrian Sandler

I. Description of the problem.
A. Definitional issues.
1. Tourette syndrome (TS).
   - TS is a disorder with multiple motor tics and one or more vocal tics (not necessarily concurrently), lasting a period of at least 1 year, in which the individual is never tic-free more than three consecutive months.
   - The tics may change in nature and severity, and are associated with distress or impairment in function.
   - Onset is before age 18 years, with peak onset around 5 to 8 years.
   - Although there is wide variability in symptoms and clinical course, there is a tendency for severity to peak around 9 to 11years, with improvement or even resolution during puberty.
2. The tic disorder spectrum.
   - *Transient tic disorders* include single or multiple motor and/or vocal tics, lasting at least 4 weeks up to 12 months.
   - Most transient tics are simple rather than complex and they do not usually cause great distress. A child with complex and distressing motor and vocal tics lasting a few months may be at risk for developing TS.
   - *Chronic tic disorders* are single or multiple motor *or* vocal tics that last more than a year. It is thought that these disorders share the same pathogenesis and occur on a spectrum.

B. Epidemiology.
1. Prevalence of tic disorder spectrum.
   - Simple tics are very common in childhood. The 3-month prevalence is 4.3% in boys and 2.7% in girls, and 6% to 13% of all children will experience a transient tic at some time during childhood.
   - The childhood incidence of chronic tic disorder is around 1% to 2%, with approximately 3:1 ratio of boys to girls.
   - TS is less common, with prevalence around 3 per 1,000 in 6- to 17-year-olds, based on the 2007 NSCH (National Survey of Children's Health) survey. TS was twice as likely for teenagers than for preteens, and the ratio of boys to girls was 3:1.
   - White children were twice as likely as black and Hispanic children to have TS, but there were no differences by parental education or household income.
2. Comorbidity of TS with obsessive-compulsive disorder (OCD) and attention-deficit/hyperactivity disorder (ADHD).
   - More than 50% of children with TS have extensive obsessions and/or compulsions, and 40% meet criteria for OCD. More than 20% of all children with tic disorders have OCD. Conversely, 18% of children with OCD also have a concurrent tic disorder.
   - Among all children previously diagnosed with TS, 64% had been diagnosed in the past with ADHD. Fifty percent of all children with tic disorders have ADHD.
   - Children with TS are 3 to 4 times as likely to have ADHD and 11 times as likely to have OCD as children without tic disorders.
   - Among all children with TS, clinical depression (36%), anxiety (40%), developmental problems (28%), and learning difficulties (80%) are common.
   - Sixty percent of children with Asperger syndrome have a tic disorder at some time during childhood.

C. Etiology/contributing factors.
1. The genetics of tic disorders and TS.
   Twin studies show fairly high heritability, but there are clearly nongenetic factors influencing phenotypic expression. Linkage studies and genome-wide association studies have indicated signals on chromosomes 2p21, 17p, 8q, and 11q, but to date no single candidate gene has been identified. Other lines of evidence suggest several vulnerable

genes plus environmental stressors causing increased fetal sensitivity in regions of the developing brain. Similar genetic and nongenetic factors appear to be operating in OCD.

2. The neurobiology of tic disorders and TS.

Specific cortico-striato-thalamo-cortical circuits have been implicated because of their role in initiating and inhibiting psychomotor activity and in harm detection/avoidance. Emotional (limbic), cognitive, and motor circuits function in integrated ways to suppress behaviors triggered by internal and external stimuli. In patients with TS, fast-spiking inhibitory (FSI) interneurons in caudate and putamen are decreased, and inhibitory striatal GABAergic (gamma-aminobutyric acid) networks may be deficient. Cortical disinhibition may be related to hypersensitivity of dopamine D2 striatal receptors.

II. Making the diagnosis.
A. Signs and symptoms.
1. What is a tic?
   - Tics are more easily recognized than precisely defined. They can be described as rapid, coordinated, isolated fragments of normal motor or vocal behaviors. Tics can be easily mimicked and sometimes are confused with normal behavior.
   - Motor tics are typically brief, nonrhythmic, repetitive movements of eyes, face, neck and shoulders, with eye blinking, facial grimacing, and head jerking the most common. Vocal or phonic tics may commonly include repetitive throat clearing, sniffing, grunting, or barking.
   - Tics may be described in terms of location, number, frequency, and duration. They may also be characterized by their intensity, forcefulness, and complexity. Although tics are most commonly *simple* (brief and meaningless), they may be *complex* (longer and more elaborate). A few specific terms have been used to describe particular recognizable kinds of tic, such as palilalia (repeating others), coprolalia (uttering obscenities), and copropraxia (making obscene gestures).
   - Children as young as 6 years describe premonitory sensory urges, a feeling of pressure or a kind of "itch." These distracting urges may contribute to attentional problems. Tics are not entirely involuntary, and may be experienced as intentional surrender to virtually irresistible sensory urges, usually accompanied by a fleeting and incomplete sense of relief.
2. Differential diagnosis: What isn't a tic?
   - Children with allergies often have recurrent throat clearing and sniffing, but tics are more repetitive and less variable.
   - Habits such as hair-twirling, nose-touching, skin-picking lack the repetitive uniformity of tics. Repetitive habits like rocking and thumb sucking are more rhythmic and continuous than tics.
   - Brief epileptic seizures and movement disorders (such as chorea, athetosis, dystonia and myoclonic jerks) are more clearly *abnormal* movement patterns than tics.
   - There is no definitive test for tics, and so there are gray areas between habits and simple tics, and between the compulsions of OCD and complex tics.
3. Evaluation of tic disorders.
   - Evaluation of tic disorders includes detailed medical and developmental history, child interview, and careful neurological examination. It is important to ask the child and family about the time course of tics, relationship to medication use, and possible exacerbating factors. The child's subjective experience of the tics and their social or emotional consequences should be explored. Specific inquiry about recent or previous streptococcal exposures or infections should be made. The history should include screening questions regarding OCD, ADHD, learning problems, anxiety and depression. In addition, the pediatrician should take a family history regarding tic disorders and these associated conditions.
   - **Physical and neurological examination** is important to rule out other movement disorders. Other than tics, children with TS usually have a normal examination. Many children effectively suppress tics during the clinic visit, and the absence of tics does not preclude a diagnosis of tic disorders.
   - **Neurodevelopmental examination** can be helpful in providing opportunities to observe attention deficits and other processing problems. Also, many children begin to have tics when stressed in this way.
   - There are no specific diagnostic tests. Electroencephalogram (EEG) and imaging studies are not routinely indicated. Standardized rating scales and checklists may be very helpful regarding ADHD symptoms and general functional impairment at home and school. Other self-report or clinician-rated measures of tics and

obsessive-compulsive symptoms may be useful both for clinical and research purposes, for example, Yale Global Tic Severity Scale (YGTSS).

B. **Pediatric autoimmune neuropsychiatric disorders associated with group A *Streptococcus* (PANDAS).**

- PANDAS are closely related to Sydenham's chorea of rheumatic fever. Circumstantial evidence suggests antineuronal antibodies are affecting basal ganglia function.
- Some children appear susceptible to abrupt onset of tics, compulsions, emotional lability, and anxiety during or following streptococcal pharyngitis. This condition may be episodic and recurrences are common.
- Children usually, but not always, have clinical evidence of tonsillopharyngitis. Anti-DNAase B titers are very high, but there is no clear relationship between titers and clinical course. If there are clinical indications, including sudden onset of symptoms or known exposure to *Streptococcus*, most clinicians obtain streptococcal culture, antistreptolysin O (ASO) titers, and anti-DNAase B. If there is confirmation of streptococcal infection, treatment with penicillin often leads to improvement in tics and obsessive-compulsive symptoms.
- Antibiotic prophylaxis with penicillin or azithromycin may help to prevent recurrences and exacerbations of neuropsychiatric symptoms.

III. **Management.**

A. **Treatment goals and modalities.**

The goals of management of tic disorders are to **minimize stress, social isolation, and functional impairment.** Education and demystification for the affected child, his/her family, and school personnel help to promote support and tolerance.

1. Behavioral techniques.
   - **Habit reversal** involves training the individual in awareness, relaxation, and establishment of a competing response. A recent NIMH (National Institute of Mental Health)-funded study of **Comprehensive Behavioral Intervention for Tics (CBIT)** demonstrated 53% positive response, with 40% reduction in tics after an eight-session, 10-week, randomized, controlled intervention.
   - **Cognitive behavior therapy** involving repeated exposures and response prevention (ERP) is of benefit in OCD, sometimes enhancing medication response or allowing responders to discontinue medications. Similar techniques may be effective treatments in tic disorders and TS.

2. **Pharmacotherapy** is the cornerstone of treatment of tic disorders, but tics should not be treated too aggressively if they are not causing major functional impairment. The presence, scope, and severity of comorbid diagnoses (ADHD, OCD, depression) should be assessed in planning pharmacotherapy.
   - **Alpha-2 norepinephrine agonists:** Clonidine and guanfacine may be useful first-line medications in tic disorders and TS. These agents tend to decrease hyperactivity, impulsivity, hyperarousal, exaggerated stress responses, and aggression, in addition to decreasing tics. Guanfacine has recently been approved by FDA (Food and Drug Administration) for treatment of ADHD. An adequate trial may be 2 months. Sedation is the major side effect, especially for clonidine.
   - **Stimulant therapy in children with ADHD and tic disorders:** Guanfacine may be helpful in treating ADHD symptoms in children with ADHD and tics, but a combination of stimulant plus alpha agonist may be necessary. In children with tic disorders, a trial of stimulant therapy may increase tics in one-third, have no effect in one-third, and lead to improvement in tics in one-third. The combination of methylphenidate and clonidine in children with TS and ADHD was more effective than either medication alone (Treatment of ADHD in children with Tic Disorder (TACT) study). Children with tic disorders and ADHD who have side effects on stimulants may respond to atomoxetine, which does not affect tic frequency.
   - **Antipsychotics/neuroleptics:** Older dopamine blockers such as haloperidol and pimozide can be very effective in treating severe tic disorders, but long-term use may cause tardive dyskinesia (TD) and other extrapyramidal side effects (EPS). Pimozide may have fewer EPS but can cause QT prolongation. The atypical antipsychotics are associated with a lower risk of TD and EPS. Risperidone, a potent D2 antagonist, has proven effective in short-term clinical trials in children and adults with TS, and pilot data with aripiprazole and other atypical antipsychotics are encouraging.
   - **SSRI antidepressants:** The selective serotonin reuptake inhibitors (SSRI) are of proven effectiveness in the treatment of OCD, and they may also help to decrease compulsions in children with tics and TS. In children with TS, OCD, and ADHD, a combination of SSRI and stimulant may be helpful.

- **Other medications:** Clonazepam, levetiracetam, topiramate, and nicotine have been effective in uncontrolled studies. Vitamin B_6, magnesium and omega-3 fatty acids have been used with anecdotal success.

B. **Clinical pearls and pitfalls.**
- Demystification is critical: Although tics are involuntary, it may be helpful for children to become more aware of their tics and to use behavioral strategies to decrease tic frequency.
- Tics should not be treated too aggressively with medications unless they are causing stress, social rejection, or other functional impairments.
- The presence of tics does not preclude the use of stimulants in children with ADHD.
- Think of PANDAS when there is a sudden emergence or dramatic increase in tic frequency/severity or obsessive-compulsive symptoms.

BIBLIOGRAPHY

For parents

Chansky TE. *Freeing Your Child From Obsessive-Compulsive Disorder. A Powerful, Practical Program for Parents of Children and Adolescents.* New York, NY: Three Rivers, 2001.

Dornbush MP, Pruitt SK. *Teaching the Tiger: A Handbook for Individuals Involved in the Education of Students With Attention Deficit Disorders, Tourette Syndrome or Obsessive-Compulsive Disorder.* Duarte, CA: Hope Press, 1995.

Haerle T. *Children With Tourette Syndrome: A Parent's Guide.* Rockville, MD: Woodbine, 2003.

Web sites/DVD

OC Foundation, www.ocfoundation.org

Tourette Syndrome Assocation, www.tsa-usa.org

Available from TSA: "I have Tourette's, but Tourette's Doesn't Have Me," Emmy award winning HBO documentary DVD.

For professionals

Leckman JF, Cohen DJ (eds). *Tourette's Syndrome—Tics, Obsessions, Compulsions: Developmental Psychopathology and Clinical Care.* New York, NY: Wiley, 1999.

Leckman JF, et al. Course of tic severity in Tourette syndrome: the first two decades. *Pediatrics* 102:14–19, 1998.

Singer HS. Tourette's syndrome: from behaviour to biology. *Lancet Neurol* 4:149–159, 2005.

Swain J, et al. Tourette syndrome and tic disorders: a decade of progress. *J Am Acad Child Adolesc Psychiatry* 46(8):947–968, 2007.

Tourette Syndrome Association. *Diagnosing and Treating Tourette Syndrome*, a comprehensive CD/DVD set.

Tourette Syndrome Study Group. Treatment of ADHD in children with tics: a randomized controlled trial. *Neurology* 58:527–536, 2002.

Woods D, Piacentini J, Chang S, et al. *Managing Tourette Syndrome: A Behavioral Intervention for Children and Adults.* New York, NY: Oxford University Press, 2008.

Woods D, Piacentini J, Walkup J. *Treating Tourette Syndrome and Tic Disorders: A Guide for Practitioners.* New York, NY: Guilford Press, 2007.

84

Toilet Training

Steven Parker
Laura Sices

I. Description of the problem. Toilet training is one of the great developmental challenges of early childhood. After 2 years of glorious indifference to social niceties regarding the process of excretion, in Selma Fraiberg's phrase, "The missionaries arrive . . . bearing culture to the joyful savage." Armed with Dr. Spock rather than the Bible, the adults try to cajole the skeptical child into making a dramatic developmental leap without clear benefits. It is a difficult sales pitch and is best attempted only after the child exhibits developmental readiness to understand and master the complex physiologic and psychological tasks of toilet training (Table 84-1). This "child-centered" approach, described by Brazelton in 1962 is the most commonly used in the United States and almost always effective. However, for situations in which immediate results are needed, the motivated parent can attempt the "toilet training in less than a day" method.

A. Epidemiology.
- In the United States, 26% of children achieve daytime continence by age 24 months, 85% by age 30 months, and 98% by age 36 months.
- Nighttime continence usually occurs within a few months after daytime control is achieved.
- The average time to successful toilet training is 3 months.
- Girls are usually faster than boys in achieving control.
- Differences exist in expectations for timing of toilet training between racial and ethnic groups in the United States; for example, on average, African American parents may expect initiation of toilet training to occur earlier than Caucasian parents. There have been secular trends in the United States toward later initiation of toilet training over time.

II. Management. Suggestions for parents on toilet training strategies are set out in Table 84-2.

A. Information for parents. The issue of toilet training is best discussed as part of anticipatory guidance at the 15- to 18-month visit. A number of key principles should be discussed with the parents:

1. **There is usually no hurry or benefit to early toilet training.** Although the process can be initiated in response to outside pressures (e.g., childcare requirements), there are good reasons to try to wait until the child is developmentally prepared.
2. Like most other developmental challenges of childhood, **it is best to empower the child to take responsibility for achieving continence**. Since control of stool and urine will be achieved sooner or later, the most important outcome of toilet training is a boost in the child's self-esteem at mastering the task. This is a long-term goal that should never be sacrificed to the short-term strategies to achieve continence.
3. **Toilet training is not a contest; it proceeds by fits and starts, with successes and frequent relapses; if the timing is wrong, it can always be postponed.**
4. **The parents should not transmit a sense of disgust toward the stool but treat it as a wonderful gift from the child.**

B. Resistance to toilet training. Some children resist toilet training, even if the parental technique is impeccable. The primary care clinician can make these suggestions to the parents:

1. **Do not fight, punish, shame, or nag under any circumstances.** Be sympathetic and try to understand the resistance from the child's point of view. (Children with difficulty toilet training are more likely to have intense or less adaptable temperament traits than children who toilet train easily).
2. **Discontinue training for a few weeks or months if the child is emphatically negative.**
3. **Continue discussions with the child** about toilet training and emphasize the maturity demonstrated by such behavior.
4. **Encourage the child to imitate parents and siblings** by inviting the child into the bathroom.
5. **Read potty training books or view potty training videos together.**

Table 84-1. Signs of developmental readiness for toilet training

Language skills

Able to follow two-step independent commands (e.g., "Take off your pants and go to the bathroom")

Uses two-word phrases (e.g., "bye-bye poop," "go potty")

Cognitive skills

Imitates actions of caregivers (e.g., sweeps the floor)

Understands cause and effect (i.e., is capable of understanding the reasons for mastering the actions involved in toilet training)

Emotional skills

Desires to please parents/caregivers by complying with their requests

Shows diminishing oppositional behaviors and power struggles

Shows drive for independence and autonomy in self-care activities (e.g., insists on feeding self, tries to take off own clothes)

Evinces pride and possessiveness toward belongings ("*my* car" and eventually "*my* poop")

Motor skills

Can ambulate with ease

Is capable of pulling pants off independently

Can sit still for 5 min without help

Has some control over urinary/anal sphincter (e.g., urinates large amounts sporadically, rather than constant wetting)

Body awareness

Shows awareness of wet or soiled diaper

Manifests signs of urge to void or defecate (e.g., facial expression, goes off into a corner)

Table 84-2. Ten steps to successful toilet training

1. Buy a potty chair, and place it in a conspicuous, convenient place. Tell the child, "This is your potty chair. This is where you will [use child's terms for urination and defecation]." Be sure to stress what a special and wonderful chair it is.
2. Allow the child to get used to the chair by sitting on it, fully clothed, for about 5 min a couple of times a day for about a week. Have the child wear loose-fitting pants such as sweat pants that s/he can pull off easily, quickly, and independently when s/he starts using the potty. Try to choose times that the child is more likely to have a bowel movement (e.g., after meals). Never force the child to sit on it.
3. Encourage the child to watch parents or siblings use the bathroom. Explain, "This is where we go potty." Let the child watch the excreta being flushed down the toilet and wave "bye-bye" to it (skip this if the flushing frightens the child).
4. Have the child sit on the potty with the diapers off. Do not urge or expect results, but if it happens, praise the child. Move the potty chair progressively closer and finally into the bathroom.
5. With the child, throw the stool from the soiled diaper into the potty. Tell the child that this is where the stool and urine should go. Then take the pail and dump the stool down the toilet. Wave "bye-bye poop" with the child.
6. Ask the child during the day, "Do you have to go potty?" to help the child recognize bodily sensations. Observe the child for signs of impending urination or defecation. Say, "Let's take off your pants and go potty." Assist the child in disrobing and going to the potty chair. Sit for as long as the child wants. Praise success, but do not criticize failure ("Oh, you don't want to go. Okay. Maybe next time").
7. Reinforce positive features of potty training to child (e.g., "just like a big boy," "just like Mommy does," "You did it by yourself!"), and praise successes as they occur.
8. Once a semiconsistent pattern of voiding/stooling on the potty is established, ask the child if he or she wants to give up the diaper "like a big boy or girl" during the day. If yes, make a show of throwing them all away in the garbage and wave "bye-bye" to them. Admire the child for putting on training "big boy or girl" pants.
9. Once training is well established, try an over-the-toilet-seat chair.
10. Nighttime continence may take a few months to acquire after daytime dryness is achieved. There is usually no special strategy needed; simply ask your child when they would like to try training pants at night.

6. **Remind the child that this task is their responsibility.** Ultimately, it is theirs, not yours.
7. **Encourage the child to change their own diapers.** Remind the child how "yucky" it feels to walk around with a wet or soiled diaper.
8. **Matter-of-factly ask the child at the first sign of impending defecation if the child wants to use the potty.**
9. **If the child appears afraid of painful stools, add prune juice or fiber to the diet to ensure soft stools.** Postpone potty training until fear of defecation subsides.
10. **Discuss what rewards the child would like in response to successful toilet training.** Try star charts to reinforce successful attempts.
11. **Take the child to settings where other children their age are successfully potty trained.**
12. **If the child is obstinately recalcitrant, is clearly capable of mastering the task, is developmentally and emotionally healthy, is more than age 3 years, and the lack of training is a significant problem for the family,** have a solemn ceremony of throwing away the diapers, announce that the child is an official big boy or girl now, give encouragement to "do your best," and allow maturational urges to overtake autonomy issues.

BIBLIOGRAPHY

For parents

Azrin NF, Foxx RM. *Toilet Training in Less Than a Day*. New York: Pocket Books, 1989.
Gomi T. *Everyone Poops*. San Diego, CA: Kane/Miller Book Publishers, 2001.
Sparrow JD, Brazelton TB. *Toilet Training the Brazelton Way*. Cambridge, MA: Da Capo Press, 2004.

Web sites

Parenting iVillage: http://parenting.ivillage.com/tp/tppotty/0,,9mx1,00.html
WebMD: http://children.webmd.com/tc/toilet-training-topic-overview

For professionals

Blum N, Taubman B, Nemeth N. Why is toilet training occurring at older ages? A study of factors associated with later training. *J Pediatr* 145:107–111, 2004.
Brazelton TB. A child-oriented approach to toilet training. *Pediatrics* 29:121–128, 1962.
Michel RS. Toilet training. *Pediatr Rev* 20:240–245, 1999.
Schonwald A, Sherritt L, Stadtler A, and Bridgemohan C. Factors associated with difficult toilet training. *Pediatrics* 113(6):1753–57, 2004.
Schum TR, Kolb TM, McAuliffe TL, et al. Sequential acquisition of toilet-training skills: a descriptive study of gender and age differences in normal children. *Pediatrics* 109(3):E48, 2002.
Stadtler AC, Gorski PA, Brazelton TB. Toilet training methods, clinical interventions, and recommendations. *Pediatrics* 103(6):1359–1368, 1999.

85

Unpopularity

Melvin D. Levine

I. **Description of the problem.** Chronic rejection by peers condemns a child to a life of isolation, extreme self-doubt, and perpetual anxiety. The unpopular schoolchild is susceptible to daily embarrassment through both passive and active exclusion by classmates. Such a child must endure the inevitable painful refrain, "Sorry, this seat is saved." In many cases, exclusionary comments and actions may be augmented by bullying and verbal abuse. It is regrettably true that many of the most popular children are able to boost their status among peers by being especially creative and demonstrative in their predatory acts against unpopular children. The victim's imposed isolation and constant fear of further humiliation is likely to take its toll on development and behavior.

A. **Contributing factors.** There are multiple pathways that may culminate in a state of unpopularity during the school years. In many instances, more than one factor may predispose a child to peer rejection. The following are among the common predisposing factors:

1. **Intrinsic social cognitive dysfunction,** such as a "learning disability," impairing social awareness, practice, and skill. Social cognitive dysfunction, probably the most common source of unpopularity, may mediate or interact with other factors to yield unpopularity in a child. Table 85-1 contains 18 of the most important subcomponents of social cognitive dysfunction. A clinician assessing a patient's social cognition can make use of such a list to pinpoint a child's troubles in specific subcomponents. This process may ultimately provide a basis for coaching the child in the social domain.

2. **Attention deficits.** Traits such as impulsivity, insatiability, and verbal disinhibition associated with attentional dysfunction engender unpopularity.

3. **Physical unattractiveness.** Children whose physical appearance is somehow displeasing to their peers have been shown to be vulnerable to social isolation.

4. **Poor gross motor skills.** Inferior athletic abilities may potentiate unpopularity.

5. **Language disability.** Children with expressive language problems may not be able to use verbal communication to control relationships and keep pace with the banter and lingo of peers.

6. **Autism spectrum disorders.** Children who show signs of an autism spectrum disorder display varying degrees of social cognitive dysfunction, which commonly incites peer rejection.

7. **Shyness.** Some youngsters who are chronically shy in their temperament and therefore avoid social contact may fail to gain the experience needed in the quest for popularity.

8. **Poor coping skills.** A lack of adaptability and problem-solving skills may cause some children to react to daily stresses and conflicts with maladaptive behaviors, such as aggression. Such behaviors alienate others and promote rejection by classmates.

9. **Eccentricity.** Children who are nonconformists or have unusual interests, speech patterns, tastes, or values may be rejected by their more conventional peers who feel more comfortable with close replicas of themselves and harbor fears of contamination with "weirdness." Thus, a child who loves to learn about spiders or enjoys listening to Handel oratorios may be ostracized by more conventional classmates.

10. **Family patterns.** There exist self-contained families that do not value generalized popularity, or the family unit itself remains isolated, either voluntarily or of necessity (perhaps due to genetic social cognitive dysfunctions).

B. **Secondary phenomena.** The clinical picture of an unpopular child is likely to be complicated by a chain of secondary phenomena, which may include extreme anxiety (or even depression), low self-esteem, and a repertoire of maladaptive defense tactics, such as excessive and inappropriate clowning, extreme controlling behaviors, or outright withdrawal. Often, these children seek relationships with adults or with much younger children because they are unable to form alliances within their own age group. In some cases, school phobic behaviors or somatic symptoms may be encountered. Finally, it is

Table 85-1. Social cognitive dysfunction: the troubled subcomponents

Subcomponent	Description
Weak greeting skills	Trouble initiating a social contact with a peer skillfully
Poor social predicting	Trouble estimating peer reactions before acting/talking
Deficient self-marketing	Trouble projecting an image acceptable to peers
Problematic conflict resolution	Trouble settling social disputes without aggression
Reduced affective matching	Trouble sensing and fitting in with others' moods
Social self-monitoring failure	Trouble knowing when one is in social trouble
Low reciprocity	Trouble sharing and trouble supporting/reinforcing others
Misguided timing/staging	Trouble knowing how to nurture a relationship over time
Poor verbalization of feelings	Trouble using language to communicate true feelings
Inaccurate inference of feelings	Trouble reading others' feelings through language
Failure of code switching	Trouble matching language style to current audience
Lingo dysfluency	Trouble using the parlance of peers credibly
Poorly regulated humor	Trouble using humor effectively for current context/audience
Inappropriate topic choice/maintenance	Trouble knowing what to talk about and for how long
Weak requesting skill	Trouble knowing how to ask for something inoffensively
Poor social memory	Trouble learning from previous social experience
Assertiveness gaps	Trouble exerting right level of influence over group actions
Social discomfort	Trouble feeling relaxed while relating to peers

not unusual for children who experience social difficulties at school to become aggressive, oppositional, and/or excessively demanding and dependent at home.

II. **Making the diagnosis.** Unpopular children merit careful clinical assessment. Their social difficulties may in fact represent the tip of an iceberg with respect to behavioral and developmental health. The causal factors and potential complications of unpopularity need to be sought through direct history taking, direct observations of the child's image and manner of relating, physical and neurodevelopmental examinations, and reports from teachers. Especially difficult cases may necessitate investigation by a multidisciplinary team.

Information can be gathered from several sources to detect the presence of subcomponents of social cognitive dysfunction listed in Table 85-1.

The unpopular child should be interviewed alone to elicit their perspective. Nonthreatening questions may be posed to acquire insight into traumatic social scenarios at school. The most common interpersonal "hot spots" are the bus stop, the school bus, the playground, the bathroom, the gymnasium, and the area around lockers. Children can often recreate vividly the stressful scenes that unfold daily against these backdrops. The patient should be reassured that many other children have such difficulties and that it is safe and important to talk about them with an adult.

III. **Management.** The management of the unpopular child must take into consideration the multiplicity of factors operating to engender peer rejection. Associated neurodevelopmental problems (such as a language disability or an attention deficit) require appropriate treatment. The complications, such as somatic symptoms or depression, also demand targeted intervention. In addition, the child's individual social cognitive dysfunction must be addressed. Some possible management approaches to deal directly with a child's unpopularity are summarized below.

A. **Explain the social skill problems carefully to the child.** These may require multiple sessions; not all affected children can process such information readily.

B. **Have the parent of the child who needs social improvement accompany that child to an activity with other children.** Then, during a calm and private interlude, the parent can discuss the social interactions (especially the *faux pas* and transgressions) that occurred.

C. **Help the child locate one or two companions with whom to relate and begin to build skills.** It can be helpful if such peers share interests and perhaps some traits with the unpopular child.

D. **Inform the classroom teacher or building principal if a child is victimized by peer abuse in school.** It is the school's responsibility to make every effort to contain this activity. A strongly worded note from a primary healthcare provider may be vital in such cases.

E. **Help the rejected child to develop skills, hobbies, or areas of expertise that can enhance self-esteem and be impressive to other children.** The management of such a child should always include the diligent quest for and development of such specialties. Ideally, such pursuits should have the potential for generating collaborative activities with other children.

F. **Never force these children into potentially embarrassing situations before their peers.** For example, an unpopular child with poor gross motor skills needs some protection from humiliation in physical education classes.

G. **Manage any family problems or medical conditions** through counseling, specific therapies (e.g., language intervention or help with motor skills), and/or medication (e.g., for attention deficits or depression).

H. **Identify social skills training programs within schools and in clinical settings.** Clinicians should be aware of local resources that offer social skills training to youngsters with social cognitive deficits. Most commonly this training makes use of specific curricula that are used in small group settings in a school or in the community.

I. **Reassure these children that it is appropriate for them to be themselves, that they need not act and talk like everyone else in school, that there is true heroism in individuality.** Clinicians, teachers, and parents need to tread the fine line between helping with social skills and coercing a child into blind conformity with peer pressures, expectations, and models.

BIBLIOGRAPHY

For parents and children

Levine MD. *All Kinds of Minds.* Cambridge, MA: Educators Publishing Service, 1993.
Osman B. *No One to Play With: The Social Side of Learning Disabilities.* New York: Random House, 1982.

Web sites for parents and professionals

All Kinds of Minds, http://www.allkindsofminds.org/index.aspx

For professionals

Asher SR, Coie JD (eds). *Peer Rejection in Childhood.* Cambridge, MA: Cambridge Press, 1990.
Cartledge G, Milburn JF (eds). *Teaching Social Skills to Children.* New York: Pergamon Press, 1980.
Coleman WL, Lindsay RL. Interpersonal disabilities: social skill deficits in older children and adolescents—their description, assessment, and management. *Pediatr Clin North Am* 39(3):551–568, 1992.
Norman F. Kafer. Interpersonal strategies of unpopular children: some implications for social skills training *Psychol Sch.* 9(2):255–259, 2006.

86

Violence and Youth

Peter Stringham

I. **Description of the problem.** Parents are anxiously searching for sensible advice to keep their children safe in what they perceive as an increasingly violent world. Pediatric practitioners can suggest behaviors that will increase nonviolent problem-solving skills in their patients.

A. **Epidemiology.**
- The murder rate of men of ages 15 to 24 years in the United States is 1/5,000 (compared to 1/80,000 in England and 1/200,000 in Japan). Murder is the second leading cause of death (after auto accidents) in this age group. The lifetime risk for being murdered in the United States is 1 in 450 for white females, 1 in 164 for African American females, 1 in 117 for white males and 1 in 28 for African American males.
- The rate of assaults outnumber fatalities by a ratio of more than 100. Adolescents' victimization rates are almost twice the rates for adults 25 to 34 years old (74/1,000 vs. 38/1,000 per year).
- For adolescents in dating relationships, rates are between 32% and 50% for females using violence and between 20% and 32% for males. Three percent of female college students admit to injuring their boyfriends; 7% of males admit to injuring their girlfriends.
- Guns are unsafely designed, so that anyone who borrows or steals a gun can easily fire a lethal cartridge. User specific guns (guns that cannot fire unless the owner gives permission), while feasible, are not part of the 50 million handguns now in circulation in the United States.

B. **Etiology/contributing factors.**
1. **Environmental.** A host of environmental factors have been shown to contribute to violent behaviors in children and adults: a cold, inconsistent child-rearing style; the experience of child abuse; excessive corporal punishment; witnessing violence in the home and community; viewing media violence; coping with socioeconomic disadvantage; and the use of alcohol and other drugs. Equally important, the presence of a gun can turn a violent impulse into a lethal event.

   Environmental factors can also protect from violence. School success, having an adult from outside the family interested in the success of the child, having a feeling of connection to something bigger than they are that is positive—such as nature, humanity or the divine are all protective.

2. **Developmental.** Constant exposure to environmental violence in an infant and young child can create a disconnected, hypervigilant style of relating to adults and peers. Witnessing violence in the home, neighborhood, and television teaches children that the "best" way to solve conflict is through violence. Some parents actively teach their children to use violence to resolve conflicts. Violent individuals tend to believe that violence is the *preferred* way to handle most conflict. They tend to experience the world as harsh and interpret ambiguous situations as laden with hostility. They view people as either victims or bullies and have few nonviolent strategies for resolving potentially violent conflicts. Many have an impulsive style of acting when assessing the situation or the consequences of their actions.

   Nonviolent teenagers experience the world as a neutral or positive place. They believe themselves to be of high value and think even potentially violent opponents are of high value. In a potentially violent conflict, they are not impulsive; they ask questions of their opponents, state their own positions, and offer to work out compromises. Their response to conflict is respectful, deliberate, and not impulsive. They feel connected to realms that are larger than they are that are positive—such as nature, humanity or the divine.

II. **Making the Diagnosis.**

A. **History: Key clinical questions.** The goal of the history is to assess the risk that the child is or will become violent. As in other aspects of clinical care, the best way to determine the risk for violence is to ask directly about violence in the home, disciplinary techniques, violent encounters in the community, and personal behaviors and attitudes. Clinical judgment must be exercised in pursuing these lines of questions; there is no need to ask all the questions at each visit or for every patient.

1. **For parents.**
    a. **Spousal abuse.**
        (1) *"How do you and the baby's father get along? How often do you have yelling or screaming fights? How about pushing or shoving fights?"* If answers are negative, no other questions are necessary. At subsequent visits, the clinician can inquire about how the couple is getting along.
        (2) *"Any injuries? What was it about? Tell me about your worst fight. Tell me about your last fight. Are you afraid? Are you safe now? Do you know what to do if you are not safe? Is there a gun in the house?"*
    b. **Gun in the house.**
        "Is there a gun in any place where your child spends time? What kind? What is it for? Is it loaded? Is it locked up?"
    c. **Discipline.**
        "How do you correct the child if he or she slaps or bites? For an older child, how do you correct your child if he or she misbehaves?"
    d. **Attitudes toward violence.**
        "If a child tries to pick on your child, what do you think your child should do?"
    e. **Street fighting.**
        "How many fights has your child had in the last year? What were they about? What did you do about it?"
2. **For older children and teenagers: The FIGHTS pneumonic.**
    F—Fights
    "How many pushing or shoving fights have you had in the last year? What were they about? How do you usually get out of a fight?" Assess their nonviolent coping skills.
    I—Injuries
    "Was anyone injured in any of these fights?"
    G—Guns
    "Is there a gun in your home? Possibly did you ever carry a weapon for self-protection?"
    H—Home
    "Has anyone hit you at home in the last year?"
    T—Threats
    "Have you ever been threatened with a weapon?"
    S—Sexual violence
    "Have you ever had a pushing or shoving fight with a boy or with a girl?"
    "Have you ever been forced to have sex against your will?" (As part of the sexual history.)
B. **Assessing the risk for violence.** In all areas, consider patients and their families on a continuum. They are at small risk, moderate risk, or severe risk for spousal abuse or street violence.

III. **Management.**
A. **Primary goals.**
    1. **To teach beliefs and skills that enhance the child's ability to respond to stress and perceived threats in a nonaggressive way.**
    2. **To help parents and patients incorporate nonviolent behavior as an integral part of their self-image.**
    3. **To decrease the environmental factors that increase violence.**
B. **Initial treatment strategies.**
    1. **Intimate partner violence.** Pediatric clinicians need basic screening skills for intimate partner violence because medical professionals may be the only adults outside the family who have any contact with a coerced or battered parent.
        The ideal clinical practice has set up a 24-hour referral service, where a trained mental health clinician can do an in-depth assessment and/or intervention after a medical clinician screens for and discovers intimate partner violence. Large medical practices can set up in a house on call schedule. A time-limited task force with professionals from mental health, pediatrics, internal medicine, OB/GYN (obstetrics/gynecology), urgent care, security, support services, and human resources can plan and implement a sensible screening and referral network. Human resources is essential so that all employees get basic intimate partner violence training; people with any patient contact get more training. Clinicians get more training, and the mental health staff that will do the deeper assessments, interventions and referrals can get intensive training. Smaller practices need to make a relationship with a mental health group or urgent care center who can help with subacute and acute assessments.

a. **Small risk.** A parent tells of physical fights in the past, but none now, and she states that she has no fear, but that sometimes her partner tells her who her friends can be and where she can go. She might be considered at low risk for spousal abuse. Advocate that coercion be stopped and that fighting be discussed with the spouse. Try to see if the mother could say to her partner, *"If you are upset and tell me you are upset, I will try to help you. If you attack me verbally or in any other way I will put a lot of distance between us—emotionally or physically."* The woman may need other counseling.

b. **Moderate risk.** A mother describes some physical fighting, but no injuries. The woman denies fear and says she is safe. The fights are not initiated by the woman, who tries to placate the partner. The clinician can come down strongly on the side of nonviolence: *"This worries me a lot"* or *"You do not deserve to be hit"* or *"This may be getting out of control. Are you safe now? Do you know what to do if you don't feel safe?"* The clinician should refer her for an indepth assessment for danger and for help. If she refuses, give the telephone number of a domestic violence hot line and attempt to refer for counseling, specifically to discuss the violence and abuse.

c. **Large risk.** A mother describes injuries from beatings, fear, a gun in the home, serious threats to the mother or children. The family should not leave the office until the clinician feels she is "safe." Other professionals will need to be involved. The clinician should not intervene with the abusing partner as this may cause more harm. The police might need to be involved. Clearly, this is best handled if you have already set up a referral network to people who deal with this frequently.

2. **Promoting nonviolent discipline.**

a. Ask about disciplinary techniques at the 9-month visit, and suggest to parents: *"Your child will soon be getting into everything. While curiosity is essential, there are some things a child should not do. I recommend that a major rule in your house be 'No hurting anyone.' They cannot hurt themselves or anyone else. If they hit you might be able to stop it by just saying 'no' and redirecting them toward another activity. Sometimes you may need to go further and use a 'time out.' We don't recommend hitting. It is confusing to a child when you say he should not hurt and then hit him yourself."* See other methods of discipline in Chapter 16.

b. If a parent prefers corporal punishment or slaps a child in the clinician's office, the clinician should not shame the parent. Behavior change comes from an alliance between practitioner and parents. *"I agree with you that discipline is very important. Children who do not know what is right can grow up insecure. There are some new ways to correct poor behavior that seem to work better or as well as hitting and I can tell you about them"* (see Chapter 16).

3. **Teenagers with street violence.** All the described interventions are in the office, but they can be adapted to larger groups and to the community. Clinicians should try to involve parents, schools, coaches, police, and community leaders to promote nonviolence as the norm in the larger community. Don't promote coercion or fear in this effort, i.e., don't conduct a "war on violence."

a. **Lowest risk**—A teenager with no or few nonserious fights, knows how to get out of a fight, does well in school, and does not have other high-risk adolescent behaviors. Teach the four steps to getting out of a fight (Table 86-1). (Note that these are the same steps we all use when dealing with an irate, out-of-control parent whose child is critically ill.)

b. **Moderate risk**—A teenager in a few fights who says he would never walk away from a fight. No weapon carrying, no major injuries, doing OK in school, and not many other high-risk behaviors.
"Your examination shows that you are strong and well, but you told me that you have been in a few fights and that you would never walk away from a fight. That worries me. Not many, but a few, kids around here carry weapons and you should not have to walk around in fear of these few kids. There are some things teenagers around here do to keep themselves safe. They go pretty much everywhere and are afraid of no one, because they know how to not fight with everyone." If they are at all amenable, go through the "how to be safe on the street" intervention (Tables 86-1 and 86-2).

c. **High risk**—A teenager in many fights, who has dropped out of school, is involved with other high risk behaviors, likes to fight, may be in a violent gang, may carry a weapon.
   (1) Express your concern or worry about his behavior.
   (2) Help teenager handle his own frustration or depression better.
   (3) Identify who he can talk to, teach meditation.

Table 86-1. Steps for getting out of a fight

I want you to stand up. Now, pretend I am a guy who wants to fight you. Start walking toward me, and tell me when you should stop. (Most patients intuitively will stop before you are within arms reach. Point this out to them.) People who might want to fight are probably afraid of you and when you get too close they think, "I think he's going to punch me, so I better hit him first." Don't crowd someone who is upset.

The guys who don't fight treat even strangers who want to fight like they are cousins. This usually works, but sometimes you have to walk away from a fight.

1. **Walk away if you feel real fear. If you walked out of your house and a bear came running at you, what would you do? You would probably go back in the house right away because you would feel fear. Fear protects us, so if you are in any situation and feel fear, you are probably right. Something is really wrong. Get away the best way you can. Things are almost certainly as dangerous or more dangerous than you think.**
2. **Walk away if you begin to lose your temper. Do you think straight when you have lost your temper? Most people don't. If you are talking with someone who wants to fight you and you think you are beginning to lose your temper, say, "I'm beginning to lose my temper. I'm leaving now. I want to make things right between us, but I can't talk to you now. I'm leaving." Most people respect that.**
3. **Walk away if the other person is acting like they are high or somewhat crazy. It is hard to talk to people who want to fight you when they are high on alcohol or other substances or if they are having severe mental problems. Get away the best way you can.**
4. **Walk away if you see an injustice, but you cannot stop it yourself. You might see two big guys beating up another guy, and you don't know them. If you don't do anything you will feel guilty, but you cannot stop the fight yourself. Leave and then get help. In school, get a teacher. On the streets, you can leave and call 911.**

If they say these strategies won't work, ask teenagers what would work for them.

For young children, particularly when they arrive with their fathers, do the above intervention in younger kid language. Since older relatives give the most influential advice about how to handle street conflict, you are trying to change the father's advice.

(4) Present dilemmas that show he handles some situations nonviolently: *"Your best friend's aunt is in the hospital. You really feel sorry for your friend and would like to help him out, but he begins to yell at you, 'You and your family always looked down on me. You always thought you were better than me. Let's step outside and settle this right now!' You don't want to hurt him, what could you do?"* After he struggles through a solution, show him how he used the six steps. Suggest that the same techniques that work with a friend can work with a stranger.

(5) Address weapon carrying. *"You told me that sometimes you carry a gun to feel safe. Have you told anyone about this? Do you think teenagers keep secrets well? So your friends might have told other kids and many people might know about this. What might happen if a kid had a genuine disagreement with you and needed to discuss it, but he worried that the disagreement might turn into a fight? Do you think he might bring a weapon or have friends bring weapons?"*

Table 86-2. How to be safe on the streets

I did not grow up in this neighborhood, so I asked kids from here who don't fight and who never get picked on how keep out of fights. This is what they tell me. See if it makes sense to you.

They say the most important thing for keeping out of street fights is a "good attitude." They treat everyone they meet like "they are a cousin."

If a cousin is upset and starts swearing at you or wants to fight you, you will step back and ask, "What is going on?" or "Why are you doing this?" Maybe you did something wrong. If you did you can apologize. If you didn't do anything wrong you can explain your side. If you disagree about what has happened, you can say, "I won't fight you to settle this, but I want things to end up 'right' between us." You might say, "I'm leaving now, but when things are calmer I will talk to you and make things right between us."

Wouldn't that make you less safe? I think teenagers are safer if they have a reputation for settling conflicts by talking about it calmly."

(6) Try to teach a deliberate nonimpulsive approach to ambiguous situations. *"When most guys are approached by a guy who wants to fight they ask themselves, 'Why is this guy trying to fight me? Is he upset? Is he high? Have I caused this in any way?' Then they ask 'Is he armed?' and then they ask, 'If I wanted to calm him down, what could I do?' After they have answered all those questions they decide whether or not to fight."*

(7) Help them with their depression, unemployment, alcoholism, or other problems and try to refer them to a program that will help address all their needs.

(8) If there is a history of violence towards a girlfriend, keep approval of the patient while expressing disapproval of the poor behavior. *Has your girlfriend begun to fear you yet?* Most will say "no." *That is really lucky, because if you ever get to the point where a woman fears you then love will surely die. You deserve support, respect and love. You can only get that when you are in a relationship with a woman who treats you like a best friend. That means you treat her like a best friend. Fear poisons all love relationships. It is mean for women, and men lose also.*

4. **After an injury.**
   a. **Acute care.** When the patient is medically stable, take a nonjudgmental history of the incident, asking yourself:
   - **Is the patient safe to leave the hospital right now?**
   - **Is there anyone else who is not safe now** (another person, other friends or relatives)?
   - **Is there anyone who can settle this dispute nonviolently?**
   b. **Postacute care.** Assess each patient to see if they need further services.
      (1) **Trivial injury by a friend—more an accident than a violent act.** (No need for further service.)
      (2) **Patient at wrong place at wrong time—an innocent victim.** (May need post traumatic stress counseling.)
      (3) **Patient put themselves in harm's way.** (May need counseling for depression or substance abuse.)
      (4) **Patient flirting with violence.** (Needs help redirecting themselves toward nonviolent life style—youth groups, school program, or violence prevention counselor. See **Moderate Risk** interventions.)
      (5) **Patient deeply committed to violence.** (See **High Risk** interventions.)

BIBLIOGRAPHY

Alpert E, Freund K. *Partner Violence: How to Recognize and Treat Victims of Abuse—A Guide for Physicians.* Waltham, MA: Massachusetts Medical Society, 1992.
American Psychological Association.*Violence and Youth: Psychology's response.* Volume 1: Summary Report of the American Psychological Association Commission on Violence and Youth. Washington, DC. American Psychological Association, 1993.
Hennes H, Calhoun A, (eds). Violence among children and adolescents. *Pediatr Clin North Am* 45:2, 1998.
Prothrow-Stith D. *Deadly Consequences: How Violence Is Destroying Our Teenage Population and a Plan to Begin Solving the Problem.* New York: Harper Collins, 1991.
Rosenberg M, Fenley MA, (eds). *Violence in America: A Public Health Approach.* New York, NY: Oxford University Press, 1991.
Sege R. Adolescent violence. *Curr Opin Pediatr* 4:575–581, 1992.

87

Visual Disability: Developmental and Behavioral Consequences

Michael E. Msall

I. **Description of the problem.** Legal blindness is defined as central visual acuity in the best eye with corrective lenses of 20/200 or worse, or a restriction in the visual field so that the widest diameter of vision subtends an angle of 20 degrees. The term legal blindness is a misnomer as approximately 75% of individuals with legal blindness have some residual visual function. In addition, the majority of adults with legal blindness can read large print. For children with vision worse than 20/400, ophthalmologists use functional descriptors such as child's ability to count fingers or detect hand motion, nearby large objects, the direction of a light source or its presence. Students can be classified as educationally visually impaired if their corrected vision is 20/70 or worse. The World Health Organization (WHO) classifies visual disability into five categories described in Table 87-1.

A. **Epidemiology.** The epidemiology of severe visual impairment is changing. Both laser surgery for severe threshold retinopathy of prematurity and advances in the prevention of congenital rubella, measles, *Hemophilus influenza*, pneumococcal, and group B β-streptococcal meningitis have substantially decreased their contributions to visual and multiple disabilities. Current estimates of the prevalence of childhood blindness are 6 per 1,000. Congenital blindness occurs with a frequency of 30 per 100,000. In developing countries, the major contributors to visual disability include gonoccocal ophthalmia neonatorum, trachoma, vitamin A deficiency, and measles. Worldwide, there are 1.5 million children who are legally blind. The United States does not keep a registry for children with severe visual disability, but 50,000 children are considered visually impaired by school systems of which 20,000 require Braille as a reading medium. Children with combined deafness and blindness number 500 per year and include 10,000 children from birth to age 21 years.

B. **Etiology.** Table 87-2 describes the major known etiologies of severe visual impairment in childhood. The timing of these etiologies is prenatal in 43%, perinatal in 27%, postnatal in 8%, and unknown in 22%. Several multiple malformation syndromes involve visual impairment and include chromosomopathies, CHARGE association (coloboma, heart disease, choanal atresia, intellectual disability, growth and genital anomalies, ear anomalies), Lowe syndrome (intellectual disability, cataracts, renal tubular dysfunction), neurocutaneous disorders (tuberous sclerosis, optic gliomas in Neurofibromatosis-1), metabolic (homocystinuria) and neurodegenerative disorders (leukodystrophies and optic atrophy, gangliosidosis and cherry red macula, Batten's disease).

1. Many syndromes affect both vision and hearing. These include Alport's, Usher's, Cockayne's, Stickler's, and Refsun's syndromes as well as congenital infections, lysosomal storage disease, and leukodystrophies.

2. Postnatal causes of blindness account for 8% to 11% of all childhood blindness. Etiologies include infections, trauma, complicated hydrocephalus, retinoblastoma, craniopharyngioma, demyelinating diseases, and leukemia with CNS (central nervous system) involvement.

3. **Blindness and associated developmental disabilities.** It is important to recognize that in more than 50% of children with visual disability, there are additional major disorders including cerebral palsy, cognitive–adaptive developmental disability, autistic spectrum disorders, recurrent seizures, hearing impairments, and learning disabilities. Among children with visual disability in a comprehensive community registry, 65% had additional disabilities. Of the children with multiple disabilities, cortical visual impairment (CVI) occurred in 50%.

C. **Developmental aspects of vision.** Pupillary light reactions and lid closure to bright light are present at 30 weeks gestation. Brief visual fixation is present at birth including brief saccades to a moving person, moving face, and dangling ring. At birth, acuity has been assessed as approximately 20/400 by optokinetic nystagmus (OKN), forced preferential looking (FPL), and visual evoked potentials (VEP). By three weeks, watching a mother speak occurs. The presence of strabismus is easily identified by an off-center asymmetry of

Table 87-1. WHO classification of visual disability

Category 1	Impaired	20/60 to 20/200
Category 2	Severe impairment	20/200 to 20/400
Category 3	Blind	20/400 to 20/2,400
Category 4	Blind	<20/2,400 and light perception
Category 5	Blind	No light perception.

reflected light, the Hirshperg reflex. Eyes that do not see well tend to deviate or drift, and this along with nystagmus may be the first indication of poor vision. Pupillary responses, an intact red reflex, and the ability of a child to track 360 degrees are indicators of globally adequate vision. Developmental consequences of these core visual skills impact on motor, manipulative, communicative, social and adaptive skills and are shown in Table 87-3.

II. Making the diagnosis.

A. **Clinical Presentation.** Infants with visual disability present in one of three clinical scenarios.

1. In the first scenario, **parents are concerned that their child is not seeing.** At 6 to 10 weeks, the child is not smiling reciprocally and does not follow faces or rings but does have a normal papillary response, red reflex, and intact globe. These children either have cortical visual impairment (CVI), delayed visual maturation (DVM), or evolving developmental disability. Both CVI and DVM have high rates of motor, cognitive, and communicative disability. However, in DVM, functional visual recovery occurs, while in CVI, some visual improvement may occur but low vision is a common sequelae. In children with severe evolving developmental disability, the children stare and are inattentive because of disorders of nonvisual higher cortical function impacting on learning, perception, communicating, and social skills.

2. In the second scenario, **children present in infancy with nystagmus, sluggish pupils, and visual inattention.** Ophthalmological findings reveal anterior segment or optic nerve disorders such as cataract, corneal opacities, glaucoma, and microphthalmia. The posterior segment abnormalities include colobomas of the optic nerve or retina, optic nerve hypoplasia or atrophy, retinal dystrophy, retinopathy of prematurity, or retinoblastoma.

3. In the third scenario, **infants show visual inattention, nystagmus, and variable pupillary responses.** Ophthalmological evaluation reveals a normal globe and intact red reflex. Strabismus may be present. Electoretinogram (ERG) testing is most helpful in revealing the nature of these disorders. The most common is Leber's congenital amaurosis, a recessively inherited retinal dystrophy with an extinguished ERG. This disorder currently accounts for 10% of childhood blindness with a range of visual function from legal blindness to no light perception. Associated findings may include renal and skeletal anomalies and cataracts, strabismus, and keratoconus. Additional differential diagnoses in this scenario are rod monochromatism, an autosomal recessive disorder with missing cone photoreceptors, congenital stationery night blindness, and retinitis pigmentosa.

B. **Acuity testing.** Teller acuity cards utilize preferential looking at standardized cards with varying width of black and white stripes. They can be used in preverbal children and have been widely used in children with retinopathy of prematurity as well as children with motor or developmental disability. By age 3 years, many children can cooperate with a variety of tasks such as Allen Cards, Multiple E Charts, and HOTV cards. If there are either parent concerns, presence of any developmental or neurological disability, or physician concern about vision screening, then referral to an ophthalmologist is warranted.

C. The **differential diagnosis** of the infant who demonstrates a reduced visual response from birth includes:

Table 87-2. The major known etiologies of severe visual impairment in childhood

Retina	Optic nerve	Lens	Posterior visual pathways
Severe retinopathy of prematurity	Optic nerve atrophy Optic nerve hypoplasia	Cataract	Periventricular leukomalacia
Retinitis pigmentosa	Leber congenital amaurosis	Corneal dystrophies	Occipital malformations

Table 87-3. Visual skills and developmental milestones

Age of child	Visual milestone present	Formal visual testing
Birth	Alertness to visual stimulus presented 8–10 inches from eyes	20/400 FPL = VEP = OKN
1 mo	Follows red ring 90 degrees, smiles in response to faces	
2 mo	Follows red ring 180 degrees, chest up in prone	20/200 FPL = OKN, 20/60 VEP
3 mo	Tracks red ring 360 degrees, begins midline hand play	
4 mo	Bats at ring, on wrists in prone, holds bottle, turns to voice	
5 mo	Attains ring, crumples paper, looks for source of sound, rolls	
6 mo	Early sitting balance, transfers blocks, lifts cup	20/150 FPL, 20/100 OKN, 20/40 VEP
9 mo	Crawls, pulls to stand, mature pincer, finger feeds, gesture language	
12 mo	Cruises, walks with support, puts cube in cup, removes socks, points	20/60 OKN, 20/50 FPL, 20/20 VEP

OKN = optokinetic nystagmus, FPL = forced preferential looking, VEP = visual evoked potentials.

1. **Persistent neurodevelopmental abnormalities** such as evolving cognitive adaptive developmental disabilities (i.e., intellectual disability), cerebral palsy, or autistic spectrum disorders.
2. The presence of **perinatal problems** including inborn errors of metabolism, sequelae of hypoxic–ischemic encephalopathy, perinatal stroke, or an evolving seizure disorder.
3. **Severe visual impairment** due to significant ocular problems
4. **Visual impairment of unknown cause.**
   D. **Developmental assessment of blind children.**
      1. **Cognitive development.** A key area to monitor in children with severe visual impairment is communicative milestones. Children who are blind and who do not have associated neurological abnormalities achieve developmental milestones at a slower pace but should not be considered motor or cognitively disabled. The slower developmental milestones are the result of different experiences of nonverbal skills, motor exploration, and understanding spatial relations. For example, the infant is unable to see details of facial expression, lip movements, gestures, object position in space, use of utensils, indoor and outdoor activities. As a result, different tactile, verbal, and orientation experience are required to help the child construct knowledge of both immediate and distant environments.
      2. **Motor development.** Fraiberg's classic longitudinal study involved 10 children with congenital blindness and demonstrated both the differences in the learning of gross motor and hand skills and the value of developmental interventions and family supports. The median age of sitting balance was 8 months, pulling to stand 13 months, walking alone 15 months and walking across a room 19 months. Over 30 years later, we are in a different era of visual disability and of premature infants who develop severe retinopathy of prematurity. Even among children with legal blindness, those whose residual vision is between 20/500 and 20/800 make better developmental progress than if their vision is 20/800 or worse.
III. **Management.**
   A. **Primary goals.** The responsibility of the clinician is to interpret and facilitate the infant's behavior and development, to coordinate diagnostic evaluations, and to understand their child's strengths, challenges, and ways of learning. In addition, referral to early intervention programs, provision of supplementary security income, visual aids, parent groups, family supports, and advocacy are required.
   B. **Emotional supports: Normal grieving, parental fears, and hope.** It is the physician's task to support parents through the stages of normal grieving, allow them to express their sadness and anger, and clarify sources of confusion. Except in neurodegenerative disorders, all children with visual disability continue to learn. It is important to also help

parents understand the importance of residual functional vision. Families are highly sensitive to feelings of isolation and abandonment by clinicians, especially if they perceive discomfort with the disability. Clinicians can also assist with anticipating some of the challenges especially if they include behavior supports for day-to-day management. This strategy includes supports for addressing sleep difficulties, feeding skills, hygiene, toileting, and demanding behaviors. Recognition of parental stress, anxiety, depression, and feelings of being overwhelmed requires empathy, appropriate counseling, and referral and advocacy for mental health services. Supports to siblings should include discussion of etiology, contagiousness, stigma, dealing with peers, and family crisis.

C. **Developmental interventions.** It is critical to remember that children with blindness are children first and benefit for proactive biopsychosocial interventions that promote use of residual vision if possible, and optimize communicative, cognitive, behavioral, and social competencies. **Several model curricula** are available to early intervention teams:

1. **Infancy.** Family supports, communicating and recognizing infants' cues, mobility, manipulation, and orientation should be the major themes. Touching, labeling, smelling, and exploring people, toys and objects encourage the infant to learn about their surroundings. Participation in small group experiences with visually impaired and non-visually impaired peers is important.
   - Fraiberg and colleagues used auditory–tactile paired cues to stimulate interactions and taught parents to recognize infant's tactile gestures for communicating basic needs.
   - Joffee program is a home-based model for orientation and mobility. Parents learn how to enrich their home environment by auditory toys that are brightly colored and have tactual cues, interactive paired verbal and tactile activities, singing, guided touch, and describing daily activities.
   - In Erwin parent-centered approach, parents are trained to teach toddlers how to ask questions, describe objects by using modifiers (e.g., hot, warm, and cold water), and to use personal social labels in speech.
   - Klein's Parent and Toddler Training emphasizes social responsiveness. Target training themes include understanding early childhood development, social development, family reactions, behavior management, enhancing infant development, family communication, and problem solving.

2. **Preschoolers.** Preschoolers can experience both small group, quality, early childhood educational experiences as well as receiving extensive consultation from a teacher of the visually impaired. A functional and developmental approach can emphasize communication, rich sensory experiences exploration, learning through play, music, adaptive, and social skills. All state educational systems receive funds to ensure appropriate educational supports and visual aids.

3. **School age.** A comprehensive individualized curriculum is essential. Both talking books and specialized computer screens are important. Physicians in partnership with families can set goals that allow the child to learn appropriate academic, social, and extracurricular skill. The school-aged child should participate in community-based classroom activities that will allow preparation for higher education, as well as for independent living. Children with visual disability and multiple additional disabilities require strategies that do not leave them and their families isolated and in only part day learning activities.

4. **Adaptations and technology:** Braille continues to be the mainstay of nonvisual communication. The use of records and tapes are critical sources for reading and information about the world. The OPTACON (Optical to Tactile Converter) was developed by the Stanford Research Institute to convert printed text to a tactual dot figuration. In many public libraries, there are print to speech converters (Kurzweil devices) that allowed printed material to be read aloud. A variety of computerized technology systems in conjunction with videocamera technology have been developed to translate environmental information to tactile or optic nerve stimuli. It is important for professionals to understand that adults with adventitious blindness (i.e., individuals with some experience of sight before they became blind) have been the initial users of these prototypes.

5. **Orientation and mobility skills (peripatology).**
   a. **Orientation** requires that a child know present position and space, their destination, and the pathway for travel.
   b. **Mobility** refers to the technique for safely and efficiently traveling to a predetermined indoor or outdoor destination. These skills can be enhanced with long canes. Guide dogs are widely used with adults. The Canterbury Child's Aid is based on sonar wave emissions that are converted to audible stimuli.

    c. There remain major gaps in the knowledge base for understanding in children both quantifiable positive outcomes and challenges with current devices, for developmentally appropriate independence, vocational opportunities, and community participation.

BIBLIOGRAPHY

For parents

American Foundation for the Blind, Louisville, KY, www.afb.org

Educational booklets and videos in English and Spanish: the Blind Children's Center, Los Angeles, CA, http://www.blindchildrenscenter.org/

Fraiberg S. *Insights From the Blind.* New York: Basic Books, 1977.

Holbrook C. *Children With Visual Impairments: A Parent's Guide* (2nd ed), Bethesda, MD: Woodbine House Inc, 2006.

National Association for Parents of Children With Visual Impairments (NAPVI). http://www.spedex.com/napvi/

National Library Services for Blind and Physically Handicapped. http://www.loc.gov/nls/

For professionals

Davidson P, Harrison G. The effectiveness of early intervention for children with visual impairments. In Guralnick MJ (ed), *The Effectiveness of Early Intervention.* Baltimore, MD: Paul H Brookes, 1997.

Fenichel GM. Disorders of the visual system. In *Clinical Pediatric Neurology* (5th ed), Philadelphia, PA: Saunders Elsevier, 2005.

Kelly DP. Sensory deficits. In Wolraich ML, et al. (eds), *Developmental-Behavioral Pediatrics: Evidence and Practice.* Philadelphia, PA: Mosby Elsevier, 2008.

Levine LM. Visual system problems. In: Maria B (ed), *Current Management in Child Neurology* (4th ed), Shelton, CT: BC Decker, 2009.

Mervis CA, Yeargin-Alsopp M, Winter S, Boyle C. Etiology of childhood vision impairment, metropolitan Atlanta, 1991–93. *Paediatric and Perinatal Epidemiology* 14:70–77, 2000.

Msall ME, Phelps DL, Digaudio KM, et al. Severity of neonatal retinopathy of prematurity is predictive of neurodevelopmental functional outcome at age 5.5 years. *Pediatrics* 106:998–1005, 2000.

Teplin SW, Greeley J, Anthony TL. Blindness and visual impairment. In Carey WB, et al. (eds), *Developmental–Behavioral Pediatrics.* Philadelphia, PA: Saunders Elsevier, 2009.

Thompson L, Kaufman LM. The visually impaired child. *Pediatr Clin North Am* 50(1):225–239, 2003.

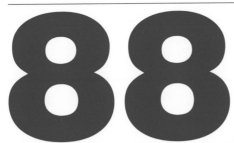

Witness/Child Exposure to Community or Domestic Violence

Betsy McAlister Groves

I. **Description of the problem.** Children who are exposed to violence in their communities or in the home are often hidden victims. Although it has been well established that children who are the *victims* of violence (e.g., child abuse and sexual abuse) suffer severe and long-lasting consequences, there is now ample evidence that *witnessing* violence is also damaging to children, and in some cases, may be more psychologically toxic than being a victim. Because their scars are emotional and not physical, the primary care clinician may not fully appreciate their distress and miss an opportunity to provide needed interventions for these children.

A. **Epidemiology.**

1. **Community violence.**
   - In one study, more than a third of school-aged children in New Orleans had witnessed severe violence; 40% had seen a dead body.
   - In a study of urban middle school students, the majority (76%) of young adolescents reported witnessing or being victimized by at least 1 violent event in the prior 6 months.
   - In a survey of parents of children aged 0 to 6 in an outpatient pediatric setting, one in ten children had witnessed a knifing or shooting; half the reported violence occurred in the home.
   - Nearly two-thirds of young children attending a Head Start program had either witnessed or been victimized by community violence, according to parent reports.

2. **Domestic violence.**
   - In a survey of parents in three SAMHSA-funded community mental health partnerships, 23% of parents reported that their children had seen or heard a family member being threatened with physical harm.
   - A recent survey of American households revealed that 15 to 17 million, or nearly 30%, of children in this country live in homes where there is some form of intimate partner violence.
   - A July 2009 analysis of more than 10,000 children served by the National Child Traumatic Stress Network found that 44.3% of the children reported exposure to domestic violence.
   - Children aged 5 and younger are disproportionately represented in households with domestic violence.

   Although exposure to community or domestic violence is the most prevalent type of child exposure to violence, a complete listing would include child exposure to war and terrorism. With the growing number of immigrant and refugee families served in most pediatric practices, it is likely that the clinician will see children who have been exposed to these types of traumas.

B. **Etiology.** Research in the past two decades has shown that children of all ages may be adversely affected by violence in their environments. Short-term symptoms include sleep difficulties, avoidance of reminders of the event, somatic symptoms, hyperarousal, helplessness, and fear, even if the child is not immediately in danger. Longer term effects include an increased risk of substance abuse, juvenile delinquency, anxiety or depression, and adverse health outcomes. Studies suggest that young children are particularly vulnerable to the impact of violence in the environment, and that chronic exposure may affect brain development and self-regulatory processes. In addition, children under the age of four may be particularly vulnerable to threats that involve the safety (or perceived safety) of their caregivers.

II. **Making the diagnosis.**

A. **Symptoms.** Children may develop a range of post-traumatic symptoms, and in some cases will meet criteria for the diagnosis of post-traumatic stress disorder (PTSD) (Table 88-1). Although young children may not fully meet these criteria, certain behavioral changes are uniquely associated with their exposure to trauma: sleep disturbances, aggressive

Table 88-1. Symptoms of post-traumatic stress disorder (DSM IV)

Re-experiencing
1. Intrusive and distressing recollections, thoughts
2. Distressing dreams of the trauma
3. Acting or feeling as if the trauma were recurring ("flashbacks")
4. Psychological distress at exposure to cues that symbolize the trauma
5. Physiological reactivity at exposure to cues that symbolize the trauma

Avoidance and numbing
1. Efforts to avoid thoughts, feelings associated with the trauma
2. Efforts to avoid activities, places, people that arouse recollections of the trauma
3. Diminished interest in activities
4. Feeling of detachment from others
5. Restricted affect
6. Sense of foreshortened future

Arousal
1. Sleep problems
2. Irritability, outbursts of anger
3. Concentration problems
4. Hypervigilance
5. Exaggerated startle response

Symptoms that are unique to children aged 6 or younger:
1. Aggressive behavior
2. Increased separation anxiety
3. Development of new fears
4. Developmental regression

behavior, new fears, developmental regression, and increased anxiety about separations from caretakers.
  B. **History: key clinical questions.** It is important for the primary care clinician to inquire about violence in the lives of all children. Questions may be prefaced by a statement that assures the family members that they are not being singled out for this line of questioning and that the clinician considers the topic of violence to be within the scope of problems to be addressed in a medical visit. By doing so, the clinician has communicated that violence and exposure to violence are a risk to the child's well-being and are a legitimate focus of concern during the clinical visit.
    1. *"I know that there is a lot of violence in our world these days. I have begun to ask all of my patients about their experiences with violence. I would like to ask you a few questions."*
       • *"Are you ever worried about your child's safety?"*
       • *"Has your child seen frightening things?"*
       • *"What does your child watch on television? Are you concerned about what your child is watching on television?"*
       • *"Has your child witnessed violence on the streets or in the neighborhood?"*
       • *"Has your child witnessed violence in the home?"*
    2. If there are disclosures of witnessing violence, the following questions will explore how the child may have been affected.
       • *"What happened? What did the child see or hear?"*
         The clinician should elicit the story from both the child and the parent. It is preferable to hear the child's story first and, if possible, separately. Children's accounts of traumatic events give important clues about how they viewed the event, how they perceive their role, and what kind of meaning they make of the event. Since children frequently misunderstand or misperceive a sequence of events, the child's account provides important information about how to correct misperceptions.
       • [To the child] *"When and how often do you think about what happened? Do thoughts come to you while you are in school? What do you do when these thoughts occur?"*
       • *"Does the child seem less interested in play or school? Does the child worry more?"*
       • *"What behavioral changes have you observed in the child? Is the child fearful of being apart from you or other caretakers?"*

III. Management.

A. Counseling the parents. The primary care clinician should include the following components of parent guidance in their intervention with the parents.

1. A careful **review** of the facts and details of the violent event.

2. **Information** about the expectable symptoms and behaviors associated with witnessing violence.

3. **Assistance** in restoring a sense of stability to the family in order to enhance the child's feelings of safety (e.g., by establishing consistent routines, assistance in accessing concrete supports such as housing, benefits).

4. **Strategies** to encourage the child to talk about the event with the parent and/or other trusted adults (e.g., verbally, through drawings, or play).

5. **Assurance** that it is not a forbidden topic for discussion. It is helpful to the child to be able to talk about it within the family. Without overfocusing on the incident, parents can communicate their willingness to talk to the child about what has happened.

   Intervention is more difficult if the child is living with ongoing domestic violence. Maximizing safety may be a difficult task because the parent may have few options in terms of leaving the batterer. In cases of domestic violence, it is necessary to help the victim assess the safety of her children and herself. This discussion should convey the clinician's concern about the impact of violence on the child and parent. The clinician should help to formulate a plan the parent can use in the event of future violence, including the telephone numbers of the local domestic violence hotline and battered women's shelter. A referral to a battered women's support service should be encouraged.

B. Counseling the child. For some children the process of telling their story in detail is in itself therapeutic. The child has a chance to reflect on the event, to try out new coping strategies, and to receive empathic and supportive feedback. By asking sensitive and detailed questions, the clinician models for the parents how to talk to children about frightening or unpleasant events. Thus, the primary care clinician's role with the child is to:

1. Review the facts and details of the traumatic event and help the child accurately understand what has happened.

2. Give the child a forum to share worries, fears, and anxieties and to help the child accommodate to the trauma.

3. Schedule a follow-up appointment within 2 to 3 weeks of the initial session. This is particularly important in cases involving domestic violence.

C. When to refer a child for counseling. The child or family should be referred for mental health intervention in the following circumstances:

- The child's symptoms have persisted for more than 3 months.
- The trauma was particularly violent or involved the loss of a parent or caretaker.
- The caretakers are unable to be empathetically attuned to the child.
- The child is in an unsafe environment.

Referrals should be made to mental health specialists familiar with treating children who have experienced trauma. If the case involves domestic violence, the clinician should also have experience with the particular dynamics of these families. Specialized treatment for these children may include psychological debriefing through play therapy, behavioral/cognitive strategies to decrease sensitivity to traumatic reminders, and pharmacological interventions.

BIBLIOGRAPHY

For parents

Books

Groves BM. *Children Who See Too Much: Lessons from the Child Witness to Violence Project.* Boston: Beacon Press, 2002.

Web sites

Child Witness to Violence Project www.childwitnesstoviolence.org
National Child Traumatic Stress Network www.NCTSN.org
The Child Trauma Academy www.ChildTrauma.org
The National Scientific Council on the Developing Child. http://developingchild.harvard.edu/topics/science_of_early_childhood

For professionals

Groves BM, Augustyn M, Lee D, et al. *Identifying and Responding to Domestic Violence: Consensus Recommendations for Child and Adolescent Health* (can be downloaded at www.endabuse.org). San Francisco, CA: Family Violence Prevention Fund, 2002.

Hurt HH, Malmud E, Brodsky NL, et al. Exposure to violence: psychological and academic correlates in child witnesses. *Arch Pediatr Adolesc Med* 155:1351–1356, 2001.

Pfefferbaum B. Post-traumatic disorder in children: a review of the past ten years. *J Am Acad Child Adolesc Psychiatry* 36(11):1503–1511, 1997.

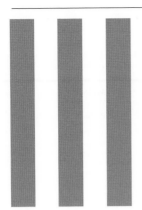

Family Issues

Adoption

Lisa Albers Prock

I. Description.
  A. Epidemiology and nomenclature.
  - Approximately 2% of the U.S. population is adopted with more than 120,000 children adopted annually since the early 1990s.
  - Federal reporting in the United States classifies adoption into three categories:
    - Domestic private agency, kinship (including step-parent) and tribal adoption (more than 50% of annual adoptions)
    - Domestic public (child welfare agency) adoption (approximately 40%)
    - International adoption (<10% of U.S. adoptions annually)
  - The legal process of adoption is widely variable between each of the 50 states with respect to waiting time for adoptive parents and notification of birth fathers. Internationally, adoption to the United States and other member countries is governed by the Hague Convention on Intercountry Adoption, which establishes ethical practices for intercountry adoption.
  - Although the exact numbers are not known, families may elect to "disrupt" an adoption in some cases, estimated to occur in less than 3% of adoptions.
    - Placement with one or two parents is equally successful.
    - In general, the younger the child is at the time of adoption, the more successful is the adoption.
  - A child's history of adoption should be considered a risk factor for later developmental and emotional disorders given preadoptive experiences and genetic risk factors.
  - Preferred terminology when discussing members of the **adoption triad** includes **birth parents, adoptive parents,** and **adopted child/person.** Terms to avoid include "real" or "natural" parents.

II. Primary care clinician's role: information gathering.
  A. Preadoption. If involved during the preadoption process, a clinician should attempt to obtain information from birth parents and medical records via the adoption agency. Children with a history of adoption are somewhat more likely than the general population to later be diagnosed with attention deficit hyperactivity disorder, fetal alcohol spectrum disorder, intellectual disability, or have congenital malformations. The clinician should specifically ask about known family history and consider the relevance for the adoptive parents and their child. The clinician should also try to obtain details about the birth parents' appearance, interests and talents, education and work, and their reason for placing the child for adoption; information that an adopted child may be interested in learning later in life.
  B. Postadoption. Studies indicate **that adoptive families may struggle with transitional problems but that adequate preadoptive preparation can decrease this risk.** All parents may have idealized expectations about their child's behaviors that may not be realized, and adoptive parents may additionally be dealing with the loss of their fantasized birth child. As a result, a clinician should plan a follow-up visit sooner after a newly adopted child joins their family rather than later, and keep close and frequent contact with the adoptive parents in order to understand parental expectations and child behavior. Especially after international adoption, children should be screened for a range of possible infections as well as having routine vision, hearing, and developmental/behavioral surveillance.
  C. Older child adoption. For children adopted beyond the newborn period, the clinician should seek additional information on the history and quality of the child's social attachments, history of adverse experiences (such as abuse, deprivation, neglect, rejections, and separations), and educational experience (including quantity, quality, and potential special needs).

III. Management.

  A. When to tell the child he is adopted. Most experts suggest that families begin discussing adoptive and birth history as soon as a child joins their family. For newborns, this allows parents to become comfortable discussing the topic of adoption without worrying about a child's response. It is imperative that all children learn the important points of their adoptive history from their adoptive parents rather than from someone else. For children adopted in toddlerhood and beyond, memories of their preadoptive experiences will need to be integrated with their story of adoption. Many adoptive children find creating a "life book" which details their history prior to and following joining their adoptive family to be a positive experience.

  B. How to tell the child he is adopted. A discussion of a child's "history of adoption" can be expected to happen many times over the years rather than in a single "disclosure conversation." A child's adoption story should be explained at an appropriate developmental level and with enough, but not too much, information. The following elements are helpful to convey to a child or adolescence about being adopted during conversation:

    1. Acknowledge the important role of the birth parents in the creation of the child.

    2. Discuss adoptive parents' motivation for adoption.

    3. Explain that the child was conceived, grew inside the birth mother, and was born just like all other children.

    4. Emphasize that the decision of the birth parents to place him or her for adoption was in no way the fault of the child.

    5. Acknowledge that there are happy (especially for adoptive parents) and sad feelings (for birth and adoptive parents as well as adopted individuals) associated with the history of adoption.

    6. A statement of the adoptive parents' love for the child and how happy they are that he/she joined their family.

    7. The specifics of each adoption story will vary according to the circumstances.

      • The adoption story might be something like, *"We could not make a baby ourselves so we decided to adopt. You were made by another man and woman, your birth parents, and born to your mother, just like all other children. But, your birth parents could not take care of a baby, so we adopted you. We're sure that they were sad that you were separated from them. You came to live with us, and we're happy we're a family."*

  C. Sequence of developmental issues. A child's understanding of adoption changes as he develops. At different ages, children will focus on different issues and need access to different information (Table 89-1).

    1. During the **preschool** age, children are interested in the facts of how they were born and came to be part of their families. A picture book that depicts the story can be very helpful. Children at this time are also increasingly aware of how "same" and "different" they are when compared with their adoptive parents and siblings.

    2. Around **age 7 to 11 years,** children begin to appreciate the uniqueness and implications of his or her adoptive status. Children's questions about the birth family may

Table 89-1. Adoption topics for children at different ages

Preschool
"Where did I come from?"
Questions about life and death issues
Adoption as a concrete fact (similar to eye color)

School age (7–11 years)
"Why was I adopted when most people aren't?"
May worry about their value as a person because they are adopted
Increasing concerns about being different
Aware that they have lost someone who played an extremely important role in their life
Fantasize that birth parents are rich, famous, and more attractive than adoptive parents

Adolescence
Identity development: discovering how they are different and how they are connected to birth and adoptive families
Wondering about birth, family history of health or mental health concerns, appearance, and aptitude
Emerging or continued interest in meeting birth parents

be viewed by adoptive parents as a potential rejection. Clinicians can prepare parents for this experience and reassure them that the emergence of the child's questioning is part of the normal development sequence and should be responded to in a factual and developmentally appropriate manner in order to maintain open communication about this important topic. Children at this age may imagine their birth parents to be richer, more famous, and otherwise more attractive than their adoptive parents. Many adoptive parents share letters from and pictures of the birth parents with children at this age to begin to introduce facts that they know about a child's history. If birth parents are known to the child (but not as his or her birth parents), the elementary school years are an opportune time to reveal this information to the child.

3. In the **early adolescent phase of identity development,** adopted children may begin to seek more specific information about their birth parents. Teenagers embark on the task of identity development by discovering how they are different from every other human being and how connected they are to their birth and adoptive families. Having more than two parents adds an additional dimension to this task. If little is known about birth parents, adolescents may continue to idealize them.

4. In the **late adolescent period,** topics of sex, marriage, and children may lead to an increased interest in birth family history. Concerns about medical and mental health concerns may increase. By adolescence, individuals should have all available information about their birth family available to help them to facilitate their making sense of their entire life story. Disclosure of difficult topics, including rape and incest, may best be facilitated by working with a therapist.

D. **Questions about birthparents.** As a child or adolescent asks more probing questions about their birth mother and why she was not able to parent him or her, adoptive parents should endeavor to provide optimistic yet realistic answers to support a child's creation of their own life history. In a discussion of this issue, a parent could say, *"Your mother chose adoption for you because she felt unprepared to raise a child, any child, at that time. She probably thinks about you and wonders about how you are doing."* An adoptive parent could explain that their child's birth mother felt unprepared for reasons related to a lack of money, maturity, and resources or illness. Adoptive parents should emphasize that adoption was not related to something the child did but related to birth parent circumstances.

Often there is little information available about birth fathers at the time of adoption. As children realize that there most certainly was a father involved, he or she also recognizes abandonment by a birth father as well. An adoptive parent could say: *"Your birth father may have been overwhelmed by the situation and thought that he was not entitled to be more involved. He probably thinks about you and wonders about how you are doing."* As with discussions about birth mothers, optimistic yet honest comments about birth fathers are best.

If birth parents were known or suspected to have had challenges such as alcoholism, drug abuse, child abuse, domestic violence, or mental illness, which contributed to child's adoption history, these circumstances need to be discussed and explained in a supportive and realistic way. For example: *"Your parents needed help, but were not getting the help that they needed. As a result, they needed someone else to care for their child."*

E. **Outsiders and adoption.** People may ask personal and at times intrusive questions about adoptive families out of curiosity or because the child looks different from the adoptive parents. Parents should never hide the fact that a child is adopted but should always respect their child's right to privacy with regard to details about birth parents and their child's adoptive circumstances. Private details might include genetic and social history or details that have not yet been shared with the child. Parents may respond by stating: "I prefer not to discuss the details of my child's history because I think it should be his or her choice at an older age as to what information will be shared and with whom."

Parents should also be aware that especially in preschool years, children may "overshare" their adoptive story. As a result, details of their adoptive history that might better not be shared with peers and strangers may best be saved until children better understand the concept of privacy. In the early elementary school years, children with a history of adoption may be teased about being adopted. Parents should prepare their children for that when this happens; it is fine to have a response that puts a positive spin on adoption. For example, children can be coached to say, "Yeah, I'm adopted, so what? So were Presidents Ford and Reagan!"

F. **Searching for birth parents.** Some children and adolescents express an interest in meeting their birth parents, others may only be interested in knowing certain information (such as what they look like). More than 40% of adopted adults report seeking for the identity of their birth parents (known as "adoption search") or seek to locate and meet them (known as "adoption reunion"). In contrast to the fears of many adoptive parents, studies show that following reunions with birth parents, the majority of adopted children/adults report similar or more positive relationships with their adoptive parents. The best time to search for or reunite with birth families is quite controversial, little researched, and may be very different for different children/families. Some experts suggest that searching and meeting with birth family members during childhood or adolescence while residing with adoptive parents can provide a safe environment to make sense of one's adoption story. Others advocate waiting until a young adult is living independently and can process information about their birth family after having become physically independent from their adoptive families.

G. **Special-needs adoptions.** Children categorized as "special needs adoptions" in the United States may have known chronic medical challenges or significant developmental challenges or may be demographically "harder to place" including children from certain minorities, older children, or part of a sibling group. It is imperative that preadoptive counseling for parents adopting older children or sibling groups explore potential challenges and provide resources to family. Adoption agencies and "adoption medicine clinicians" (see AAP Section on Adoption and Foster Care in bibliography) may be particularly helpful in these situations.

H. **Transracial or mixed racial adoption.** In concert with international consensus and children's right advocates, the American Academy of Pediatrics supports children being placed with a family of the same racial and cultural background whenever possible. However, as minorities are over represented in the group of children available for adoption, clearly this is not necessarily realistic. With respect to identity development, between 3 and 7 years of age, children are becoming aware of difference in skin color and racial groupings. Since every child needs a positive sense of racial and ethnic identity, adoptive parents have a responsibility to acquaint a child with his or her heritage and to integrate aspects of the child' heritage into the family's life (e.g., celebrating the holidays of the child's ethnic origin, making foods from the child's country of origin). Positive role models and family friends who share an adopted child's racial and ethnic identity are very helpful in supporting healthy racial identity development for all children including those with a history of transracial adoption.

I. **Open adoption.** "Openness in adoption" occurs along a continuum of information sharing between and in-person meetings with birth and adoptive families prior to and following the adoption of a child. One advantage of openness in adoption is immediate access to information as the child feels a need for it. In some cases, such as significant parental mental illness or active substance use, current research suggests that openness in adoption is associated with long-term positive experiences for adopted individuals as well as their birth and adoptive families.

J. **International adoption.** For several decades prior to 2007, international adoptions to the United States included more than 20,000 children per year. Ninety percent of these children were born in Asia, South America, and Eastern Europe. Given the poor health and economic conditions in most birth countries, many children joined their families following international adoption with treatable or chronic disease, developmental delays, and growth retardation; the American Academy of Pediatrics provides extensive guidance regarding postadoptive screening (see A Healthy Beginning in the bibliography). All medical records must be scrutinized and laboratory tests should be performed in the United States in most situations.

BIBLIOGRAPHY

For parents and professionals

Books

Eldridge S. *Twenty Things Adopted Kids Wish their Adoptive Parents Knew.* New York, NY: Dell Publishing, 1999. (Explores common emotions that adoptees experience through vignettes and case examples. Gives practical advice for helping children to understand and resolve their feelings.)

Pavao JM. *The Family of Adoption.* Boston, MA: Beacon Press, 1998. (An adult adoptee and lifelong therapist working with birth families, adoptive families, and adult adoptees discusses her model of adoption, with the use of anecdotes from her own life and practice. A MUST read for anyone—family, friend or professional—touched by adoption.)

Magazine

Adoptive Families: http://www.adoptivefamilies.com/

Web sites

A Healthy Beginning: Important Information for Parents of International Adopted Children http://www.aap.org/sections/adoption/healthtopic/COECADCBrochure.pdf

American Academy of Pediatrics – Section on Adoption and Foster Care www.aap.org/sections/adoption

U.S. Department of State Office of Children's Issues: http://adoption.state.gov/

The Joint Council on International Children's Services: www.jcics.org

Evan B. Donaldson Adoption Institute: http://www.adoptioninstitute.org/index.php

Organizations

North American Council on Adoptable Children http://www.nacac.org/about/about.html

National Adoption Center http://www.adopt.org/assembled/home.html

For professionals

Albers LH, Barnett EB, Jenisa JA, et al. International adoption: medical and developmental issues. *Pediatr Clin North Am* 52(5):1221–1532, 2005.

American Academy of Pediatrics. Coparent or second-parent adoption by same-sex parents. *Pediatrics* 109(2):339–340, 2002.

American Academy of Pediatrics. Medical evaluation of internationally adopted children for infectious diseases. In Pickering LK, Baker CJ, Kimberlin DW, Long SS (eds). *Report of the Committee on Infectious Diseases* (28th ed).Elk Grove Village, IL: American Academy of Pediatrics, 2009:177–179.

Borchers D and Committee on Early Childhood, Adoption, and Dependent Care. Families and adoption: the pediatrician's role in supporting communication. *Pediatrics* 112(6):1437–1441, 2003.

90

Bereavement and Loss

Benjamin S. Siegel
Maria Trozzi

I. **Description of the problem.** It is estimated that 5% of all children will experience the death of a parent by age 15 years, and 40% of junior and senior high school students have experienced the death of a friend or an acquaintance their age.

   A. **Coping with loss.** The task of children who experience a great loss is to attempt to understand what happened and why the death occurred, to mourn the lost person in their own way and at their level of cognition and affective development, and to construct an enduring inner reality of that lost person and the lost relationship.

   Long-term mental health outcomes of bereaved children are influenced by:
   - The age at which death takes place
   - The person who has died (parent, sibling, friend, or relative)
   - The nature of the relationship between that person and the child
   - The nature of the death (illness, suicide, SIDS, AIDS, murder, accident; was it witnessed by the child)
   - The child's history of losses

   It is useful to divide childhood into four major age categories to understand the child's knowledge of and emotional reaction to death and loss (Table 90-1).

   B. **Communication issues.** Most adults in our culture feel uncomfortable talking with children about death. Death is viewed as outside the normal cycle of life, something to be fought against and to be denied. This attitude is problematic when the adults who are most needed by children are in the midst of their own mourning and grief, so that their grief intensifies when their children question them or discuss the death. Other times, adults may wish to protect children from emotional distress by denying the loss altogether. Well-meaning adults may use euphemisms to explain about death, such as "going to sleep," which may be confusing to children and make them afraid to go to sleep or fearful when a loved one is sleeping.
   - Adults must help children to come to terms with difficult questions: "What is death? Can it happen to me? Can it happen to some other loved one? Am I responsible for the death? Who will take care of me now? Why did the person die? Where is the dead person now? Why won't the dead person come back?"

II. **Role of the primary care clinician.** The primary care clinician, especially one who has had a long-term relationship with the patient and family, is in an excellent position to provide initial counseling and appropriate referral (Table 90-2). Competence in this area requires not only the willingness to explore these issues with families but also an honest appraisal of one's own thoughts and feelings about the meaning of death.

III. **Management.** The most important goal for the clinician is to help the parents address their thoughts and feelings about the loss and to encourage them to be emotionally available to their children. The clinician should encourage the adult caretakers to communicate with the children and remember that accommodation and adaptation to the death of a loved one are a continual process, often lasting a lifetime. Children confront the loss at each stage of development as they gain a greater understanding of the world and themselves, and they experience new feelings at each stage of development. Since it is a developmental process, children grieve *longer* than adults, as they apparently re-grieve at each developmental stage. Clinicians need to remind parents of this phenomenon. Nurturing and support over time by family and friends are the best healing experiences for the bereaved child.

   A. **Very young children (to age 2 years).**
   1. **Encourage parenting figures to provide consistent care in a familiar environment** since children at this age react to death primarily with feelings of separation and loss.
   2. **Familiar toys, appropriate transitional objects, and consistent caretaking are crucial.** Frequently, family members are involved in their own grief and have little energy to spend with the infant or toddler. A close relative or even a babysitter well known to the child could be engaged to provide the support of which others may be incapable.

Table 90-1. Cognitive and affective stages of grief and loss

Age	Cognitive understanding	Emotional/affective	Potential symptoms
Young children less than age 3	Death is separation, abandonment, change	Feelings of loss	Sadness Fearfulness Poor feeding Sleep problems Irritability Developmental delay Regression Increased crying
Preschool (3–6 yr)	Realization that death exists	Guilt (I am responsible)	Delayed grief
Preoperational (prelogical)	Reversibility of death (3–5)	Shame	Enuresis
Magical thinking	Death equals sorrow of others	Fear of punishment because of my thoughts, feelings, and actions	Encopresis
Fantasies	Death is temporary	Fear of catching whatever caused the death	Sleep disturbances
Causation of thought*	Death is catching	Fear of other loved one dying	Nightmares
Egocentric	Fear that sleep = death	Anger at loved one	Temper tantrums
	Loving someone is dangerous	Denial	Hyperactivities
	Dead people still eat and breathe		Loss of control of behavior
School age (6–11 yr)	Death is permanent	Anger, sadness	
Concrete operations (logical)	Death will not happen to me	Guilt	
Problem solving	Biologic understanding of death	Some fear of retribution	Somatic complaints
	Death is universal	Denial	Resistance to going to school
	Dead people do not think, feel		Decreased school performance
	Dead people can sometimes look alive		Inattention, fighting, daydreaming, failure to complete work
			Acting-out behavior
Adolescence (12+ yr)	Death as an inevitable universal process	Strong denial of death	Delinquency
Formal operations (abstract logical)	Death as irreversible	Anger	Drug and alcohol abuse
	Death can happen to me	Guilt	Somatic complaints
	Idealization of dead person	Sadness	Depression
		Embarrassment	Suicide ideation
		Wanting to join loved one	Sexual acting out
			School failure

*The idea that one's thoughts or wishes can cause something to happen.

Table 90-2. Role of primary care clinician

To acknowledge one's own feelings of sadness and loss

To demystify and explain the reasons for death at a level the child can understand

To encourage the child to ask questions and explore his fear and fantasies

To encourage the child to see the body of the person who has died if the child and adults feel comfortable, and to participate in the religious or cultural rituals of grief and mourning as practiced by the family

To explore hidden feelings and memories of the dead person

To explain to parents different stages of cognitive and affective development of children and anticipate specific kinds of grief reactions

To deal with and accept any of the displaced anger family members may have. To monitor the grief reaction and refer for mental health consultation when appropriate

To support the child and family over time

To consult with the school or other community institutions as appropriate

B. **Preschool (ages 3–6).**
1. **The child's understanding.** Since children at this age are egocentric, they believe they may have caused the death. It is important to emphasize that the loved one really has died, that they did not cause the death, and that they will be taken care of. Often children at this age appear not to acknowledge the death. However, their behavior often belies this, as their grief is often expressed through aggressive, mischievous behavior. Sometimes the pain of the loss is simply too great for children to comprehend, and they behave as if nothing has happened. Or they become angry with whomever brought the bad news or angry with family members because they were not strong enough to prevent the death.
2. **Explanations.** Because children at this age believe that death is reversible they may ask such questions as, "When is Daddy coming home?" or questions of bodily functioning, such as, "If Grandma is in the coffin underground, won't she get cold?" or "How will she breathe if she is all covered up?" These questions may be upsetting for grieving adults, who need to be encouraged to be quite direct and honest: *"He is dead. We will never see him again. We are all very sad." "I will try to answer your questions and would like to know what you think or feel when someone dies. I also want you to know that you will be taken care of at all times."* Sometimes referring to a dead pet (if that had been in the child's experience) is a useful way to link the child's past lost to the present. Reading selected stories can also be useful.
3. **Participation in rituals.** The child's participation in rituals can be helpful, *assuming* that the child is able to understand a concrete explanation of the event; e.g., the wake, sitting Shiva, the funeral, a visit to the graveside. The adult should ask the child what he is curious about, as well as what concerns he may have in order to uncover fantasies prior to the child's participation. Children should be accompanied by an empathetic adult who is well known to them and emotionally available to meet their needs. The direct experience about what happens at funerals prevents unrealistic fears and fantasies from developing and enhances long-term adaptation. If a child does not wish to go to the funeral or is overwhelmed by the crowd and the communal grief reaction, special times may be established for later visitation to the funeral home or gravesite. If children choose not to participate, a clear, concrete description of what happened should be provided.

C. **School age (ages 6–12 years).**
1. **The child's understanding.** At this age children can understand biologic functioning. Adults should be encouraged to give more information about the reasons for the death (e.g., *"His body stopped working completely,"* or *"Her heart stopped,"* or *"The lungs no longer worked,"* or *"He died of cancer"*).
2. **Explanations.** Honesty, even about suicide or homicide, usually facilitates long-term adaptation. Explanations regarding what will remain the same, and what will be different as a result of this death, can be particularly useful. Some children may require more detailed explanations, regarding both the death as well as what will happen to the person's body after death. Let the child lead the discussion. Questions such as *"What do you know?"* or *"Tell me what you think happened,"* are helpful.

3. **Grieving.** Parents should be encouraged to acknowledge their emotions to their children and give their children permission to express their own feelings. Grieving of parents and children may be dyssynchronous. The child's grief reaction may appear just at the time that adults are getting over the acute mourning stage.

4. **Participation in rituals.** Children at this age should be encouraged to participate in all formal events, such as funeral services, burial services, memorial services, and other rituals dictated by religion or culture. The child needs an empathic person present and should not be forced to participate if he does not wish to.

D. **Adolescence.**

1. **The adolescent's understanding.** Adolescents understand death as adults do; however, they are new to the philosophical "why's" involved in any death. Although they have a mature understanding of death, they fantasize about their own immortality and may engage in risk-taking behavior, as though they are invincible to death. Many choose to create their own rituals with their peers in addition to/instead of participating in traditional rituals.

2. **Adolescents can sometimes harbor guilt** that they may have been responsible for the death.

3. Peer relationships are very strong and **adolescents often prefer to be with their friends** rather than family members. The death of a peer may shatter their fantasies of immortality and their grief reaction often appears excessive to adults. Denial of their feeling from adults in their lives may prolong their grief reaction.

4. **Sometimes they develop idealized images of the loved one, occasionally want to "join" the loved one,** and have thoughts of suicide. Although suicidal ideation is a common symptom in bereaved adolescents, it is rare for adolescents actually to attempt suicide.

E. **School.** The school is a natural environment for groups of children to face the death of a teacher or classmate. Trained teachers, who already know the students, have an increased capacity to assist them with the tasks of mourning: understanding, grieving, commemorating, and moving on. The school itself naturally creates a safe, structured environment for teachers to model their own grief response, normalize individual grief reactions, particularly when the death is stigmatic, and assist students who choose to informally commemorate through activities; such as planting a tree, drawing pictures, making a memory book, talking about the "friend" who dies. As school resumes its regular activities, counselors should be sensitive to those youngsters who require a professional referral. When a youngster returns to school after a death in his family, his teacher should be informed so that she can facilitate the child's return. Again, the classroom setting provides an inclusive environment for strengthening and mastering the coping skills required to face future losses.

F. **Support Groups.**

Grief isolates. A child whose parent or sibling has recently died often experiences a difficult adjustment as s/he creates a 'new normal' without that loved one. Support groups can mitigate the isolation that children experience.

A good child bereavement support program will group children by their age/stage; for example, a group for children ages 5–8 and another for children ages 9–13 years. Children under the age of five are not likely to benefit from the psycho-educational activities that further a child's accomplishing the four psychological tasks of understanding what happened, grieving, commemorating and adapting the loss within the context of the child's life. Likewise, teen groups are often successful when facilitated in the school context.

Bereavement camps accomplish a similar purpose. While engaging children and adolescents in fun, camp-like activities, the camp agenda sets aside times to discuss, share, do psycho-therapeutic art projects, etc. Just knowing that every camper has suffered a loss of a parent or sibling mitigates the isolation that is the hallmark of loss.

IV. **Criteria for referral.** In order to help the child and the family, time needs to be set aside to address many of the issues mentioned. Some primary care clinicians feel that their role is to obtain a history and to refer to a mental health clinician. Others, especially if there has been an ongoing relationship and they enjoy the role of counseling and education, can use that relationship to address immediate issues of grief and follow the child and family through the grief process. After the initial consultation at the time of the death, a 2- to 4-week and 4- to 6-month follow-up consultation are appropriate. A mental health referral is advisable when the clinician feels uncomfortable by the feelings or generated during the consultation. Other reasonable criteria include distress for more than 6 months; intense, inconsolable grief; and poor functioning at home, in school, or with peers.

BIBLIOGRAPHY

For children

Books for ages 3–6 (preschool)

Brown L, Brown M. *When Dinosaurs Die: A Guide to Understanding Death*. Boston: Little, Brown, 1996.

Brown M. *The Dead Bird*. New York: Dell, 1939.

Bryan M, Ingpen R. *Lifetimes: The Beautiful Way to Explain Death to Children*. New York: Bantam Books, 1983.

Clifton L. *Everett Anderson's Goodbye*. New York: Holt, 1983.

Cohen M. *Jim's Dog Muffins*. New York: Greenwillow, 1984.

Cohn J. *I Have a Friend Named Peter*. New York: William Morrow, 1987.

de Paola T. *Nana Upstairs and Nana Downstairs*. New York, NY: Penguin Books, 1978.

Johnston T. *Day of the Dead*. New York: Harcourt, Inc., 1997.

Kohlenberg S. *Sammy's Mommy Has Cancer*. New York: Imagination Press, 1993.

Lanton S. *Daddy's Chair*. Rockville, MD: Kar-Ben Copies, 1991.

Rogers F. *When a Pet Dies*. New York: Putnam & Sons, 1988.

Thomas P. *I Miss You (A First Look at Death)*. New York: Barrons, 2000.

Vigna J. *Saying Goodbye to Daddy*. Morton Grove, Ill.: Albert Whitman and Co., 1991.

Viorst J. *The Tenth Good Thing About Barney*. New York: Atheneum, 1971.

Wilhelm H. *I'll always Love You*. New York: Crown Publishers, 1985.

Wintrop E. *Promises*. New York: Clarion Books, 2000.

Books for ages 6–9

(Many of the above books are also appropriate)

Alexander A. *A Mural for Mamita*. Omaha, NE: Centering Corp., 2002.

Alexander A. *Sunflowers & Rainbows for Tia – Saying Good-bye to Daddy*. Omaha, NE: Centering Corp., 1999.

Bahr M. *If Nathan Were Here*. Grand Rapids, MI: Eerdman Books, 2000.

Egger B. *Marianne's Grandmother*. New York: E.P. Dutton, 1978.

Girard L. *Alex, the Kid with AIDS*. Morton Grove, Ill.: Albert Whitman and Co., 1991.

Jukes M. *Blackberries in the Dark*. New York: Knopf, 1985.

Machenski M. *Some of the Pieces*. Boston: Little, Brown, 1991.

Miles M. *Annie and the Old One*. Boston: Little, Brown, 1971.

Powell S. *Geranium Morning*. Minneapolis: Carol Rhoda Books, 1990.

Schwiebert P, DeKlyen C. *Tear Soup*. Portland, OR: Grief Watch, 1999.

Sims A. *Am I Still a Sister?* Albuquerque, N.M.: Big A and Co., 1986.

Tiffault B. *A Quilt for Elisabeth*. Omaha, NE: Centering Corp., 1992.

White EB. *Charlotte's Web*. New York: Harper, 1952.

Books for ages 9–12 (preadolescents)

Aub K. *Children Are Survivors Too*. Boca Raton, FL: Grief Education Enterprises, 1995.

Baur MD. *On My Honor*. New York: Bantam Doubleday, 1986.

Creech S. *Walk Two Moons by*. New York: Harper Collins, 1994.

Krementz J. *How It Feels When A Parent Dies*. New York: Knopf, 1983.

Krementz J. *How It Feels When Parents Divorce*. New York: Knopf, 1988.

Lowry L. *A Summer to Die*. New York: Bantam, 1970.

Mann P. *There Are Two Kinds of Terrible*. New York: Avon, 1979.

Park B. *Mick Harte Was Here*. New York: Scholastic Inc., 1995.

Paterson K. *Bridge to Terebithia*. New York: Harper and Row, 1977.

Smith D. *A Taste of Blackberries*. New York: Crowell, 1973.

Books for ages 13+ (adolescents)

Agee J. *A Death in the Family*. New York: Grosset & Dunlap, 1938.

Blume J. *Tiger Eyes*. New York: Macmillan, 1981.

Dower L. *I Will Remember You*. New York: Scholastic Inc., 2001.

Fitzgerald H. *The Grieving Teen*. New York: Simon & Schuster, 2000.

Gravelle K. *Teenagers Face to Face with Bereavement*. New York: Messner, 1989.

Grollman E, Malikow M. *Living When a Young Friend Commits Suicide*. Boston: Beacon Press, 1999.

Grollman E. *Straight Talk About Death for Teenagers*. Boston: Beacon Press, 1993.

Guest J. *Ordinary People*. New York: Ballentine Books, 1976.

LeShan E. *Learning to Say Good-Bye When a Parent Dies*. New York: Macmillan, 1975.

Richter E. *Losing Someone You Love: When a Brother or Sister Dies.* New York: Putnam, 1986.
Scrivani M. *When Death Walks In.* Omaha, NE: Centering Corp., 1991.
Shakespeare W. *Romeo and Juliet. [Various editions.]*

For parents and adults

Gravelle K. *Teenagers: Face to Face With Bereavement.* Messner: New York. 1989.
Grollman E (ed). *Bereaved Children and Teens.* Boston, MA: Beacon Press, 1995.
Grollman EA. *Talking about Death. A Dialogue Between Parents and Child* (3rd ed), Boston: Beacon Press, 1990.
Kubler-Ross E. *On Children and Death.* New York: Macmillan, 1983.
Rando T. *How To Go On Living When Someone You Love Has Died.* New York: Bantam Books, 1991.
Ross EK. *On Children and Death,* (Reprint edition) New York: Scribner 1997.
Trozzi M, Massimini K. *Talking with Children About Loss: Words, Strategies and Wisdom to Help Children Cope with Death, Divorce and Other Difficult Times.* New York: Penguin Putnam, 1999.

For professionals

Committee on Psychosocial Aspects of Child and Family Health. The pediatrician and childhood bereavement. *Pediatrics* 89:516–518, 1992.
Siegel B. Helping children cope with death. *Am Fam Physician* 31:175, 1985.

Web sites

Centering Corporation: www.centering.org
Crisis, Grief, and Healing (links to hundreds of online resources): www.webhealing.com
The Good Grief Program of Boston Medical Center: http://www.bmc.org/pediatrics-goodgrief.htm
Grief Watch: www.griefwatch.com
Bereavement Camp for Children: www.comfortzonecamp.org

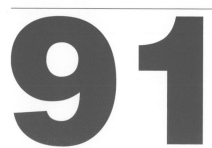

Bilingualism

Naomi Steiner

I. **Description and definition.**
   A. **The importance of foreign language mastery is being increasingly recognized** in the global economy.
   B. **Bilingualism** is the mastery of two languages, and encompasses different levels of proficiency as follows:
      1. **Level 1: Ability to understand a second language (passive bilingualism).** Children who are learning a second language often understand the language before they can speak it.
      2. **Level 2: Ability to speak a second language fluently.**
      3. **Level 3: Ability to read and write in two languages (biliteracy).**
         Each level should be considered as **a stepping stone** to the next. So that a child who has level 1 passive understanding can quite rapidly with increased exposure attain level 2 and start speaking the language. For instance if a child speaks with her parents in English, but understands her parents and grandparents speaking Spanish together, she could rapidly start speaking in Spanish if placed in a Spanish-speaking only child care.
         Parents should expect that a child will have a **dominant language,** which is the stronger and mostly used language, along with a weaker and less used language. **Balanced bilingualism,** which is high proficiency in two languages, is the exception rather than the rule. The dominant language can flip throughout childhood as quantity of exposure between the languages also shifts. This often happens at preschool or kindergarten entry when English starts to develop more rapidly and becomes the dominant language.
II. **Epidemiology.**
   A. **The National U.S. Census 2000** shows that 18% of people living in the United States speak a language other than English at home. After English, Spanish is the most frequently spoken language in the United States with 28 million speakers, followed by Chinese (2.0 million speakers), and then French (1.6 million speakers).
   B. **Worldwide** there are more bilinguals than monolinguals. Bilingualism is the norm.
III. **Learning theory.**
   A. **What affects the proficiency level of language in bilingualism?** In order of importance:
      1. **Priority placed by the family to raise a bilingual child,** which may not be related to the parents' own level of proficiency in the second language. As children grow older, it is important for parents to affirm their beliefs and to discuss this with their children.
      2. **Consistency and amount of exposure.**
      3. **Child's attitude towards language learning and speaking another language,** which includes temperament and is also affected by family dynamics.
      4. **Ability towards learning foreign languages.**
   B. **Second language development and the brain.**
      1. How children develop separate language systems in order to master expression in one language versus the other is a matter of debate. However, most scientists agree that **language functions of both languages are more intertwined than previously thought.**
         • As children learn language concepts in one language (such as the concept of plurals) the **theory of transfer,** explains that they then do not have to be re-learnt in the other; rather this knowledge can be transferred directly from one language to another.
         • The **theory of suppression** describes how a bilingual person is constantly suppressing one language in order to speak the other. Bilinguals are constantly flipping between two languages.

2. **Bilingualism is considered a natural ability.** Children do not need to have above average intelligence to become bilingual. All typically developing children can become bilingual. Babies are able to learn sounds from all languages, and can tell the difference between two languages within a few months of age. The brain is primed to learn more than one language.

3. **Supporting second language development.**
   - **The earlier the better.** It seems common sense that learning a second language takes years, so it is better to start early. However, from a neurological perspective, the younger brain is more plastic and better able to adapt to a new language environment and learn a second language. Scientists believe that the younger brain requires less language input to learn the second language. **There is no critical period.** False beliefs around second language learning relate that after a certain age it is impossible to learn another language. This misconception comes from the fact that around puberty one should not expect to learn to speak a new language with a native-like accent. However, there is more to language learning than the accent, such as the vocabulary, expression, and understanding of the language. So, it is more exact to say that a child's brain will adapt to her environment, and that there will be a gradual decline over the span of a lifetime. Adults too can learn a foreign language.
   - **The greater the language input the faster the acquisition and the greater the language proficiency.**
   - Contrary to the myth, **children do not learn languages "like a sponge."** They require **ongoing quality language input in both languages in order to become bilingual**. The ultimate proficiency level will depend on the level of the language exposure. Children who receive poor language input in their heritage language and have difficulty learning English at school are at **risk of developing poor language proficiency in both languages.**
   - **Consistency of language input should be the goal.** This leads to increased input and to success. The **One Parent One Language (OPOL)** approach is when each parent chooses in which language they are going to speak to their children and stick to it. Parents can either both speak the same language to their children or speak in different languages, *but they should always stick to that language.* This method is highly successful towards raising a bilingual child, because it guarantees ongoing consistency and ongoing language input. Additional support comes when grandparents or other extended family members or caretakers also speak with the child a fixed language.
   - **The brain is able to learn from different sources.** For some parents the OPOL approach does not fit their family dynamic. These parents should know that the child's brain can successfully learn languages even if they are exposed in a more scattered way, though the consistency will probably be decreased and therefore the level of proficiency also.
   - **Use it or lose it.** As many adults have experienced, it requires ongoing language input to maintain a language. If the exposure stops, the language fades rapidly. This is what often happens when children from expatriate families return to the United States. Families should be encouraged to make plans to keep up the language even before returning, such as buying books, DVDs, and other materials that would be needed.
   - **Monolingual parents can raise a bilingual child.** Monolingual parents are a new force in the United States interested in raising their children bilingual. Monolingual parents often feel that schools do not prioritize foreign or world language curricula, and that their children will be at a disadvantage in the global world. Monolingual parents might have minimal language proficiency, such as high school remnants, yet they can learn a language along with their children. When children are young, this technique can be very successful. Later as children progress to higher levels, they will usually need increased outside support, such as Saturday language school, or a tutor.
   - **Children will mix both languages as they learn them.** Being raised bilingual follows a developmental course, where children will use one language, usually the dominant one, to support expressive fluency in the other as they strive to communicate in a language that they might not fully master. This does not mean to say they are confused; they are not. In fact, children even very young will not speak to someone in a language that they have not heard them use. Facts to keep in mind about mixing of languages are the following:

(1) **When parents mix children mix.**
(2) **Parents mix even if they do not think that they are mixing.**
(3) **Parents should try their best to speak only one language.** In this manner children have the opportunity to extend their vocabulary and the complexity of their sentence structure in that language.

- There is no scientific evidence that bilingualism leads to language delay. However, because speech and language delay is the most prevalent developmental condition in early childhood (incidence 5%–10%), bilingual children will also present with language delay.

IV. **Risks and advantages of bilingualism.**
   A. **Risks.**
      1. **Poor language development in both languages.** Continued input in both languages is necessary for a child to be raised bilingual. Many children who have just arrived in the United States are struggling at school to progress in English as well as academically. Additionally their home environment might not offer high level language input in their heritage language. These children are at risk of limited bilingualism, when a child fails to progress and attain native-like proficiency in either language.
      - **The expressive language debate.** Recent research suggests that bilingual children might learn words at a slower pace than monolingual children. When each of the languages of the bilingual child is considered separately, vocabulary in each language will develop slower in bilingual children compared to monolingual children. However, total combined vocabulary from both languages in the bilingual child compares similarly to the vocabulary of the monolingual child. Recent studies also suggest that bilinguals might have decreased verbal fluency.
   B. **Benefits.** Constant shifting between languages is suggested to explain the possible decreased verbal fluency, but also the numerous advantages of the bilingual brain. Bilingual children are constantly trying to figure out what different words mean, to explain sentences even if they might not fully understand all the content, and to figure out language. Recent studies in bilingual infants point towards a more flexible brain, primed to learn new information, as compared to monolinguals.
      - **Language benefits.** Compared to monolinguals, bilingual children show increased phonemic awareness. Phonemic awareness is the ability to breakdown words into sounds and is a precursor for reading and writing.
      - **Academic benefits.** Bilinguals show increased ability in math, to understand how language works, and to figure out what words mean.
      - **Other cognitive advantages** include benefits in abstract thinking, grasping rules, processing information, creativity, and cognitive flexibility towards learning new information.
      - **Cultural advantage.** Bilingual children describe themselves as a "bridge between two cultures." They have enhanced cultural awareness, which is important in this global world.

V. **Making the diagnosis of speech and language delay in a bilingual child.**
   A. **Understand that in general bilingualism is both under-referred and misunderstood.** Professionals that the pediatric clinician might typically reach out to for support with a language question, such as speech and language therapists, might not be trained in the area of bilingualism. Teaching staff in schools is also often poorly equipped to guide families and practitioners. Therefore, professionals might give well-meant, however, incorrect advice to parents, and do not take into consideration the long-term bilingual goals of parents.
   B. When faced with a bilingual child who presents with possible language delay, "following the process" will help you take steps towards decision making.
      1. **Take a history** of the child's language milestones and languages spoken at home. Do not assume that a child is being raised bilingual.
      2. **Take advantage of the many questionnaires that have been translated into other languages.** Examples of questionnaires in Spanish include the PEDS (Parents' Evaluation of Developmental Status), Ages and Stages, and the M-CHAT (Modified Checklist for Autism in Toddlers).
      3. **Observe and interact with the child even if he is speaking another language.** Do not be intimidated by a child or family speaking another language, attempt to interact with the child, or ask the parent to converse with the child. Use a trained interpreter or ask the parent to translate as well as she can.
   C. **Speech and language assessments.** The golden standard for a speech and language assessment in a bilingual child is a bilingual speech and language assessment by a speech and language pathologist who can assess both of the languages that the child speaks. However, this could lead to significant delay in the assessment. Therefore, realistically the

bilingual child should be referred to a speech and language pathologist with experience in working with bilingual children. Not all speech and language pathologists have training or experience with bilingual children, so it is good for practitioners to have a list at hand.

   D. Speech and language therapy can be delivered in English because of transfer. Transfer is the ability of the brain to learn a language concept in one language and use it in the other.

VI. From birth to graduation: fostering the heritage or second language learning in your practice.

   A. Discuss bilingualism, starting at the prenatal visit or at birth. Though parents want to transmit their language, they might not feel that their language is valued or would make a difference for their child. The pediatric clinician is in a unique position to answer questions at birth or during a prenatal visit. This is a window of opportunity, because starting to speak two languages at birth is the easiest way for parents. Starting to raise a child bilingual can happen at any age, however, the transition requires an increased effort for the parents and should be done in an incremental way.

   B. Recognize that the decision to raise a child bilingual often feels overwhelming to parents who might strive towards perfection. **Parents raising a bilingual child usually have questions.** Clinicians can explain that all levels of bilingualism are stepping stones to the next level. This reassures parents and validates their efforts.

   C. Because of the risk of limited bilingualism, **language enhancement should be raised at each surveillance visit** of a child being raised bilingual. This translates into proactively speaking to parents about how to booster language, such as through reading out loud, head start, library visits. Parents who *successfully* raise bilingual children usually have a supportive community of friends and/or family and are constantly searching for materials in their language in order to ensure a language-rich environment at home.

   D. Around preschool or kindergarten entry, parents often wonder if they should switch from speaking their heritage language to English. **There is no evidence that dropping the heritage language and switching to English is going to speed up the English language learning.** On the contrary, parents should not speak to their children in broken language, which transmits poor vocabulary and grammar to their children. **Parents should speak in a language in which they are fluent** to their children, in order to assure continued progress in higher language skills. Because of transfer, strong language skills in the heritage language will support the learning of English. Additionally, children need strong language skills in order to develop and discuss ideas and concepts. Strong heritage language skills enable continued higher level thought process in a child who is an English Language Learner (ELL).

   E. Children will typically want parents to speak with them in English around kindergarten age. If parents feel strongly about transmitting their heritage language or a second language they should follow their convictions. They can enhance their success by explaining to their children why it is so important for them all in continuing to speak to them in their language and requesting response back in their language.

   F. Consistency of input is key, so that the OPOL should be seriously considered, if raising a child bilingual is a priority for a family.

   G. As children enter school, a third language option is usually offered at school. Parents should know that not only bilingual children "still have enough space" in the brain for another language but that bilingual children **learn their third language with greater ease than monolingual children learn their second.**

   H. Children with learning disabilities can learn a second language too. Because of logistics, children with learning disabilities are often scheduled for academic support during foreign/world language classes. Monolingual parents are often concerned about this because of the importance of foreign/world language mastery in the global world. There is no "brain" reason why children with learning disabilities should not learn a second language, though they might require accommodations (which they require for their other subjects too), thus giving them the opportunity too to be included in the classroom and progress in this important area of development.

BIBLIOGRAPHY

For parents

Steiner NJ, Hayes SL. *7 Steps to Raising a Bilingual Child*. NY, NY: Amacom, 2008.
Harding-Esch E, Riley P. *A Bilingual Family: a Handbook for Parents*. Cambridge, England: Cambridge University Press, 2003.

Web sites

www.spanglishbaby.com
www.bilingualfamiliesconnect.com

For teachers

Center for Applied Linguistics. Ellis R. Principles of Instructed Second Language Acquisition. http://www.cal.org/resources/Digest/digest_pdfs/Instructed2ndLangFinalWeb.pdf
ERIC Digest. A Global Perspective on Bilingualism and Bilingual Education. http://www.eric.ed.gov/ERICDocs/data/ericdocs2sql/content_storage_01/0000019b/80/15/eb/59.pdf
Baker C. *Foundations of Bilingual Education and Bilingualism*. Bristol, UK: Multilingual Matters, 2006.

For professionals

Bialystok E. *Bilingualism in Development: Language, Literacy, and Cognition*. Cambridge University Press, 2001.
Bialystok E, Hakuta K, Wiley E. Critical Evidence: a test of the critical period hypothesis of second-language learning. *Psychol Sci*. Cambridge, England: Oxford University Press, 14:31–38, 2003.
Lesaux NK, Siegel LS. The development of reading in children who speak English as a second language. *Dev Psychol* 39(6):1005–1019, 2003.
Kroll JF, De Groot AMB. *Handbook of Bilingualism: Psycholinguistic Approaches*. Oxford Press, 2005.

92

Child Care

Margot Kaplan-Sanoff
Wilhelmina Hernandez

I. **Description.** For a majority of today's young children, spending time in the care of someone other than a parent is now part of their daily life experience. Second only to the immediate family, child care has become the context in which early development unfolds. Coupled with the growing body of research suggesting that early childhood experiences play a significant role in shaping future life outcomes, child care serves as an important arena for addressing the diverse needs of children and parents and for promulgating public policy and advocacy initiatives. Given the diverse work hours and shift patterns of working parents, child care is not just "day" care, and it is not just "care." Quality child care provides nurturance and support for enhancing child development and learning, in addition to offering services for families, including parent support and education, poverty reduction through vouchers allowing families to return to school or work, and respite care for child welfare cases. While state child care regulations often mandate minimal involvement from pediatrics, the opportunity for powerful and meaningful collaboration between child care and pediatric care is enormous.

A. **Epidemiology.**
- More than 20 million families in the United States have either a single working parent or two working parents and, as a result, rely on some form of nonparental child care; 11.3 million children younger than 5 years need care while their parents are at work. Yet, child care costs continue to rise and, for many families, child care has become their second largest expense, surpassed only by housing.
- Sixty-one percent of children younger than 6 years have parents in the labor force, and 73% of these children are cared for by someone other than a parent.
- Children are enrolled in child care very early in life; the average age of entry into care is 3.31 years for an average of 30 hours a week of care and 1.7 million infants younger than 1 years are currently in child care.

B. **Types of care.** The term *child care* has come to represent a wide variety of options from a quality developmental program for children to a basic support service for working parents. Within this spectrum, child care programs can be for-profit or nonprofit, faith-based or nondenominational, company-based or employer-supported/affiliated, private or public. Most child care options fall into the following major categories:
1. **Home-based care.** This category includes care either in the home of the child or in the home of the caregiver, where the care is provided by relatives or nonrelatives.
   a. **In-home care.** This type of care involves a caregiver, such as a relative, babysitter, or nanny, coming to or living in the child's home. Such an arrangement can be costly but does offer children the familiarity of their home environment, as well as added convenience and flexibility for parents, especially those working long hours or variable workday schedules. Approximately 4% of children younger than 5 years are currently in-home child care while their parents work.
   b. **Family child care.** Family child care is care provided in someone else's home. According to the National Association for Family Child Care (NAFCC), there are approximately 1 million family child care providers providing care for 4 million children in the United States. For regulation purposes, family-based care is subcategorized into small (less than seven children) and large (seven or more children). Many parents are attracted to the home-like atmosphere and the potential for close bonding with a single child care provider that family-based care offers. Family-based care may offer greater flexibility in hours and be less expensive than center-based care but can also be less reliable when the caregiver becomes ill or goes on vacation. Provider training and credentials/certification, as well as program quality, is regulated by individual states and thus tends to be far more variable than center-based care. While most family child care homes are licensed by the state, there exists an "underground" network of unlicensed family child care homes that do not comply with any state health, safety, or educational standards.

Approximately 7% of children younger than 5 years are currently in family child care while their parents work.

2. **Center-based care.** *Center-based child care* refers to care provided in a nonresidential facility. For regulation purposes, it also includes residential-based, family child care facilities that serve more than 12 children. Center-based programs include nursery/preschools, child care centers, prekindergarten programs, church-based centers, and Early Head Start/Head Start programs. While most programs are open year-round and are licensed by the state, center-based child care offers less flexible hours, is more expensive than family child care, and may provide less opportunity for close bonding with caregivers because of large class sizes, changing classrooms, and high staff turnover. On the positive side, centers often attract high-quality, well-trained teachers who provide a stimulating curriculum and learning environment for young children, allowing children the opportunity to interact with a greater number of peers. Finally, center-based programs have many adults and parents who can observe the program and individual interactions between children and between children and staff, offering parents additional sets of eyes on their child's safety and well-being. A majority (60%) of the 3- to 5-year-olds in child care are enrolled in some form of center-based care.

3. **School-aged care.** Included in this category are before- and after-school programs and vacation programs. School-aged child care settings include both school-based facilities and other community locations. They offer an alternative to unsupervised after-school time and provide children with the opportunity to interact with peers, but they introduce added cost, their structure can be quite variable, and not all programs are regulated.

C. **Ratios, licensure, and accreditation**
1. **Ratios.** Although not a guarantee of quality, lower child to staff ratios, as well as total group size, have been deemed to be very important indicators in the setting of national standards for quality child care. Research indicates that child–provider ratio is the most sensitive indicator of quality care. (See Table 92-1 for child–provider ratios.)

2. **Licensure.** Regulated by state agencies, licensure of child care programs and certification of child care providers can vary significantly from state to state. Criteria for licensure typically include standards relating to child to staff ratios, staff qualifications and training, supervision and discipline, administration of medication, emergency planning, and hand-washing and diapering procedures. In some states, certain types of care (such as faith-based, school-aged, or summer programs) may be exempt.

3. **Accreditation.** Some child care programs voluntarily undergo a process of accreditation to demonstrate their commitment to and delivery of quality child care above and beyond what is required for licensure. Accreditation offers parents and caregivers a useful way to assess quality, and the process of attaining and maintaining accreditation may actually improve quality of care and increase professionalism. There are 7170 programs serving 667,728 children currently accredited by the National Association for Early Childhood Education. Once approved, accreditation is granted for 5 years. Organizations such as the NAFCC have also developed quality standards for family care accreditation.

II. **Role of the clinician.**
A. **Parental support and guidance.** Although 79% of pediatric clinicians have reported that they want to be involved in child care decisions made by the families in their care, only 32%

Table 92-1. Recommended child to adult ratio and group size for large family child home care and centers

Age	Child to staff ratio	Maximum group size
Birth–12 mo	3:1	6
13–30 mo	4:1	8
31–35 mo	5:1	10
3 years olds	7:1	14
4–5 years olds	8:1	16
6–8 years olds	10:1	20
9–12 years olds	12:1	24

American Public Health Association and American Academy of Pediatrics. *Caring for Our Children: Guidelines for Out-of-Home Child Care Programs, a Collaborative Project.* Copyright 2002 by the American Public Health Association, the American Academy of Pediatrics, and The National Resource Center for Health and Safety in Child Care.

Note: Group size refers to number of children in a room or other well-defined space.

actually offered parents resources and information on the subject. Pediatric clinicians should be willing and able to discuss a family's child care options and arrangements, address any concerns that might arise, and offer guidance on how to find safe, affordable, child care that is developmentally, educationally, and nutritionally sound. Table 92-2 offers a list of potential factors that parents should consider when deciding on the best child care option for their family. The following is a sample list of some of the key questions that pediatric clinicians can discuss with parents to guide them in their search for quality child care:

1. *"Is it a stimulating and nurturing environment?"* Parents must feel comfortable that the caregiver(s) they choose is caring and able to provide a nurturing environment. Parents should be encouraged to ask about licensure and accreditation, the training and experience of the staff, the rate of turnover, and references. In addition, parents should look for child care programs that exceed ratio requirements, that are structured so that children can bond either with a single caregiver or with only a few primary caregivers, that have established routines that still allow for appropriate exploration, that have adequate time, space, and supplies for age-appropriate play, and use appropriate discipline techniques with which the parents are comfortable. Recommendations—whether from a child care referral agency, other parents, or a clinician—can help parents feel more secure in their decision.

2. *"Is it safe?"* The Consumer Product Safety Commission, which has studied the prevalence of potential safety hazards in child care, recommends that parents assess for several specific areas of risk, including:
   - Appropriate sleep position, with infants placed on their backs
   - Crib safety, that is, no soft bedding, pillows, or comforters
   - Play area safety, that is, surfacing made of safe materials and well maintained; toys of appropriate size according to the age of children; clean, uncluttered space for infants to explore
   - Large furniture securely attached to floor or walls to avoid falling on children
   - Windows, blinds, and doors should be safely secured
   - Safety gates properly installed and used

3. *"Does it fit the family's financial and scheduling limitations?"* The quality of child care programs is quite often directly correlated with expense, and parents should consider how much they are willing and/or able to pay. Location and accessibility to work or home factor into many parents' selection, and scheduling considerations should also be taken into account—ask about earliest drop-off and latest pick-up times, vacation time and holiday programs (as well as whether or not parents must pay extra for them), summer-time program schedules, and part-time options.

B. **Provide health consultation.** In some states, the affiliation of child care programs with a health consultant is mandated. The national standard is for center-based child care facilities to be visited by a healthcare professional at least monthly, with all others to receive quarterly visits. By establishing relationships with child care providers, either informally or in the role of an official health consultant, pediatric clinicians can help to improve and ensure the health, safety, and quality of care for young children. Child care providers and the families utilizing child care can benefit from such basic contributions from pediatric clinicians as the dissemination of accurate health and medical information, the appropriate administration of commonly used medications, principles of first aid, cardiopulmonary resuscitation (CPR), safety and injury prevention, and discussion of special care plans for children with special health needs. The publication *Caring for Our Children National: Health and Safety Performance Standard: Guidelines for Out-of-Home Child Care Programs, 2nd Edition,* consists of national child care health and safety standards that are endorsed by the American Academy of Pediatrics.

C. **Advocacy.** Involvement by pediatric clinicians at the local, state, or national level can help effect change in areas such as access to quality care and the establishment and/or enforcement of healthy and safe standards of care.

III. **Common issues in child care.**

A. **Communicable diseases.** Attending a child care program has been implicated as a cause of more frequent illnesses in early childhood. Anecdotal evidence from clinicians and parents suggests that while children attending preschool programs do tend to get sicker more often, they are less vulnerable to typical childhood illnesses later in elementary school, having already been exposed to these diseases in child care. Pediatric clinicians can counsel parents and providers on the prevalence, methods of prevention, and appropriate management of commonplace childhood. "Universal precautions" with good hygiene and infection control measures—particularly as it pertains to diaper-changing,

Table 92-2. Questions when selecting child care

- **Licensing/accreditation:** Is the home or facility licensed or registered with the appropriate local government agency? Are there any outstanding violations? Is the program accredited by a nationally recognized professional child care association such as the National Association for Family Child Care or the National Association for the Education of Young Children?
- **Location:** Is it located close to your home or work? Can you get there quickly in case of emergency?
- **Accessibility:** Can you visit the center before your child is enrolled? Does the provider welcome parent visits during normal operating hours, including after enrollment? Can you see all the areas that your child will use? Are visitors screened or is their identification checked so that only approved adults can visit the center and pick up children?
- **Hours of operation:** Do the hours of care fit your needs given your schedule? What is their policy regarding parents who are late picking up their children?
- **Communication:** Do you have access to the caregiver during the day or by phone/e-mail on a regular basis? Can you talk with staff on a regular basis? If there was something sensitive you needed to bring up, would you feel comfortable talking to them?
- **Staff experience and training:** Are the caregivers trained and experienced? What is the caregiver's educational and professional background? What type of additional training has the staff had during the past year? Has staff received any outside training from qualified experts in the past year? Is CPR/first aid training required of the staff? Do they conduct CORI checks on all staff members prior to employment?
- **Adequate staffing ratio:** Do the child–staff ratios and the size of the groups of children fall within nationally recognized standards? Are there enough trained adults available on a regular basis? What happens if staff members are ill or on vacation? Are there enough permanent staff members per number of children so that staffing is sufficient to cover those absences? Are children supervised by sight and sound at all times, even when they are sleeping?
- **Quality:** Are children cared for in small groups? Do the children in the program seek out the staff when they are upset? Does the staff talk to the children throughout the day? Is there a daily schedule? Is there daily indoor and outdoor play time? If children can watch TV, what is watched and for how long?
- **Curriculum:** Are there age- and developmentally appropriate activities for your child? Are there books available for the children to look at throughout the day? Are there quiet and noisy play areas? Does the staff screen children's development on a regular basis?
- **Policies:** Check the center's written policies. Are the program's policies on meals, napping, and issues such as toilet training the same as yours? What is the discipline policy? Do they have all infants sleeping on their backs? Do the children go on outings? If they travel by car, van, or bus, are the proper child safety seats, booster seats, and seat belts used? Is there someone besides the driver supervising the children during transport?
- **Illness:** What is the sick child policy? What are the policies when children are mildly ill? Are the center's policies available in writing, and are they consistent with your own? When your child becomes sick in child care, will you be notified in a timely manner?
- **Healthcare:** Does the program have a qualified healthcare professional such as a doctor or a nurse who serves as a consultant? Do children need a medical examination before they can enroll? Have staff members been checked by a doctor to be sure that they are healthy?
- **Cleanliness:** Are there sinks in every room, and are there separate sinks for preparing food and washing hands? Are children and staff instructed to wash their hands throughout the day? Are the toilets and sinks clean and readily available for the children and staff? Are disposable paper towels provided so that each youngster will use only his own towel and not share with others? Are the child care rooms and equipment cleaned and disinfected at least once a day? Are toys that infants and toddlers put in their mouths sanitized before others can play with them?
- **Nutrition:** Does the program provide healthy snacks? Do they provide nutritious lunch or does the parent provide the child's food? How is the food heated? Do they have a plan for food allergies, especially nuts? Is food handled in areas separate from the toilets and diaper-changing tables?
- **Breast/bottle-feeding:** How do they support breast-feeding mothers? Is breast milk labeled and stored correctly? How are bottles warmed? What is the policy on when children can have their bottle? Do they provide juice, water, formula, or does the parent bring it in daily?
- **Fees and services:** What is the cost? How are payments made? Are there other services available in addition to child care? Do these services cost extra?
- **Backup plans:** What happens if your child is sick or the child care program is closed?
- **References:** Ask for references and contact information from parents who use the program, as well as at least 1 parent whose child was in the program during the past year.

hand-washing, and food handling—should be reinforced for child care providers. Written explanations or instructions regarding specific illnesses and medication administration are helpful for child care providers as well as parents. Establishing channels of communication between child care programs and local pediatric practices, through parental consent and healthcare consultation, can provide valuable information from pediatric clinicians to child care providers and vice versa.

B. Behavioral concerns. Behavioral issues rank high on the list of concerns for both parents of children in child care and their child care providers.

    1. Parent–child relationship. A decade of research on the developmental outcomes of child care has confirmed that the effects of child care derive not from its use or nonuse but from the quality of the experiences it provides to young children. The attachment relationship between the parent and the child appears to be largely protected from any possible negative effects emanating from early entry into and extensive hours of care. The primary influence on the attachment relationship is not from child care per se but from the sensitivity of the care that the parent provides. Thus, the influence of child care is not as large as the influence of the family environment, although child care can foster resilience and protect children from such negative family risks as maternal depression, child abuse and neglect, and extreme poverty.

    2. Separation. Introducing young children to new settings and/or unfamiliar caregivers can cause separation challenges that vary considerably in duration and extent based on the child's age, temperament, previous experiences in care, and individual response to change. Pediatric clinicians can help families transition their children into child care by routinely discussing age-appropriate handling of separation, such as allowing adequate time for children to adjust to the transition, facilitating bonding with a single caregiver, providing the child with a transitional object such as a blanket or stuffed animal or a picture of the parents to help with separations, establishing predictable times of parental departure and return, and the establishment of well-defined routines.

    3. Aggression. Aggression, typically in the form of hitting, pinching, and/or biting, is a common challenge for both providers and parents of young children in child care. Recent research suggests that prekindergarteners are expelled for aggressive behavior at a rate that is more than three times that of their older peers in kindergarten through high school, whereas at the individual classroom level, prekindergarten expulsion is not uncommon, with 10.4% of prekindergarten teachers expelling at least one preschooler in a given year. Child care programs should have access to mental and behavioral healthcare consultants who can provide help to child care staff when dealing with children whose challenging behaviors threaten their expulsion and impact the entire program. Pediatric clinicians can also educate parents and child care providers on reasonable expectations for play, sharing, and communicating between young children, potential causes of aggressive behavior such as poor language skills, low tolerance for frustration, and exposure to toxic stress at home, and recommend methods of age-appropriate management/discipline.

C. Quality of staff. Research suggests that it is the quality of the daily transactions between the child and the child care providers that carry the weight of the influence of child care on child development. Exposure to language and the verbal environment created in the child care setting are particularly critical for positive cognitive and language outcomes in young children. High-quality staffing of child care with low ratios is associated with such positive outcomes as children's cooperation with adults, ability to initiate and sustain positive exchanges with their peers, and early competence in math and reading. Child–provider ratio is the most sensitive indicator of quality care. Yet, child care providers are often inadequately trained and supervised, poorly paid for their work, undervalued, and overwhelmed, all of which contribute to a workforce with high turnover and less provider consistency for children.

D. Long-term outcome. There continues to be research and debate on the developmental implications on child care, particularly focusing on quality, duration, and time of initiation. Child care is neither the inevitable risk factor that some have portrayed it to be nor does it replace parents as the major influence on early development. To date, the findings suggest that quality of care is inherent in the child care provider whether it is a family member, family child care provider, or center-based provider. Variables that sustain high-quality child care are the providers' education, specialized training, and their attitudes about work and the children in their care. The features that enable them to excel in their work and remain in their jobs include small ratios, small groups, and adequate compensation.

BIBLIOGRAPHY

For parents

American Academy of Pediatrics. *Making Child Care Choices Count for Your Family.* Elk Grove Village, IL: American Academy of Pediatrics, 2007. http://www.healthychildren.org/English/family-life/work-play/pages/Making-Child-Care-Choices-Count-for-Your-Family

National Association for the Education of Young Children. www.naeyc.org

National Resource Center for Health and Safety in Child Care. http://nrc.uchsc.edu/

U.S. Consumer Product Safety Commission. *Child Care Safety Checklist for Parents and Child Care Providers.* Document #242. www.cpsc.gov/cpscpub/pubs/child care.org

Zero to Three: Choosing Quality Child Care. http://www.zerotothree.org/choose_care.html

For professionals

Caring for Our Children: National Health and Safety Performance Standards: Guidelines for Out-of-Home Child Care Programs (2nd ed). Elk Grove Village, IL: American Academy of Pediatrics and Washington, DC: American Public Health Association, 2002. http://nrc.uchsc.edu/CFOC/index.html; also available at http://nrckids.org

Gilliam WS, Shahar G. Prekindergarten expulsion and suspension: rates and predictors in one state. *Infants Young Child* 19(3):228–245, 2006.

Moving Kids Safely in Child Care, 2002. An American Academy of Pediatrics/The National Resource Center for Health and Safety resource serving as the first national occupant protection curriculum for child care providers and administrators. www.healthychildcare.org

National Child Care Information Center. www.nccic.org

NICHD Early Child Care Research Network. The NICHD Study of Early Child Care: contexts in development and developmental outcomes over the first seven years of life. In Brookes-Gunn J, Berlin LJ (eds), *Young Children's Education, Health and Development: Profile and Synthesis Project Report.* Washington, DC: U.S. Department of Education, 2000.

NICHD Study. http://www.nichd.nih.gov/od/secc/pubs.htm

The Pediatrician's Role in Promoting Health and Safety in Child Care. Elk Grove Village, IL: AAP Bookstore, ID#: MA0175, 2001. www.aap.org/bookstore

93 Cultural Issues

Lee M. Pachter

I. **Description of the issue.** A cultural group is a **collective of individuals who share common beliefs, values, attitudes, and behaviors.** Individuals may consider themselves members of many different groups based on shared identity, for example, ethnic heritage, geographic region, occupation, sexual orientation, lifestyle, or any other collective to which the individual feels connected to. Cultural identity and group identity are fluid concepts that may change with time and context.

In the clinical context, all interactions may be considered "cross-cultural"—between the culture of "medicine" and the culture of "patients." Clinicians enter into the clinician–patient relationship with our own set of values, beliefs, and assumptions. As the cultural distance between individuals increases—as when traditional beliefs and practices of a family may be discordant with the mainstream biomedical view—it becomes crucial to find ways to bridge the gap between the two belief systems.

Ethnocultural beliefs and practices regarding childrearing and child behavior and development are based on a group's adaptation to specific environmental, economic, social, and family contexts. These beliefs and practices have formed over many years and many generations and although they change over time, they do so at varying rates and degrees. Traditional beliefs and practices are often reinforced by older family members, as well as recollections of parents, when they were growing up.

A. **Culture versus class and minority status.** In many industrialized countries individuals from minority cultural groups are overrepresented in low-socioeconomic strata of society. This socioeconomic and material disadvantage results in differential access to services. The effects of (1) **traditional cultural beliefs,** (2) **poverty and access to material goods,** and (3) **being a minority** on health and healthcare are distinct but often interlinked. The clinician needs to be aware of these distinctions and try to tease out whether clinical issues that come up may be, in part, related to any or all of these three separate but interrelated issues.

B. **Intracultural variability.** *There is as much variability in beliefs and practices within cultural groups as between cultural groups.* Any one individual's approach to parenting and child development is an amalgamation of personal beliefs, past experiences, media and expert influence, *and* traditional cultural beliefs (as well as other factors). Nonetheless, it is important to have a general understanding of traditional beliefs and practices as a background and a starting point for discussion and communication.

C. **Cultural change.** One source of intracultural variability is the effect of **acculturation,** or the changes that take place over time in individuals and groups due to continuous contact with other cultures and living environments. Modern theories of acculturation stress that it is not a unidirectional process; individuals do not acculturate "from" a traditional culture "to" the host culture. Instead, the process is one better described as becoming "bicultural" or "multicultural." Individuals retain certain aspects of their traditional culture while incorporating beliefs and values of other groups, including the majority culture. Cultural change occurs in areas such as traditional practices, ethnic pride, self-identity, and language use. Not all of these dimensions change at the same rate or degree.

II. **Ways that culture affects child behavior and development.**

A. **Parenting practices and beliefs about childrearing.** For example, norms regarding sleeping arrangements (e.g., co-sleeping), discipline practices, infant and child feeding practices, parental interactions with teachers and the role of the parent in a child's education, specific parenting roles of the father and the mother, and discussions about topics such as sexuality, all may be influenced by traditional beliefs and practices.

B. **Family composition/structure.** In some cultural traditions, different family structures may be the norm, such as the reliance on or cohabitation with extended family or fictive kin (e.g., godparents or nonrelated cousins).

C. **Culturally normative values.** A major aspect of child development includes the learning of acceptable and "normal" behaviors, values, and ideals. This includes the foundations of beliefs that may not be specific to parenting or child development but nonetheless create the milieu in which children live, grow, and learn. They comprise the "models" of behavior to which children are taught to conform. Styles of communication and interaction among individuals, for example, are culturally constructed to some extent. Some cultures put high value on an interactive style that is warm and personal, whereas others prefer styles that are more reserved during interpersonal communication and interaction. Sometimes the style of interaction is based on the relative social position of the individuals involved, and different cultures employ different "rules" to do this.

The value system that underlies proper personal behavior is in part culturally mediated as well. For example, some cultures put a high value on individualism (e.g., independence, self-confidence), whereas other cultures put a higher value on the attainment of social competencies based on collectivism (e.g., interdependence, respectfulness). Acceptable physical distance between individuals in different social settings, physical touch, and eye contact are other examples of belief systems that are in part culturally mediated.

D. **Perceptions about normal child behavior.** The Victorian concept of "children should be seen but not heard" is an example of one such culturally derived model of child behavior. A physically active child may be seen as "a problem" in one system and "naturally inquisitive" in another. A quiet child may be seen as "slow, dull, or unmotivated" in one context but "quiet and respectful" in another. These different expectations about child behavior may become an issue as the growing child begins spending time in multiple settings (such as at home, at school, and in the community) where the cultural beliefs may clash.

E. **Perception about normal child development.** Studies have shown differences in both perceptions and expectations. The Digo people in Kenya believe that infants are ready to learn developmental tasks such as toilet training at a very early age. They begin training in the first month and have some degree of bowel and bladder control by 4–6 months of age. This is accomplished by maternal sensitivity to infant cues, positioning the infant to facilitate elimination, and behavior modification.

In another study from the United States, parents from four different ethnocultural groups (African American, West Indian/Caribbean, Puerto Rican, and European American) were asked about their beliefs regarding the ages at which infants and children were able to attain specific developmental milestones. While most of the responses from all the groups were within what would be considered appropriate range of developmental expectations, there were group differences even after controlling for other variables such as socioeconomic status, education, and maternal age. The greatest differences were found in the person and social domains of development. Specific differences (e.g., in tasks such as sleeping throughout the night, or age at which an infant could be fed from a spoon) could be explained by difference in core cultural values, childrearing practices, or the physical environment of family life.

In all of these examples, culture is but one of many factors that moderate child development and behavior. Other variables such as the physical environment, socioeconomic conditions, and intergroup relationships have important effects. It is also necessary to recognize that cultural beliefs and practices are not static but are constantly changing as a result of interaction with other groups and differing living contexts.

III. **Racial/ethnic disparities in health and healthcare.** The last decade has seen growth in the study of health and healthcare disparities based on race, ethnicity, and class. A *disparity* is defined as an inequitable and potentially avoidable difference in health, healthcare, or developmental outcome. A growing literature is documenting the specific disparities in child behavioral and developmental health. For example, Latino youth report higher scores on depression inventories than do European American youth, even when socioeconomic status is controlled for. Similar findings are seen with African American boys (although not with African American girls). Latino, African American, and Asian American youth have been shown to have higher scores on anxiety scales as well. It must be noted that in *some* studies, racial/ethnic disparities in internalizing symptoms diminish or become insignificant when other demographic variables (such as parental education) are controlled for.

With regard to attention-deficit/hyperactivity disorder (ADHD), studies show that African American and Latino children have less ADHD symptoms by parent report but greater positive screening rates by teacher report. These discrepancies may be attributed to differences in context (school environment vs. home), differences in perceptions of behavioral norms, or personal/institutional discrimination. For those diagnosed with ADHD, African American and Latino youth have lower rates of prescribed stimulant treatment than European Americans, although the response to stimulant treatment does not differ among these groups. For autism spectrum disorders (ASDs), studies show that autism is diagnosed later in African

American children than in European American children (due to entering the mental health care system later as well as having a longer time in the system before diagnosis). African American children meeting surveillance criteria for ASD are also less likely to receive a diagnosis of ASD than European American children.

IV. Clinical approaches.

A. **Screening/testing.** *Most questionnaires and instruments used to assess behavior and development were created and tested on white, middleclass children.* Although they may have "face validity" for use in minority children, be aware that differences in cultural beliefs and practices, perceptions of normal and abnormal behavior, and even scoring style differences need to be taken into account when evaluating responses. Translations of questionnaires are helpful for limited English-proficient families, but **mere translation does not guarantee cross-cultural conceptual or measurement equivalency.** Clinicians who use screening and diagnostic surveys often in their practice should try to choose instruments that have some data on validity and reliability for diverse populations.

B. **Health beliefs history.** A health beliefs history is a way of getting the perspective of the patient or family regarding the clinical issue at hand. By inquiring into the parent's "ethnotheories" about children, one may be able to ascertain whether or not the specific clinical issue is being viewed by the parent as problematic. What might be considered "a problem" from the clinical standpoint may not be a problem from the perspective of the parent.

C. **Key clinical questions.** Examples of questions eliciting the patient's or family's perspective include the following:

- *"Do you think that this behavior is a problem? Why (or why not)?"*
- *"What is most concerning to you about this?"* (Sometimes the issues that is most important for the family is not the same as the issue that is most important from the clinical standpoint.)
- *"Why does he or she have this problem?"* (You may get to some beliefs about causation that need to be addressed before intervention)
- *"How should a __-year-old act?"* (This may also uncover attitudes and knowledge about child behavior and development that will need follow-up education.)
- *"What problems does it create for your child?"*
- *"Are there other people who you have spoken with, and have they given you opinions and ideas about it?"* (Other family members may have strong opinions and influences.)
- *"Sometimes there are ways of treating problems that physician do not know about. They might be effective. Have you tried anything yet to help solve this?"* (Approach alternative treatments and practices in a nonjudgmental fashion.)
- *"What do you expect from the treatment?"*

D. **Clinical communication.** The goal of a culturally informed approach to clinical pediatrics is to try to **gain an understanding of the patient's or family's understanding of a clinical issue.** Often, children present either because the parents are concerned about a problem with the child's development or behavior or because another agent (usually the school or child care) has identified a potential issue. Be aware that families from different cultural backgrounds may interpret child behavior and development with different underlying frameworks.

The **Awareness-Assessment-Negotiation** approach may help to work through cultural and individual differences in the clinical setting. This approach recommends the following:

- The clinician become *aware* of any general beliefs and practices concerning parenting and child behavior/development in the groups commonly seen in a particular practice. This information provides only a general orientation that should not be used in clinical practice until validated by the direct discussion with particular families.
- In the *assessment* phase, assess the likelihood that a particular family subscribes to the beliefs and practices, keeping in mind the importance of intracultural diversity.
- If there are discrepancies between parent-held beliefs and practices and biomedical/clinical point of view, attempt to *negotiate* between models. Negotiation allows a common ground to be created that acknowledges and respects the family's views and beliefs and builds upon them whenever possible. Incorporate family-held beliefs into patient education and culturally acceptable treatments into the care plan, whenever possible. It may be helpful to include other individuals such as grandparents, godparents, or other family-identified support individuals in the plan. When modifications to the family's beliefs or practices are necessary, do it in an open way that allows for discussion and feedback. Recognize that behavioral change usually does not occur in a brief 15- to 30-minute visit, but laying the groundwork for an ongoing relationship

that includes bidirectional and respectful communication may result in such a change over time.

BIBLIOGRAPHY

For parents

Beal AC, Villarosa L, Abner A. *The Black Parenting Book.* New York, NY: Broadway, 1999.
Comer JP, Poussaint AF. *Raising Black Children.* New York, NY: Plume, 1992.
Powell Hopson D, Hopson DS. *Different and Wonderful: Raising Black Children in a Race-Conscious Society.* New York, NY: Fireside, 1990.
Rodriguez G. *Raising Nuestros Ninos: Bring Up Latino Children in a Bicultural World.* New York, NY: Fireside, 1999.

For professionals

Anderson ER, Mayes LC. Race/ethnicity and internalizing disorders in youth: a review. *Clin Psychol Rev* 2010. doi:10.1016/j.cpr.2009.12.008.
Arnold LE, Michael Elliott M, et al. Effects of ethnicity on treatment attendance, stimulant response/dose, and 14-month outcome in ADHD. *J Consult Clin Psychol* 71(4):713–727, 2003.
Mandel DS, Wiggins LD, Arnstein Carpenter L, et al. Racial/ethnic disparities in identification of children with autism spectrum disorders. *Am J Public Health* 99(3):493–498, 2007.
National Center for Cultural Competence. http://gucchd.georgetown.edu//nccc/.
Nolan EE, Gadow KD, Sprafkin J. Teacher reports of *DSM-IV* ADHD, ODD, and CD symptoms in schoolchildren. *J Am Acad Child Adolesc Psychiatry* 40(2):241–249, 2001.
Pachter LM, Dworkin PH. Maternal expectations about normal child development in 4 cultural groups. *Arch Pediatr Adolesc Med* 151:1144–1150, 1997.
Pachter LM, Harwood R. Culture and child behavior and psychosocial development. *J Dev Behav Pediatr* 17:191–198, 1996.
Stevens J, Harman JS, Kelleher KJ. Ethnic and regional differences in primary care visits for attention-deficit hyperactivity disorder. *J Dev Behav Pediatr* 25:318–325, 2004.

94

Death During Childhood

David J. Schonfeld

I. **Description of the problem.** When a child is dying, the child and the family need reassurance, support, and guidance. The primary care provider who has a supportive and ongoing relationship with the child and the family is in a unique position to provide them with that support throughout this difficult period. Some general principles to consider in providing care to dying children and their families are presented in Table 94-1.

II. **Issues in helping the dying child.**

A. **Healthcare providers must attend to the immediate physical needs of these children.** It is crucial to relieve pain and suffering and to assure the children that adults are always available. Children should be told by both the parents and the healthcare providers, "We want you to tell us whenever anything is bothering you. I will always be here (or be able to be reached) anytime you want me. We will all do our best to make sure that you feel as comfortable as possible."

B. **Children at different developmental stages have different conceptual understandings of the meaning of death.** This will affect their ability to understand and adjust to their impending death (see Chapter 90). Children with a terminal illness usually do appreciate the seriousness of their illness and may develop a precocious understanding of death and their personal mortality.

C. **Many parents and clinicians are uncomfortable when children openly acknowledge an awareness of their impending death.** Children often feel that it is their task to provide emotional support to their parents and to carry on the mutual pretense that they are unaware of their health status. This conspiracy of silence isolates the child from available supports. Most children, in fact, fear the *process* of dying more than death itself.

D. **To the extent possible, children should be informed about their health status.** Children often turn to members of the healthcare team to ask questions, directly or indirectly, about their illness and impending death. Children who are dying may also directly ask family members and staff, "Am I going to die?" Adults should initially clarify the motivation for such questions: Is the child seeking reassurance that all efforts will be made to minimize pain, that parents and family members will remain available, or that every reasonable effort will be made to treat the underlying illness? Is the child merely attempting to determine the seriousness of his illness? Once the motivation for the question is identified, the adult family member or healthcare provider can provide the necessary reassurances or information. Prohibitions on informing children about their condition force parents and professionals to lie, thereby jeopardizing a caregiving relationship built on mutual trust and respect. The principles to consider in informing children about a terminal illness or impending death are summarized in Table 94-2.

E. **Facilitating discussion about children's concerns often involves projective techniques** such as play or picture drawing. Many children choose not to discuss their impending death directly. It is rarely necessary (or appropriate) to confront children with the reality that they are dying after they have been appropriately informed. Instead, clinicians should remain available and offer indirect outlets for addressing the child's concerns. Children will avail themselves of these opportunities when, and if, they are ready.

F. **Clinicians are often anxious that they will not know what to say to a child who is dying.** The goal of counseling children who are dying is not to take away their sadness or to find the "right" answers to all their questions. Rather, it is to listen to their concerns, to accept and empathize with their strong emotions, to offer support, and to assist them in finding their own coping techniques (e.g., "Some children find it helpful to talk to others about what is worrying them; other children prefer to draw pictures or keep a diary. Whatever you decide to do is fine. I'm always available to talk with you about your feelings, or just to sit and talk about something else."). In many cases, the best approach is to talk about a topic of interest to the child or merely to sit quietly and hold the child's hand.

G. **Children must be allowed, even encouraged, to continue to have hope and to go on with their lives.** These children should be regarded less as children who are dying and

Table 94-1. General principles for practitioners in the care of dying children and their families

Physical context
Minimize physical discomfort and symptoms
Optimize pain management

Emotional context
Provide an opportunity for the expression and sharing of personal feelings and concerns for both the children and their families in an accepting atmosphere
Tolerate unpleasant affect (e.g., sadness, anger, despair)

Social context
Facilitate communication among members of the healthcare team and the children and their families
Encourage active participation of the children and their families in the treatment decisions and the management of the illness

Personal context
Treat each child and family member as a unique individual
Form a personal relationship with the child and the family
Acknowledge your own feelings as a healthcare provider and establish a mechanism(s) to meet your personal needs

more as individuals living with a serious and/or life-threatening condition. The goal must be to optimize the quality of their remaining life and not merely to prolong its duration. Important routines should be continued with as little disruption as possible, such as allowing them to attend school or to do schoolwork in the hospital. Although regressive behavior may be normative and appropriate at times of stress, excessively regressive behavior (e.g., a 6-year-old who begins biting staff) should be addressed supportively but firmly, often employing a behavioral management approach developed by the treatment team and the family.

H. **Many children and adolescents feel guilty and ashamed about their illness.** Children who rely on magical thinking and egocentrism to explain the cause of illness may assume that terminal illness and death are the result of some perceived wrongdoing ("immanent justice"). Children need to be reassured frequently that they are not responsible for their illness.

I. **To the extent possible, children should be informed about and participate in the decisions regarding their healthcare.** Older children and adolescents may possess the intellectual and emotional maturity to allow them to play a significant role regarding critical and difficult decisions (e.g., whether to discontinue aggressive treatment). All children need to be aware of the nature and rationale of planned treatments and should be active participants in the treatment process even if they are able to make only seemingly minor decisions (e.g., whether they should take the pill with juice or with soda).

Table 94-2. Principles involved in informing children about a terminal illness or impending death

Inform the child over time in a series of conversations. During the initial conversation, it is important to convey that the child has a serious illness.

If the child asks directly whether he or she is going to die, initially explore the reason for the question and the child's concerns (e.g., "Are you afraid that you might die?" "What are you worried about?"). Do not provide false reassurances ("No, don't worry, you're going to be okay.") but always try to maintain hope ("Some children with your sickness have died, but we are going to do everything we can to try and help you get better.").

Focus initial discussions on the immediate and near future. Young children have a limited future perspective. Dying "soon" to them may mean minutes, hours, or days and not months or years.

Answer questions directly, but do not overwhelm the child with unnecessary details.

Assess the child's understanding by asking him or her to explain back to you what you have discussed.

Reassure the child of the lack of personal responsibility or guilt. For this reason, avoid the use of the term bad in the description of the illness (e.g., "You have a bad sickness.").

III. **Issues in helping the parents.**
   A. **Parents faced with the impending (or actual) death of their child may demonstrate shock, denial, anxiety, depression, or anger.** Almost any reaction can be seen; there is no "correct" way to deal with the death of a child. In addition, parents may alternate among these emotional states without demonstrating any clear pattern of progression. In general, it is important to accept parents' reactions without making judgments about whether or not they are appropriate, unless there are concerns related to personal safety (e.g., drinking and driving, suicidal or homicidal threats, etc.).
   B. **The response of family members to the death may be affected by the duration of the illness.** Anticipatory grieving allows family members to experience graduated feelings of loss while the child is still alive. In the setting of open communication, many families will take advantage of this time to resolve conflicts with the dying child and to express love. Clinicians should appreciate that other families may approach this impending loss with a different coping style and may not choose to engage in this form of leave-taking behavior.
   C. **Members of the family may proceed with anticipatory grieving at different rates.** Conflicts may result when one family member's course of grieving is not synchronous with that of another member of the family. Primary care clinicians can help families to identify when someone (either a family member or a healthcare team member) has abandoned the child after having prematurely reached resignation and acceptance of the child's death.
   D. **As part of anticipatory grieving, family members and healthcare professionals may wish for the death of a terminally ill child.** This wish may result in excessive guilt and cause the individual to compensate by becoming overly protective or indulgent with the dying child. The healthcare provider can assist parents with such comments as: *"Many parents of children who have been critically ill for a prolonged period sometimes find themselves wishing their child would just die quickly. This is a common and normal feeling, even for parents who love their children dearly."*
   E. **Family members should be allowed, even encouraged, to continue to have hope and to go on with their lives.** While the desire for second opinions should be honored, excessive searches for cures that compromise the health of the child or the financial well-being of the family should be discouraged. Parents must be actively assured that they have done everything reasonable to ensure the highest quality of care for their child and that they have no reason to feel guilty.
   F. **To the extent possible, parents should be informed about and participate actively in decisions regarding their child's care. The healthcare providers must provide families with clear professional recommendations and be willing to discuss alternate options when appropriate options exist.** When families are faced, for example, with the difficult decision of whether to continue aggressive therapy when little hope of cure remains, the clinician must provide information on the likelihood of success and the anticipated morbidity associated with the treatment process. Palliative and supportive care should always remain available even if children and their families choose a management plan that is not the preferred option of the provider. For terminally ill children maintained on life support at the time of death, the clinician should elicit and honor the parents' wishes about the timing of termination of life support. Care should be taken so that parents do not infer that they are being asked about whether to allow their child to die.
   G. **Sudden or unexpected death requires an immediate recognition of the loss.** In this setting, families often initially use denial to cope. Family members should be allowed additional time to hold or be with the child's body in a quiet and private area of the hospital and should be given an opportunity to express their shock, disbelief, and anger before further and more detailed explanations of the cause of death are provided.
   H. **Support systems for families of dying children are often hospital-based and frequently withdrawn at the time of the child's death.** Providers should remain available to families after the death has occurred and should help the family establish ties, prior to the death, with community-based support systems, such as parent groups, clergy, and counseling services. Hospital support networks should not become an additional loss coincident with the death of the child.
   I. **At the time of the child's death, parents and other family members should be offered assistance with immediate and pragmatic needs.** Such diverse needs include ensuring safe transportation home for grieving family members at the time of the death, making funeral and burial arrangements, and deciding how to notify family members and friends. Families should be given an appointment for a follow-up meeting (often 2–6 weeks after the death, earlier if necessary) to answer remaining questions about the illness and death (e.g., to review the autopsy report) and to inquire about adjustment of family members. A

meeting can also be arranged later on with the siblings either individually or with their parents.

J. **Families in grief may feel immobilized and incapable of making even simple decisions.** Complex and emotionally laden decisions such as those regarding autopsy or organ donation may seem especially overwhelming at this time. When death is anticipated, the primary care provider may suggest that family members consider their personal feelings about such decisions before the fact. In sudden and unanticipated deaths, families may need a period of time (1–2 hours) to adjust to the reality of the loss before such questions are asked.

IV. **Issues in helping the siblings.**

A. **The needs of the siblings are often neglected when a child in the family is dying.** Parents have limited reserves of energy, time, and money and strained emotional and psychological resources. Providers must ensure that outreach is provided to siblings to meet their needs.

B. **The siblings should be included in receiving information about the child's health status and treatment plan and should participate to some extent in the provision of care for the ill child.** Young children may be given simple tasks such as bringing and opening mail, watering plants in the room, or bringing toys to a child in bed. Parents must be careful not to overburden the siblings, especially the older children and adolescents, with unreasonable chores or responsibilities. Siblings should be encouraged to maintain their peer groups and continue involvement in activities outside the family.

C. **Siblings respond to the death with the same diversity of emotional responses seen in adults.** They may be angry at the child who has died or experience guilt over having survived. Primary care clinicians need to monitor how families reorganize after the death of a child so that siblings are not made a scapegoat or the focus of projected defenses. For example, parents who continue to feel guilty about their child's death may overprotect the surviving siblings and interfere with normative attempts to achieve independence.

V. **Helping the healthcare providers.**

A. **Healthcare providers must understand their personal feelings about death to be effective in providing support to others.** Often this will involve some introspection about one's own losses and an awareness of the impact of the deaths of their patients on their professional and personal lives.

B. **Providers must extend the same quality of care to themselves, as they would offer to patients.** The death of a patient is one of the most stressful personal and professional experiences faced by healthcare providers. It triggers a similar, albeit less intense, grief response as would a personal loss. Permission and tolerance for professionals to discuss and have their personal needs met regarding bereavement (e.g., for support or reassurance for lack of personal responsibility for a patient death) is necessary. Psychosocial rounds (especially in intensive care settings), retreats, and other support services dealing directly with providers' responses to patient death are important aspects of professional development.

C. **All members of the healthcare team should be involved in important decisions regarding the care provided to a dying child.** Conflicts that arise when one or more members of the team disagree on the appropriateness of care being provided can seriously undermine the clinical care. For example, physicians who avoid clarifying do-not-resuscitate orders with the family of a dying child may place the nursing staff in the uncomfortable position of having to initiate resuscitation efforts when the death occurs. House staff forced to continue treatment that they feel is not in the best interest of the child or family may be angry if they were not involved in the decision. Often staff differences are best resolved through team meetings.

D. **Primary care providers should avail themselves of the expertise and skills of members of related disciplines,** such as the clergy, child life, nursing, psychiatry, psychology, and social work, when responding to the needs of the child and family members, as well as their own personal needs.

BIBLIOGRAPHY

For parents

Organizations

Candlelighters Childhood Cancer Foundation. For information and referral for parents, families, and professionals working with children with cancer. www.candlelighters.org

Children's Hospice International. For information and referral regarding local hospice care and bereavement counseling services. www.chionline.org

Compassionate Friends. For referral to a self-help group for families who have experienced the death of a child. www.compassionatefriends.org

National Sudden and Unexpected Infant/Child Death and Pregnancy Loss Resource Center. http://www.sidscenter.org

The Dougy Center for Grieving Children and Families. www.dougy.org

Publications

Information on how to support grieving children

Emswiler M, Emswiler J. *Guiding Your Child Through Grief.* New York, NY: Bantam Books, 2000.

Schonfeld D, Quackenbush M. *After a Loved One Dies—How Children Grieve and How Parents and Other Adults Can Support Them.* New York, NY: New York Life Foundation, 2009. May be freely downloaded as PDF or hardcopies ordered at cost at http://www.nylgriefguide.com

For professionals

Organizations

National Center for School Crisis and Bereavement. For assistance to schools related to the death of a student. www.cincinnatichildrens.org/school-crisis

Publications

Adams D, Deveau E. When a brother or sister is dying of cancer: the vulnerability of the adolescent sibling. *Death Stud* 11:279–295, 1987.

Glazer J, Schonfeld DJ. Life-limiting illness, palliative care, and bereavement. In Martin A, Volkmar F (eds), *Lewis' Child and Adolescent Psychiatry: A Comprehensive Textbook* (4th ed), Baltimore, MD: Lippincott Williams & Wilkins, 2007:971–980.

Greenham D, Lohmann R. Children facing death: Recurring patterns of adaptation. *Health Soc Work* 7(2):89–94, 1982.

Schonfeld D. Talking with children about death. *J Pediatr Health Care* 7:269–274, 1993.

95

Divorce

Margot Kaplan-Sanoff

I. **Description of the problem.** Divorce is not a single event. Rather, **divorce is a process** that begins in an unhappy marriage, extends through the separation, and continues into the new postdivorce life. Long before a marriage ends, children have begun the process of coping with the parental coldness and hostility that leads to or is the consequence of an unraveling relationship between their parents. It has been said that "it is not divorce per se that makes kids crazy but the craziness of divorcing parents that disrupts the orderly process of their children" (Hetherington, 1989).

A. **Incidence.**
- Approximately 50% of all marriages end in divorce, usually within the first 8 years of marriage.
- Eighty-five percent of parents who divorce remarry, and 40% of these new marriages also end in divorce.

B. **Stages of divorce for the parents.** In many divorcing families, each parent is in a different stage of the process. Often one parent is ready to let go of the relationship while another is still holding on. For parents, the timeline for moving through the stages is thought to be 1 year for every 5 years of marriage. During this difficult period, parents are often preoccupied by their own problems, but for their children, they remain the most important people in the children's lives.

1. **Holding on.** In this first stage, one or both parents are in denial, looking backward to determine what went wrong. Even 12–18 months after filing for divorce, parents report feeling angry, guilty, humiliated that the marriage did not last, depressed, anxious, and afraid to move forward, often with little energy to attend the needs of their children.

2. **Letting go.** This stage brings an acceptance of the loss of the relationship, with parents feeling relief, exhilaration, and grief at the ending of the marriage, often without much emotional availability for their children.

3. **Starting over.** Parents in this stage are ready to take risks and find a new identity as a single person. They tend to be future oriented and quite enthusiastic as they try out new lifestyles and begin dating.

4. **Building a new life.** This final stage represents stabilization for families as they begin to feel "back to normal."

C. **Emotional tasks for children during the divorce.** The basic task for children is to integrate, without psychic damage, the loss of the parenting relationship and the change in their social status. Children need to perceive events as being under their control, even though the divorce was not their decision. They need to avoid constructing a view of divorce and its consequences as random and one in which they view themselves as the hapless targets of external forces.

   Thus, the tasks for the children are to:

1. **Understand the divorce.** Children must understand the immediate changes that the divorce brings and sort out their fantasies and fears from the reality of the divorce. They may respond with blaming, sadness, anger, guilt, and/or anxiety to the separation and decision to divorce. How children are told about the divorce and the way the family separates in part determines the nature of the postdivorce year. Children may blame themselves for the divorce and try to be the "perfect child" in hopes of reuniting the family.

2. **Strategically withdraw.** Children need to get on with their own lives and to have permission to remain children by continuing to join extracurricular activities, such as sports or art programs. Very young children are unable to avoid the anger and hostility of the divorce, whereas older school-aged children and adolescents often simply escape from the house.

3. **Cope with loss.** In a divorce, children often lose daily contact with one of their parents and they lose the family into which they were born. Other loses and changes for many

children include a decrease in financial resources and a move to a new neighborhood, school, and peer group.

    4. Deal with anger. Although divorce is a voluntary action for at least one of the adults in the marriage, it is an event completely out of control of the children who feel cheated out of family experiences and exposed in front of peers.

II. Factors that affect children's adjustment to divorce.

    A. Temperament. Children with difficult temperaments may receive more negative attention and become the object that distracts the family from the real issue of conflict—the divorce. Shy, inhibited children may become even more withdrawn and reclusive, but because they do not demand parental attention, their confusion, sadness, and anger are often ignored or misinterpreted as adjustment.

    B. Developmental level. As Table 95-1 shows, the age and developmental level of children at the time of the divorce greatly affects their response to the event.

Table 95-1. Responses of child to parent's divorce within the first year

Developmental status	Child's response	Primary care clinician's role
Preschool	Regressive behavior	Encourage stable, predictable meal and bedtime routines
	Sleep disturbance	Help parents develop consistent patterns of joining and separating from child
	Bowel and bladder difficulties	Encourage continued contact with noncustodial parent
	Tantrums, aggressive behavior	Provide reassurance
	Fears of abandonment, clinging	Promote parental understanding of child's coping mechanisms
Younger school age	Sadness, anger, fearfulness	Empathize with child's feelings
	Loyalty conflicts	Provide regular opportunities for child to talk
	Attempts to determine responsibility for divorce	Support child's continuing relationship with both parents
	Hopes for family reconciliation	Offer reassurance
	Declining school performance	Encourage open communication with teachers
Older school age/prepubertal	Grief, intense anger	Express interest in and availability to the child
	Declining school performance	Support child's school and peer involvement
	Disrupted peer relationships	Provide clear acknowledgment and support for child's working through feelings on the divorce
	Attempts to clarify responsibility for the divorce	
	Provide referrals for therapeutic interventions as appropriate for the child's needs	
	Caretaking of a parent	
Adolescence	Depression, anger	Provide opportunities for discussion
	Increase in adolescent acting out	Encourage parents to support appropriate independence in their teens
	Premature emancipation	
	Sleeper effects, particularly in females	

Adapted from Wallerstein JS. Separation, divorce, and remarriage. In Levine MD, Carey WB, Crocker AC (eds), *Developmental-Behavioral Pediatrics* (2nd ed), Philadelphia, PA: Saunders, 1992.

C. Predivorce developmental achievements. Although we cannot predict what developmental progress children *might* have made had their parents stayed together, their achievements prior to the divorce continue to impact their abilities postdivorce.

D. History of previous loss. For children who may have experienced earlier losses such as the death of a grandparent or pet or the loss of a beloved child care provider prior to the divorce, the new loss experienced as a result of the divorce will trigger memories of old losses.

E. Gender. Consistently, **boys have been found to be more disrupted by divorce.** Boys often receive less positive support and nurturance and are viewed more negatively, particularly by their mothers, which then exacerbates their acting out, dependency, and immature behaviors. Girls, on the other hand, tend to be more compliant immediately following the divorce but experience "sleeper effects" 5–10 years later as they begin to confront the commitment, intimacy, and loyalty demands of young adulthood.

F. Extent of parental hostilities before and after the divorce. The prime determinant of adverse outcomes for children, regardless of age or gender, is ongoing parental hostility. Parents involved in a conflictual relationship are less emotionally available and less effective disciplinarians to their children.

G. Level of economic stress. For many women, divorce brings a dramatic change in their financial security. They may have to return to school or work, work longer hours, and/or move to a less expensive home and neighborhood, necessitating more changes in the children's lives.

H. Emotional stability of the custodial parent. Although both parents may experience emotional lability, depression, emotional dependence or disengagement with their children, overindulgence, the excitement of a new active social life, or the risk for alcohol or substance abuse, it is the custodial parent upon whom the child relies to create a stable, familiar environment.

I. Stability of visitation. Seeing where and how the noncustodial parent lives can help a child create a new image of family, whereas inconsistent visitation offers children no such relief from their anxiety and fear of abandonment.

J. Support systems. Children who can access social supports outside the home, especially a consistent, empathic relationship with another family member, supportive adult, friend, or sibling are better able to manage their anxieties and anger about the divorce. Many schools offer support groups for children of divorcing parents within the structure of the school day.

III. Management.

A. Help families develop a plan. Helping parents develop a plan for how to tell the children is invaluable. Children who experienced the most precipitous regressions were those children who had been given no explanation for the separation or for their parent's departure. Children need to be reassured clearly and repeatedly that *"divorce is a grown-up problem"* and that they were not responsible for the breakup of the marriage. They need to be told explicitly about what will stay the same for them and what will change. Help parents to determine whatever was steady in their child's life and problem solve with them about how to try to keep that aspect intact. Use trigger questions to ask each parent about discipline problems and changes in the child's sleep and play patterns to generate information about each one's style of parenting and their level of concern about the child's behavior. Talking to children about a divorce is difficult. The following tips can help both children and parents with the challenge and stress of these conversations:

- Do not keep it a secret or wait until the last minute.
- Tell the children together, with both parents participating in the conversation.
- Keep things simple and straightforward.
- Tell the children that the divorce is not their fault.
- Admit that this will be a hard and upsetting time for everyone and that it is OK to feel sad, angry, or confused.
- Reassure the children that both parents still love them and will always be their parents.
- Do not discuss the other parent's faults or problems with the children.

B. Advise parents to inform their child's pediatric clinicians and teachers about the divorce. Both parents should sign a "consent to treat" form so that medical decisions can be made quickly if necessary. Ask parents whether they each want to receive copies of medical reports. Suggest that they each request in writing to receive school reports and notices so that they can be equally informed about their children's progress.

C. Maintain structure and organization. All children have difficulty exerting self-control and organizing their lives when their family arrangement is changing; they need more external control and structure during the stress of a divorce. Regardless of the custodial parent's feelings about the other parent, continuity of the child's relationships with both parents should be promoted.

D. Answer children's concerns. Parents should be informed that when children ask questions about the divorce, they should try to give truthful answers, even if they need to omit certain information. It can be extremely confusing and painful for parents to acknowledge their child's wish for reconciliation. Parents should acknowledge their child's hope for reunion while making it clear that the request will not happen—"You really wish that Daddy and Mommy would live together again in this house. That is not going to happen, but you will see Daddy in his new house every weekend." Reassure parents that it is expected that children will feel sad and that they should give their children permission to grieve and to cry, regardless of their age and gender.

E. Avoid conflictual interactions around the children. Watching parents argue without a positive resolution is particularly difficult for children. They bear the guilt of thinking that they are the reason for the conflict. Encourage parents to seek mediation and/or therapy to help them resolve their conflicts without the children needing to witness their anger.

F. Should we stay together for the sake of the children? Although there is never a good time for a family to divorce, growing up in a family in which there is an "emotional divorce" characterized by high levels of tension and low levels of warmth between parents, parents who discredit each other, where one parent aligns with the children to form a coalition against the other parent, or where the child manipulates the parents is also not in the best interests of the child. Staying together for the children places an enormous burden on the children to fill the emotional void between the parents.

BIBLIOGRAPHY

For children

Annie Ford, and Jann Blackstone-Ford. *My Parents Are Divorced Too: A Book for Kids by Kids.* New York, NY: Imagination, 1998. (Ages 9–12).

Holyoke N. *A Smart Girl's Guide to Her Parents' Divorce: How to Land on Your Feet When Your World Turns Upside Down.* Middleton, WI: American Girl Publishing Inc, 2009. (Ages 8–11).

Masurel C. *Two Homes.* Somerville, MA: Candlewick Press, 2003. (Ages 2–5).

Rogers F. *Let's Talk About Divorce.* New York, NY: Putnam, 1996. (Ages 3–7).

Thomas P. *My Family's Changing.* Happauge, NY: Barron's Education Series, 1999. (Ages 3–8).

For parents

Books

Gardner RA. *The Parents Book about Divorce* (rev. ed). New York, NY: Bantam, 1991.

Jones-Soderman J, Quattrocchi A, Steinberg S. *How to Talk to Your Children about Divorce.* Scottsdale, AZ: Family Mediation Center Publishing Co LLC, 2006.

Lewis J, Sammons W. *Don't Divorce Your Children: Parents and Children Talk about Divorce.* Chicago, IL: Contemporary Books, 1999.

Teyber E. *Helping Children Cope with Divorce.* New York, NY: Lexington Books, 1992.

Web sites

Divorce and Children. www.divorceandchildren.com

DivorceInfo. http://www.divorceinfo.com/children.htm

For professionals

Publications

Hetherington EM. Marital transitions: a child's perspective. Special issue: children and their development: knowledge base, research agenda, and social policy application. *Am Psychol* 44(2):303–312, 1989.

Lewis J, Sammons W. *Don't Divorce Your Children: Parents and Children Talk about Divorce.* Chicago, IL: Contemporary Books, 1999.

Teyber E. *Helping Children Cope with Divorce.* San Francisco, CA: Wiley Jossey-Bass, 2001.

Wallerstein JS, Blakeslee S. *Second Chances: Men, Women, and Children: A Decade after Divorce.* New York, NY: Ticknor & Fields, 1989.

Web sites

American Academy of Child and Adolescent Psychiatry. http://www.aacap.org/publications/factsfam/divorce.htm

Divorce Source. http://www.divorcesource.com/info/children/children.shtml

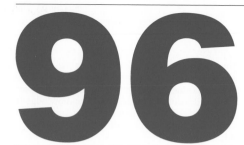

Foster Care

Moira Szilagyi

I. **Description of the problem.** Foster care **is government subsidized and regulated temporary care for children who have been removed from their families for reasons of abuse and neglect**. The goals of foster care are health, safety, and permanent caretaking for children. The main types of care are family foster care, placement with relatives (kinship care), and residential group care. For brevity, the term *foster care* will be used for all three types of care.

A. **Epidemiology. (See Table 96-1.)**

B. **Contributory factors.** Children entering foster care have typically endured multiple and chronic adverse life experiences, including abuse and neglect, inconsistent and chaotic parenting from multiple caregivers, severe emotional and financial deprivation, and limited access to appropriate services. Removal from their families and all that is familiar is often a traumatizing event and the uncertainty inherent in the foster care system may further erode a child's sense of well-being. The impact of foster care on individual children depends on their personal strengths and coping skills, prior life experiences, developmental abilities, and the availability of protective environmental factors.

II. **Identifying problems.**

A. **General issues.**

1. The periodicity schedule of the American Academy of Pediatrics (AAP) for child health supervision may need to be adjusted to reflect the more intensive support and monitoring necessary because of the many junctures in foster care that may adversely affect a child's health and well-being. A checklist that includes the crucial aspects of the health assessment and healthcare for children in foster care is available through the AAP (www.aap.org/advocacy/HFCA).

2. Intensive healthcare management to guarantee access to an appropriate array of developmental, mental health care, medical, and dental services is essential to good health outcomes for children in foster care.

3. The single greatest health need of children in foster care is for mental health care services and support.

B. **Specific issues.** Healthcare practitioners should consider children in foster care as a population with special healthcare needs.

1. **Primary pediatric care.** Children in foster care should have a "medical home." The AAP recommends visits

   - Monthly until 6 months of age, particularly if born prematurely
   - Every 3 months from 6 to 24 months of age
   - Every 6 months from 24 months to 21 years

   Primary care clinicians should address the adjustment of the child to the foster care placement, emotional and behavioral issues, school functioning, and the capacities of all the child's families to meet the child's needs. As thorough a history should be taken as possible to include information about the child's reason for placement, legal status, and the names and roles of the child welfare workers who are responsible for the child (e.g., foster parents, caseworker, law guardian). On physical examination, it is important to follow-up growth parameters, skin findings, and vision, hearing, dental, musculoskeletal, and neurological assessment. Clear communication and collaboration with the other professionals involved in the child's care is essential. Frequent follow-up visits and a high index of suspicion for emotional and psychological problems are fundamental to providing appropriate healthcare for this population.

   Mental health is the most significant health concern for children and adolescents in foster care. Children in foster care may have to deal with issues of separation and loss and may feel unloved or abandoned by their parents or experience anger, anxiety, and depression. It may help children to describe their parents as *unable*, rather than *unwilling*, to care for them. Children with a history of maltreatment may have extreme behaviors and difficulty trusting others. Clinicians can play a valuable

Table 96-1. Dimensions of foster care

Relevance

A total of 542,000 children are in foster care (an increase of 90% since 1982); 130,000 freed for adoption, about half of whom are in preadoptive placement

Types of care
72% in regular (including kinship) care
18% in group or residential care
8% in other arrangements

Age of foster children
4% infants
24% 1–5 years of age
24% 6–10 years of age
41% teenagers

Race; ethnicity of foster children
37% white, non-Hispanic
38% African American, non-Hispanic
17% Latino
6% Other

role by supporting and educating foster parents and engaging the child in a consistent and caring manner during more frequent office visits.

2. **Transitions in foster care.** Placement changes, sibling separation or reunion, changes in visitation patterns, and the termination of parental rights are but a few of the instances during which children in foster care need special support. The primary care clinician can advocate for appropriate preparation for the child to facilitate these transitions and provide anticipatory guidance to the foster parent about ways to support the child. The clinician should emphasize the need for abundant patience, affection, consistency, and nurturance during these difficult junctures.

3. **Screening questions for foster parents to assess how the transition is progressing include:**
   - *"How do you think your child is doing? How does this child fit in with your family?"*
   - *"Are there some behaviors you are worried about?"*
   - *"What has it been like for others in your home since your foster child moved in?"*
   - *"How are you coping?"*
   - *"Have there been any other significant changes in your family?"*

4. **The child's view of being in care.** Depending on a child's maturity and expressive abilities, it may be possible to ascertain directly how he or she perceives foster care. Useful questions, without the caregiver present, include
   - *"What is it like for you living in this home?"*
   - *"What do you like best? Least?"*
   - *"How do you get along with the people in your new home?"*
   - *"What would you like to change?"*
   - *"Do you feel loved and cared for where you are living?"*

5. **Visitation with parents.** Visits with birth parents can evoke strong, ambivalent emotions and difficult behaviors in children. Practitioners should encourage foster parents to maintain a positive view of the birth parents, at least, in front of the child. For example, foster families should help the child prepare for visits and rehearse their response to potentially difficult situations. Occasionally, the clinician may need to recommend a change in visitation that is clearly stressful to a child; for example, the clinician might recommend that the child go for a visit only if the parent calls ahead if there has been repeated failure by the parent to show up for visits. The clinician has to be careful to avoid simplistic explanations for children's responses to visits (e.g., interpreting aggressive behavior after a visit as reflecting a child's negative feelings toward his or her parents when, in fact, it is due to the anxiety of separating from them).

6. **Discipline in substitute care.** Foster caregivers are not allowed to use corporal punishment for children placed in their care. Disciplinary techniques should focus on using positive words and instructions, distraction techniques, teachable moments, and rewarding positive behaviors. Healthcare professionals should inform foster parents that children might experience emotional difficulties during the transitional period

into foster care; providing consistency and support in the foster home environment may help with this adjustment. Understanding a foster caregiver's parenting skills and abilities is fundamental to offering them parenting advice (e.g., *"How do you cope when your child is acting this way?"*)

7. **Abuse and neglect in substitute care.** Abuse and neglect occasionally occur in substitute care. Primary care clinicians need to remain alert to the physical and behavioral markers of maltreatment and assess whether these resulted from abuse or neglect prior to or during placement. Weight loss or poor weight gain in a young child is often the first sign of a neglectful foster care placement.

8. **Discontinuous healthcare.** Children in foster care have had frequent changes in healthcare providers or inadequate access to healthcare. Health information is often sparse or unavailable, and the primary care clinician should be mindful of gathering and maintaining medical documentation that will be useful to future clinicians. Communication with child welfare professionals about health information is crucial to appropriate permanency planning for children in foster care.

9. **Support for substitute caregivers.** Many children in foster care have serious problems, especially emotional and behavioral, that their foster parents and caseworkers are not equipped to handle. Primary care clinicians can help through more frequent visits for education, emotional support, and counseling. Many foster parent groups have newsletters for which some clinicians write a column on health issues. Timely referral to appropriate mental health care, developmental, and home health services may stabilize a foster care placement for a child. The clinician can offer foster parents support and respect by expressing admiration for their parenting skills and the stability and consistency they are providing children in their care.

10. **Involvement with birth parents.** Birth parents retain legal custody of their children unless they have been freed for adoption. Consent and confidentiality issues are complex in foster care, and the clinician should clarify who has the capacity to consent for a given child with the foster care agency. Involvement of the birth parents in the healthcare of their child is encouraged when deemed appropriate by the agency.

11. **Support for caseworkers.** Casework staff are often overwhelmed, undertrained, and underpaid. As the case managers for children in foster care, caseworkers are mandated to work with the birth family toward reunification while ensuring the health, safety, and well-being of children. Often, the latter involves the development of an alternative permanency plan. Clinicians can help casework staff by maintaining clear and open lines of communication, providing useful clinical information, and acknowledging their efforts (e.g., *"You're really making a big difference in his life by finding all the services he needs"*).

12. **Children preparing for independence.** In almost every state, children in foster care are expected to assume increased responsibility for themselves as they reach 18 years of age. Since very few have the experience to manage independently, this raises complex ethical and practical issues. The clinician can suggest measures to prepare the adolescent for independent living. (Materials to assist caregivers and youth in this task are available from the National Foster Care Resource Center.) Ideally, the pediatric clinician will continue caring for the young adult or make a referral to another healthcare provider.

BIBLIOGRAPHY

For parents

Organizations

American Professional Society on the Abuse of Children. www.apsac.org
Child Welfare League of America. www.cwla.org
National Foster Parent Association. http://nfpainc.org

For professionals

Publications

American Academy of Pediatrics; Committee on Early Childhood, Adoption and Dependent Care. Developmental issues for young children in foster care. *Pediatrics* 106:1145–1150, 2000.
Dubowitz H, Feigelman S, Zuravin S, et al. The physical health of children in kinship care. *Am J Dis Child* 146:603–610, 1992.
Jee SH, Antonucci TC, Aida, M, et al. Emergency department utilization by children in foster care. *Ambul Pediatr* 5:102, 2005.

Jee SH, Szilagyi M, Ovenshire C, et al. Improved detection of developmental delays among young children in foster care. *Pediatrics* 125:282, 2010.

Pilowsky DJ, Wu LT. Psychiatric symptoms and substance use disorders in a nationally representative sample of American adolescents involved with foster care. *J Adolesc Health* 38:351, 2006.

Simms M, Dubowitz H, Szilagyi M. Health care needs of children in the foster care system. *Pediatrics* 106:909–918, 2000.

Web site

The Future of Children. http://www.futureofchildren.org/pubs-info2825/pubs-info.htm?doc_id=209538

97

Health Literacy

L. Kari Hironaka

I. **Description of the problem/issue:** *Health literacy* is defined as "The degree to which individuals have the capacity to obtain, process, and understand basic health information and services needed to make appropriate health decisions."
  - Health literacy skills can affect one's ability to navigate through the healthcare system, share pertinent health-related information with medical providers, and engage in self-care and disease management.
  - The Institute of Medicine has identified health literacy as one of the key factors influencing patient safety, health disparities, and quality improvement.

II. **Epidemiology**
  A. Approximately one of three adults (36%) in the United States have limited health literacy skills.
  B. Limited health literacy skills can be divided into "basic" and "below basic." Examples of "basic" health literacy skills include understanding a growth chart or associating medication administration with food intake. Examples of "below basic" health literacy skills include dosing an over-the-counter medication or reading a clinic appointment card. Individuals with limited health literacy are less likely to obtain health-related information from newspapers, books, magazines, and the Internet. They are more likely to acquire health-related information from TV or radio. Limited literacy skills are often associated with a significant amount of shame and embarrassment.
  C. Health-related outcomes
  In adults, the relationship between limited health literacy and poorer health outcomes have associated limited literacy skills with the following:
  - Decreased utilization of preventive health services
  - Poorer understanding of medical conditions and disease-specific knowledge
  - Suboptimal self-management skills
  - Higher rates of hospitalization and emergency department visits
  - Poorer outcomes for specific chronic conditions
  - Increased risk of mortality
  Limited **parental** health literacy has been associated with the following:
  - Decreased health-related knowledge
  - Decreased disease management for specific chronic conditions
  - Decreased rates of exclusive breast-feeding
  - Use of a nonstandardized dosing instrument for measuring liquid medications
  D. Specific challenges for pediatric patients
    1. **Maturation and the developmental change of children over time.** Understanding the evolving role and significance of a child's own health literacy and self management skills on health-related behaviors and outcomes is one of the challenges of assessing the impact of health literacy in the pediatric population. The transition from a child's complete dependence on a parent to independent decision-making by the adolescent or young adult is a process that evolves over time and varies significantly between different families, individuals, and cultures.
    2. **Multiple caregivers.** Children are often cared for by multiple caregivers who share in the responsibility for health-related decisions. Parents, grandparents, child care providers, and teachers may transfer this responsibility from one caregiver to another multiple times throughout a day. Therefore, it may be important to consider the health literacy skills of all the adults involved in a child's care. Furthermore, these "handoffs" may be critical periods for errors or confusion to occur.

III. **Making the diagnosis.** There are a number of standardized instruments for measuring health literacy. Most of the commonly used instruments assess reading recognition, reading comprehension, and/or numeracy. Examples of such measures include the Rapid Estimate of Adult Literacy in Medicine (REALM) and the Test of Functional Health Literacy in Adults (TOFHLA). The REALM-Teen is also available for adolescents.

IV. Addressing the issue: Universal approach to effective communication. Given that even individuals with sophisticated health literacy skills can find the healthcare environment difficult to navigate and health-related information complicated or confusing, a universal approach to utilizing clear communication techniques should be implemented. This is particularly important in times of illness when pain, high emotion, and sleep deprivation may contribute to a decreased capacity to process health-related information.

V. Management
- **A. Improving health literacy and effective functioning.**
  1. **Ask Me 3.** This is a patient education campaign designed to promote clear communication by having patients ask three questions in every healthcare encounter.
     - "What is my child's main problem?"
     - "What do I need to do?"
     - "Why is it important for me to do this?"
- **B. Accommodations for families with limited health literacy.**
  1. "Teach Back." Confirm comprehension with the "teach back" technique
     - The parent/patient is invited to "teach back" information to the healthcare provider in his or her own words.
     - For example, pediatric provider might say, *"We went over a lot of information today. Would you mind telling me what you are going to do for Jane's wheezing, so I am sure that I didn't leave anything out?"*
  2. Using an iterative process, the provider corrects misunderstandings and has the parent/patient restate information until comprehension is confirmed.
  3. Reduce the complexity of health-related information
     - Use plain language and avoid jargon
     - Limit discussion to the two or three of the most important topics
     - Focus on desired behaviors rather than medical principles
  4. Provide low-literacy information
     - Much of the health-related printed material is written at or above the 10th-grade level.
  5. Utilize multiple forms of communication
  6. **Perform a "literacy walk through" in your practice.** Consider the skills needed to navigate to the front desk, complete the sign-in process, participate in the visit, and check out. Attention should be devoted to signs, written information, or instructions that families with limited health literacy skills may find challenging.

BIBLIOGRAPHY

Web sites

Harvard School of Public Health—Health Literacy Studies. http://www.hsph.harvard.edu/healthliteracy

Health Literacy. U.S. Department of Health and Human Services/HRSA. http://www.hrsa.gov/healthliteracy/

Ask Me 3 Campaign sponsored by the Partnership for Clear Health Communication. www.npsf.org/askme3

For professionals

Abrams MA, Dreyer BP. *Plain Language Pediatric Patient Education: Health Literacy Strategies and Communication Resources for Common Pediatric Topics.* Elk Grove Village, IL: American Academy of Pediatrics, 2009.

Hironaka LK, Paasche-Orlow MK. The implications of health literacy on patient–provider communication. *Arch Dis Child* 93:428–432, 2008.

Nielsen-Bohlman LT, Panzer A, Kindig D. *Health Literacy—A Prescription to End Confusion.* Washington, DC: Institute of Medicine, National Academies Press, 2004.

Sanders LM, Federico S, Klass P, et al. Literacy and child health—a systematic review. *Arch Pediatr Adolesc Med* 163(2):131–140, 2009.

Schwartzberg J, Van Geest JB, Wang CC. *Understanding Health Literacy: Implications for Medicine and Public Health.* Chicago, IL: AMA Press, 2005.

98 Incarceration of Parents

Stephanie Blenner

I. **Description of the issue.** Parental incarceration is an experience shared by an increasing number of children in the United States. Having a parent incarcerated can impact family structure and functioning, as well as a child's behavior and development. Pediatric clinicians have the opportunity to help support children and families affected by a parent's incarceration.

   A. **Epidemiology**
   - According to the Department of Justice, 2.3% of children younger than 18 years (1.7 million children) have a parent in prison. This statistic does not include children who have a parent confined in the nation's jail system.
   - The number of children impacted grew by 80% between 1991 and 2007.

   B. **Terminology.** Parents may be confined in jails or prisons. Jails are local or county facilities that typically house inmates serving shorter sentences or awaiting transfer to prison. Prisons are state or federal institutions where inmates serve longer sentences; prisons are often located distant to communities where offenders' families live.

   C. **Characteristics of incarcerated parents.** The majority of parents are fathers (92%), though maternal incarceration is increasing more rapidly. African American fathers compose the largest percentage of those incarcerated, whereas inmate mothers are more likely to be white. Many inmates have their own childhood histories involving risk factors such as parental substance use, foster care involvement, abuse, and family members who were also involved with the criminal justice system. Drug offenses, often accompanied by chronic substance abuse, are a common reason for incarceration. Almost half of inmates lived with their children prior to arrest; this percentage is higher for parents in local or county jails or when the mother is incarcerated. Most inmate parents maintain some contact with their children during incarceration.

   D. **Affected children.** The majority of affected children are 14 years or younger. African American children are six and a half times more likely and Hispanic children two and half times more likely than white children to have a parent in prison. Like their parents, children often have multiple risks that may potentially impact their developmental outcome.

II. **Impact of parental incarceration.**

   A. **Custodial status.** The child's custodial status during a parent's incarceration varies depending upon whether it is the father or the mother who is incarcerated. Most children with an incarcerated father are cared for by their biologic mother. When the mother is incarcerated, children typically are cared for by relatives, often a grandparent. Involvement with the child welfare system is more likely when the mother is incarcerated.

   B. **Socioeconomic consequences.** Affected children often grow up in impoverished households and are impacted by additional incarceration-related financial strains. More than half of inmates report having provided primary financial support for their children prior to incarceration. Not only does the household lose this income when a parent is incarcerated but also relatives caring for the children may incur substantial cost in trying to maintain the parent–child relationship through visitation or phone contact. Recurring costs can include transportation to distant facilities, food and lodging, commissary deposits for prisoners, and collect phone calls. A history of incarceration may also be stigmatizing, making postrelease employment difficult.

   C. **Behavior.** Studies based on caregiver report have identified a range of child behavioral responses to a parent's incarceration. Common reactions include sadness, withdrawal, and acting out behavior. Boys more typically display externalizing behaviors, whereas girls are more likely to manifest internalizing behaviors. Social support is critical, with children who have lower levels of support demonstrating more behavioral difficulties. Children who are less hopeful, after accounting for stress and social support, also have more behavioral difficulties.

   D. **Development.** There has been limited study of the impact of parental incarceration on a child's development. Younger children and those experiencing maternal incarceration may be particularly vulnerable to developing a pattern of insecure caregiver attachment, with subsequent developmental consequences. In one study of children $2\frac{1}{2}$ to $7\frac{1}{2}$ years of age experiencing maternal incarceration, almost half scored at or below 84 on the Stanford-Binet Intelligence Scale. Poorer cognitive outcomes were associated with higher caregiver risk status and mediated by the family environment.

E. **Longitudinal effects.** An often-asked question by both professionals and caregivers concerns the long-term impact of a parent's incarceration. In longitudinal studies, parental incarceration has been found to be associated with depression, alcohol use, and delinquency in the teenage years and with offending behavior in adulthood. In several studies, these associations were partly or fully attenuated after controlling for familial and social risk factors other than incarceration.

III. Management

A. **Identify affected families.** Caregivers may not readily share a parent's incarceration with pediatric clinicians, though most caregivers report not doing so because they were not asked. Effective screening can be incorporated into standard care by inquiring about household composition and changes at each visit. For example, *"Have there been any changes in your family or in who is living at home?"* Using nonjudgmental language and focusing on a willingness to help support the child and family will help facilitate disclosure.

B. **Provide developmentally appropriate information**
- Caregivers may need guidance in how to talk with children about incarceration. In what has been called a "conspiracy of silence," many children are not told about the incarceration or are given other reasons for a parent's absence such as being told that the parent is at work, at school, or traveling. It is important to provide developmentally appropriate, truthful demystification to help the child understand the situation, emphasizing that the circumstances are not the child's fault. In the absence of such information, children will often invent their own explanation that may differ significantly from reality. Solicit questions from children and clarify misinformation. "Bibliotherapy" (see bibliography below) can often be helpful.
- The age of the child will determine the details included in the explanation. When dealing with younger children, the caregiver may simply explain that the parent needs to be away but is safe and misses the child very much. As children get older, additional explanation about what a prison/jail is and why the parent is there may be appropriate depending on the specifics of each case. With school-aged children, it is also critical to discuss with whom, under what circumstances, and how a child would share information about the parent's situation.
- Contact with the incarcerated parent is frequently a concern for caregivers. When in the child's best interest, visitation, telephone contact, or letters can help support the parent–child relationship. Some facilities have programs in which inmates tape-record themselves reading a child's favorite bedtime book to share with the child. When bringing a child to visit a correctional facility, the caregiver should be prepared with child care items, toys, and snacks. Younger children should visit only if rested and healthy. School-aged children will benefit from a detailed explanation of what to expect. For example, what type of contact is allowed, how long will the visit last, and when will the child see the parent again.

C. **Address co-occurring developmental and behavioral problems.** Developmental, behavioral or emotional concerns should be identified and the child and/or family referred for appropriate intervention.

D. **Support caregiver and cultivate protective factors.** Family/caregiver stress may be decreased by referring eligible families for financial support, legal advocacy or housing, energy, and child care assistance. A child's social support can be enhanced by involvement with after-school programs, athletics, or religious or civic groups. Some communities have targeted programs for children dealing with parental incarceration or for grandparents raising grandchildren.

E. **Recognize that incarceration often is a cycle** and that children and families may need support at each stage—arrest, confinement, and reintegration.

BIBLIOGRAPHY

For professionals and caregivers

The Center for Children of Incarcerated Parents. www.e-ccip.org
The Family and Corrections Network. www.fcnetwork.org

For children

Brisson P. *Mama Loves Me from Away.* Honesdale, PA: Boyds Mills Press, 2004. (Ages 7 and up).

Hodgkins K, Bergen S. *My Mom Went to Jail.* Madison, WI: The Rainbow Project, 1997. (Written at two levels: right pages for preschoolers; left pages for children 6–10 years).

McGuckie CJ. *What Is Jail, Mommy?* Centennial, CO: Lifevest Publishing, 2006. (Ages 4–8). www.whatisjailmommy.com

Woodson J. *Visiting Day.* New York, NY: Scholastic Press, 2002.

99

Gay and Lesbian Parents

Ellen C. Perrin

I. Description of the issue.

A. Epidemiology.

- About 2 million children in the United States younger than 18 years have a (or two) parent(s) who is/are lesbian or gay. Most children with a lesbian and/or gay parent were conceived in the context of a heterosexual relationship. A parent (or both parents) in a heterosexual couple may recognize, acknowledge, and/or disclose his or her homosexuality, after which some parents divorce and others continue to live as a couple. Increasing social acceptance of diversity in sexual orientation has allowed more gay men and lesbians to form committed intimate relationships and to embark on parenthood as a couple. Most of the considerations that exist for heterosexual couples when they consider having children are also faced by lesbians and gay men: concerns about time, finances, how children will affect their relationship, their own and their children's health, and their ability to manage new parenting roles.
- Lesbians and gay men undertaking parenthood face additional challenges, including deciding whether to conceive or adopt a child, obtaining donor sperm, or arranging for a surrogate carrier, finding an accepting adoption agency, making legally binding arrangements regarding future parental relationships, creating a substantive role for the nonbiologic or nonadoptive parent, and confronting emotional pain and restrictions imposed by heterosexism and discriminatory regulations.
- Lesbians who wish to conceive a child may do so by alternative insemination techniques using sperm from a completely anonymous donor, from a donor who has agreed to be identifiable when the child becomes an adult, or from a fully known donor (e.g., a friend or a relative of the nonconceiving partner). Lesbians also can become parents by fostering or adopting children, as can gay men. These opportunities are increasingly available, though local legal statutes in some states and countries may still impose limitations. A growing number of gay men have chosen to become fathers through the assistance of a surrogate carrier who bears their child and possibly also an egg donor. Others have made agreements to participate as sperm donors in the conception of a child (often with a lesbian couple) and arranged to have variable levels of involvement with the child.
- When a lesbian or a gay man becomes a parent through alternative insemination, surrogacy, or adoption, the biologic or adoptive parent is recognized legally as having full and more or less absolute parental rights. Despite the biologic or adoptive parent's partner functioning as a co-parent, he or she has no formal legal rights with respect to the child unless he or she formally adopts the child. Such co-parent (or second-parent) adoption has important psychological and legal benefits.

B. Psychological adjustment and parenting attitudes of parents.
Empirical evidence obtained over the last three decades reveals few differences between lesbian and heterosexual parents' self-esteem, psychological adjustment, attitudes toward child rearing, anxiety, depression, social support, and parenting stress. Much less is known about gay fathers and their children, but early research suggests that these families function in much the same manner as other successful families.

C. Children's gender identity and sexual orientation.
The gender identity of preadolescent children raised by lesbian mothers or gay fathers has been found repeatedly to be consistent with their biologic sex. No differences have been found in the toy, game, activity, dress, or friendship preferences of prepubertal boys or girls who had lesbian mothers compared with those who had heterosexual mothers. Young adults who had homosexual parents have more often reported feelings of attraction toward someone of the same sex and were slightly more likely to consider the possibility of having a same-sex partner. Limited longitudinal research suggests that adult men and women whose parents are heterosexual are as likely to identify themselves as gay or lesbian as are adults who had a homosexual parent.

D. Children's emotional and social development. Because historically most children whose parents are gay or lesbian experienced the divorce of their biologic parents, descriptions of their subsequent psychological development have to be understood in that context. Whether they are subsequently raised by one or both separated parents and whether a stepparent has joined either of the biologic parents are important factors for children.

- A considerable body of research reveals that children of divorced lesbian mothers grow up in ways that are very similar to children of divorced heterosexual mothers. Several studies comparing children after divorce whose mothers were lesbian versus heterosexual have failed to document any differences in personality, peer group relationships, self-esteem, behavioral difficulties, academic success, or the quality of family relationships. Adult children of divorced lesbian mothers have recalled more teasing by peers during childhood than have adult children of divorced heterosexual parents, but they also report satisfaction with their friendships and social relationships.
- Children born to and raised by lesbian couples appear to develop quite normally. Ratings by their mothers and teachers have demonstrated good social competence and self-esteem, and the prevalence and types of behavioral difficulties they demonstrate are comparable with population norms. Some reports suggest that these children may be less aggressive and more tolerant of diversity than children who grow up with heterosexual parents. Children whose lesbian parents report greater relationship satisfaction, more egalitarian division of household and paid labor, and more regular contact with grandparents and other relatives have been rated by parents and teachers to be better adjusted and to have fewer behavioral problems.
- Although gay and lesbian parents may not, despite their best efforts, be able to protect their children fully from the effects of stigmatization and discrimination, parents' sexual orientation is not a variable that, in itself, appears to predict their ability to provide a home environment that supports children's development. Overall, it appears that children are more powerfully influenced by their own biology and family relationships than by family structure.

E. Legal issues. As long as the permanence and full legal status of marriage are not uniformly available to gay and lesbian parents, it is important for them to consider obtaining "power of attorney" for their children and/or seeking full parental rights for both parents via co-parent adoption. Decisions about custody and visitation for children whose parents are separating should be made independent of either parent's sexual orientation.

II. Pediatric management.
A. The office context. The pediatric office settings should be made explicitly welcoming to families of diverse constellations. Posters, books, and magazines and relevant information posted on the waiting room bulletin board can signal to gay and lesbian parents and their children that families such as theirs are expected and appreciated. The language on office handouts and forms should be checked to eliminate heterosexist bias (e.g., be sure they have spaces for "parent" and not "mother" and "father"). Signs and policies should emphasize confidentiality and a respect for diversity, as well as a policy of "zero tolerance" regarding homophobic jokes and comments.

B. Clinical care.
1. Healthcare for children whose parents are gay or lesbian differs little from healthcare that is appropriate for all children. Just as for all children, both parents should be invited to prepare for and to participate in healthcare visits. Discussions about family and peer relationships are always an important part of health supervision. Parents and children should be invited to discuss their family's structure and functioning, including any concerns they may have about it. Information about helpful reading materials as well as about national and local groups of families in which one or both parents is or are gay or lesbian may help parents to build social relationships with other families in which parents are gay or lesbian, as it is helpful for children to know others in similar circumstances.
2. In addition to the developmental tasks and challenges that all children face, children growing up in a family in which one or both parents is or are gay face some predictably challenging transitions.
   - Gay and lesbian parents have to consider how they wish to respond when their child around *3 to 4 years of age* begins to be interested and curious about her or his social/biological origins. Of prime importance to children of this age is security and permanence.
   - For many parents, the impact of *social stigma* is of paramount importance, especially as their *5- or 6-year-old* child ventures out into school life. Parents should exercise some caution with regard to passing on their worry to their children, who may have an easier time introducing themselves and their families than their parents fear.

Parents may be advised to prepare their children with constructive responses to questions or teasing about their family.

- In *early to middle adolescence*, children are likely to be particularly concerned about their own heritage and family history. In most circumstances at this stage, it is helpful for parents to be fully open about the history of the child's conception and family background.
- During *later adolescence*, all children are exploring their own sexuality and romantic attractions. Teenagers who have grown up in a family that includes one or more gay parents may find that unique assets and impediments coexist in their families just as among those of their peers who have heterosexual parents.

3. **Coping with stigma.** Parents may need encouragement and/or advice regarding how to help their child(ren) recognize, discuss, and cope with stigmatization or embarrassment that arise as a result of their parent(s)' sexual orientation or their family constellation. Pediatric providers may be able to help parents to identify strategies to help their children to manage painful encounters with homophobia. It is often helpful for children to be prepared for such experiences in advance and to know how to respond to some predictable questions from curious peers. These strategies may change as children grow up and should be reassessed and discussed repeatedly.

Adolescents may find their parents' sexual orientation of more concern, and discussion with a professional may help to make the home environment comfortable for teenagers and their friends. Older children may not reveal their feelings of marginalization or embarrassment about their homosexual parent(s), in part, out of a concern that knowledge of their stigmatization might be hurtful to the parent(s).

To prepare children, parents have to make difficult and complex decisions about disclosure. How freely are they willing to allow their child to describe their family? Are there risks to the child or the parents? Can they give children guidelines about "selective secrecy" and help them to understand how to make good decisions about disclosure? If the community is supportive, full disclosure to schools and other organizations and individuals important in children's lives will be easiest for children. Parents of older children and adolescents can be helpful by describing their own encounters with homophobia and the strategies they have used to counteract it.

4. **Discussing the family's history.** Parents may ask for assistance in initiating discussions about the child's original family or about her or his conception. Reading children's books together may help parents to explain the process of their becoming a family. If children are preoccupied or worried about the absent parent or donor or if the relationship between divorced parents is strained, a short series of meetings with a family therapist may be helpful in ensuring open communication among family members and support for the child(ren).

5. **Information control.** Many parents are comfortable in letting healthcare providers know about their sexual orientation and family constellation, but for others, this may represent too great a risk. Before recording this information in the office chart, parents should be asked their preference. It is especially important in referring a child to a specialist to be sure what information about the family constellation the child and parents wish to have shared.

C. **Beyond the office walls.** Healthcare professionals can help to support parent groups and/or groups for children whose parents are gay or lesbian, advise schools and libraries, provide information and advocacy to local and national legislators, and facilitate education via the public media and through professional organizations. They should encourage their local school and community libraries to have available a wide variety of books for children from preschool through adolescence that describe families in which the parents are gay or lesbian. An annotated list of selected books for children and adults can be found in Perrin (2002) listed in the bibliography.

As advisers to schools, child healthcare professionals have an opportunity to advocate for presentations of diverse family structures and to address issues related to sexuality and sexual orientation at every age level from kindergarten through high school. Explicit statements by healthcare professionals and evidence of their acceptance of a broad range of sexual orientation and behavior carry an important message to counteract the pervasive stigma that surrounds homosexuality.

BIBLIOGRAPHY

Organizations

Gay, Lesbian, and Straight Education Network (GLSEN). www.glsen.org
Children of Lesbian and Gays Everywhere (COLAGE). www.COLAGE.org

Family Equality Council. www.familyequality.org
Human Rights Campaign. www.hrc.org/issues/parenting

Books for parents

Bernstein RA. *Families of Value: Personal Profiles of Pioneering Lesbian and Gay Parents.* New York, NY: Marlowe Publishers, 2005.

Clunis DM, Green GD. *The Lesbian Parenting Book,* Emeryville, CA: Seal Press, 2003.

Drucker J. *Lesbian and Gay Families Speak Out: Understanding the Joys and Challenges of Diverse Family Life.* New York, NY: Perseus Books Group, 1998.

Howey N. *Out of the Ordinary: Essays on Growing Up with Gay, Lesbian, and Transgender Parents.* New York, NY: Stonewall Inn Editions, 2000.

Johnson SM. *For Lesbian Parents: Your Guide to Helping Your Family Grow Up Happy, Healthy and Proud.* New York, NY: Guilford Press, 2001.

Lev AI. *The Complete Lesbian and Gay Parenting Guide.* New York, NY: Berkley Trade, 2004.

Priwer S, Phillips C. *Gay Parenting: Complete Guide for Same-Sex Families.* Far Hills, NJ: New Horizon Press, 2006.

Snow JE. *How It Feels to Have a Gay or Lesbian Parent: A Book by Kids for Kids of All Ages.* Binghamton, NY: Routledge, 2004.

For professionals

American Academy of Pediatrics Policy Statement. Co-parent or second parent adoption by same-sex parents. *Pediatrics* 109(2):339–344, 2002.

Goldberg AE. *Lesbian and Gay Parents and Their Children.* Washington, DC: American Psychological Association Press, 2010.

Pawelski JG, Perrin EC, Foy JM, et al. The effects of marriage, civil union, and domestic partnership laws on the health and well-being of children. *Pediatrics* 118:349–364, 2006.

Perrin EC. *Sexual Orientation in Child and Adolescent Health Care.* New York, NY: Kluwer/Plenum Academic Press, 2002.

Schorzman C, Gold M. Gay and lesbian parenting in "homosexuality in child health care." *Curr Probl Pediatr Adolesc Health Care* 34(10):355–98, 2004.

Tasker F. Lesbian mothers, gay fathers, and their children. *J Dev Behav Pediatr* 26(3):224–40, 2005.

100 Media

Victor C. Strasburger

I. **Description of the issue.** Children and teens spend more time with media than in any other activity except for sleeping—an average of more than 7 hours per day. By the time today's children and teenagers reach 70 years of age, they will have spent 7–10 years of their lives watching TV alone. The presence of a TV set or an Internet connection in the bedroom increases screen time and the risk of adverse health effects. Despite this, most parents are reluctant to control their children's media use and are relatively clueless about what media they are using. New media (the Internet, social networking sites, video games) allow teens and preteens to download violent videos, post risqué sexual photographs, send sexual text messages ("sexting"), engage in anonymous bullying behaviors, and even buy prescription drugs, alcohol, and cigarettes.

- Despite the Internet and cell phones, TV remains the predominant medium for children and adolescents. Young children are especially vulnerable to the influence of TV. According to the social learning theory, children and adolescents learn from watching their parents and other adults model certain behaviors. Certainly, there are no more attractive role models than those on TV, discussing everything from sex and alcohol to food and careers. TV gives young people secret glimpses into the adult world and serves as a powerful teacher, shaping attitudes and influencing behavior.
- New media *are* important, however. Studies show that a majority of youth have accessed pornography on the Web, and many teens reference their own risky behaviors in their on-line profiles. Internet bullying occurs, and violence Web sites and pro-Ana (pro-Anorexia Nervosa) Web sites are potentially dangerous. First-person shooter video games desensitize players and can actually teach teens how to shoot a gun.
- Super-peer theory states that the media function very much like an especially powerful peer group, particularly when risky behaviors are concerned. TV, movies, and social networking sites often make it seem like that all teenagers are engaging in sexual intercourse, drinking alcohol, and engaging in other risky behaviors.
- According to the cultivation effect, heavy media users tend to believe that the media world is real and that people in everyday life should behave accordingly. Media also exert a powerful displacement effect: 3 hours a day spent viewing TV, for example, are 3 hours a day lost from schoolwork, reading, and exercise.

II. **Areas of concern.** Practitioners should familiarize themselves with the specific areas of concern with regard to TV content.
   A. **Baby Videos and TV.** Studies show the 70% of American infants younger than 2 years currently watch 1–2 hours of TV and videos per day. Yet, there are now seven peer-reviewed studies that document potential language delays, and *no* studies that document benefit. Early brain development research indicates that babies learn best from interacting with live humans and not inanimate screens.
   B. **Violence.** According to the National TV Violence Study (which examined nearly 10,000 hours of American TV in the mid-1990s), children's TV is more violent than adults TV. In addition, one quarter of the violent interactions features guns. The average child views 10,000 murders, rapes, and assaults per year on TV. Violence is frequently portrayed either as humorous or as an acceptable solution to a complex problem, particularly for the "good guy." The notion of justified violence—so prevalent on American TV and movie screens—is perhaps the most powerful reinforcement for aggressive behavior. Scientific studies suggest that a heavy exposure of TV violence may lead to aggressive behavior in certain susceptible children and teens. In one study, for example, children became more violent in their play after TV was introduced into their community. They also exercised less and were less creative in their play. In another remarkable 22-year study, a heavy exposure of violent TV programs aimed at those 8 years or younger correlated significantly with more aggressive behavior at 19 and 30 years of age. Nearly everyone who views media violence is *desensitized* to real-life violence, and very young children may be frightened by what seems perfectly acceptable to older children or adults.

C. **Commercialism.** Children view more than 25,000 commercials per year. This is especially problematic for children younger than 8 years, who do not understand the difference between programming and commercials or do not understand that commercials do not always tell the truth. The American economy spends $250 billion a year on advertising—more than twice the amount spent by any other country.

   Clearly, advertising works. Children exposed to advertising request more toys, fast food, and junk food. Digital advertising (Internet, cell phones, interactive TV commercials, etc.) will soon become commonplace.

D. **Overweight and Eating Disorders.** Numerous studies demonstrate a link between the amount of TV viewed and the prevalence of overweight in children. The mechanism remains unclear: TV may (1) displace more active activities, (2) give children and teens unhealthy ideas about nutrition, (3) influence eating patterns and habits, and (4) interfere with sleep. Snack food, fast food, and heavily sugared cereals are most frequently advertised. TV characters rarely engage in nutritious eating practices. The average child or teen sees between 4400 and 7600 food advertisements per year on TV alone. Media are also critical in influencing many young girls' body self-image. The average American model or movie star is a size 0 or 2 compared with the average American woman who may be a size 12–14. A naturalistic study of Fiji teenagers, before and after the introduction of American TV shows, documented that symptoms of eating disorders increased dramatically within 3 years afterwards.

E. **Sex and Sexuality.** American media have become the leading sex educator in America today. This occurs in part because parents are reluctant to discuss sex or birth control with their children and in part because the majority of schools no longer offer comprehensive sex education programs. On prime-time TV, 75% of shows contain sexual content, but only 10% mention the risks or responsibilities of sexual activity or the need for contraception. Children and teens view an estimated 14,000 sexual references and innuendoes a year. Advertisements for condoms or birth control pills are rarely seen on national network TV and never mention pregnancy prevention. Experts attribute the high teenage pregnancy rate in the United States to three key factors: (1) inadequate access to birth control, (2) ineffective sex education in school, and (3) inappropriate media portrayals of human sexuality. There are now several cause-and-effect longitudinal studies documenting that exposure to sexual content in a variety of different media may lead to earlier onset of sexual intercourse during adolescence.

F. **Drugs.** Of the $250 billion spent on advertising annually, nearly 10% is spend advertising drugs—$13 billion on cigarette advertising and promotion, $5 billion on alcohol, and $4 billion on prescription drugs. American children and teens view 2000 beer commercials per year. Most of the advertisements try to create the illusion that drinking alcohol is a normative behavior and that people who do so are more successful, happier, and sexier. For every antidrug public service announcement (PSA) on TV, there are estimated 25–50 beer commercials. Most PSAs deal only with marijuana, cocaine, inhalants, or heroin and not with alcohol—the leading killer of American teenagers today.

   Several researchers have documented Web sites that seem to encourage alcohol use by underage drinkers, and teens have been known to purchase cigarettes, alcohol, and even prescription drugs online. New research also indicates that exposure to scenes of cigarette smoking or drinking in the movies may be the leading cause of early adolescent smoking or drinking.

G. **Rock music and music videos.** Despite the fact that rock music lyrics have become sexier and more violent since the 1950s, there are no data to show that such lyrics have a negative behavioral impact (although a preference for heavy metal or rap music may be a marker for risky behaviors). Indeed, in one study, only 30% of young people even knew the lyrics to their favorite songs and their ability to decipher the meaning of the lyrics was age dependent. Music videos, on the other hand, are more likely to have a demonstrable impact. Although many music videos are harmless "performance videos" (of the band playing), others are concept videos that often tell a story replete with sexual imagery, violence, drug use, and sexism.

H. **The Internet and social networking sites.** Nearly all teenagers (93%) are online, and 71% have a cell phone. Internet use includes watching videos (57%), visiting social networking sites such as MySpace and Facebook (65%), making online purchases (38%), and getting health information (28%). Research shows that online communication and self-disclosure can increase adolescents' social connectedness and their well-being, but it comes at a price. Online bullying occurs, but its true frequency is unknown. Similarly, while parents fear online sexual predators, most recent studies suggest that sexual solicitation of minors occurs more often by other minors. One national survey of cell phone "sexting" found that 20% of 13- to 19-year-olds had sent a sexual message and nearly half had received one.

I. **Other areas of concern.** Heavy media use has also been associated in correlational studies (i.e., not necessarily cause-and-effect studies) with poor academic performance in school, hyperactivity, hypertension, hypercholesterolemia, depression, and mood disorders.

III. **Advice and guidance for families.**

A. **The American Academy of Pediatrics (AAP) recommends that parents limit their children's total media screen time to no more than 1–2 hours per day and that parents should avoid letting infants younger than 2 years routinely watch TV or videos.** The easiest way to accomplish this is to counsel parents of 6- to 12-month-olds about the potential harmful effects of TV on children and to advise them to set strict limits from the outset.

B. **The AAP recommends that parents control which shows their children watch and that they watch TV with their children.** Studies show that parents can override any potentially harmful effects of TV programming and other media by discussing objectionable material with their children.

C. **Primary care clinicians should counsel parents to avoid placing a TV set or an Internet connection in a child's bedroom.** Currently, one fourth of young children, one third of older children, and more than half of teenagers have a TV set in their own bedroom. Control over TV viewing or Internet use is impossible when the TV or Internet connection is in the child's or teen's bedroom. Studies show that the presence of a bedroom TV increases the risk of obesity and adolescent substance abuse (since children are exposed to more PG-13 and R-rated movies).

D. **Advising parents not to use the TV as "an electronic babysitter" is probably unrealistic. Rather, parents should be counseled to use the videocassette recorder or DVD player to control what and when their child is viewing.** An easy way to put the issue into perspective for parents is through the following analogy: *"No parent would allow a stranger into his or her home to teach his or her child for 3–5 hours a day (especially a stranger who is obsessed with sex, violence, and commercialism). Yet that is precisely what TV is doing."*

E. **Primary care clinicians should consider asking two simple questions: (1) *Is there a TV set or an Internet connection in the child's bedroom?* (2) *How much total screen time does the child view per day?*** Brief office counseling has been shown to be effective in getting parents to limit screen time.

F. **Clinicians and parents need to familiarize themselves with children's media.** For preschoolers, the Rabbit Ears series of classic children's stories, narrated by Hollywood stars, with music by well-known performers, is an outstanding alternative to the usual network fare. Many organizations have Web sites that can help parents decide what media are appropriate for their children. Parents need to look carefully for prosocial media for their children. Parents should also avoid taking young children to see PG-13 and R-rated movies that often may contain violence, alcohol use, or cigarette smoking.

G. **Clinicians need to work both with schools and with parents to emphasize the need for media education.** Teaching children how to view media can help mitigate many of the negative effects, and such programs are common in other developed countries.

H. **Feedback—both negative and positive—to the networks, the cable companies, and the Federal Communications Commission is critically important in trying to improve the quality of programming for children.** The networks estimate that one letter represents 10,000 viewers.

BIBLIOGRAPHY

For professionals and parents

Organizations

American Academy of Pediatrics, Council on Communications and Media. http://cocm.blogspot.com/
Center on Media and Child Health. www.cmch.tv
Center for Media Literacy. www.medialit.org
Common Sense Media. www.commonsensemedia.org
Federal Communications Commission (FCC). www.fcc.gov
Interactive Food & Beverage Marketing. www.digitalads.org
National Institute on Media & the Family. www.mediafamily.org
New Mexico Media Literacy Project. www.nmmlp.org
Parents' Choice Foundation. www.parents-choice.org
Rudd Center for Food Policy and Obesity. www.yaleruddcenter.org

Media

Rabbit Ears videos/DVDs/tapes. http://www.greattapes.com/gt/series.phtml/rabbitears

Publications

American Academy of Pediatrics. Policy statements (all published in *Pediatrics*): Media violence, *Pediatrics* 124:1495–1503, 2009. Impact of music, music lyrics, and music videos on children and youth, *Pediatrics* 124:1488–1494, 2009. Sexuality, contraception, and the media (2010, in press); Media education (2010, in press); Media use in children under 2 (2010, in press); Children, adolescents, substance abuse, and the media (2010, in press); Children, adolescents, obesity, and the media (2010, in press).

Christakis DA, Zimmerman FJ. *The Elephant in the Living Room*. Emmaus, PA: Rodale Books, 2006.

Strasburger VC, Jordan AB, Donnerstein E. Health effects of media on children and adolescents. Manuscript under review, *Pediatrics* 125:756–767, 2010.

Strasburger VC, Wilson BJ, Jordan A. *Children, Adolescents, and the Media* (2nd ed).Thousand Oaks, CA: Sage, 2009.

101

Military Families and Deployment

Molinda Chartrand

I. Description.

A. Military deployment. Deployment is the short-term assignment of military service members to a duty location other than the one to which they are assigned. Deployments may be planned or unexpected, to a combat or noncombat zone, and can last from 1 to 18 months. The current average length of deployment across all military services is 12 months. One thing that all deployments have in common is the separation of service members from their family. Both active duty and reserve military members experience deployment. These deployments may have significant repercussions for every member of the military family.

B. Military culture. The military, in the broadest sense, encompasses everyone that wears a military uniform as well as his or her family members. This includes both active duty (full-time) military service members and the reserve/guard component members. In general, the military community tends to be close-knit and supportive. On top of shared day-to-day and life experiences, there are strong core values for each service (Army, Air Force, Navy, and Marines) that help to bring a sense of purpose and meaning through difficult times. Among those are patriotism, duty, honor, and courage.

Military families routinely face many stressors such as frequent moves, separation from extended family support systems, and significant job-related hazards. They are typically resilient to these various challenges. The factors that contribute to military family resilience are not different from those for civilian families; that is, the health, mental health, and functioning of the mother, the father, and the family contribute to the development and well-being of children.

II. Demographics.

A. Active duty members. In 2009, there were 1.4 million active duty military members in the Army, Air Force, Navy, and Marines. They are accompanied by 700,000 spouses and more than 1.2 million children (0–5 years: 40%; 6–11 years: 32%). They typically live on or near a military base, have relatively easy access to a wide variety of military support services including family-readiness center, military family life consultants, mental health care providers, spousal support groups, and child care.

B. Reserve members. In 2009, the reserve component had more than 1.1 million members, 455,000 spouses, and 720,000 children (0–5 years: 24%; 6–14 years: 47%). Service members and their families who are serving in the reserves face unique challenges. These "citizen soldiers" are rarely located near a large military base and as a result have limited access to military-specific resources that are related to deployment. These service members and their families often receive their medical care in the civilian community from clinicians who may not be as aware of military unique circumstances or the impact of deployments on families.

III. Deployment.

A. Emotional cycle of deployment. Every family handles deployments differently. For some families, deployment is a part of the "military lifestyle"; they are resilient and able to cope with minor hiccups. For other families, deployment can be a catastrophe. A family's response to deployment can be complicated and is not limited just to the time of separation. The emotional cycle of deployment (Fig. 101-1) is a typical and predictable pattern of emotional response when a military member is deployed. The cycle can provide a guide for intervention. The framework divides deployment into five phases: predeployment, deployment, sustainment, redeployment, and postdeployment. Each stage is characterized by a defined set of emotional changes and different stressors.

- During **predeployment,** the family has been notified that the family member is leaving. Family members may not know where, and it may also be short notice. Accompanied by this notification is an immediate anticipation of loss that is balanced by denial. Military service members often spend long hours away from the family training and getting

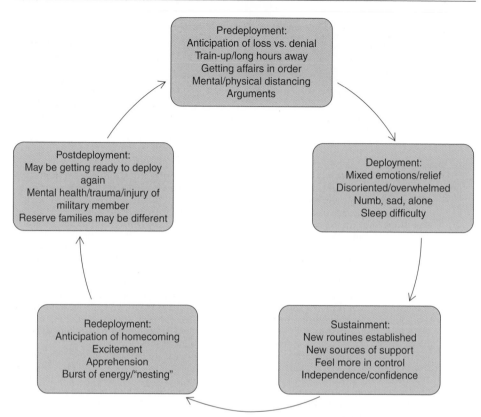

Figure 101-1. The Emotional Cycle of Deployment. Adapted from Logan KL. "Emotional Cycle of Deployment," Logan KV. The Emotional Cycle of Deployment. *Proceedings*, Feb 1987:43–47.

affairs in order. There can be a mental/physical distancing. Emotional stress may lead to arguments and saying things you wish you had not on the part of everyone.
- With **deployment,** there can be mixed emotions, even a sense of relief. The remaining parent can feel overwhelmed with new duties. There may be difficulty with sleep.
- After some time, the family members enters the **sustainment** phase. They settle into new routines, and new sources of support are found (may be more difficult for reserve families). There also may be a sense of independence and confidence.
- With **redeployment** home of the service member, the anticipation of homecoming is a new emotional whirlwind: excitement, apprehension.
- Finally, the member has returned home in the **postdeployment phase:** there is the joy of having him or her home safe and sound, but there is a loss of independence, disruption of routines, and the challenge of reintegrating the military member back into the family. Because of the recent trend toward back-to-back deployments, some have begun to speak of deployment as a "spiral" rather than a "cycle" because there is never a return to normal life.
B. **Risk factors during deployment.** Research conducted during the first Gulf War and the current conflicts has identified certain characteristics that can place a family at greater risk for adverse response to deployment. They are as follows:
  - Young and recently married (<5 years), lower-ranking soldier families
  - Younger children (<5 years old)
  - Families that have experienced multiple deployments
  - Families with prior mental health stresses and families that were not functioning well before deployment for any reason
  - Reserve/guard families
  1. **Typical child responses during deployment.** In general, children take their emotional cues from their parents. If their parent is anxious, irritable, or frightened, young

children will respond and mirror these emotions. Children cope best when the adults in their life can be supportive and available. All family members will experience emotions during the cycles of deployment that are a normal response to an abnormal situation that is unique to the military—deployment. Some "normal" responses of children to deployment are as follows:

- **Preschoolers.** They may be clingy and irritable. They may be more aggressive and act out. They may have more somatic complaints and have fears about their parents or others leaving. They may also seem to regress behaviorally—potty accidents, thumb sucking, baby talk, or refusing to sleep alone. When service members return home, their preschooler may be shy and fearful or talkative and clingy.
- **School age.** Despite support, school-aged children may be shocked, angry, or in denial. They may have a greater understanding of world events and their military parent's job and so may be fearful for their parent's well-being. These emotions may manifest with angry outburst, lots of "what if" types of questions, and limit testing. Sleep disturbances are common. Children of reserve/guard families may have a sense of isolation and loneliness because they may be the only child in their neighborhood/community who is experiencing a deployment. When the service member returns home, school-aged children will be excited and crave their parent's attention or they may still have some anger at being left.
- **Teenagers.** For teenagers, deployment can be a time of personal growth during which they take on additional roles and responsibilities within the family. On the flip side, it can also be a difficult time that adds stress to an already developmentally turbulent time. Teens may become emotionally distant, moody, depressed, angry, and disrespectful. They may become very worried and anxious about their deployed parent, especially in the setting of a combat deployment. School, friends, and homework may suffer. Teens can often become "parentified," taking on the deployed parents roles and responsibilities, which can create a challenging transition at homecoming.

IV. Epidemiology.

Since the start of the conflicts in Iraq and Afghanistan, more than 1.6 million military members have served at least one deployment, with 34% having served more than one deployment. Currently, almost 2 million children are living in military families during a time of war. While most military families and children weather deployments, some detrimental effects of military deployments are as follows:

A. Impact on military members.

- Since 2003, tens of thousands of service members have been injured, and thousands have died in military service.
- One in five service members meets screening criteria for posttraumatic stress disorder (PTSD) 1 year after return, and injured soldiers have higher rates. More soldiers screen positive for PTSD at 7 months than at 1 month, indicating that the posttraumatic effects may be delayed.
- National Guard members and Reservists screen positive for mental health concerns at slightly higher rates than active duty members.

B. Impact on the military spouse.

Military spouses are more likely to experience depression during a spousal deployment as well as lower marital satisfaction and the perception of less social support than civilian wives.

When husband and wife perceive an upcoming deployment in positive terms, spousal relationships are also more positive.

Social support predicts a positive mental health outcome for wives and children of deployed fathers.

C. Impact on children in military families.

Children with a deployed father had:

- More behavioral problems
- Higher levels of depression and anxiety
- Twofold increase in rates of child neglect during combat deployments
  Adolescents with a deployed parent had higher heart rates, systolic blood pressures, and higher self-perceived stress.

Approximately 30,000 United States children have experienced the return of an injured parent or the death of a parent. The impact of living with a parent who may be suffering with PTSD, other mental health disorder, or significant physical injury is unclear.

V. Supporting military families.

The most important step in supporting military families is identifying them in your practice. Screen your families for military involvement and deployment history. Some questions that will help you support military families are as follows:

A. If you have a military family in your practice:
- Active duty or reserve component?
- Where is the family in the "cycle of deployment"?
- Ask about possibility of deployment
- Obtain a deployment history—how many previous deployments have happened, how did the family function? What was easy and what was hard?
- Screen for predeployment risk factors

B. If a family member is deployed:
- Ask about his or her job, where is he or she, how often he or she is able to communicate?
- Are there worries about the service member's safety?
- How are the nondeployed spouse and the children doing? Screen for typical responses to deployment and provide reassurance when typical responses occur.
- Is there support in the area—families, friends, community, and military base? Become knowledgeable about available community resources.

C. If a family member has been deployed and has returned
- Ask about the reunification adjustment, how is everyone reconnecting?
- How is the service member doing? Any concerning behaviors?

D. Provide routine support for military families that are doing well. Make them aware of available resources. If a child is having extremely disruptive behaviors, the symptoms last longer than 2 weeks, or threats of injury to themselves or others occur, a referral for mental health care provider is warranted.

BIBLIOGRAPHY

For parents

Talk Listen Connect. http://www.sesameworkshop.org/initiatives/emotion/tlc. Talk, Listen, Connect is a multiphase, bilingual, multimedia initiative that guides families through multiple challenges, such as deployments, homecomings, and changes that occur when a parent comes home.

NMFA—Operation Purple Camps. http://www.nmfa.org/site/PageServer?pagename??op_default. The goal of these free summer camps is to bring together youth who are experiencing some stage of a deployment and the stress that goes along with it. Operation Purple® camps give children the coping skills and support networks of peers to better handle life's ups and downs.

Military One Source. http://www.militaryonesource.com/skins/MOS/splash.aspx or call 1-800-342-9647). Military One Source is provided by the Department of Defense at no cost to active duty, guard, and reserve (regardless of activation status) and their families to help with child care, personal finance, emotional support during deployments, relocation information, and resources needed for special circumstances. The service is available by phone, online, and face-to-face through private counseling sessions in the local community. Highly qualified, master's degree-prepared consultants provide the service.

Military Child Education Coalition. www.militarychild.org. The Military Child Education Coalition is a nonprofit organization that identifies the challenges facing the highly mobile military child, increases awareness of these challenges in military and educational communities, and initiates and implements programs to meet these challenges.

Tragedy Assistance Program for Survivors. www.taps.org or call 800959TAPS. The Tragedy Assistance Program for Survivors, Inc, is a nonprofit Veteran Service Organization offering hope, healing, comfort, and care to thousands of American armed forces families each year who experience the death of a loved one.

Zero to Three—Coming Together Around Military Families. www.zerotothree.org/about-us/funded-projects/military-families. Military Projects at Zero To Three has launched Coming Together Around Military Families, a program aimed at strengthening the resilience of young children and their families who are experiencing deployment and separation.

Mental Health Self-Assessment Program. DOD sponsored anonymous mental health/alcohol screening and referral program offered to families and service members affected by deployment or mobilization—available online 24/7 at www.MilitaryMentalHealth.org.

For kids

Ferguson-Cohen M. *Daddy, You're My Hero!* // *Mommy, You're My Hero!* 2005. (For kids ages 4–8)

LaGreca A, et al. *Helping Children Cope with the Challenges of War and Terrorism.* (Kids ages 7–12). 7-Dippity. Entire Book is available for download: www.7-dippity.com/other/UWA_war_book.pdf Supplement (for using with school classes or groups): www.7-dippity.com/other/Supplement.pdf.

Robertson R. *Deployment Journal for Kids.* St. Paul, MN: Elva Resa Publishers, 2005.

Spinelli E, Graef R. *While You Are Away.* New York, NY: Hyperion Books for Children, 2004. [Picture book for children whose parents are deployed; ages 4–8]

For teens

Sherman MD, Sherman DM. *My Story: Blogs by Four Military Teens* is a series of blogs by four military teens that highlights their feelings and experiences before, during, and after parental deployment. www.seedsofhopebooks.com

For professionals

American Academy of Pediatrics (AAP) Military Youth Deployment Support Web site. http://www.aap.org/sections/uniformedservices/deployment/index.html

Caring for America's children military youth in a time of war. *Pediatr Rev* 30:e42–e48, 2009.

Zero to Three—Coming Together Around Military Families. www.zerotothree.org/about-us/funded-projects/military-families

102 Maternal Depression

Prachi E. Shah

I. **Description of the problem.** Depression and depressive disorders are among the most prevalent mental health problems in the United States. For women 15–44 years of age, depression is the leading cause of disease burden worldwide. The effects of maternal depression on child development are well documented. Children of depressed parents are at risk for developing significant psychological, social, learning, and behavioral problems. The mechanisms by which maternal depression affects child development are multifactorial and may be related to a transaction between genetics, parent–child interactions, parenting behaviors, and child characteristics. Maternal mental health issues often go undetected, and pediatric clinicians are in an optimal position both to screen and to refer mothers at risk for further evaluation and treatment.

- Maternal depression is a significant psychosocial risk factor with serious adverse implications for child development.
- Adverse child health outcomes include increased risk of developmental delay, behavior problems, mental health disorders, including depression, poorer cognitive, social, and emotional functioning, asthma, and injuries.
- Children may be at higher risk for adverse outcomes if both parents are in poor mental health. Alternatively, a father with better mental health can buffer the effects of maternal depression on the child's behavioral and emotional outcomes.
- Depressed mothers are more likely to utilize emergency department services and specialty health services and are less likely to engage in preventive parenting practices and utilize well-child care visits.
- Increased rates of depression are seen in families with several young children or with a child with a chronic illness in the household.
- Higher rates of depression are associated with living in the inner-city, lower socioeconomic status, immigrant status, poor marital relationships, drug and alcohol usage, and lower levels of education.
- Estimates of maternal depressive symptoms in a variety of pediatric practice settings has ranged from 12% to 47%.
- Postpartum depression has a reported incidence of 8%–15%.

II. **Classification of Maternal Depression.**

A. **Depression (or major depressive disorder)** is defined by the following *Diagnostic and Statistical Manual of Mental Disorders, Fourth Edition* criteria: Five (or more) of the following symptoms have been present during the same 2-week period and represent a change from previous functioning and at least one of the symptoms is either (1) depressed mood or (2) loss of interest or pleasure.

- Significant weight loss when not dieting, or weight gain, or decrease or increase in appetite nearly every day.
- Insomnia or hypersomnia nearly every day.
- Guilt (excessive or inappropriate) or feelings of worthlessness nearly every day.
- Energy loss or fatigue nearly every day.
- Concentration diminished or indecisiveness, nearly every day (by either subjective account or observation made by others).
- Agitation (psychomotor) or retardation nearly every day.
- Pleasure lost (anhedonia) in all, or almost all, activities most of the day, nearly every day as indicated by either subjective account or observation made by others.
- Suicidal ideation or recurrent thoughts of death without a specific plan, or a suicide attempt, or a specific plan for committing suicide.

B. **Postpartum mood disorders.**

1. **Postpartum blues** is experienced by 40%–80% of new mothers and is characterized by rapid mood swings, emotional lability, anxiety, decreased concentration, and sleeping difficulties that occur within the first 2–3 days of delivery and that **resolve by 2 weeks**

postpartum. If symptoms persist for more than 2 weeks, a diagnosis other than postpartum blues must be considered.

2. **Postpartum psychosis.** Prevalence: 0.1%–0.2% and is characterized by severe sleeping disturbances, rapid mood swings, anxiety, delusions, hallucinations, racing thoughts, rapid speech, and thoughts of suicide or infanticide.

3. **Postpartum depression.** Prevalence: 8%–15% and is characterized by sleep disturbances, changes in appetite, profound lack of energy, anxiety, anger, guilt, feeling overwhelmed, sense of being unable to care for baby, or feelings of inadequacy. For a diagnosis of postpartum depression, depressive symptoms must occur **within 4 weeks of childbirth.**

III. **Effects of maternal depression.**
The symptoms of maternal depression are demonstrated in the mother but are also manifested in the children.

A. **Mothers.** The symptoms of depression interfere with effective parenting:
- Mothers with depression may have increased negative and intrusive behaviors.
- They may have emotional disengagement and demonstrate a lack of responsivity to a child's cues
- They often manifest a lack of warmth, irritability, and aggression, which can contribute to disordered parent–child interactions.
- They may use increased punitive attitudes and criticism and have inaccurate expectations of child development.
- They often have a lower tolerance for child behavior and demonstrate negative attributions for their child's behavior, for example, behavior is attributed to child "being a bad kid" or "being mean or spiteful."
- They are more likely to use ineffective discipline techniques with their children and exhibit more negative appraisals of their children's behavior.
- They often have lower level of confidence in their caregiving abilities.

B. **Children of mothers with depression** may demonstrate numerous signs of emotional and behavioral dysregulation, but symptoms will vary with developmental age:
1. **Infants.**
   - Difficulties with sleep
   - Demonstration of depressive, withdrawn behavioral styles
   - Greater difficulty in soothing, decreased capacity to regulate emotions, increased fussiness
   - Increased risk for insecure attachment
2. **Toddlers and preschoolers.**
   - Decreased exploratory behaviors
   - Lower Bayley Mental and Motor scores
   - Increased aggression, noncompliance, temper tantrums, and externalizing behavior
3. **School-aged children.**
   - Higher levels of internalizing and externalizing symptoms: increased dysphoria and passivity
   - Higher levels of treatment of psychiatric disorders
   - Increased deficits in social competence and academic functioning
   - Increased vulnerability to psychiatric disorders later on
4. **Adolescents.**
   - Increased risk of depression, substance abuse, and conduct disorder
   - Maternal depression can interfere with the adolescent's ability to form a healthy separation from the parent and develop a healthy, separate, autonomous identity.
5. **Gender.**
   - Boys of depressed parents often exhibit more externalizing behaviors (aggression and oppositionality)
   - Girls of depressed parents often exhibit more internalizing behaviors (anxiety and depression)

IV. **Screening for maternal depression in primary care. Validated screening tools for maternal depression.**
Formal screening tools exist to assess for the presence of depressive symptomatology. The following screening tools are suggested because of their widespread availability, well-established psychometric properties, existence in multiple languages, and ready accessibility from the Internet:

A. **Edinburgh Postpartum Depression Scale.** The 10-question Edinburgh Postnatal Depression Scale is a validated screening tool to identify mothers at risk for perinatal depression. The scale queries how the mother felt during the previous week. Scores range from 0 to 30, with scores of more than 13 suggestive of the presence of a depressive illness for which further clinical assessment is indicated.

B. Center for Epidemiologic Studies Depression Scale (CES-D). The CES-D scale is a short self-report scale designed to measure depressive symptomatology in the general population. Scores range form 0 to 60, with scores of more than 16 suggestive of the presence of depressive symptomatology for which further clinical assessment is indicated.

C. Brief 2-question screener for maternal depression. A brief 2-question screener has also been shown to have a high sensitivity for detecting maternal depression compared with longer questionnaires:

- *"During the last 2 weeks have you often been bothered by feeling down, depressed, or hopeless?" (Yes/No)*
- *"During the last 2 weeks, have you been bothered by having little interest or pleasure in activities?" (Yes/No)*

However, despite its high sensitivity, the 2-question screener has a low specificity for detecting maternal depression. If positive results are obtained on the two-question screener, a follow-up questionnaire, such as the PHQ-9, may be used. In addition, follow-up questions can address other somatic symptoms such as changes in sleep, appetite, or activity levels. "Has your depression made it hard for you to do your work, take care of things at home, or get along with other people?"

V. Treatment/interventions of suspected depression.

A. The role of the pediatric clinician. Pediatric clinicians are in a unique position to discuss family issues, probe for depressive symptoms, and possible triggers and to counsel families about the effects of depression on the child's health and well-being. The pediatric clinician is also poised to provide support, comfort, and help to a mother who is suffering and vulnerable.

1. **Acknowledge the mother's perceptions of the problem.** Mothers with depression will often present to the pediatrician with complaints/concerns about their child's behavior. This can be an opportunity to probe further about her experiences of stress and support in the parenting role. A helpful framework to provide a therapeutic alliance and address the mother's affective risk factors in the context of the pediatric encounter can be conceptualized by the mnemonic: **SHARE:**

   - **S:** *Support* the parent and the child: building a therapeutic alliance by joining with the mother in her experience of the child.
   - **H:** *Hear* the parents' concerns about their child's behavior and use the responses to the screening questions as starting point for a conversation about her mood and symptoms.
   - **A:** *Address* the concern for maternal depression and explore with the mother her feelings about the diagnosis and her readiness for treatment.

     Acknowledge that the child is also experiencing the mother's depression and that you will work with her and the child to help the child understand and cope.
   - **R:** *Reflect* with parent how depression may be affecting her experience of the child and her level of functioning.

     Reframe child behavior in terms of the parent–child relationship and the child's ability to self-regulate.

     Reinforce your alliance with the mother and your commitment to help her and her child and their relationship.
   - **E:** *Empower* the parent by formulating an "action plan" to address the concerns identified in the visit that can include individual support for her, intervention for her child, and dyadic interventions to address vulnerabilities or areas of strain in the parent–child relationship.

2. In addition, for older children, it may also be important to help the school-aged and adolescent children know that they did not cause their mother's depression but that their mother has a medical condition for which she needs treatment.

3. Because of the known effects of maternal depression on child development, evaluate the child for the effects of maternal depression (e.g., perform social-emotional and behavioral screen).

B. Initial treatment strategies. Caregivers with unremitting depressive symptoms should be referred to a mental health care provider for further evaluation and treatment. Treatment may include a trial of antidepressants as well as psychotherapy.

1. **Schedule a follow-up visit with the mother.** A scheduled follow-up visit to monitor the quality of her affective symptoms can reinforce your commitment to the mother with depression, and to her mental health, and can underscore your commitment to supporting her in the parenting role.

2. **Consider a referral for parent–child therapy.** Maternal depression often contributes to a child's ability to regulate his emotions, and many children of depressed mothers may demonstrate behavior problems and parent–child relational difficulties. A referral to a child mental health care provider may also be of assistance to address any child affective concerns raised and to provide the mother with techniques and strategies to address any areas of stress or perturbation in the parent–child relationship.

BIBLIOGRAPHY

For Professionals

Center for Epidemiologic Studies Depression Scale. Downloadable from http://www.chcr.brown.edu/pcoc/cesdscale.pdf

Edinburgh Postnatal Depression Scale. Downloadable from http://www.fresno.ucsf.edu/pediatrics/downloads/edinburghscale.pdf

Gjerdingen D, Crow S, McGovern P, Miner M, Center B. Postpartum depression screening at well-child visits: validity of a 2-question screen and the PHQ-9. *Ann Fam Med* 7(1):63–70, 2009.

Useful Web site for maternal depression resources. http://www.medicalhomeportal.org/clinicalpractice/screening-and-prevention/maternal-depression.

103 Sibling Rivalry

Robert Needlman

I. **Description of the problem.** The life-altering impact of sibling rivalry has been recognized since biblical times. At the extreme, sibling relationships are marked by high levels of verbal aggression and physical violence (sibling abuse). Negative sibling relationships predict internalizing disorders (e.g., depression) in adolescence, independent of the parent–child relationship. Conversely, cooperative play, negotiation, and friendly competition between siblings enhance social skills; positive sibling support decreases acting-out behaviors, and affection between siblings blunts the deleterious effects of stress. Parents care deeply about their children getting along. Sibling relationships are often the most enduring relationship, and filial solidarity often provides lifelong social support.

A. **Epidemiology.**
   - 80% to 90% of people have siblings. In childhood, sibs spend on average 13% of their waking time together, often more time than with anyone other than with their parents.
   - Following the birth of a sibling, some degree of upset and behavioral regression (e.g., bed-wetting) is almost universal. One third of children also show developmental gains after a sibling's birth, such as increased self-care and language sophistication.
   - Among younger siblings, negative interactions occur on average eight times per hour, including struggles over toys, hitting or pushing, teasing, name-calling, and verbal threats. The rate decreases with age.
   - Violent acts occur in 49%–68% of sibling pairs, with boy–girl pairs having the most, and girl–girl pairs the least. In one study, 40% of children had hit a sibling with an object.
   - Older siblings are more likely to engage in verbal (as opposed to physical) antagonism; in most surveys, the frequency of positive sibling interactions is greater still. Girl siblings are often closer during the teen years; boy siblings are often closer before or after their teens.

B. **Etiology/contributing factors.**
   1. **Loss of exclusive relationship.** Children with the closest relationships to their mothers may show the greatest upset after the birth of a sibling. In contrast, a close relationship with the father may be protective.
   2. **Spacing of siblings.** Siblings spaced about 2 years apart may experience the most intense rivalries, perhaps because the older child must deal with increased separation from the mother at a time when separation is particularly difficult. Twins, in contrast, seem less prone to rivalry, as do children born 3 or more years apart.
   3. **Temperament and developmental differences.** Siblings with very different behavioral styles may irritate each other or simply not develop common interests. Behavioral disorders (e.g., attention-deficit/hyperactivity disorder) are associated with sibling conflict. Children with developmental disabilities evoke disparate responses in siblings, either pride and protectiveness or intense resentment.
   4. **Role uncertainty.** Older children are often required to take leadership or managerial roles vis-à-vis their younger siblings. At other times, children are expected to play together as equals, with no identified boss. Moving back and forth between these quite different relationships generates friction.
   5. **Family organization and parenting.** High levels of family chaos as well as harsh or emotionally cold parental discipline foster sibling conflict.
   6. **Favoritism and fairness.** Parental favoritism, real or perceived, exacerbates sibling conflicts and fosters anxiety, depression, and acting out in the nonfavored child. In contrast, a belief in parental fairness reduces jealousy.

II. **Making the diagnosis.**
A. **Signs and symptoms.** Sibling fighting may be the chief complaint, or it may emerge during the assessment of other problems, such as aggression, school failure, or acting out. Naughty behavior and mild regression after the birth of a new baby are expected; withdrawn, listless behavior signals more serious psychological strain. Jealousy may also

underlie perfectionism, obsessive worries ("What if the baby gets hurt?"), or overly grown-up (parentified) behavior. It is safe to assume that ambivalent feelings exist whether or not they are apparent.

B. History: Key clinical questions.

1. *[to the child] "Tell me about your brother(s) and sister(s)."* Most children find this question nonthreatening. Invite the child to draw a picture of everyone in the family ("functional family drawing"). "What do they like to do together? When do they get mad at each other?"

2. *[to the child] "What happens when you and . . . fight?"* To get beyond generalizations, ask about specific, recent events. Elicit a play-by-play account, focusing on the antecedents, behaviors, and consequences (ABCs). "What were the children doing before the conflict began? How did it start? What did the parent do? How did it end? Was it typical?"

3. *[to the parent] "How have you handled sibling fights in the past?"* Before offering advice, find out what the parent has already tried.

4. *"Tell me about the children in the family."* Listen for typecasting ("my touchy one; my peacemaker"), stereotyping ("She's always the first to get into an argument"), and siblings with special problems or accomplishments. How does the parent–child relationship vary among the siblings?

5. *"Do the children have separate bedrooms?"* Conflicts may be greater in families in which privacy and personal possessions are not respected.

6. *"How did your child respond to the birth of his or her younger siblings?"* Jealousy may not arise until the older child realizes the baby is staying; or until the baby becomes more interactive around 4 months; or begins to take the older child's toys around a year.

7. *"Tell me the history of your family, from the start."* When the child was born were the parents beginning careers and trying to make ends meet? What was life like in the family with the addition of each child? External changes—for example, a promotion, a move, and death of a grandparent—can greatly affect a child's experience growing up, exacerbating differential treatment by parents and thus sibling jealousy.

8. *"In your family, how are arguments usually settled?"* Sibling conflicts tend to be more violent in the context of marital hostility. Children may fight either in response to built-up anger and tension or to draw attention away from simmering marital conflicts. Where sibling conflict is part of a larger pattern of dysfunction, family intervention may be necessary.

III. Management.

A. Primary goals.

1. **Insight.** Parents may respond with greater empathy, less anger, and more firmness if they recognize in themselves the strong emotions that drive sibling conflicts. To encourage this perspective taking, ask parents how they would feel if their spouse brought home a second husband/wife one day and wanted everyone to live happily together.

2. **Reasonable expectations.** Parents need reasonable expectations for sibling coexistence. Ambivalence is normal; friction may be inevitable. Draw attention to the positive aspects of the relationship (e.g., loyalty). It may not be reasonable to expect an older sibling to take on a supervisory or custodial role if the behavior of the younger sibling is challenging.

3. **Appropriate intervention.** Parents may need to step in to prevent physical harm. Young siblings left to their own devices fight more, at times viciously. Older siblings may be better able to work out their differences on their own. A parent who always comes in on the side of one child (the identified victim) may be inadvertently fueling future attacks. Parents should intervene as much as they have to, but no more.

B. Specific strategies.

1. **Let older siblings help.** With a new baby in the house, a toddler (male or female child) may benefit from having a baby doll to take care of (or drop head first). Advise parents to involve the older child, such as by saying, "The baby is crying! What do you think? Should we try getting a new diaper?"

2. **Avoid comparisons and labels.** Sensitize parents to listen for typecasting statements ("my problem child"). Even positive labels such as "my good listener" or "my little helper" can lead the child to misbehave in order to assert his individuality or can imply to the other children that they are not expected to show those positive qualities.

3. **Fairness, not equivalence.** Parents should explain that everyone in the family is different and everyone needs different things. Children do not get the same thing, but they each get what they need. It helps to refer to fairness: "I pay attention to you when you need me, but right now your sister needs my attention."

4. **State principles.** The perception of parental unfairness fuels sibling resentment. To demonstrate fairness, parents need to set forth principles and refer to them when making their judgments. For example, it is a good principle that every child has the right to privacy in his or her own room or space; siblings have to go away, if asked.

5. **Separate young children.** For siblings, playing together is a privilege, not a right. Let children try to work out their differences but step in and separate the combatants before fighting breaks out. This may mean time-outs for both children, either in opposite corners or in separate rooms.

6. **Challenge the victim–aggressor roles.** While it is true that an older child may consistently dominate a younger one, often the "innocent victim" is actually needling the other sibling to the point of explosion and then basking in parental sympathy while watching the rival being punished.

C. **Follow-up/backup strategies.** Schedule repeated visits to reinforce new patterns of parenting. In particular, after parents limit their intervention, sibling conflicts may temporarily increase. Have parents role-play management strategies (e.g., praising a child's behavior without commenting on the general goodness of the child or making covert sibling comparisons). The following features should suggest referral for subspecialist care.

1. **Multiproblem children.** When sibling jealousy accompanies other problems, such as oppositionality to parents or teachers, aggression toward nonsibling peers, or school failure, the problem is unlikely to resolve without attention to the whole picture.

2. **Multiproblem families.** Parental anger, violence, disorganization, depression, or disengagement may require family or individual therapy, or legal assistance; the sibling relationship may improve as a result.

3. **Physical abuse.** A pattern of repeated injury inflicted by one sibling against another signals a family emergency. The risk of psychological damage is high to both the aggressor and the victim. Parents need to establish the family as a zone of safety, if not tranquility. If they cannot, then more intensive intervention is called for.

BIBLIOGRAPHY

For parents

Faber A, Mazlish E. *Siblings Without Rivalry: How to Help Your Children Live Together So You Can Live Too.* New York, NY: Avon Books, 1988. (An excellent guide designed to help parents understand their children's behavior and make the necessary changes in their own. It presents sound principles using wonderfully clear examples. The cartoon scenarios are particularly helpful.)

Reit S. *Sibling Rivalry.* New York, NY: Ballantine Books, 1985. (A good review of the subject, written for parents, full of useful information.)

Web sites

KidsHealth. http:kidshealth.org/parent/emotions/feelings/sibling_rivalry.html
PBS Kids. http://pbskids.org/itsmylife/family/sibrivalry.html
University of Michigan. http://www.med.umich.edu/yourchild/topics/sibriv.htm

For professionals

Dunn J. *Sisters and Brothers.* Cambridge, MA: Harvard University Press, 1985. (Dunn has carried out some of the best and most relevant longitudinal research on siblings, well summarized here.)

Kim JY, McHale SM, Crouter AC, Osgood DW. Longitudinal linkages between sibling relationships and adjustment from middle childhood through adolescence. *Dev Psychol* 43(4):960–973, 2007.

Newman J. Conflict and friendship in sibling relationships: a review. *Child Study J* 24(2):119–152, 1994. (A thorough review of decades of studies.)

104

Single Parents

J. Lane Tanner

I. **Description of the issue.** A variety of family reconfigurations have become prevalent over the past two decades, but no change has been more dramatic than the shift toward families headed by a single parent. While single-parent status does not represent a problem in itself, single-parent families as a group are significantly more strapped for personal, social, and economic resources and are more likely to have experienced significant losses and change. This chapter is intended to alert the clinician to the stressors and special needs that commonly confront the single-parent family.

A. **Demographics.**
- At least 50% of U.S. children born in the last two decades will spend a substantial period of time living in a home headed by a single parent or guardian.
- Between 1970 and 2007, the number of single-mother homes has more than doubled, from 12% to 26%, whereas single-father homes have increased from 1% to 5.8% during the same interval.
- In 2007, single mothers were living alone with their children in 65% of single-family homes and with another adult, not the father, in 35% of homes.
- Dramatic variations exist in the proportion of families headed by single parents according to race. In 2007, the percentiles of children living with a single parent were as follows:

Age of child	0–2 years	12–17 years
White	6%	17%
Black	35%	42%
Hispanic	10%	22%

- 86% of children in one-parent families live with the mother.
- Single-parent status is the result of parental divorce (37%), a never-married single parent (36%), parental separation (23%), and parental death (4%).

B. **Problems of single-parent families.**
1. **Limitations of available resources.**
   a. **Money.** With 34% of mother-only families living below national poverty levels, the clinician is increasingly obliged to inquire regarding the family's financial resources, the parent's employment status, and the family's dependency on contributions from others.
   b. **Time.** Single parents who are employed are likely to feel that they are continually in a race to provide adequate time to the family, the job, and the endless details of daily life, from groceries to taxes. Unpredictable events, such as an important school activity, a household emergency, or a child's illness, further intrude on this tightly stretched schedule.
   c. **Physical and emotional energy.** In addition to providing the tangible goods and supplies needed by the family, the single parent is called on to provide almost 100% of the emotional support and sustenance for the children. Alone, this parent must shoulder the responsibility for decisions, great and small, that shape their lives.
2. **Network of social support.** Mapping the sources of social support for the single parent requires an awareness of the availability of those sources and the frequency with which the parent actually uses them. Are there other adults (relatives, friend, lover) living in the home? Are they emotionally or responsibly involved with the family? Who is dependent on whom? Are there other people who are emotionally close to the parent who can offer understanding and support? What about institutions (such as the school, workplace, church, or clinic) that can provide support for both the parent and the child?
3. **Major life events, losses, or transitions.** Single-parent status is often born out of crisis (e.g., separation or divorce or the partner's death). These events may also bring

a cascade of secondary losses, which may include changes in the family home, the child's school, friends, or community. Grief, anger, guilt, and depression regularly follow the trauma of such changes. The subsequent transitional period is likely to be disorganized and tumultuous until a realignment of schedule, roles, expectations, and feelings can permit a new and stabilized family life. Such events may have meanings for the child that are very different from those for the parent. For example, divorce and the loss of the family home may bring desired independence and relief for the parent but an unmitigated sense of loss for the child. The clinician must assess these differential meanings and be aware of the time course of adaptation displayed by each family member.

4. **Shifts in relational dynamics.** Family dynamics are substantially different when children are oriented to a single parent as the sole authority and provider and when the parent has only the children as main companions at home.

C. **Common clinical issues.** As with other risk factors, single-parent status by itself confers no predictable condition on the child. The following clinical issues are thus presented as common concerns and should not be understood as applicable to single-parent families across the board.

1. **The single parent who feels off balance and uncertain regarding parenting and child management.** While self-doubt in parenting is surely felt by all parents from time to time, single parents are even more susceptible. The parent seeks advice from the clinician but also "reality testing" and reassurances that her efforts, responses, and feelings (especially negative feelings) are warranted, or at least understood.

2. **The helpless, overwhelmed single parent.** The clinician becomes aware that this parent is not simply looking for good advice but for someone else to lean on in order to make the hard decisions and to take over the responsibility that has become incapacitating. Parental isolation and depression are especially frequent concomitants.

3. **Child behavioral disorders.** These are particularly likely to emerge when the child is pushing the parent to provide unmet needs or when the parent's sense of concern, guilt, or exhaustion regarding the child renders behavioral management ineffective. Behavior disorders in the child may also be symptomatic of ongoing conflict between separated parents.

4. **The child who takes on a "parentified helper role."** The child's adoption of a parental role may be necessary and adaptive for the family while providing rewards for the child connected with his or her new and special position with the parent. On the other hand, such a role may infringe on the individual sociodevelopmental needs and growth of the child.

5. **The child who becomes the parent's companion and confidant.** The key issue here concerns the boundaries between the parent and the child—whether each has her or his own friends, activities, rights of privacy, and freedom to disagree or express anger with the other.

6. **Issues related to the absent parent.** Children must come to terms with developmentally staged personal dilemmas regarding who the absent parent was, is, and will be to them. Special difficulties and challenges exist for the child when the parents' relationship remains conflictual, as well as when the child has entirely lost contact with a parent who was formerly close.

7. **The adolescent single parent and the three-generation household.** This "kinship family" provides crucial social support, shared child rearing, and other resources. There are, however, likely to be intrinsic tensions between the grandparent(s) and the teenage parent. These most predictably center on issues of parental authority for the young child and personal autonomy for the adolescent. The nature of the grandparents' support for their daughter or son and whether they realistically and flexibly encourage the growth of her or his competencies is an important question to address.

8. **The introduction of a new adult into the household.** Whether a friend, relative, or potential future mate, the arrival of a new adult into an established single-parent household is a major event. Its meaning to the child is shaped by his or her own developmental stage and past events and patterns. The potential for the child to feel displaced, intruded on, or disregarded is substantial. Long-term adaptation requires that the parent display her or his intention to remain the head of the household, in charge not only of the children but also in overseeing the authority and responsibilities that are delegated to the new adult.

II. **Management.**

A. **Empathy with the issues.** The primary care clinician is often called on to hear, understand, and validate the concerns and responses of the single parent. Most common to these parents is the sense of aloneness in the consuming and awesome task of child rearing.

It is an attitude of respect for this experience that becomes the clinician's first and most important tool.

- The clinician's direct inquiry of the parent (e.g., *"You have a lot to juggle. How is it going?"* or *"How are you doing balancing everybody's needs? How about your own?"*) opens the door to establishing this basis of understanding and respect.

B. Monitoring the needs of the child. To monitor the needs of the child in the single-parent family, the clinician must remain mindful of the challenges confronting the child and assess his or her adaptation to them. As always, behavioral patterns, school performance, social functioning, and overall sense of happiness and confidence are the best indicators of the child's adaptation to stress. However, in some children, signs of difficulty may not be obvious. For example, the child's anxious loyalty to a single parent or the parent's own urgent or unmet needs may keep either from acknowledging the stressful influences that impinge on the child. The child's needs may come into direct conflict with those of his or her parent (e.g., a parent's new adult relationship that takes away time with the child). Thus, it falls to the clinician to initiate, with the child as well as the parent, an exploration of the potential problems and issues. Directly asking the child about daily routines such as sleep patterns, home responsibilities, daily schedule, and school achievement will often open the door to an exploration of stress and poor adaptation.

C. Supporting the parent. With rare exceptions, support for the child requires support for the parent. The clinician can encourage and support a parent by simply valuing her or his efforts. Advocacy for clearly established generational boundaries and effective parental authority may help clear away some of the hesitancy and doubt the parent is experiencing. Concern for the parent as a person, with individual needs and goals, may encourage him or her to seek an effective network of social support. For the single parent who comes across as helpless and overwhelmed and seems to be pushing for a truly dependent relationship, simple empathy, validation, and good advice are not enough. The clinician may experience the urge to rescue the parent in some way or, alternatively, to run away from such expressed neediness. Advice and helpful ideas offered by the clinician may be met with a disparaging "yes, but" response from the parent.

- For such parents, redescribing expressions of helplessness in terms of particular dilemmas introduces the possibility of choice and action (e.g., *"It sounds as if you are dealing with a lot, and your child's behavior sounds particularly difficult right now, for both of you. Tell me your ideas for handling it"*). By resisting the impulse to provide the answers and by encouraging and organizing the parent's own efforts at problem solving (e.g., *"What will be the effect on your child of such a plan? How about on you and on your goals for yourself as a parent in the short term and in the long term?"*), the clinician's role shifts from that of the fantasized rescuer to that of an understanding yet realistic coach. In addition, reminding the parent of her or his demonstrated competencies, especially those that contradict the current perceptions of helplessness, may bolster self-efficacy and hopefulness.

BIBLIOGRAPHY

For parents

McLanahan S, Sandefur G. *Growing Up with a Single Parent: What Hurts, What Helps.* Cambridge, MA: Harvard University Press, 1994.

Wallerstein J, Blakeslee S. *What About the Kids? Raising Your Children Before, During, and After Divorce.* New York, NY: Hyperion Press, 2003.

For professionals

American Academy of Pediatrics. Family pediatrics. *Pediatrics* 111(suppl):1541–1587, 2003.

Tanner JL. Separation, divorce, and remarriage. In Carey WB, Crocker AC, Coleman WL, et al (eds), *Developmental-Behavioral Pediatrics* (4th ed). Philadelphia, PA: Saunders Elsevier, 2009.

U.S. Census Bureau. America's families and living arrangements: 2007, September 2009. www.census.gov/population/www/socdemo/hh-fam.html. Accessed December 15, 2009.

105

Stepfamilies

Margorie Engel*

I. Description of the problem.

A. Epidemiology.

- Almost 16 million children live in a stepfamily relationship according to the 2000 U.S. Census Bureau. This number does not include the many stepfamilies formed by a child's noncustodial parent, stepfamilies with college-aged and adult stepchildren, and families in which an unwed mother married a man who is not the biological father of her child, as well as the growing number of cohabiting stepfamilies or gay and lesbian households in stepfamily-like relationships.
- The prefix "step" denotes connection between members of a family by the remarriage of a parent and not by blood. Approximately 65% of all remarriages create a stepfamily, whereas 35% of all remarriages are created by childless couples. Therefore, it is important to note that the words "remarriage" and "stepfamily" are not synonymous, especially when reading redivorce statistics.
- It is estimated that by the year 2010, the stepfamily relationship will constitute the most common type of American family.

B. Stresses for children.

1. **Multiple changes.** Stepchildren come into their stepfamily with a history of multiple changes related to their parents' divorce that may put some of the children at risk. Life in a stepfamily brings another set of changes. When a residential move occurs, some obvious ones include leaving a familiar home, neighborhood, school, and best friends. More subtle changes include the new status of being the eldest or youngest child in the family, of no longer being the only child, and of sharing time, attention, and intimacy with a parent who previously had no competing emotional ties.
   - The new stepfamily adults, often caught up in their own personal happiness, may not be fully aware of their children's feelings about all of these changes. Processing change postdivorce usually takes 3–5 years; the remarriage occurs on average 2–3 years postdivorce and may explain the child's heightened resistance to the new set of changes.
   - In the short run, divorce is usually painful for a child, although new and extensive research indicates that the long-term effects may have been exaggerated. Comprehensive studies indicate not all children experience change and loss to the negative degree often implied. In terms of general well-being, a significant percentage of children not only survive the breakup and remarriage but also thrive. As young adults, they emerge from divorce and stepfamilies with enhanced functioning—not despite the things that happened to them during the divorce and after but because of them.
2. **Loyalty conflicts.** Loyalty conflicts are inevitable. An emotional connection to a stepparent may be experienced as a betrayal of the parent who is not living in the household. The absent parent is usually considered to be physically available to the child on a periodic basis. Loyalty conflicts are also present following parental abandonment or death when a child's parent remains present only in memory.
3. **Loss of control.** Feeling a loss of control may be at the root of much of the anger and depression in children and often predates life in a stepfamily. The adults have chosen to make major changes in their lives, oftentimes for the better; the children have had those changes imposed on them.
4. **Stepsiblings.** The presence of stepsiblings may exacerbate the stresses that accompany stepfamily life. Feelings of sibling rivalry, jealousy, insecurity, and the fear that

---

* Prior to their deaths, Emily and John Visher contributed portions of this stepfamily information to chapters in the 1st and 2nd edition of this book.

a sibling may be more loved are often more intense in a stepfamily. Noncustodial children may be offered special treats or exempted from the house rules that resident children must follow. Grandparents may give their grandchildren more lavish gifts than those to their stepgrandchildren. If a baby is born into the stepfamily, sibling jealousy might be magnified by the fear that the "mutual child" may be more loved by the adults. Conversely, the birth may help to solidify the stepfamily because the new baby is biologically related to all of the children and adults. It is certainly true that many stepsiblings develop close bonds, united by their common experience of many family changes.

C. Children's responses.

1. **Preschool.** The stress of a remarriage may cause some preschoolers to cling to parents and to regress behaviorally. In the stage of magical thinking, they may believe that their angry thoughts already have led to or will lead to family disruption. They may also harbor thoughts that they can magically reunite the divorced parents.

2. **School age.** School-aged children are often angry about their powerlessness to halt the changes in their lives. They may counter these feelings of helplessness by imagining that they caused the breakup of the marriage—a fantasy that at least offers some influence over a situation they cannot control. They may still wish that their parents were together and fantasize that if they are "good," their parents will be reunited or that if they are "bad" or "sick," their parents will come together to help. As a result, when divorced parents do work together for the benefit of their child, he or she may unrealistically anticipate that short-term togetherness will lead to long-term reunion.

   • Children at this stage are rarely able to express these feelings verbally and are likely to act out their anger and guilt. They may have tantrums at home, fight with siblings or classmates, develop psychosomatic symptoms, become accident prone, start failing in their schoolwork, or even try to break up the new marriage. Conversely, they may respond by behaving with an angelic virtue, following all the rules and making no obvious waves, so that their inner turmoil remains concealed.

3. **Adolescence.** Adolescents present special difficulties for the stepfamily. They are caught up in their own issues of identity and autonomy, making the new relationships even more difficult to accept. Teen sexuality is burgeoning at the very time they enter a household that is, inevitably, highly sexualized by the newness of the adult marriage. The residential presence of close-in-age stepsiblings or stepparent of the opposite sex can also create sexual tensions.

   • Often an independent teenage child of a single parent is pressured, after the parent's remarriage, to return to a more childish stage of dependency. Teenagers who are used to being a parent's confidant and the "man" or "woman" of the house find themselves losing that favored status when they are expected to become "children" again. This may accelerate their drive to separate from the parents or a desire to live in the home of the other parent.

D. Stress for couples in stepfamilies. Adult couples in stepfamilies must also deal with many strong emotions. Loyalty to their children predates the stepfamily and may create conflicts with the new spouse. Parents may attempt to please the children at all costs in order to compensate for the many family changes. They may also avoid forming a solid bond with a new spouse because they mistakenly feel that to do so would be experienced as a betrayal of their relationships with their children. This, in turn, frequently conflicts with the needs of the new spouse, who may understandably feel like an outsider in an established household.

II. Helping children.

A. General principles.

1. **Accept the child's feelings.** While always validating a child's feelings, from a developmental perspective, children can be taught empathetic skills from early childhood onward and are cognitively capable from around the age of 5. The research on adolescent stepchildren's initiation of conflict with stepparents prescribes emphasizing empathetic skills on the part of children, just as we emphasize this with adults.

2. **Reassure the child (repeatedly, if necessary) that he is not responsible for the dissolution of the parents' marriage.**

3. **Stress that the child is a worthwhile, special person, no matter what decisions parents have made about their own lives.**

4. **Help the child put feelings into words rather than into negative behaviors.** Encourage verbal expression. For example, "A lot of children feel very angry when they have to share a room with stepbrothers or stepsisters. Maybe you feel that way sometimes."

5. **Encourage the child to communicate with parents and stepparents.** The clinician can do this by talking to the family as a group or by asking a child privately for permission to communicate specific information to the adults. For example, discussing with the parents a child's feeling that a stepsibling is being favored, or distress over parents' fighting.

6. **Provide support to the parents and stepparents.** Research strongly suggests that the psychological well-being of children depends more on the functioning of the family than the type of family.

B. **Teenagers.**

1. **The acting out of sexual attraction between stepsiblings can be minimized by having the family adopt a dress code, making appropriate bedroom arrangements, and providing adequate supervision.** Adults also need to be aware of and deal with their sexual feelings toward a stepchild who may appear to be a younger version of their spouse.

2. **Adolescents are often reluctant to become an active member of the stepfamily because of their developmental drive for independence and autonomy and the primacy of their peer relationships.** While remaining open to shared activities, the adults need to allow adolescents to maintain their independence from the stepfamily and to integrate at their own pace. In some cases, the teenager chooses to move out in order to find his or her identity. It is important to remember and acknowledge that children living in stepfamilies are integral members of two separate households.

3. **Divided loyalties may make the adolescent act out in a negative way toward the stepparent.** The parent must emphasize to the adolescent the need to always act in a respectful, if not warm, manner toward the stepparent.

4. **The stepparent may never be able to serve as a parent to the adolescent.** Other types of relationships, such as with an adult friend or a confidant, can play equally important and rewarding roles for both adolescent and stepparent.

III. **Helping adults.**

A. **The couple.**

1. **The adults almost always have unrealistically high expectations of what their new family will be like.** Such misconceptions can be avoided both by anticipatory guidance and by directing them to sources of information that provide realistic information about stepfamily life, especially in the early phases. They can also talk with other, more experienced remarried parents and stepparents. Stepfamily life education, especially the comprehensive program *Smart Steps for Adults and Children in Stepfamilies*, is recommended for all stepfamily members.

2. **Communicate to stepfamily members' acceptance of their family as a valid entity and not a flawed version of the nuclear family.** Reassure them that their struggles are not unique but are an expected part of the complex task of creating a stepfamily, a task that usually takes several years. The first couple of years are typically chaotic!

3. **Remind the parent and the stepparent that a strong relationship with one another is not a betrayal of their children.** All children need a solid bond between the adults in the household, especially to allay fears that the stepfamily will dissolve in the way that their previous family did. They also need a model of a couple working well together, including appropriate conflict resolution, to help them as they grow up and begin to form adult relationships of their own.

B. **Stepparenting.**

1. **The best advice is, "Don't try to be an instant parent."** The foundation of good relationships is a supply of positive, shared memories. Authoritative parental relationships need time to build; with older children, there may not be enough time for this to fully materialize before they leave home as young adults.

2. **While stepparents often serve as parents in significant ways, they are additional parent figures and not replacements for a deceased or absent parent.** A stepparent is another reliable adult who can fill some of the child's needs for economic and emotional support along with child-rearing tasks at home and in the child's world outside the home. Stepparents may be relieved to learn that there are many different yet satisfactory roles they can play in their stepchildren's lives, support system roles that depend on the ages and needs of the children as well as the desires of the stepparent. For example, a stepparent can be a parent to a young child, a friend to an older child, or a confidant to a teenager and adult stepchild.

3. **Adults may come into a new marriage with very dissimilar parenting experiences.** It is helpful to supply information about child development, correct misconceptions, and, in some cases, recommend that the couple take parenting and stepfamily dynamics courses together.

IV. Questions frequently asked by stepfamily adults.

    A. What do children call a new stepparent? "Mother" and "father" (or variations on these) are more than just names; they describe relationships. It is not helpful to encourage or insist on such terms when a relationship has not yet developed or when the child feels uncomfortable using the name. All but the youngest children may initially feel that by calling the stepparent "Mommy" or "Daddy" they are forsaking the absent parent. What children call their stepparents often progresses through different stages. At first, the child may call the stepparent by his or her first name. Later, it might become "Daddy John" or "Mommy Mary." The important point is that for both the child and the adult, the name feels comfortable and does not imply a rejection of the absent parent. Many stepfamilies find that nicknames for stepparents are a comfortable compromise for everyone.

    B. What do stepparents do about discipline? Discipline is a major source of tension in most stepfamilies with young children. Frequently, a parent unrealistically expects a new spouse to discipline the children effectively. Children, however, do not view a new stepparent as someone with the instant authority to set limits on their behavior. The best approach is for the two adults to work out house rules together and, at least initially, leave the enforcement of those rules to each child's parent. It may take several years with young children (longer with older children) for the stepparent to have sufficient emotional authority to discipline the child effectively.

    C. How do stepfamilies deal with the absent parent? When adults criticize a child's other parent or use children as messengers or spies in unresolved hostilities, it prevents the development of successful stepfamily relationships. Children feel that criticism and anger toward any parent are also directed at them. It hurts them to hear negative comments about a parent they love. The clinician can help by showing parents how this behavior harms children and by supporting the children's desire not to be involved in conflicts between their parents. Encourage parents to verbally give children permission to care about *all* of the adults in their lives, with no need to choose sides, take part in a battle, or be responsible for the happiness of a parent who is left behind while they spend time in their other home.

    D. How long does it take to feel like a family? Adults and children feel like a family when they identify themselves as part of a system to which they all belong, where they feel comfortable, and where their basic needs are met. The time it takes to feel that way varies but is almost always much longer than the adults expect. With young children, the process of settling down takes at least 18–24 months; with older children, it may take 5–7 years.

    E. Should children continue to see the noncustodial parent? Children in stepfamilies usually do better if they can maintain ties with both of their parents as long as no physical or emotional risk is involved. When children move back and forth between households, it is easier if the adults collaborate as a parenting coalition. A parenting coalition is a limited alliance that is formed to promote the welfare of the children. It is a cooperative rather than a competitive relationship and is based on an understanding that all the adults are important to the children. Another successful parenting style is parallel parenting, which is used when the divorced parents are unable to collaborate. When each household has distinct yet consistent ways of functioning, the child adjusts to the different behaviors, activities, and expectations.

    F. What can make the children's "dual citizenship" easier? When children have just returned from visiting their other parent, they need transition time. It usually works better if the adults inform children about what happened while they were away instead of interrogating them about what happened in their other home. In each home, children need a space of their own: a separate room, part of a room, or even a closet or drawer where personal belongings are kept. Particularly helpful is a house rule that nothing in a child's private space can be touched without that child's permission.

        Some children might be disturbed over the differences in rules between the two households, and others may use those differences as a weapon to play one household against the other. Nevertheless, children do eventually learn that codes of acceptable behavior differ between households (just as they differ between home, school, and the homes of friends). What matters is to know the rules in each location and to abide by them. Children accept this most readily if they have some input into the creation of rules in the stepfamily household and if the parents are not defensive about the rules the adults have established. Finally, it is important to keep the consequences for misbehavior within the household where it occurred. An infringement of one household's rules should not affect time spent or activities in the other household.

BIBLIOGRAPHY

For stepfamilies

Organizations and programs

National Stepfamily Resource Center (developed by the Stepfamily Association of America), a Division of the Center for Children, Youth, and Families, Auburn University. Questions? Use the NSRC e-mail: stepfamily@auburn.edu or visit the Web site at www.stepfamilies.info

Adler-Baeder F. *Stepfamily Life Education Program. Smart Steps for Adults and Children in Stepfamilies*. A 6-week research-based educational program designed for use in a professional or support group environment.(Program also available in Spanish. Christian supplement: *Growing in Wisdom*.) Purchase from the National Stepfamily Resource Center, www.stepfamilies.info

Web sites

National Stepfamily Resource Center (developed by the Stepfamily Association of America). Research-based information, education, support, and advocacy to stepfamily members and the professionals who serve them; home page includes a search feature. www.stepfamilies.info

Stepfamilies-International. Stepfamily information and resources including popular conference presentation and discussion topics. www.stepfamilies-international.org

Stepping Stones Counseling Center. www.stepfamilies.com

Books on general stepfamily dynamics

Bernstein AC. *Yours, Mine, and Ours: How Families Change When Remarried Parents Have a Child Together*. New York, NY: Scribner, 1989.

Bray JH, Kelly J. *Stepfamilies: Love, Marriage, and Parenting in the First Decade*. New York, NY: Broadway Books, 1998.

Deal RL. *The Smart Stepfamily: Seven Steps to a Healthy Family*. Bloomington, MN: Bethany House, 2002.

Lauer R, Lauer J. *Becoming Family: How to Build a Stepfamily That Really Works*. Minneapolis, MN: Augsburg Fortress, 1999.

Visher E, Visher J. *How to Win as a Stepfamily*. New York, NY: Brunner/Mazel, 1991.

Books for children

Berman C. *What Am I Doing in a Stepfamily?* Secaucus, NJ: Lyle Stuart, 1982.

Holyoke N. *Help! A Girl's Guide to Divorce and Stepfamilies*. Middleton, WI: The Pleasant Company Publications, 1999. (Ages 9–12)

Lumpkin P. *The Stepkin Stories: Helping Children Cope with Divorce and Adjust to Stepfamilies* Wilsonville, OR: Book Partners, 1999. (Age under 10).

Rogers F. *Let's Talk About It: Stepfamilies*. New York, NY: GP Putnam's Sons, 1997. (Ages 4–8; by Fred Rogers of *Mr. Rogers' Neighborhood*)

For adolescents

Block JD, Bartell SS. *Stepliving for Teens*. Los Angeles, CA: Price Stern-Sloan, 2001.

Prilik PK. *Becoming an Adult Stepchild: Adjusting to a Parent's New Marriage*. Washington, DC: American Psychiatric Press, 1998.

Webber R. *Split Ends: Teenage Stepchildren*. Camberwell, Victoria, Australia: Australian Council of Educational Research, 1997. SAA 800-735-0329.

For stepparents

Annarino KL. *Stepmothers and Stepdaughters: Relationships of Chance, Friendships for a Lifetime*. Berkeley, CA: Wildcat Canyon Press, 2000.

Burns C. *Stepmotherhood: How to Survive Without Feeling Frustrated, Left Out, or Wicked*. New York, NY: Three Rivers Press, 2001.

McBride J. *Encouraging Words for New Stepmothers*. Ft. Collins, CO: CDR Press, 2001.

Oxhorn-Ringwood L, Oxhorn L (with Krausz MV). *Stepwives: 10Steps to Help Ex-wives and Stepmothers End the Struggle and Put the Kids First*. New York, NY: Fireside/Simon & Schuster, 2002.

For professionals

Hetherington E. *For Better or for Worse: Divorce Reconsidered*. New York, NY: Norton, 2002.

Mahoney MM. *Stepfamilies and the Law*. Ann Arbor, MI: University of Michigan Press, 1994.

Papernow P. *Becoming a Stepfamily*. Melbourne, Victoria, Australia: Routledge, 1993.

Visher E, Visher J. *Old Loyalties, New Ties: Therapeutic Strategies with Stepfamilies*. New York, NY: Brunner/Mazel, 1988.

106

Twins

Aasma A. Khandekar

I. **Description of the issue.**
   A. **Epidemiology.**
      1. The twin birth rate is approximately 32 in 1000 births.
      2. Monozygotic twins occur with uniform frequency (3.5/1000 births) and are not appreciably influenced by race, maternal age, or other known factors.
II. **Advice to parents of twins.**
   A. **Infant twins.** Parents of infant twins need support and advice regarding organization, feeding, individualization and separation issues, and stress management. Ideally, discussion of the more relevant issues should begin *before* the birth of the twins. It is an excellent idea to refer expectant parents to a local Mother of Twins Club for advice and support both before and after delivery.
      1. **Organization.** Efficient organization of the household and anticipatory preparation for caregiving tasks are essential for twin families. Parents should try to recruit outside help in the first weeks after the birth.
         - Parents can buy either a twin stroller or two less expensive umbrella folding-type strollers, which can be clamped together. Two infant car seats will be necessary. Infant twins can sleep in bassinets or even in a bed with bolsters rather than in two expensive cribs. Many baby retailers offer twin discounts on items such as clothing and other gear.
         - Organizing daily activities is very important to reduce stress. It may be helpful to make charts for feeding and other essential daily activities (a daily bath for the babies is not essential).
         - Parental time, both alone and spent with other family members, should be planned. It is also important to set aside separate time for parents to spend with the twins' other siblings.
      2. **Feeding.** Feeding infant twins can be very stressful. This may be due to specific feeding problems with premature or small-for-gestational-age twins or simply because it takes so long to feed two babies.
         - Oversized feeding pillows designed for twins can be helpful with formula- or breast-feeding both infants at the same time.
         - Twins may be breast-fed simultaneously ("tandem nursing"), which will cut down on feeding time. This may not be practical until the infants/mother have mastered latching and effective nursing.
         - Modified demand feeding, in which the baby who wakes to feed is fed first and the second one is awakened to feed after that, is another preferred option.
         - Breast-feeding mothers may also choose to pump in the immediate postpartum period to stimulate milk supply. A lactation specialist may be able to advise and/or assist the mother in alternative feeding methods including cup feeding and supplemental nursing systems. Breast-feeding mothers can be reassured that with adequate stimulation, it is possible to supply enough milk for both babies.
         - Babies should be alternated on both breasts to ensure even milk production and vary visual stimulation.
         - Many mothers will elect to bottle-feed their twins at least some of the time. Whenever possible, two adults should be enlisted so that both twins are held for feedings. When this is not possible, the mother or other caregiver could prop one twin up against a leg or across the lap while holding the second infant so that both may be fed simultaneously.
         - When babies advance to solid foods, freezing large quantities of food at one time will cut down on the work of meal preparation. Parents should be counseled to avoid comparing how much one twin eats with the other.
      3. **Sleep.** Promoting good sleep habits is as important in twins as singletons. Twins who sleep better also allow for more well-rested parents.

Table 106-1. Parental behavior promoting individualization of twins

Choose different-sounding names.
Do not dress twins alike all of the time.
Use individual names when referring to twins.
While twin pictures are appealing, take several pictures of each child individually.
Take twins on separate excursions.
Spend quality time alone with each twin.
Refer to other twin as "your brother/sister" or by his or her name.
Praise individually.
Discipline individually.
Encourage frequent opportunities for individualized contact with other adults, siblings, and peers.
Provide toys according to individual preferences, needs, and interests.
Expect that twins' behavior and thinking will differ most of the time, and approve of differences.
Encourage relatives and friends to treat twins as two individuals (e.g., individualize gifts and social activities).

- Parents may find that setting a schedule (around the timing of naps and nighttime sleep) for both twins to sleep at the same time may be challenging initially but helpful in the long term.
- Encourage parents to establish a sleep routine from an early age. Bathing, cuddling, and singing can be performed together, as can be storytelling. One parent can read to each twin, or both can be propped up on the lap and read to by one parent.
- During or after transitions, illnesses, or vacations, temporary disruptions are expected, but it is important to maintain and reestablish, when necessary, elements of the bedtime routine as soon as feasible.

4. **Separation and individuation.** Facilitating separation and individuation of twins is important. Whereas a single infant bonds primarily to his or her mother, a twin also develops a strong tie to his or her twin. Problems with separation and individuation may be compounded if twin children are always treated as a single unit by family and friends (this is particularly the case with monozygotic twins). Table 106-1 outlines parental behaviors that will promote successful individualization of twins, and Table 106-2 presents questions for assessing the level of individualization of each twin.

5. **Stress.** Most parents of twins report that the first year is very exhausting and difficult. While it is tempting to shuttle the family with two crying infants out of the clinician office as quickly as possible, it is important to allow sufficient time to discuss stress and coping ability carefully with parents. This may require having someone take the twins out of the examining room to provide a quiet environment to discuss parental needs and other issues involving care and management of the twins.

Table 106-2. Assessment of twins' level of individualization

Does he or she cry if the other twin cries?
Who is his or her main source of comfort? (It should be the parents.)
Does he or she think his or her mirror image is the twin (after 15–18 months of age)?
Does he or she engage in excessive imitation games with the twin?
Does he or she respond only to his or her own name (not the twin's) when called?
Is he or she frequently upset when the other twin is disciplined or upset?
Is there a "twin language"?
Is he or she excessively upset when separated from the twin?

School-aged twins
Are the twins afraid to be separated (e.g., at school, overnight stay)?
Do the twins enjoy dressing differently?
Does one twin tend to serve as the "spokesperson" for the other?
Are the twins excessively jealous of the co-twin's friends?
Do the twins exhibit either excessive competition or total lack of competition with each other?
Do the twins have age-appropriate peer relationships and social activities?
Does each twin have individual interests, hobbies, and goals?

6. **Acute illness.** Common childhood infectious illnesses frequently occur in both twins concurrently. It is advisable to warn the family of the inevitability of the other twin becoming ill if one twin develops an infectious disease. Consequently, caregivers should give instructions for both twins, even if only one is ill. The clinician can minimize additional stress by counseling against the use of separation measures, which can be extra work and are not likely to prevent disease spread.

B. Preschool twins.

1. **Language delays.** Monozygotic twins (in the absence of perinatal risks) should achieve developmental milestones at about the same time. Young twins may be delayed in many aspects of speech and language including delayed onset of speech, poor articulation, decreased speech production, and deficient sentence construction and usage. The reasons for language delay in young twins are unclear and do not seem to be due to perinatal biologic complications. Theories include reduced opportunity for extended verbal interaction with parents, increased interaction between twins, and competition for adult attention leading twins to speak quickly and omit whole syllables to get their information across more quickly.

2. **Discipline.** Disciplining twins poses a unique challenge. However, the type of discipline used should be no different from that suggested for singleton children.
   - Remind parents to discipline each twin appropriately and separately.
   - There is a temptation to discipline both twins even when only one misbehaves, particularly as the "good" twin will often attempt to do what the "bad" twin just got punished for.
   - Twins should not be compared with each other in terms of behavior (e.g., "Why aren't you good like your twin?").
   - Biting is a particularly common observation among twins.
   - If twins are fighting, it is sometimes helpful to give both a "time out" in order to give both an opportunity to settle down. Attempting to determine "who started it" is counterproductive and promote blaming and rivalry in the long term.

3. **Toilet training.** Twins may toilet train at a somewhat later age than singleton children. Parents should delay toilet training until the twins are truly interested and can indicate this interest. Some twins will prefer to train together; others will do better when trained separately.

4. **Siblings.** Parents should be encouraged to set up outings that include only one twin and the nontwin sibling(s) or siblings alone. Activities should be planned in which all siblings can interact equally together (e.g., music, sport activities).

C. School.

1. **Classroom placement.** Separating twins in school (may be the first time they are separated) is a controversial subject, with some studies suggesting improved performance with separation and others suggesting poorer performance and a higher incidence of internalizing problems for twins who are separated. The outcomes may depend on the twins' individual temperaments and the nature of their relationship. Some studies suggest that zygosity may also play a role in the effects of separation on behavior and cognition. Issues to consider in the decision are as follows:
   - Parents should be consulted on their preferences regarding separation into different classrooms, as they may have more insight into their children's level of individuation and ability to cope with separation. Consideration should be given for separating twins with very different abilities because problems may occur when one twin performs better than the other. Assigning to different classrooms may help to decrease intertwin dependency; accelerate individual independent, academic, and social growth; and discourage excessive comparison by teachers and peers.
   - Children who have not been separated before school may experience more difficulty if assigned to different classrooms. Also, one twin may become less confident in the absence of his sibling, affecting school performance. A partial separation, such as placement into separate work groups within a classroom, may encourage independence.
   - If twins seem anxious about classroom separation, having them carry a picture of their twin or permitting occasional visits to their twin's classroom may be helpful. If twins experience significant academic and emotional problems because of classroom separation, placement in one classroom for a period of time may be necessary.
   - The decision to separate or to not separate should be a flexible one. Parents and teachers should work together to determine the appropriateness of classroom placement and review periodically on the basis of twins' behavior and academic performance.

2. **Social relationships.** School is an important place for social growth and peer relationships. The initiation of separate social relationships may be particularly difficult for

twins and for their parents. Twins should be encouraged to have their own friends and develop individual and separate social experiences. Decisions about individual dress and hairstyles should be left to the twins themselves. It must be emphasized to parents and to schools that the social and educational processes must be individualized for each twin. Comparisons should be actively discouraged.

BIBLIOGRAPHY

For parents

Organization

National Organization Mother of Twins, Club P.O. Box 23188, Albuquerque NM 87192-1188, 505-275-0955. www.nomotc.org

Publications

Double Talk (published bimonthly); P.O. Box 412, Amelia OH 45102; 513-231-8946

Flais SV. *Raising Twins: From Pregnancy to Preschool.* Elk Grove Village, IL: American Academy of Pediatrics, 2010.

Gromada K. "Breastfeeding Multiples," NEW BEGINNINGS, Vol. 23 No. 6, November-December 2006, pp. 244–249

La Leche League International. www.llli.org

Twins Magazine. www.twinsmagazine.com

Two Four Six Eight. Educating twins, triplets, and more. www.twinsandmultiples.org

For professionals

Hay DA, Preedy P. Meeting the educational needs of multiple birth children. *Early Hum Dev* 82:397–403, 2006.

Hay DA, Prior M, Collett S, et al. Speech and language development in preschool twins. *Acta Genet Med Gemellol (Roma)* 36:213–223, 1987.

Klein BS. *Not All Twins Are Alike: Psychological Profiles of Twinship.* Westport, CT: Praeger, 2003.

Siegel SJ, Siegel MM. Practical aspects of pediatric management of families with twins. *Pediatr Rev* 4:8–12, 1982.

107

Vulnerable Children

Carol C. Weitzman

I. **Description of the problem.** The term *vulnerable child* is used to refer to children who have an increased, atypical, or exaggerated susceptibility to disease or disorder due to medical, socioeconomic, psychological, biological, genetic, and environmental risk factors. The term *vulnerable child syndrome* (*VCS*) was coined by Green and Solnit (1964) to describe children who have often experienced a real or imagined life-threatening incident or illness and are now viewed by their parents as being at greater risk for behavioral, developmental, or medical problems. Although these children appear to have recovered from their initial illness, their parents continue to view them as especially prone to illnesses and death. Perceiving both an essentially healthy child and a chronically ill child as exceedingly vulnerable has been shown to adversely influence many aspects of children's health, development, and adaptation. The VCS represents a transactional relationship between child and parent factors.

- The VCS represents the extreme end of a spectrum. The severity of any individual contributing factor will influence how fully the syndrome is expressed and how fixed the beliefs of the family system will be. The term *VCS* should be reserved only for cases meeting the criteria in Table 107-1.

A. **Epidemiology.** The percentage of parents who perceive their child as vulnerable is unknown, as is the extent to which the VCS underpins child problems. The literature on outcomes related to perceptions of child vulnerability is limited but suggests that children's development may be adversely influenced in a number of ways.

- In a community-wide study of 1095 children aged 4–8 years, 10% of children were categorized as "perceived vulnerable." In that study, 21% of all the mothers reported that they had had prior fears that their child might die.
- Studies have shown that 64% of infants born prematurely continued to be viewed as vulnerable by their parents when they were preschoolers.
- In a cohort of 116 premature infants, those children whose parents had high perceptions of child vulnerability were more likely to have lower adaptive development at 1-year adjusted age.
- In a cohort of 69 children with chronic rheumatologic and pulmonary diseases, those children whose parents had increased perceptions of child vulnerability had greater social anxiety.
- A number of studies have demonstrated an increased sense of vulnerability among mothers who are unmarried, of younger age, and of lower socioeconomic status. The influence of maternal education has been less clear on the development of VCS across different studies.
- The persistence of parental perception of child vulnerability remains unclear. In some studies, it has been shown to decrease over time as the child's health improves and parents are able to reshape their views of their child's health and resilience. Other studies have shown that early perceptions continue to predict later perceptions.
- Children with chronic and serious illnesses, such as diabetes, cancer, and asthma, whose parents perceive them as vulnerable have been shown to have poorer behavioral and social adjustment, and greater uncertainty about their illness, than children whose parents do not hold these beliefs.

B. **Etiology.** Child, parent, and sociodemographic factors can all contribute to a parent perceiving his or her child as vulnerable. Parent risk factors may relate to problems with fertility, pregnancy, or birth, as well as parental psychopathology or mental health (Table 107-2). In general, the earlier that an event occurs in a child's life, the more likely it is to enhance the parent's perception of the child as vulnerable. The transformation of parental fears into childhood problems is a complex process that is transactional in nature. Perceptions of vulnerability reflect parents' cognitions, attitudes, and beliefs related to their child's health and well-being. These perceptions may lead to a pattern of parents' behaviors including overprotection, reluctance to allow the child to have typical separation and individuation experiences, and a need to maintain control. The child, in

Table 107-1. Diagnostic criteria for the vulnerable child syndrome

1. A real or imagined event in the child's life that the parent considered to be life-threatening.
2. The parent's continuing unrealistic or disproportionate belief that the child is especially susceptible to illness or death (often associated with a high frequency of healthcare use).
3. The presence of symptoms in the child that appear disproportionate to the apparent level of illness or impairment.

turn, sensing parents' concerns and their need or desire to keep the child close may begin to behave in ways that reinforce these beliefs, such as acting frailer and having more illness complaints. Conversely, children may act out in ways to defy these perceptions.

II. **Making the diagnosis.**
   A. **Presentation.** The hallmark of VCS is in the high healthcare utilization rates seen in these children and what frequently seems to be the misperception by parents of the severity of the child's illnesses and risks. In addition, many parents who experience VCS will be refractory to standard pediatric interventions such as reassurance. These features may be among the most important clues to identifying a family system grappling with VCS. Vulnerable child syndrome can also present with a number of both specific and nonspecific parent and/or child behaviors (Table 107-3).
   B. **History: Key clinical questions.** Sensitive history taking begins the therapeutic process by conveying support and empathy to the parents. The clinician should ask questions that lead to an understanding of the parent's sense of vulnerability.
      1. *"To understand your child better, I need to know more. Let's go back to the beginning. Let's start with your getting pregnant."* This allows a more complete history that can focus on factors contributing to perceptions of vulnerability.
      2. *"What did the doctors tell you might happen? Did you at any time fear that the child might not make it or worry that this was more serious than what was being told to you?"* This type of question should be asked whenever a parent reports a problem, particularly during the pregnancy, delivery, and childhood, no matter how minor it might appear and allows the clinician to understand more about parents' cognitions and beliefs.

Table 107-2. Antecedents of the vulnerable child

Child factors
- Newborn period
  - Prematurity
  - Neonatal illness or complications
  - Congenital abnormalities
  - Hyperbilirubinemia
  - False-positive results of screening (e.g., phenylketonuria)
- Early childhood
  - Excessive crying, colic, spitting up
  - Any serious illness
  - Admission to hospital for such things as "to rule out sepsis"
  - Self-limited infectious illnesses (e.g., croup, gastroenteritis)

Parent factors
- Fertility related
  - Difficulty getting pregnant
  - Recurring stillbirths or miscarriages
  - Concern for fetal loss during the pregnancy
- Pregnancy related
  - Pregnancy complications such as vaginal bleeding
  - Abnormal screening results (e.g., abnormal alpha-fetoprotein)
  - Delivery complications
- Death of a relative or a previous child early in life
- Parent psychopathology and mental health
  - Depression
  - Negative portrait of child
  - Anxiety
  - Displacement of intense emotions onto the child
- High levels of parental stress

Table 107-3. Presentation of vulnerable child syndrome

- Parental attitudes and behaviors
  - Reluctance to separate from the child
  - Difficulty setting appropriate limits
  - Tolerance of physical aggression by the child towards them
  - Overvigilant toward the child
  - Overdirective toward the child
  - Overindulgence of the child
  - Disproportionate concern for seemingly minor illnesses or health risks
  - Description of the child as less developmentally competent than other children
  - Frequent visits to the pediatrics clinician for seemingly minor illness
- Child behaviors
  - Recurring symptoms of minor illness such as stomachache and headache
  - Regulatory problems including sleep and eating difficulties
  - Dysregulation of attention
  - School underachievement
  - Reluctance to separate from parents
  - Learning challenges

3. *"That must have been very frightening for you."* Whenever parents report something that might have been particularly worrisome to them, an empathic response will encourage them to talk further about their fears.

4. *"How often are you and your child apart? How does that typically go?"* Try to assess the parents' level of comfort in separating from their child by asking questions about the use of babysitters and their level of worry when separated from the child. Other questions should include information about other separation difficulties (e.g., when the child first started child care or school).

5. *"Overall, how stressful has it felt to parent this child particularly in light of their earlier or current difficulties?"* Parental stress has been shown to moderate the relationship between perceptions of child vulnerability and child reported symptoms of depression and adjustment.

6. *"Tell me more about your discipline strategies and how easy or hard it is to enforce them?"* Parents who perceive their child as vulnerable may have more difficulty in setting and enforcing appropriate limits and have also been reported to be overindulgent.

7. *"Have you ever experienced symptoms of worry or depression unrelated to your child's health?"* Questions such as these may help the clinician to understand a parent's mental health profile and risks for psychopathology. Parents with high levels of anxiety have been linked in some studies to having a higher likelihood of VCS.

C. **Assessment.** A number of standardized measures exist that can provide a fuller understanding of the complex beliefs and attitudes of parents that may accompany the VCS. The Vulnerable Child Scale and the Child Vulnerability Scale are brief measures with cut points above which VCS should be suspected. The Vulnerable Baby Scale is a 10-item measure that is a modification of the Child Vulnerability Scale and may be more suitable in detecting parent perceptions of vulnerability in infants and young children.

III. **Management.**

A. **Prevention.** The clinician must realize that any event or illness, even one considered to be medically insignificant, may have a very different meaning and implications for the parent. The clinician needs to take time to understand parents' beliefs and fears and address these appropriately. This may occur, for example, when a colicky infant's formula is changed. Some parents might interpret the change as implying that the child has a gastrointestinal abnormality. By explaining that colic is a self-limited condition affecting normal infants and by reinforcing this concept by changing back to the original formula within a few weeks, the clinician can help to prevent the development of perceptions of vulnerability. When a child who is hospitalized for an acute but treatable illness is ready for discharge, the clinician should emphasize to the parents that recovery is or will be complete, that no special precautions will be necessary after a certain time, and that the child is no more vulnerable to illness than other children. For some children, such as preterm infants, who have had lifethreatening illness and/or children with chronic illness, the clinical course may remain unclear. Clinicians must be honest with parents and be clear about current risks and a predicted time course for symptoms if known. It is helpful for pediatricians to explore episodically parents' worries, beliefs, and attitudes about the health risks they perceive for their child. Clinicians need to be attentive to signs of parental anxiety and stress or the presence of other risk factors that may place this child at greater risk of being seen as vulnerable.

B. Treatment. Once it is recognized that parental perceptions of vulnerability are affecting a child's behavior or development, the following approach should be taken:

1. **After taking a complete history and performing a conspicuously meticulous physical examination, if the child is well, the clinician should give a clear statement that the child is physically sound.** He or she should not use equivocal comments, such as "He doesn't look too bad" or "I can't find anything wrong."

2. **Assist parents by explaining that it is a natural tendency to worry about a child after a serious illness or event.** This explanation may begin a discussion of the adverse effects of viewing the child as vulnerable and the effects this can have on everyone in the family.

3. **Allow parents of chronically ill children to express their worries and help them to identify a child's coping skills and resilience.** These types of conversations can help parents not only articulate their worries but also construct a more robust profile of their child.

4. **Support the parents in dealing with the child more appropriately** by setting consistent limits, discontinuing patterns of infantilization and overprotectiveness, dealing more effectively with problems of separation, and being less panicked about the child's somatic complaints. It may be necessary to schedule additional visits to reinforce parents' efforts, provide reassurance, and address anxious worries before they escalate. It needs to be emphasized to parents, however, that the purpose of these extra visits are not due to the child's illness or the clinician's worries.

5. Although these problems can usually be managed by the primary care clinician, a mental health referral may be necessary if the parents are unable to make the link between past events and current beliefs and attitudes and are unable to adjust their current perceptions of the child.

BIBLIOGRAPHY

Forsyth BW, Horwitz SM, Leventhal JM, et al. The Child Vulnerability Scale: an instrument to measure parental perceptions of child vulnerability. *J Pediatr Psychol* 21(1):89–101, 1996.

Gleason TR, Evans ME. Perceived vulnerability: a comparison of parents and children. *J Child Health Care* 8(4):279–287, 2004.

Green M and Solnit A. The Threatened Loss of A Child: A Vulnerable Child Syndrome. *Pediatrics* 34:58–66, 1964.

Kerruish NJ, Settle K, Campbell-Stokes P, et al. Vulnerable Baby Scale: development and piloting of a questionnaire to measure maternal perceptions of their baby's vulnerability. *J Paediatr Child Health* 41(8):419–423, 2005.

Pearson SR, Boyce WT. Consultation with the specialist: the vulnerable child syndrome. *Pediatr Rev* 25(10):345–349, 2004.

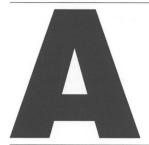

Pediatric Symptom Checklist

Clinicians interested in using the Pediatric Symptom Checklist (PSC) should obtain detailed information at http://psc.partners.org/psc_order.htm about administration, scoring, and interpretation before using it in practice.

The standard parent-completed PSC form consists of 35 items that are rated as never, sometimes, or often present and scored 0, 1, and 2, respectively. Item scores are summed, with a possible range of scores from 0 to 70. If one to three items are left blank by parents, they are simply ignored (score = 0). If four or more items are left blank, the questionnaire is considered invalid. The total score is recorded into a dichotomous variable indicating psychosocial impairment or not. For children aged 6 through 18, the cut-off score is 28 or higher (28 = impaired; 27 = not impaired). For children aged 3 to 5, the scores on elementary school related items 5, 6, 17, and 18 are ignored

Pediatric symptom checklist for school-aged children

Please mark under the heading that best fits your child:	Never	Sometimes	Often
1. Complains of aches or pains	–	–	–
2. Spends more time alone	–	–	–
3. Tires easily, little energy	–	–	–
4. Fidgety, unable to sit still	–	–	–
5. Has trouble with a teacher	–	–	–
6. Less interested in school	–	–	–
7. Acts as if driven by a motor	–	–	–
8. Daydreams too much	–	–	–
9. Distracted easily	–	–	–
10. Is afraid of new situations	–	–	–
11. Feels sad, unhappy	–	–	–
12. Is irritable, angry	–	–	–
13. Feels hopeless	–	–	–
14. Has trouble concentrating	–	–	–
15. Less interest in friends	–	–	–
16. Fights with other children	–	–	–
17. Absent from school	–	–	–
18. School grades dropping	–	–	–
19. Is down on himself or herself	–	–	–
20. Visits doctor with doctor finding nothing wrong	–	–	–
21. Has trouble with sleeping	–	–	–
22. Worries a lot	–	–	–
23. Wants to be with you more than before	–	–	–
24. Feels he or she is bad	–	–	–
25. Takes unnecessary risks	–	–	–
26. Gets hurt frequently	–	–	–
27. Seems to be having less fun	–	–	–
28. Acts younger than other children his or her age	–	–	–
29. Does not listen to rules	–	–	–
30. Does not show feelings	–	–	–
31. Does not understand other people's feelings	–	–	–
32. Teases others	–	–	–
33. Blames others for his or her troubles	–	–	–
34. Takes things that do not belong to him or her	–	–	–
35. Refuses to share	–	–	–

Adapted from Jellinek MS, Murphy JM, Robinson J, et al. Pediatric symptom checklist: screening school-age children for psychosocial dysfunction. *J Pediatr* 112:201–209, 1988.

and a total score based on the 31 remaining items is completed. The cutoff score for younger children is 24 or greater. A positive score on the PSC suggests the need for further evaluation by a qualified health (e.g., M.D., R.N.) or mental health (e.g., Ph.D., L.I.C.S.W.) professional. Both false positives and false negatives occur, and only an experienced health professional should interpret a positive PSC score as anything other than a suggestion that further evaluation may be helpful.

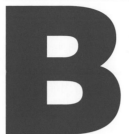

Early Language Milestone Scale

James Coplan

The Early Language Milestone Scale, second edition (ELM Scale-2) is designed primarily as a structured history of speech and language development, to be used by clinicians with varying degrees of expertise in early child development. The scale may be administered by either a pass–fail or a point-scoring method. The pass–fail method separates children into two groups: the slowest 10% with respect to speech and language development ("fail") and everyone else ("pass"). The point-scoring method yields age-, percentile-, and standard score equivalents for all possible point scores. The pass–fail method is recommended when screening large numbers of low-risk subjects; the point-scoring method is recommended when examining children who are at high risk for the presence of developmental delay or when evaluating a child with a known developmental disability. Complete instructions and pads of scoring forms are available from PRO-ED, 8700 Shoal Creek Boulevard, Austin, TX.

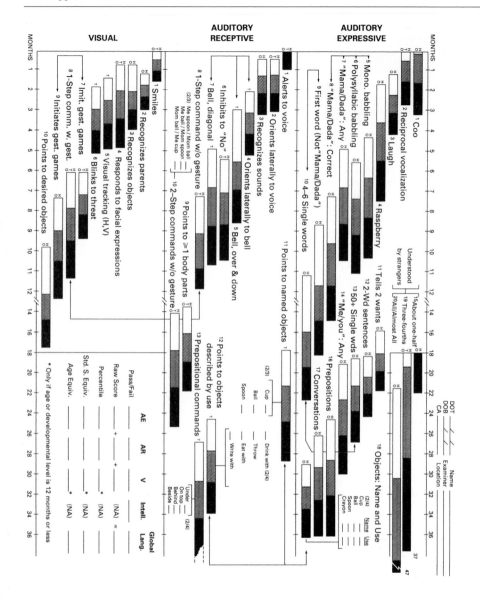

I. **General instructions.**

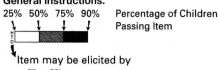

25% 50% 75% 90%   Percentage of Children
Passing Item

Item may be elicited by
H = History
T = Direct Testing
O = Incidental Observation
- Always start with H, where allowed.
- Child passes item if passed by any of the allowable means of elicitation for that item.
- Basal = 3 consecutive items passed (work down from age line).
- Ceiling = 3 consecutive items failed (work up from age line).

II. **Auditory Expressive (AE).**

A. **Content**

AE 1. Prolonged musical vowel sounds in a sing-song fashion (ooo, aaa, etc.), *not* just grunts or squeaks

AE 2. H: Does baby watch speaker's face and appear to listen intently, then vocalize when the speaker is quiet? Can you "have a conversation" with your baby?

AE 4. H: Blow bubbles or give "bronx cheer"?

AE 5. H: Makes isolated sounds such as "ba," "da," "ga," "goo," etc.

AE 6. H: Makes repetitive string of sounds: "bababababa," or "lalalalala," etc.

AE 7. H: Says "mama" or "dada" but uses them at other times besides just labeling parents.

AE 8. H: Child *spontaneously, consistently*, and *correctly* uses "mama" or "dada," *just* to label the *appropriate* parent

AE 9, AE 10, AE 13. H: Child *spontaneously, consistently,* and *correctly* uses words. Do not count "mama," "dada," or the names of other family members or pets

AE 11. H: Uses single words to tell you what he/she wants. "Milk!" "Cookie!" "More!" etc. Pass = 2 or more wants. List specific words

AE 12. H: Spontaneously, novel 2-word combinations ("Want cookie" "No bed" "See daddy" etc.) *Not* rotely learned phrases that have been specifically taught to the child or combinations that are really single thoughts (e.g., "hot dog")

AE 14. H: Child uses "me" or "you" but may reverse them ("you want cookie" instead of "me want cookie," etc.)

AE 17. H: "Can child put 2 or 3 sentences together to hold brief conversations?"

AE 18. T: Put out cup, ball, spoon, & crayon. Pick up cup & say "What is this? What do we do with it? (What is it for?)" Child must *name* the object and give its use. Cup: Pass = "drink with," etc., *not* "milk" or "juice." Ball: Pass = "throw," "play with," etc. Spoon: Pass = "eat" or "eat with," etc., *not* "food," "lunch." Crayon: Pass = "write (with)," "color (with)," etc. Pass item if child gives *name and use* for 2 objects.

B. **Intelligibility.**

AE 15, AE 19, AE 20. "How clear is your child's speech? That is, how much of your child's speech can a stranger understand?"

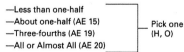

—Less than one-half
—About one-half (AE 15)   Pick one
—Three-fourths (AE 19)   (H, O)
—All or Almost All (AE 20)

To score:
If less than one-half: Fail all 3 items in cluster
If about one-half: Pass AE 15 only
If three-fourths: Pass AE 19 and AE 15
If all or almost all: Pass all 3 items in cluster

III. **Auditory Receptive (AR).**

AR 1. H, T: Any behavioral change in response to noise (eye blink, startle, change in movements or respiration, etc.)

AR 2. H, T: What does baby do when parent starts talking while out of baby's line of sight? Pass if any shift of head or eyes to voice

AR 3.   H: Does baby seem to respond in a specific way to certain sounds (becomes excited at hearing parents' voices, etc.)?

AR 4.   T: Sit facing baby, with baby in parent's lap. Extend both arms so that your hands are behind baby's field of vision and at the level of baby's waist. Ring a 2″-diameter bell, first with 1 hand, then the other. Repeat 2 or 3 times if necessary. Pass if baby turns head to the side at least once.

AR 5.   T: (See note for AR 4.) Pass if baby turns head first to the side, then down, to localize bell, at least once. (Automatically passes AR 4.)

AR 6.   H: Does baby understand the command "no" (even though he may not always obey)? T: Test by commanding "(*Baby's name*), no!" while baby is playing with any test object. Pass if baby temporarily inhibits his actions

AR 7.   T: (See note for AR 4.) Pass if baby turns directly down on diagonal to localize bell, at least once. (Automatically passes AR 5 and AR 4.)

AR 8.   H: Will your baby follow any verbal commands *without* you indicating by gestures what it is you want him to do ("Stop," "Come here," "Give me" etc.)? T: Wait until baby is playing with any test object, then say "(Baby's name), give it to me." Pass if baby extends object to you, even if baby seems to change his mind and take the object back. May repeat command 1 or 2 times. If failed, repeat the command but this time hold out your hand for the object. If baby responds, then pass item, V 8 (1-step command with gesture)

AR 9.   H: Does your child point to at least 1 body part on command? T: Have mother command baby "Show me your ..." or "Where's your ..." without pointing to the desired part herself.

AR 10.   H: "Can child do 2 things in a row if asked? For example 'First go get your shoes,' then 'sit down'?" T: Set out ball, cup, and spoon, and say "(Child's name), give me the spoon, then give the ball to mommy." Use slow, steady voice but do *not* break command into 2 separate sentences. If no response, *then* give each half of command separately to see if child understands separate components. If child succeeds on at least half of command, then give each of the following: "(Child's name), give me the ball and give mommy the spoon." May repeat once but do not break into 2 commands. Then "Give mommy the ball, then give the cup to me." Pass if at least two 2-step commands executed correctly. (Note: Child is credited even if the order of execution of a command is reversed.)

AR 11.   H: Place a cup, ball, and spoon on the table. Command child "Show me/where is/give me ... the cup/ball/spoon." (If command is "Give me," be sure to replace each object before asking about the next object.) Pass = 2 items correctly identified

AR 12.   T: Put cup, ball, spoon, and crayon on table and give command "Show me/where is/give me ... the one we drink with/eat with/draw (color, write) with/throw (play with)." If the command "Give me" is used, be sure to replace each object before asking about the next object. Pass = 2 or more objects correctly identified

AR 13.   Put out cup (upside down) and a 1-inch cube. Command the child "Put the block under the cup." Repeat 1 or 2 times if necessary. If no attempt, or if incorrect response, then demonstrate correct response, saying, "See, now the block is *under* the cup." Remove the block and hand it to the child. Then give command "Put the block *on top of* the cup." If child makes no response, then repeat command 1 time but do not demonstrate. Then command "Put the block *behind* the cup," then "Put the block *beside* the cup." Pass = 2 or more commands correctly executed (*prior to* demonstration by examiner, if "underneath" is scored)

IV. Visual.

V 1.   H: "Does your baby smile—not just a gas bubble or a burp but a real smile?" T: Have parent attempt to elicit smile by any means

V 2.   H: "Does your baby seem to recognize you, reacting differently to you than to the sight of other people? For example, does your baby smile more quickly for you than for other people?"

V 3.   H: "Does your baby seem to recognize any common objects by sight? For example, if bottle or spoon fed, what happens when bottle or spoon is brought into view *before* it touches baby's lips?" Pass if baby gets visibly excited or opens mouth in anticipation of feeding

V 4. H: "Does your baby respond to your facial expressions?" T: Engage baby's gaze and attempt to elicit a smile by smiling and talking to baby. Then scowl at baby. Pass if any change in baby's facial expression

V 5. T: Horizontal (H): Engage child's gaze with yours at a distance of 18?. Move slowly back and forth. Pass if child turns head 60° to left and right from midline. Vertical (V): Move slowly up and down. Pass if child elevates eyes 30° from horizontal. Must pass both H & V to pass item

V 6. T: Flick your fingers rapidly towards child's face, ending with fingertips 1–2? from face. Do not touch face or eyelashes. Pass if child blinks

V 7. H: Does child play pat-a-cake, peek-a-boo, etc., in response to parents?

V 8. T: (See note for AR 8.) Always try AR 8 first; if AR 8 is passed, then automatically give credit for V 8

V 9. H: Does child spontaneously initiate gesture games?

V 10. H: "Does your child ever point with index finger to something he/she wants? For example, if child is sitting at the dinner table and wants something that is out of reach, how does child let you know what he/she wants?" Pass *only* index finger pointing *not* reaching with whole hand.

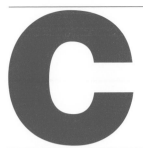

Temperament

Your child's temperament

1. **Sensitivity:** is your child sensitive to noises, temperature changes, lights, smells, and the texture of things? Does your child react strongly to loud noises or bright lights? Does he/she startle when the phone rings?

1	2	3	4	5

Usually not sensitive / Very sensitive

2. **Regularity:** does your child normally eat and sleep the same amount each day?

1	2	3	4	5

Always / Never

3. **Activity:** does your child have lots of energy? Is your child always on the go?

1	2	3	4	5

Quiet / Active

4. **Intensity:** does your child have strong dramatic reactions to situations? When happy, does your child laugh loudly or does he smile and giggle softly and briefly?

1	2	3	4	5

Mild reaction / High intensity/ dramatic

5. **Approach/Withdrawal:** what is your child's first and usual reaction to new people, new situations, or new places?

1	2	3	4	5

Outgoing / Slow to warm-up

6. **Adaptability:** does you child adapt quickly to changes or new places, like visiting friends or relatives? Is it difficult for your child when there is a new routine, new person, or new activity?

1	2	3	4	5

Adapts quickly / Adapts slowly

7. **Persistence:** does your child stick with things even when frustrated?

1	2	3	4	5

Gets "locked in" / Can stop

8. **Distractability:** is your child very aware and easily distracted by noises and people? Can you distract your child from playing with things he/she shouldn't touch by giving a different toy?

1	2	3	4	5

Easily distracted / Not easily distracted

9. **Mood**: how often is your child happy and in a good mood vs. feeling negative or serious?

1	2	3	4	5

Usually positive / Often negative or serious

Page numbers followed by f and t refer to figures and tables